CONTEMPORARY WOMEN'S HEALTH

Issues for Today and the Future

THIRD EDITION

Cheryl A. Kolander, HSD
Department of Health and Sport Science
University of Louisville

Danny Ramsey Ballard, EdD, FAAHE
Department of Health and Kinesiology
Texas A&M University

Cynthia K. Chandler, EdD, LPC
Department of Counselor Education
University of North Texas

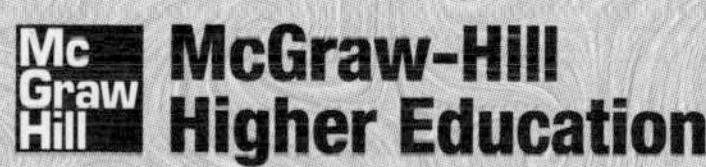

Boston Burr Ridge, IL Dubuque, IA New York San Francisco St. Louis
Bangkok Bogotá Caracas Kuala Lumpur Lisbon London Madrid Mexico City
Milan Montreal New Delhi Santiago Seoul Singapore Sydney Taipei Toronto

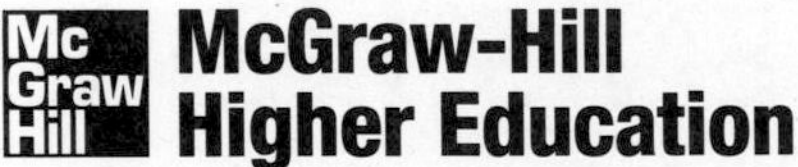

Published by McGraw-Hill, an imprint of The McGraw-Hill Companies, Inc., 1221 Avenue of the Americas, New York, NY 10020.

This book is printed on acid-free paper.

3 4 5 6 7 8 9 0 CCI/CCI 0 9 8

ISBN: 978-0-07-352965-3
MHID: 0-07-352965-6

Editor in Chief: *Emily Barrosse*
Publisher: *William Glass*
Sponsoring Editor: *Joseph Diggins*
Executive Marketing Manager: *Nick Agnew*
Director of Development: *Kathleen Engelberg*
Developmental Editor: *Beth Baugh, Carlisle Publishing Services*
Developmental Editor for Technology: *Julia D. Akpan*
Production Editor: *Holly Paulsen*
Manuscript Editor: *Margaret Moore*
Design Manager: *Violeta Diaz*
Text Designer: *Amy Evans McClure, Glenda King*
Cover Designer: *Ayelet Arbel*
Art Editor: *Emma Ghiselli*
Illustrators: *Ayelet Arbel, Katherine McNab, Cenveo, Emma Ghiselli*
Photo Research: *Alexandra Ambrose*
Production Supervisor: *Randy Hurst*
Composition: *9/12 Stone Serif by International Typesetting and Composition*
Printing: *PMS 2736, 45# New Era Matte, Courier, Inc.*

Cover: Getty Images

Credits: The credits section for this book begins on page C-1 and is considered an extension of the copyright page.

Library of Congress Cataloging-in-Publication Data

Kolander, Cheryl A.
Contemporary women's health : issues for today and the future / Cheryl A. Kolander, Danny Ramsey Ballard, Cynthia K. Chandler. —3rd ed.
p. cm.
Includes bibliographical references and index.
ISBN-13: 978-0-07-352965-3 (alk. paper)
ISBN-10: 0-07-352965-6 (alk. paper)
1. Women—Health and hygiene. I. Ballard, Danny, J. II. Chandler, Cynthia K. III. Title.
RA778.K7245 2008
613'.04244—dc22

2007020631

www.mhhe.com

Dedication

◇ *With gratitude to Kristina, Patricia, Barb, Kim, Carol and Stefanie for modeling healthy living and for their dedication to improving the health status of others.* —CAK

◇ *I dedicate this book to my beloved late mother, Fay Jones Ramsey, a woman of strength and indomitable spirit and to my precious granddaughter, Brynn Ramsey Ballard, God's gift of pure love and joy to her family.* —DRB

◇ *To my loving and supportive family, my mother and father Billie and Orbie Chandler; my sisters Betty Bush and Bonnie Thomas and brother-in-law Sam Thomas; my brother Charlie Chandler and sister-in-law Vicki Chandler; my nieces Rachel Thomas Little (and husband Tommy), Terra Chandler, and Niki Chandler; and my nephews, Lonnie Bush (and wife Heather), Brandon Bush (and wife Shasta), and Rowdy Bush (and wife Jessica); and Jason Thomas.* —CKC

Brief Contents

Contents

List of Boxes

Assess Yourself

FYI

Health Tips

Her Story

Journal Activity

Viewpoint

Women Making a Difference

Preface

The landscape of women's health has changed considerably since the first edition of this text was published. There are now specialized clinics that focus exclusively on women's health, and many hospitals have entire units dedicated to women. A plethora of goods and services related to women's health is on the market, and books, journals, and professional conferences devoted to women abound. Research on women's health issues has expanded as a result of increased federal funding, providing women with the information they need to make informed health decisions. Improving the health status of women and children is now understood around the world as a means of moving countries toward stability.

At the same time, much remains to be done. Further research and expanded funding are crucial to a broader understanding of women's health issues. Wage inequities, the undervaluation of women-dominated careers, violence against women, infant mortality disparities, female genital mutilation, a lack of available family planning, increasing rates of HIV in heterosexual women, and teen pregnancy are just a sampling of the issues that must be addressed if all women are to achieve the healthy and satisfying lives they deserve. Women need to advocate for representation on decision-making boards and in the political arena in order to continue to improve the lives of women everywhere. *Contemporary Women's Health: Issues for Today and the Future* has been written and revised with these concerns in mind.

APPROACH

In the third edition of *Contemporary Women's Health* we continue to emphasize health promotion and the impact of multicultural and diversity issues on women's health. Although we focus on "women-only" topics, we believe that both women and men can benefit from discussions of women's issues in the context of societal concerns, and our experiences in diverse classrooms have supported this belief. In the third edition we keep the applied approach of the previous editions, with a format that encourages students to examine their health-related preconceptions, attitudes, and behaviors and to explore new ways of thinking, feeling, and behaving. We believe the classroom can and should be a dynamic environment for empowering and strengthening women's positive health behavior, and our text is designed to support that goal.

Contemporary Women's Health may be used by instructors and students in health education, general education, and women's studies courses that emphasize a holistic approach to health. The text is written from a woman-centered perspective and is appropriate for both nontraditional and traditional students. The personal pronouns used throughout the text assume a female reader; we have found that men as well as women understand and appreciate this convention.

ORGANIZATION

Contemporary Women's Health is organized into five distinct parts. Part One, "Foundations of Women's Health," emphasizes the scope of women's health issues and introduces students to wellness and prevention concepts, as well as methods for facilitating lifelong changes in health behaviors. Chapters devoted to making wise consumer choices are also included in this section. Part Two, "Mental and Emotional Wellness," focuses on strategies for enhancing emotional well-being and managing stress. Part Three, "Sexual and Relational Wellness," addresses building and maintaining healthy relationships and gynecological health and designing a reproductive life plan. Part Four, "Contemporary Lifestyle and Social Issues," offers comprehensive information about nutrition, exercise, and the negative effects of tobacco, alcohol, and other drugs. Part Five, "Communicable and Chronic Conditions," includes information about AIDS, sexually transmitted infections, and important communicable diseases as well as cardiovascular health and cancer.

FEATURES AND UPDATES

The third edition of *Contemporary Women's Health* retains a variety of boxed features that support the text's approach and extend its coverage.

- *Assess Yourself* boxes provide interactive exercises and inventories to help students determine their own level of wellness and need for behavior change. Assessments include an inventory for improving your chances for accurate test results, a stress checklist, and a quiz to determine what you know about the foods you eat, among many others.

- *FYI* boxes succinctly highlight key information. They cover such topics as the discrepancies between women's and men's salaries, types of eating disorders, tips for reading food labels, yoga, and more.
- *Health Tips* boxes provide practical, helpful recommendations intended to enhance each student's personal health journey. These boxes cover a broad range of topics, such as questions to ask when taking prescription medicines, calculating fat intake, and tips for successful smoking cessation.
- *Her Story* boxes are based on real-life women confronting such challenges as postpartum depression, negative self-image, and alcoholism. In some instances, the names of the women whose lives are being discussed have been changed to protect their identity, but in other cases real names are used. Each box concludes with follow-up questions that allow students to apply the chapter content to the situation being discussed.
- *Journal Activity* boxes provide opportunities for students to record their thoughts and feelings about their health as well as the social issues affecting the health of all women. These boxes present questions for students to consider, such as "How do you handle stress?" and "Do you know someone in an abusive relationship?" They also give students tips on activities like managing time and browsing the Internet for AIDS research.
- *Viewpoint* boxes highlight controversial issues and ask students to reflect on and form their own opinions about those issues. Topics addressed by these boxes include state laws that discriminate against homosexuality, women's health versus giant pharmaceutical companies, and surrogate grandmothers.

A new feature has been added to this edition:

- *Women Making a Difference* boxes feature real-life women who have faced and overcome challenges in their lives and have assumed leadership roles. Included in these boxes are such women as Maggie Kuhn and Dana Reeve.

The third edition has been thoroughly updated with the most current health information and statistical data available. Key content updates and additions to each chapter are listed below.

Chapter 1 Introducing Women's Health

- Expanded material on sexual discrimination and sexual harassment
- Landmark legislative and legal actions related to sexual discrimination

Chapter 2 Becoming a Wise Consumer

- Updated information on nurse practitioners, benefits of massage, home health tests, and moisturizers
- Additional information about combining Western medicine and complementary and Alternative medicine
- New discussion of BOTOX in cosmetic surgery section
- Addition of sections on prescription and OTC drugs

Chapter 3 Developing a Healthy Lifestyle

- Comprehensive data on women's life expectancy in countries around the globe
- Updated statistics on women's cause of death in the United States by race and age

Chapter 4 Enhancing Emotional Well-Being

- Additional in-depth material on understanding and enhancing self-esteem
- Expanded coverage of eating disorders
- New section on family of origin issues and depression
- Discussion of emotional health theories specific to women

Chapter 5 Managing the Stress of Life

- Most recent research connecting stress with illness and connecting migraine attacks with hormonal fluctuations
- Updated research on age differences in the numbers and types of stressors for women
- Increased coverage of research on the prevalence and treatment of clinical anxiety disorders
- New research on women's greater susceptibility to posttraumatic stress disorder

Chapter 6 Preventing Abuse against Women

- New overview of the Violence against Women and Department of Justice Reauthorization Act 2005

- Revised discussion of why women stay in abusive relationships
- Newly revised section on same-sex domestic violence

Chapter 7 Building Healthy Relationships

- New sections on the biochemistry of love, sexuality, and relationship satisfaction
- Discussion of Sternberg's Triangular Theory of Love
- Expanded discussion of attributes of a successful relationship
- New in-depth discussion of positive parenting relationships
- Updated statistics on marriage rates

Chapter 8 Examining Gynecological Issues

- Added sections on benign breast conditions
- Updated American Cancer Society instructions for breast self-exam
- New discussion of polycystic ovarian syndrome and uterine fibroids
- Updated statistics on PMS

Chapter 9 Designing Your Reproductive Life Plan

- Added information on the contraceptive sponge, transdermal patch, NuvaRing, and Implanon
- New statistics on pregnancy rates and live birth rates for women over 40 using assisted reproductive technology
- Updated statistics on birth control, abortion, and adoption
- New sections on midwifery and fertility

Chapter 10 Eating Well

- New information on nutritional concerns for Americans
- Updated food label information
- Inclusion of the 2005 USDA Dietary Guidelines for Americans
- Inclusion of the new MyPyramid
- Updated benefits of vegetarianism
- New discussion of portion distortion, fast-food choices, and food allergies

Chapter 11 Keeping Fit

- Updated test standard data
- New information on exercise and breast cancer
- Expanded discussion of benefits of exercising during pregnancy
- New discussion of yoga

Chapter 12 Using Alcohol Responsibly

- Updated information on binge drinking
- New information on date rape drugs
- Updated statistics on drinking patterns and ethnicity

Chapter 13 Making Wise Decisions about Tobacco, Caffeine, and Drugs

- Updated information on nicotine replacement products
- Updated statistics on the rate of lung cancer deaths in women
- New American College of Obstetricians and Gynecologists recommendation for consumption of caffeine by pregnant women
- Expanded discussion of the effect of drug use on pregnancy

Chapter 14 Preventing Sexually Transmitted Infections and Other Infectious Diseases

- Updated discussion about sexually transmitted infections
- Updated statistics on race/ethnicity of U.S. women with HIV/AIDS
- New discussion of prevalent infectious diseases (e.g., hepatitis A, B, and C, chicken pox and shingles, West Nile virus)

Chapter 15 Managing Cardiovascular Health and Chronic Health Conditions

- Additional information on differences between men and women in symptoms of heart attacks and stroke
- Revised guidelines for high blood pressure
- New section on fibromyalgia and recognition of tender points

Chapter 16 Reducing Your Risk of Cancer

- Expanded information on benign and malignant tumors

- Updated statistics on incidence of cancer and deaths related to cancer
- New discussion of the TMN staging system for cancer
- Updated treatment options for lung cancer
- Discussion of stem cell transplantation in section on treatment options

PEDAGOGY AND LEARNING AIDS

To maximize its usefulness to students and instructors, *Contemporary Women's Health* provides these learning aids in every chapter:

- *Chapter Objectives* provide students with a succinct overview of the material in the chapter and may be used as a self-check prior to quizzes and exams.
- *Chapter Summaries* reinforce chapter content.
- *Review Questions* help students apply the concepts learned in the chapter and may be used by students to study for exams.
- *Resources* sections list a variety of information sources related to chapter content, including national organizations and hotlines, Web sites, books and articles, and videotapes and audiotapes.
- *References* list the research citations included in the chapter, giving students the opportunity to access key supporting information.

SUPPLEMENTS

The third edition of *Contemporary Women's Health* features an Instructor's Web site (www.mhhe.com/kolander3e) that offers a variety of resources, including an Instructor's Manual and PowerPoint lecture slides. Additional information is available from your McGraw-Hill sales representative.

ACKNOWLEDGMENTS

We would like to thank the reviewers of all three editions for their excellent comments and suggestions. Our text has benefited significantly from their input.

Linda Bernhard
The Ohio State University

Rebecca Brey
Ball State University

Linda C. Campanelli
American University

Susanne Christopher
Portland Community College

Susan Craddock
University of Minnesota

Sandra K. Cross
University of North Carolina at Pembroke

Becky Damazo
California State University, Chico

Rosalie DiBrezzo
University of Arkansas

Gloria C. Essoka
Hunter College

Eileen R. Fowles
Illinois Wesleyan University

Emogene Fox
University of Central Arkansas

June M. Goemer
St. Cloud State University

Shelley Hamill
Winthrop University

Donna G. Knauth
Georgetown University

Becky K. Koch
The Ohio State University

Raeann Koerner
Ventura College

Richard C. Krejci
Columbia College (Columbia, SC)

Susan Cross Lipnickey
Miami University (Oxford, OH)

Susan Ann Lyman
University of Louisiana at Lafayette

Margie Maddox
University of Scranton

Deborah A. Miller
College of Charleston

Sue Moore
University of Central Oklahoma

Willena Pearson
Indiana University–Bloomington

Margaret V. Pepe
Kent State University

Vibeke Rutzon Petersen
Drake University

Laurie Pilotto
Formerly of Hawkins County Health Department

Michelle Salisbury
Vanderbilt University

Ellen D. Schulken
University of Maryland

Felicia Taylor
University of Central Arkansas

Lori Turner
University of Arkansas

Barbara A. Tyree
Valparaiso University

Deborah VanBuren
Dutchess Community College

Jean Worfolk
Fitchburg State College

Diane Kholos Wysocki
University of Nebraska at Kearney

Jenny K. Yi
University of Houston

We appreciate the care and attention to detail provided by the knowledgeable and experienced editorial, marketing, and production teams at McGraw-Hill. Special thanks to Beth Baugh for her unwavering encouragement, gentle prodding, and kind reminders to help us meet deadlines. We have also had the pleasure of working with some incredible women in the past editions, and for that we are greatly thankful to McGraw-Hill.

Special appreciation to the women who provide more in-depth support during this edition: Kristina Dunham, graduate assistant at the University of Louisville, for her research support; Barbara Mercer, instructor at the University of Louisville, for her expertise in nutrition; and Donna Julian, health consultant, College Station, Texas.

We want to recognize the many women and students who touched our lives with their personal stories. Thank you for sharing your stories and providing further insight, encouragement, and support. Your personal stories and insightful comments have enriched our lives and the lives of others, and we hope that the content of this textbook reflects that information sharing. We know that the contributions of women and students have and will continue to make a difference in the lives of others.

About the Authors

Cheryl A. Kolander

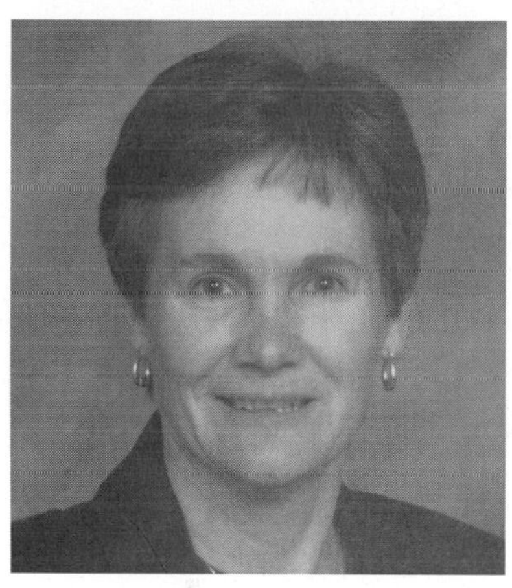

Cheryl Kolander is the associate dean for Academic Affairs in the College of Education and Human Development, University of Louisville. She is a professor in the Department of Health and Sport Sciences and previously served as a program director for health education. She received her baccalaureate degree from Luther College, Decorah, Iowa, and her master's and doctoral degrees from Indiana University, Bloomington. She is a strong advocate for social justice and equity, and has a particular interest in advancing health equity for women. Her primary research focus is prevention science, with an emphasis on women's health, school health education, and accreditation. She directs the Center for Health Promotion and Prevention Science Research, a center for collaborative studies and advocacy related to prevention science. She is a member of the performance team for UofL collegiate athletics, serves on the advisory board for Get Healthy Now, and chairs the curriculum committee for Fit4Me, an after-school program for at-risk girls.

Danny Ramsey Ballard

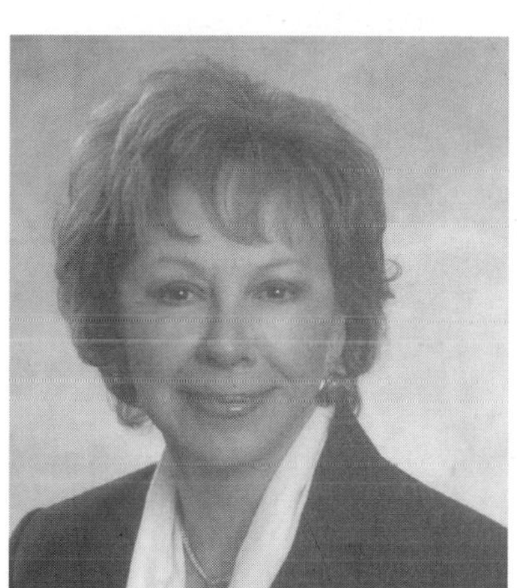

Danny Ramsey Ballard, a professor in health education at Texas A&M University, has taught graduate and undergraduate TAMU students since 1985 and is the coauthor of nineteen health-related textbooks. Dr. Ballard conducts research in multiple dimensions of women's health and delivers presentations about women's health throughout the United States. She has published more than thirty research papers and other professional materials; has delivered more than 200 national, regional, and state presentations; and has been the co–principal investigator of more than $1.72 million in funded projects. Dr. Ballard has been named fellow for the American Association for Health Education and for the American School Health Association. She is currently president of the American Alliance for Health, Physical Education, Recreation and Dance (AAHPERD).

Cynthia K. Chandler

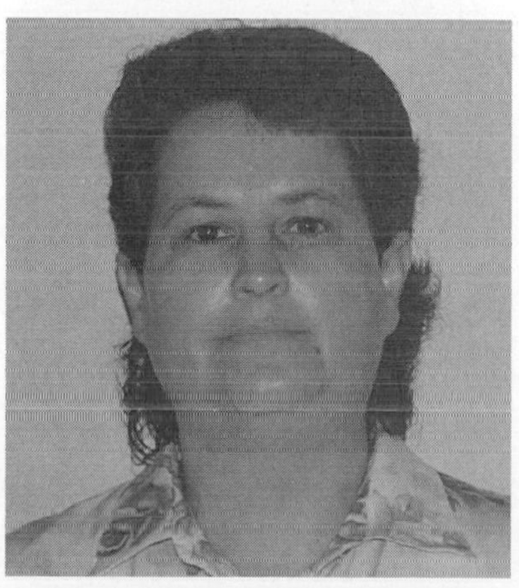

Cynthia K. Chandler, a professor of counseling at the University of North Texas, received her doctoral degree in educational psychology from Texas Tech University in 1986 and has served on the graduate faculty at UNT since 1989. Every year, Dr. Chandler teaches nine counseling graduate courses, organizes and leads a variety of institutes and workshops, and supervises an abundance of counseling interns. She is the founder and director of the UNT Biofeedback Research and Training Laboratory and the UNT Center for Animal Assisted Therapy. Dr. Chandler is a Licensed Professional Counselor, a Licensed Marriage and Family Therapist, a nationally certified Biofeedback and Neurofeedback Therapist, and an Animal Assisted Therapist. The coauthor of four books and numerous journal articles, she has given professional presentations in the United States, Korea, Austria, Greece, and Canada.

FOUNDATIONS OF WOMEN'S HEALTH

CHAPTER ONE
Introducing Women's Health

CHAPTER TWO
Becoming a Wise Consumer

CHAPTER THREE
Developing a Healthy Lifestyle

Part One

Chapter One

Introducing Women's Health

CHAPTER OBJECTIVES

When you complete this chapter, you will be able to do the following:

- Discuss the relevance of having a text dedicated to women's health concerns
- Describe three common types of health action
- Explain the significance of cultural and international diversity and women's health
- Cite important events in the history of the women's social movement and in the history of women's health
- Identify sexual discrimination in diverse settings and situations

WHY FOCUS ON WOMEN'S HEALTH?

Why do we need a text on women's health? An obvious reason is that women and men are different. In addition, many general health texts tend to relay information from studies based primarily on the male standard. A text geared specifically to women's health concerns will help to ensure that women's health issues are fairly represented.

By dedicating an entire text to women's health, we have an opportunity to provide a comprehensive presentation of the vast number of issues and concerns that affect women. Many health texts focus only on physiological conditions, whereas this text incorporates the mental, emotional, and spiritual health dimensions as well.

A text dedicated to women's health sends a message to the public that women are important. Too often, issues regarding the welfare of women are completely ignored, and when they are given consideration, it is often as an afterthought. Through long and difficult struggles women have made some progress toward being given equal consideration by the larger society, yet significant discrimination toward women still exists.

A text dedicated to women's health is not meant to subjugate the importance of men's health concerns. It is meant to serve as a forum through which a presentation of issues regarding women's health can be understood and viewed as important and significant in and of themselves. Many aspects of women's health are different from those of men and need to be given ample consideration. Through a text specific to women's issues, information regarding women's status can be shared, examined, and addressed.

Education is the keystone to progress. Education about women is the door through which women can be empowered. The performance of research studies regarding women must be emphasized. Information about the status of women must be made public, and the public must pressure politicians to make women's issues a priority. The health of the world, a country, a city, or a community rests on the health and well-being of its women and children as well as its men.

EMPHASIS ON HEALTH PROMOTION

Why is the concept of **health promotion** so important to the women's health field? The concept of health promotion is not limited to the idea that health is a condition we lose from time to time and try to gain back. Rather, health promotion includes the idea that health is something to be nurtured and by doing so we can prevent the onset of much illness and disease. Three common types of health action are proactive care, health care maintenance, and reactive care. **Proactive care** involves designing and living a lifestyle that reduces the risks of illness and also improves one's current health status. **Health care maintenance** is the continuation of what one is doing to maintain one's current health status. **Reactive care** is the treatment of any illness, disorder, or disease that may develop. The greatest emphasis in health promotion is placed on proactive care.

Proactive health care serves to reduce health care costs by preventing the onset of many illnesses, disorders, and diseases, thereby avoiding the great expense involved in their treatment. Proactive health care is a holistic lifestyle model as opposed to a medical model. The traditional medical model is primarily reactive and attends to the individual's needs after an unhealthy condition has developed. Holistic health care considers the interaction of the mind, body, and spirit: One area cannot be affected without the other areas also being affected. Understanding this interactive process is vital in providing proactive care to yourself and to others. Holistic health care incorporates all that we know about health and utilizes this information to keep the body, mind, and spirit healthy. A proactive, holistic focus empowers women to have a strong voice in their own health care.

WOMEN'S HEALTH IN A GLOBAL SOCIETY

Our text is based primarily on studies of women in the United States of America; however, women around the globe share many of the same concerns. All over the world women are living in poverty, experiencing discrimination and violence, having limited access to birth control information and materials, lacking accessible child care services, developing diseases and disorders specific to women, suffering with low self-esteem and distorted body image, and facing serious gynecological health concerns.

Women in many countries experience significant suppression of their civil rights. They may have no right to vote, to dress as they please, or to divorce. Even the slightest hint of premarital sex or adultery can lead to their death by a family member; this is referred to as "honor killing." Some women and girls as young as 10 years old are sold by their parents into pornography or to be used as sex slaves. According to the World Health Organization (WHO), more than 130 million girls worldwide are at risk of being subjected to genital mutilation, which can cause lifelong pain and medical problems. Women worldwide are dying of HIV/AIDS and cannot afford proper medical treatment. Women in countries at war are gang-raped by troops occupying their territory or are forced into prostitution or pornography to survive.

Many issues are specific to the time, place, and culture in which women live. Countries may have differing policies and attitudes toward women. In addition, religious or family traditions of certain countries place a special emphasis on certain images and roles women are expected to fulfill. The level of economic and technological development, the threat of international terrorism, or the state of war versus peace in a country may also influence the status of women and their health. It is our special obligation to pay attention to world events regarding the health and well-being of women and of all persons in the world community.

Two important concepts to consider when studying issues and events that impact women's health are sexism and misogyny. **Sexism** is an attitude of bias or an act of discrimination against a person because of his or her gender that usually involves economic exploitation or social domination. The most common practice of sexism is by men toward women. One example of sexism commonly practiced today is paying a woman less than a man for the same job. Another example is the practice of a financial lending institution, such as a bank, giving fewer loans to women because they are viewed as less capable than men of repaying the debt.

Misogyny is a hatred of women. An example of misogyny would be how the women of Afghanistan were treated in the two decades prior to the Taliban being overthrown in 2001. Women were required to wear burkas in public. These floor-length, dark veils cover every inch of a woman's body and have only a small mesh-covered opening for a woman's face. Women under Taliban rule were not allowed to get an education, hold a job, go anywhere in public alone, or wear makeup. To break the Taliban's rules meant a public flogging with sticks, death by stoning, or a rifle shot to the head. A 1999 report by Physicians for Human Rights revealed shocking statistics regarding Afghan women: 97 percent had major depression, 42 percent suffered from posttraumatic stress disorder, and 21 percent had suicidal thoughts. Sexist and misogynistic attitudes are held by people throughout the world, including here in the United States, but the impact of these attitudes

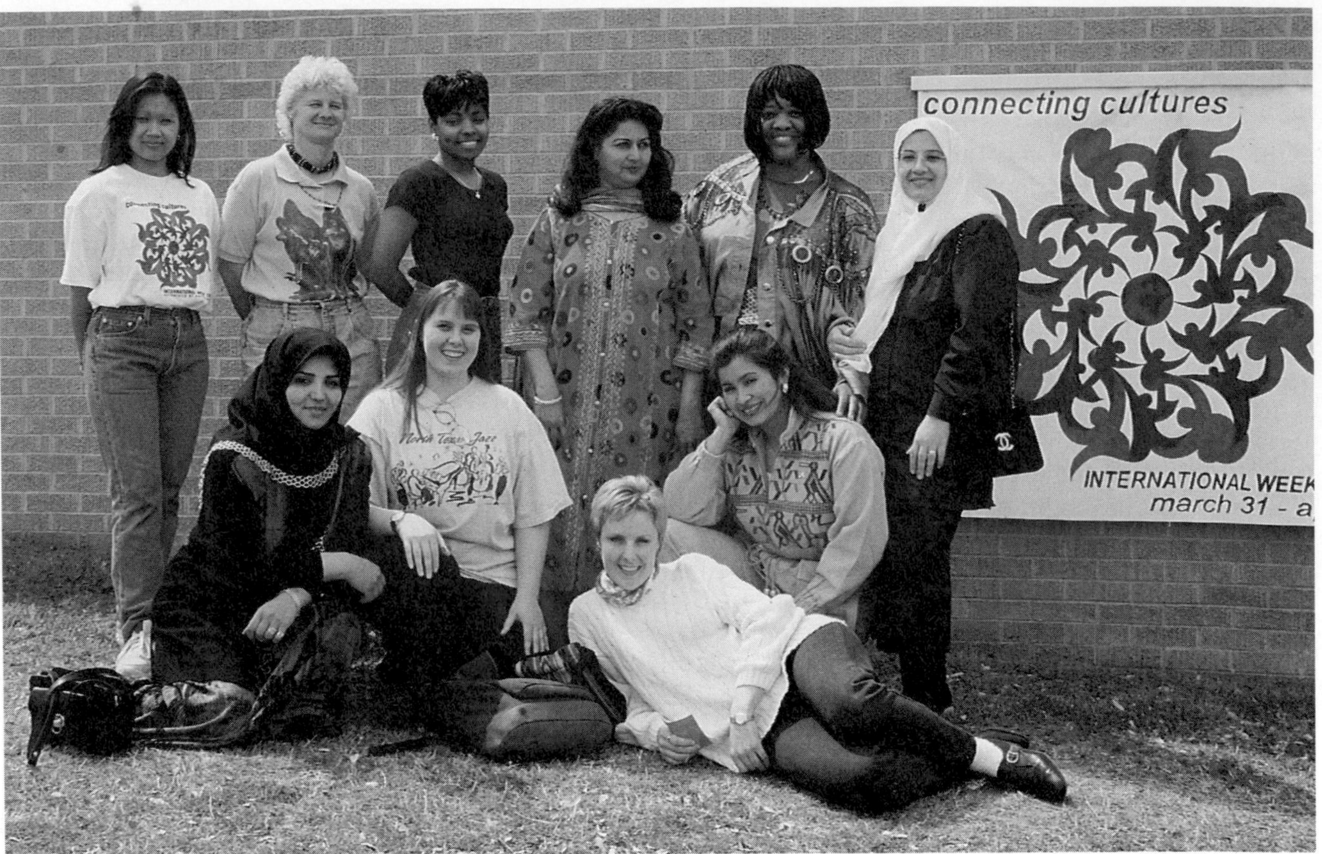

Women represent many different cultures.

and the practices they inspire are more obvious in some cultures than in others.

THE WOMEN'S HEALTH MOVEMENT IN THE UNITED STATES

The branch of medicine that specializes in female health is **gynecology.** This term is derived from the Greek *gyneco* (or *gyne*), meaning "woman," and from the suffix *ology,* meaning "the study of."[1] Gynecology deals with all female reproductive health issues. Obstetrics is a branch of medicine concerned with the treatment of women during pregnancy, labor, childbirth, and the time after childbirth. Obstetrics is often combined with gynecology as a medical specialty.

The care of women during childbirth was originally in the hands of women called midwives, and for centuries these women were the overseers during the process of birthing. In ancient Greece and Rome midwives received some formal training, but the medical arts declined during medieval times. The skills a midwife possessed then were gained only from experience and were passed down via oral storytelling from generation to generation.

In sixteenth-century Europe physicians grew interested in the field of childbirth and began to practice this form of medicine.[2] As physicians began to formalize the training and licensing of medical practitioners, midwives also began to formalize their training and licensing practice. Professional schools of midwifery were established in Europe at this time. However, midwifery did not become recognized as an important branch of medicine until the practice of obstetrics was formally established in the 1800s.

The physician largely responsible for gaining acceptance of gynecology as a medical and surgical specialty was an American, James Marion Sims (1813–1883).[3] Until then there had been opposition to it on moral grounds from midwives, the clergy, and the medical profession. Sims, a surgeon of international repute, introduced new operations and instruments (including a vaginal speculum) and in 1855 founded Woman's Hospital in New York City. He also wrote an important work, *Clinical Notes on Uterine Surgery,* in 1866. Surgical gynecology was very dangerous prior to the 1800s, but anesthesia (introduced by William Morton in 1846 at the Massachusetts General Hospital in Boston) and antiseptic use (introduced by Joseph Lister in 1865 in London) paved the way for many advances.

The first woman to receive a medical degree in the United States was Elizabeth Blackwell (1821–1910), an American physician who was born in London.[4] The degree was granted in 1849 by Geneva Medical College, now known as Hobart College. With her sister Emily Blackwell (1826–1910), who was also a doctor, and Marie Zackrzewska, she founded the New York Infirmary for Women and Children in 1857, which was expanded in 1868 to include a Women's College for the training of doctors, the first of its kind. In 1869 Elizabeth Blackwell settled in England, and in 1875 she became a professor of gynecology at the London School of Medicine for Women, which she had helped to establish. She wrote *Pioneer Work in Opening the Medical Profession to Women* in 1895 and many other books and papers on health and education.

One of the best-known early American nurses was Dorothea Dix (1802–1887), who was dedicated to reforming the institutions that cared for the mentally ill.[5] This work led her to be appointed superintendent of nurses for the Union Army during the Civil War. The first U.S. schools for the training of nurses were established in 1873, and Linda Richards (1841–1930) was the first recipient of a nursing diploma. Richards dedicated her life to the creation of training schools for nurses. She spent some time learning from Florence Nightingale in England, and she was the first president of the American Society of Superintendents of Training Schools.[6]

The first nurse to earn a PhD in the United States was Louise McManus (1896–1993).[7] She was central to establishing schools of nursing in colleges and universities, which provided the fundamental basis for a nursing science to evolve. She was a committed patient advocate and developed a "Patient's Bill of Rights," which was adopted by the Joint Commission in Accreditation of Hospitals.

The hospice movement, nursing care for the terminally ill, was brought to the United States from Europe by Florence Wald (1916–).[8] She received her nursing degree from Yale University in 1941 and later taught nursing at Yale and served as the dean of Yale's prestigious School of Nursing.

The American leader in the birth control movement was Margaret (Higgins) Sanger (1883–1966).[9] As a public health nurse, she dealt with many health and welfare issues that affect the family, such as poverty and an abundance of children for each family. She studied in London with Havelock Ellis, an English psychologist and physician whose landmark work, titled *Studies in the Psychology of Sex* (7 volumes, 1897–1928), was initially banned on charges of obscenity. Sanger returned to the United States to campaign for the legalization of birth control and practice. She was indicted in 1915 for sending birth control information through the mail and was arrested in 1916 for conducting a birth control clinic in Brooklyn. Her tireless efforts succeeded, however, and a clinic opened in 1923 in New York City and functioned until the 1970s. She organized the first American (in 1921) and international (in 1925) birth control conferences and formed (in 1923) the National Committee on Federal Legislation for Birth Control. She was president of this committee until its dissolution in 1937, once birth control under medical direction had been legalized in most states. Sanger visited many countries in Europe, Africa, and Asia, lecturing and helping to establish clinics.

The first U.S. effort to establish midwifery as a profession was undertaken by Mary Breckinridge (1881–1965).[10] A trained nurse and midwife, she established the Frontier Nursing Service (originally named the Kentucky Committee for Mothers and Babies) in 1925 at Wendover, Kentucky. Until the 1930s an American woman was more likely to die in childbirth than from any other disorder except tuberculosis. Breckinridge chose rural Kentucky as the site for her organization because she believed rural women ran a higher risk of complications and death than urban women. Breckinridge was able to organize existing midwives, recruit new ones, formalize their training, and coordinate their efforts to serve more than 1,000 families in 700-plus square miles of Kentucky. Designed around a central hospital and one physician with many nursing outposts, the nurses traveled on horseback to reach the most remote areas.

Over time more hospitals were built in smaller towns and transportation improved, making it easier for expectant mothers to travel to a physician for obstetric care. However, there was a resurgent interest in midwifery in the 1970s as a response to rising health care costs and an interest in natural childbirth. Today, contemporary midwives attend births in hospitals, birthing centers, and private homes.

Women had very little voice in the arena of women's health until the end of the 1960s. Women's advocacy groups had formed during the civil rights movement, and in 1969 a group of women angry about the way the medical establishment viewed women and their bodies gathered at a workshop in Boston and spent the summer studying the health care system and giving courses on women's health.[11] This group came to be known as the Boston Women's Health Collective, and they authored the landmark work *Our Bodies, Ourselves.* Little information on women's health issues was available at that time, and this book encouraged many women to explore health issues. This was followed by *The New Our Bodies, Ourselves* in 1984 and 1996; *Our Bodies, Ourselves: A New Edition for a New Era* in 2005; and *Ourselves, Growing Older,* which was published in 1987 and again in 1994. These works empowered women by giving them the information they needed to make informed choices about their own bodies.

The efforts of the Boston Women's Health Collective resulted in a national women's health movement. In March 1971, 800 women gathered in New York City for the first women's health conference in the United States.[12] Here, women challenged the traditional treatment of women by the medical profession, including radical mastectomies and the high incidence of cesarean deliveries and hysterectomies. The work of the women at this conference contributed to the agenda of the National Women's Health Network, founded in 1975, and advanced considerably the treatment of women's health.

THE WOMEN'S SOCIAL MOVEMENT

The social stigmas attached to being a woman have significant influence on a woman's life development, including areas such as self-image, career choices and advancement, family relations, and personal significance. The personal well-being of an individual woman cannot be isolated from the context of being a member of the larger culture of women. Therefore, it is important to address the social transitions women have passed through in recent history.

The U.S. women's rights movement was born during the drive for the abolition of slavery during the nineteenth century and owes much to the publication of Mary Wollstonecraft's *A Vindication of the Rights of Women* in 1792.[13] At that time, women were mostly considered in the context of their husbands or fathers. In almost all instances, only the male head of the household was allowed to own property, borrow money, sign legal documents, initiate divorce, or obtain legal custody of children after a divorce.

U.S. women today owe a great debt of gratitude to political activists Elizabeth Cady Stanton (1815–1902) and Susan B. Anthony (1820–1906), who energized the women's rights movement in the 1800s.[14] Stanton, along with Lucretia Mott (1793–1880) and three other women, organized the first women's rights convention in Seneca Falls, New York, in July 1848. Many sentiments for the cause of women's rights were presented at the convention, but the most controversial was Stanton's call for women's right to vote. Even Mott thought this was asking for too much too soon and encouraged Stanton not to persist. Mott feared that asking for the vote would make the whole convention a laughingstock to the public. But Stanton persisted and after great debate this sentiment was adopted by the convention. At the convention's end women went back to their own communities to advocate for the rights of women, giving birth to the women's suffrage movement.

Stanton met Anthony soon after the Seneca Falls convention, and they began a lifelong friendship and partnership for the cause of women's rights. In the early years of this friendship, Stanton wrote the speeches and stayed home to care for her children while Anthony traveled the country delivering Stanton's eloquent and moving words. Stanton and Anthony were among the first **feminists** in the United States, advocating for equal rights for all persons with a special focus on women's concerns. **Liberal feminism** is a philosophy that sees the oppression of women as a denial of equal rights, representation, and access to opportunities.[15] Stanton and Anthony's initiatives changed laws for women, first in New York and later in other states, helping women to gain the right to own property, hold wages, initiate divorce, and retain custody of their children. They also advocated for a woman's right to equal pay for equal work and a woman's right to vote, but neither lived to see these laws passed. Seventy-two years passed between the time U.S. women organized to ask for the vote in 1848 and the time they eventually received it in 1920. (See *FYI:* "Women Get the Vote!")

A second U.S. feminist movement took place during the civil rights era of the 1960s and 1970s. Betty Friedan (1921–2006) was a significant contributor to this women's rights movement.[16] Friedan surveyed classmates from her fifteenth college reunion and asked them to describe their lives since college. From their answers she wrote *The Feminine Mystique*, published in 1963. It was a national best seller. In her book, Friedan suggested that middle-class housewives were not necessarily fulfilled by housework and childbearing. She criticized politicians, health professionals, educators, businesspeople, and social scientists who pressured women to stay at home and play the stereotypic roles of mother and wife. Any inclination by a woman to do otherwise was considered by these professionals to be emotionally abnormal and socially irresponsible. Friedan helped found the National Organization for Women (NOW) in 1966 and served as its president for the first 3 years. She led the organization in its decision in 1967 to support the Equal Rights Amendment for women and to support legalized abortion.

The ERA declared, "Equality of rights under the law shall not be denied or abridged by the United States or any State on account of sex." The amendment was approved by the requisite two-thirds vote of the House of Representatives in October 1971 and by the Senate in March 1972. But it ultimately failed to achieve ratification by the required thirty-eight states by the extended deadline of June 30, 1982. Despite its defeat, public support for the ERA never fell below 54 percent, and as late as 1976 support for its passage was included in the platforms of

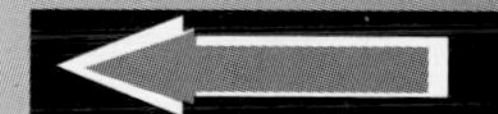

FYI

Women Get the Vote!

While men in various self-governing countries already had the vote, do you know when women first received the same right? Match the countries listed with the date that women received the right to vote.

	Country	Year
____	1. United States	a. 1917
____	2. Great Britain	b. 1906
____	3. Japan	c. 1947
____	4. France	d. 1939
____	5. Switzerland	e. 1920
____	6. Brazil	f. 1928
____	7. Mexico	g. 1971
____	8. New Zealand	h. 1942
____	9. China	i. 1917
____	10. Finland	j. 1902
____	11. Salvador	k. 1946
____	12. Soviet Russia	l. 1937
____	13. Philippines	m. 1945
____	14. Norway	n. 1913
____	15. Australia	o. 1943
____	16. Belgium	p. 1893
____	17. Guatemala	q. 1940
____	18. Canada (except Quebec)	
____	19. Quebec (Canada)	
____	20. Argentina	
____	21. Dominican Republic	

Answers: 1. e; 2. f; 3. m; 4. m; 5. g; 6. o; 7. k; 8. p; 9. c.; 10. b; 11. d; 12. i; 13. l; 14. n; 15. j; 16. k; 17. m; 18. a; 19. q; 20. k; 21. h.

Information for these answers was obtained from the Web site www.historychannel.com.

both major political parties. Technically the ERA is still alive and with thirty-five of the required thirty-eight states having already ratified it, the ERA needs only three more states to become an amendment to the Constitution.

Women continued to actively challenge the traditional domestic role assigned to them and rallied for sexual freedom. During this period, lesbians began "stepping out of the closet" and challenging society's bigoted attitudes of heterosexism. The civil rights movement gave birth to women's advocate groups all over the nation as women banded together to promote their cause. The feminist movement is spurred on today by organizations such as the National Organization for Women and the international Feminist Majority Foundation. Many women's advocate groups exist today around the world.

Over the years legislation designed to protect the rights of women and minorities in the United States has been passed, including these major legislative acts:

- The Nineteenth Amendment to the U.S. Constitution passed in 1920 awarded women the right to vote in government elections.
- Title VII of the Civil Rights Act of 1964 prohibits employment discrimination based on race, color, religion, sex, or national origin (for companies with fifteen or more employees).
- The Civil Rights Act amendments of 1991 allow for awarding damages when discrimination is proved.
- The Age Discrimination in Employment Act of 1967 protects individuals who are 40 years of age or older.
- The Equal Pay Act of 1963 requires an employer to pay all employees equally for equal work, regardless of gender.
- Title I and Title V of the Americans with Disabilities Act of 1990 prohibit employment discrimination against qualified individuals with disabilities, in the private sector and in state and local governments.
- Sections 501 and 505 of the Rehabilitation Act of 1973 prohibit discrimination in the federal government against qualified individuals with disabilities.
- The Family and Medical Leave Act of 1992 requires employers of fifty or more employees within a 75-mile area to provide up to 12 weeks of unpaid, job-protected leave for certain family and medical reasons.
- Title IX of the Education Amendments of 1972 prohibits sex discrimination, including sexual harassment in schools. This act especially opened avenues for women in schools by requiring equal opportunities in education and sports.
- Title X of the Public Health Service Act was created in 1970 and is the only federal program solely dedicated to family planning and reproductive health. Title X is administered by the Office of Family Planning, although its budget is located within the Health and Human Services Administration. The program is designed to provide access to contraceptive supplies, family planning information, and preventive health services to all who need them, with a priority given to low-income persons.

> Preventive health services include patient education and counseling; breast and pelvic examinations; cervical cancer, sexually transmitted disease and HIV screenings; and pregnancy diagnosis and counseling. For many clients, Title X clinics provide the only continuing source of health care and health education.

It is important legislation such as this that helps to protect the rights of those who might otherwise be exploited. Because of this legislation, **sexual discrimination** in wages and salaries became illegal in 1963 and sexual discrimination in employment decisions became illegal in 1964.

The Pregnancy Discrimination Act of 1978 was passed as an amendment to Title VII of the Civil Rights Act of 1964 to protect a woman against discriminatory practices at the workplace because of her pregnancy. A woman could no longer legally be denied employment or be fired because of her pregnancy, and health care coverage for her pregnancy was protected. It states that "women affected by pregnancy, childbirth, or related medical conditions shall be treated the same for all employment related purposes, including receipt of benefits under fringe benefit programs, as other persons not so affected but similar in their ability or inability to work." In 2004, the U.S. Equal Employment Opportunity Commission (EEOC) received 4,512 charges of pregnancy-based discrimination. The EEOC resolved 4,512 pregnancy discrimination charges in 2004 and recovered $11.3 million in monetary benefits for charging parties and other aggrieved individuals (not including monetary benefits obtained through litigation).

Even with legislation in place designed to protect women from wage and salary discrimination, there remains a significant gender pay gap in the United States (see *FYI:* "Women in Higher Education Make Less Money than Men," *FYI:* "Women's Salaries in Life Sciences One-Third Less than Men's," and *Viewpoint:* "Women Athletes' Salaries Unequal to Men's). In 2001 the Department of Labor's Current Population Survey showed that for full-time wage and salary workers, women's weekly earnings were about three-fourths of men's. However, the Department of Labor report states that this difference does not reflect key factors such as work experience and education that may affect the level of earnings individuals receive," so the U.S. Government Accountability Office published an investigative report in 2003 to try and explain the gender pay gap. According to this report:

> [Of] the many factors that account for differences in earnings between men and women. . . . work patterns are key. Specifically women have fewer years of experience, work fewer hours per year, are less likely to work a full-time schedule, and leave the labor force for longer

FYI

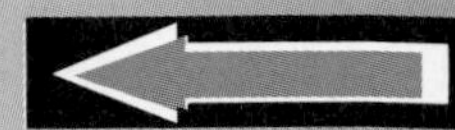

Women in Higher Education Make Less Money than Men

The American Association of University Professors *Fact Sheet 2000–2001* reported that women account for 36 percent of college and university faculty overall and make up only 31 percent of faculty at doctoral-level institutions. Women earn on average 93 percent of what men earn at the ranks of assistant professor and associate professor and 88 percent of what men earn at the rank of full professor. The discrepancy between the numbers of females working in higher education compared to males is thought to be a result of differential or discriminatory hiring practices, lack of support for women faculty for maternity and child rearing responsibilities, discrimination in promotion opportunities, a harsh or harassing work atmosphere, and discriminatory wages.

With fewer women faculty in higher education, how will women students find role models and equal opportunities for mentoring?

FYI

Women's Salaries in Life Sciences One-Third Less than Men's

A 2001 survey of 9,000 life scientists completed by the American Association for the Advancement of Science demonstrated that men have a significantly higher salary than women.[17] The survey indicated that the salary differences build throughout lengthy careers: The salary gap for postdoctoral researchers and assistant professors was moderate between $6,000 and $8,000, but at the level of university administrators and chief executive officers it increases to about $40,000. Factors that could contribute to the discrepancy include the following: Men have been working in science longer than women, more men practice in the field of medicine (a high-paying field), and women tend to work in academic settings (which pay less than industry). Even with these factors accounted for, men still make significantly more than women in the fields of life sciences. Why do you think men in life sciences make significantly more than women in these professions?

Viewpoint 

Women Athletes' Salaries Unequal to Men's

Female professional athletes receive lower salaries and get less television broadcast time than male athletes. In a 1999–2000 study of professional athletes' salaries, women professional basketball players in the WNBA made 2 cents for every dollar made by male players in the NBA.[18] Women bowlers made 70 cents for every dollar earned by male bowlers. In tennis, the proportion was 67 cents to a male's dollar, and in golf 36 cents to a male's dollar. According to the WNBA Players' Association, the average player salary is $43,000 (the league claims it is closer to $60,000 with benefits). The average NBA salary is $4.5 million. When women bowlers of the PWBA were informed that they would receive a purse of only $187,500 as compared to the men's $350,000, and no television airtime as compared to the men's scheduled 90 minutes, the women boycotted the U.S. Open. The tactic worked, and they got their own open with the same purse and airtime as the men. Do you believe women athletes should receive equal salaries and broadcast time as male athletes in the same sport? If salary inequities do not improve, do you think women will be discouraged from pursuing sports careers? What needs to take place for women's sports careers to be as recognized as men's sports careers?

FYI 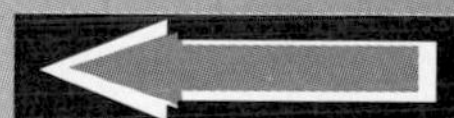

Sexual Discrimination Leads to Lawsuits

The following are high-profile sexual discrimination class action lawsuits. How important is it that women have the right to seek compensation after discrimination at the workplace? Should there be a limit placed on how much compensation can be awarded to plaintiffs?

- Women filed a class action suit against MetLife in March 2001 for gender discrimination in hiring, promotions, and compensation as well as retaliation against women who complain.[20]
- Women employees filed a class action suit against Costco Wholesale Corporation in August 2004 for gender discrimination in promotion practices.[21]
- Women filed a class action suit against Wal-Mart Stores, Inc., in June 2004 for gender discrimination in salary and promotion practices. As many as 1.6 million current and former female employees could be represented making this the largest civil rights case in U.S. history.[22]

periods of time than men. . . . When we account for differences between male and female work patterns as well as other key factors, women earned, on average, 80 percent of what men earned in 2000. . . . Even after accounting for key factors that affect earnings, our model could not explain all of the differences between men and women.

When the Equal Pay Act was passed in 1963, women made 58 cents for every dollar earned by men and in the year 2002, women were paid 73 cents for every dollar earned by men.[19] On December 1, 2003, the EEOC published a new code of practice on equal pay that explains to employers what they have to do to comply with equal pay law that was established in 1963. All employers were encouraged to perform an audit to make sure women were being paid equally to the men doing the same job or work of equal value. As a response to the continuing existence of a gender pay gap, on April 19, 2005, the Paycheck Fairness Act was introduced in both houses of Congress by Senator Hillary Rodham Clinton and Representative Rosa DeLauro. This act, if passed, would strengthen enforcement of the Equal Pay Act of 1963. It would work to improve Equal Pay Act remedies, make it easier to bring about class action claims, improve collection of pay information, prohibit employer retaliation, develop voluntary guidelines, increase training and education, and recognize model employers.

Businesses are aware that sexual discrimination is wrong and illegal, yet they do it anyway (see *FYI:* "Sexual Discrimination Leads to Lawsuits"). This is why it is necessary to have a legal system that allows persons to seek help to stop sexual discrimination. Of great concern is the proposed Class Action Fairness Act of 2003 that is currently being considered by Congress.

> The so-called Class Action "Fairness" Act of 2003 threatens to unfairly prevent victims of discrimination from seeking legal justice. If this bill is enacted, women's ability to seek redress in a court of law will be severely restricted. If passed, the bill will allow the removal of almost all state class actions to the federal courts. This process will overload the federal courts, delaying the resolution of cases and making it more difficult for federal civil rights cases to be heard. The bill will also prohibit courts from granting settlements that award a named plaintiff a greater share of relief than is awarded to all other members of the class. In effect, this

> forces the named plaintiffs to forego full relief and compensation as the price for attempting to protect others in the class. . . . The changes that this bill attempts to make in the class action process will most seriously affect the marginalized and disadvantaged members of society, including women, as it seeks to deny them access to relief from discrimination and injury.[23]

Another form of sexual discrimination that is of great concern is the denial of prescription drugs to women for reproductive health concerns (see *Viewpoint:* "Pharmacists Refuse to Fill Prescriptions Related to Reproductive Rights"). Reports of pharmacists refusing to fill legally prescribed prescriptions for birth control, including emergency contraceptives ("morning after" pill), have surfaced in several states, including California, Georgia, Illinois, Louisiana, Massachusetts, Minnesota, Missouri, New Hampshire, New York, North Carolina, Ohio, Texas, Washington, and Wisconsin.[24] These refusals appear to be based on a pharmacist's personal religious beliefs, not on legitimate medical or professional concerns about safety and the welfare of the customer. On April 14, 2005, Senator Frank Lautenberg and Representatives Carolyn Maloney and Christopher Shays introduced to both houses of Congress the Access to Legal Pharmaceuticals Act (ALPhA), which, if passed, will protect the rights of customers to obtain legal prescriptions. Under the ALPhA, pharmacists cannot prevent or deter an individual from filling a legal prescription for drugs or devices; cannot refuse to return a prescription or refuse to transfer a prescription to another pharmacist; cannot harass, humiliate, or intentionally breach the confidentiality of the individual attempting to fill the prescription; and must fill the prescription without delay, in a reasonable amount of time.

Sexual harassment is recognized as a form of sex discrimination that violates the Civil Rights Act of 1964 (and the 1991 amendments to that act). Sexual harassment is described as unwanted sexual advances, requests for sexual favors, and other verbal or physical conduct of a sexual nature that negatively affects the work environment.

The U.S. EEOC received 13,136 charges of sexual harassment in 2004, with about 85 percent of those charges filed by women. The EEOC resolved 13,786 sexual harassment charges in 2003 and recovered $37.1 million in monetary benefits for charging parties and other aggrieved individuals (not including monetary benefits obtained through litigation). A 1999 survey by the Society for Human Resource Management reported that 62 percent of companies offer sexual harassment prevention training programs and 97 percent have a written sexual harassment policy. A 2006 telephone poll by Louis Harris and Associates of 782 workers showed that 100 percent of female workers claimed their harasser was a man; and of these female workers 43 percent were harassed by a supervisor, 27 percent were harassed by an employee senior to them, 19 percent were harassed by a coworker at their level, and 8 percent were harassed by a junior employee.[26] This poll revealed that 62 percent of targets of sexual harassment took no action. Thus, the actual number of sexual harassment incidents is likely to be much higher than the number of charges filed with

---

Viewpoint

Pharmacists Refuse to Fill Prescriptions Related to Reproductive Rights[25]

On March 28, 2004, a pharmacist working at a CVS store in the north Texas town of Richland Hills refused to refill a prescription for birth-control pills for a 32-year-old woman. A spokesperson for CVS stated that the pharmacist's actions were not part of store policy. In January 2004, three Eckerd pharmacists in the north Texas town of Denton wouldn't sell the "morning after" emergency contraceptive to a woman identified as a rape victim. The Eckerd pharmacists were later fired. "This could become a serious problem, particularly if it spreads to rural areas where there are fewer drugstores," said Suzanne Martinez, vice president for public policy for the Planned Parenthood Federation of America, the nation's largest supporter of reproductive health. However, the largest professional society of pharmacists, the American Pharmacists Association, supports a "pharmacist's right to exercise conscientious refusal" in not filling certain prescriptions, said spokesperson Michael Stewart. In 22 years at the Texas State Board of Pharmacy, Executive Director Gay Dodson said she had never heard of a pharmacist refusing to fill prescriptions on moral or religious grounds before this year. South Dakota, in 1998, became the first state to adopt a "conscience clause" protecting a pharmacist's right to refuse to fill a prescription in certain cases: if the prescription would cause an abortion, destroy an unborn child as defined by state law, or cause the death of a person by any means of assisted suicide or euthanasia. Several other states are considering similar laws.

Do you think a pharmacist has the right to refuse to fill legal prescriptions related to reproductive health because of personal, moral, or religious beliefs? How does the refusal to fill these prescriptions translate into a denial of rights for women?

the EEOC. A 2006 online survey of 18- to 24-year-old college students conducted by the American Association of University Women reported that of the 2,000 who responded to the survey, 62 percent had received a comment or gesture while on campus that they found inappropriate. The survey found that women and men are "almost equally likely to say that they had been sexually harassed on campus but in different ways. Men are more likely to be called anti-gay slurs, and women are more likely to receive sexual comments or looks. Women are more likely to be uncomfortable about such incidents, and men are more likely to laugh harassment off."[27] A 2006 survey conducted by the Hyde Square Task Force "found that of 500 Boston high school students, 80 percent had experienced some form of sexual harassment during school hours. Nearly half of the survey respondents—49 percent—reported being touched, pinched, or grabbed by other students or teachers."[28]

The creation of the term "sexual harassment" dates back to 1975, and it gradually evolved into a legal precedent based on several court rulings over time.

> In 1975, a forty-five-year-old university secretary named Carmita Wood quit working for a Cornell [University] physicist after the stress of his repeated sexual advances made her physically ill. When Wood filed for unemployment compensation claiming that it was not her fault that she could no longer work, her case was discovered by Lin Farley, who taught a course at Cornell about women being forced to leave their jobs to avoid their boss's unwanted sexual advances. Farley and two of her colleagues coined the term *sexual harassment* to describe the phenomenon. That spring, she accompanied Wood to a feminist "speak out" in Ithaca, where the term *sexual harassment* found its first public airing.[29]

Later that same year, Lin Farley testified at hearings by the New York City Commission on Human Rights on the topic of women in the workplace.

> When the *New York Times* ran an article about the hearings titled "Women Begin to Speak Out Against Sexual Harassment at Work," the term entered the national lexicon for the first time.[30] (p. 70)

After the publication of the *Times* article, Lin Farley and her colleagues received a flood of reports from women who had had a similar experience as Carmita Wood. Yet, lacking a legal precedent for sexual harassment, the legal world framed early cases as unemployment insurance or workmen's compensation claims. Gradually, courts began to recognize sexual harassment as a form of sexual discrimination under Title VII of the Civil Rights Act of 1964.[31]

Protection against sexual discrimination and sexual harassment under Title VII of the Civil Rights Act of 1964 was actually a historical accident because the act did not originally include language that would offer protection based on gender. A major opponent of the bill to establish the Civil Rights Act was Virginia congressman Howard Smith, the leader of the southern conservatives who opposed the bill. Smith inserted the word "sex" into the act in hopes that including protection for women in Title VII of the Civil Rights Act would lead to its demise. But the move backfired on Smith and his constituents when the Civil Rights Act passed along with his "sex" amendment.[32]

Because the insertion of the "sex" amendment was actually a ploy meant to sink the Civil Rights Act of 1964, no one in Congress had thought through its potential ramifications. And it would take 12 years for the act that was established in 1964 to be recognized by the courts as a legal protection against sexual harassment. In 1976, two courts rejected sexual harassment as a form of gender discrimination under Title VII of the Civil Rights Acts of 1964, but one U.S. District Court in Washington, D.C., became the first federal court to hold otherwise, in *Williams v. Saxbe.*

> In that case, a woman named Diane Williams was fired from her job with the community relations department of the U.S. Department of Justice after she refused her supervisor's sexual advances. She claimed that this was a violation of Title VII, because she had been denied equal employment opportunities. If she had been a man, she argued, her boss would never have propositioned her. It was her turning down the proposition that led to her firing. . . . The court found that, in firing Williams for refusing to have sex with him, the supervisor had imposed a condition of employment on Williams that he did not impose on other workers, and that he did so because she was a woman. Therefore, the court reasoned it was a violation of Title VII. . . . That precedent stuck, and by 1977 three federal courts of appeals and a number of district courts had held that sexual harassment could be a form of sex discrimination under Title VII.[33]

In 1979 a treatise titled, *Sexual Harassment of the Working Woman* was published by a young law professor at the University of Michigan, Catharine MacKinnon, in which she stipulated that "quid pro quo" harassment, meaning "this for that" (or "put out or get out"), was not the only form of sexual harassment. MacKinnon argued that "subjecting women to a hostile work environment, including repeated exposure to sexually offensive or denigrating material, as a condition of employment could also constitute a violation of Title VII."[34] In 1980 the EEOC issued federal guidelines on sexual harassment in the workplace that incorporated both the "quid pro quo" and "hostile work environment" concepts, and these federal guidelines, though not a binding legal force, "became a benchmark for courts and employers in sorting out what conduct violated Title VII."[35] The EEOC guidelines stated:

> Unwelcome sexual advances, requests for sexual favors, and other verbal or physical conduct of a sexual nature constitute sexual harassment when (1) submission to such conduct is made either explicitly or implicitly a condition of an individual's employment, (2) submission to or rejection of such conduct by an individual is used as the basis for employment decisions affecting such individual, or (3) such conduct has the purpose or effect of unreasonably interfering with an individual's work performance or creating an intimidating, hostile, or offensive working environment.[36]

In 2002, Clara Bingham and Laura Leedy Gansler published *Class Action: The Landmark Case That Changed Sexual Harassment Law.* This book describes the true story of Lois Jenson and her female coworkers at Eveleth Mine of Minnesota who experienced repeated acts of sexual harassment in a work environment that was extremely hostile to women—a story that inspired the major motion picture *North Country* (Warner Bros. Pictures, 2005). The book details the 12-year journey, 1987–1999, of the case of *Jenson v. Eveleth* that set the most important precedent of certifying sexual harassment as a class action lawsuit. "That decision elevated sexual harassment from an individual complaint by one, usually a powerless person against another, more powerful one—a complaint that could easily be ignored or swept under the rug—to a significant civil rights issue. . . . *Jenson v. Eveleth* did not eradicate sexual harassment in the workplace. But it made corporate America take real note of it for the first time, and established once and for all that women who are subjected to a hostile work environment need never stand alone."[37]

Two additional constructs that are related to discrimination against women are **homophobia** and **heterosexism.** Homophobia is the fear or dislike of a person who is homosexual. Many people in the United States are homophobic, and thus, many homosexual women hide their lesbian orientation to avoid being ostracized or rejected by others (see *Women Making a Difference:* "Professional Basketball Star Sheryl Swoopes Comes Out as a Lesbian"). Heterosexism is a belief or attitude that results in bias or discrimination toward anyone who is not heterosexual (see *Assess Yourself:* "Gay and Lesbian Rights"). Heterosexism is highly prevalent in the United States. As of November 2005, Massachusetts was the only state that allows legal marriage for same-sex partners, and many states actually have laws that (a) prevent recognition of out-of-state same-sex marriage, (b) prohibit benefits for a state employee's unmarried partner, (c) amend the state's constitution to ban same-sex marriage, or (d) prohibit adoption of children by homosexuals (see *Viewpoint:* "State Laws That Discriminate Against Homosexuals").[38] These laws are perceived by many to be unconstitutional yet they exist as legal justification for discrimination against an entire group of U.S. citizens.

Discrimination against homosexuals is a worldwide phenomenon. However, the countries of Canada and Spain have become social justice role models for the rest of the world regarding equal rights for gays and lesbians.[40] In 1996 Canada amended the national Human Rights Act to provide protection from discrimination based on

---

Women Making a Difference

Professional Basketball Star Sheryl Swoopes Comes Out as a Lesbian

High-profile WNBA star Sheryl Swoopes publicly revealed that she was a lesbian in 2005. The story was first reported by *ESPN Magazine* on October 26. Swoopes is a three-time Olympic gold medalist and a four-time WNBA champion with the Houston Comets where she started as a rookie in 1997, and she led Texas Tech University to a national basketball championship in 1993. In coming out to the public about her relationship with former Comets assistant coach Alisa Scott, which she had kept hidden for 7 years, Swoopes said, "I feel like I've been living a lie. . . . I'm at a place in my life right now where I'm very happy, very content. I'm finally OK with the idea of who I love, who I want to be with. . . . I don't want to have to hide from the world anymore. . . . [My mother] doesn't think it's right. She'll probably never accept it. . . . But she's dealing with it. . . . I worry about the reaction throughout the country, but I really worry about Brownfield [her home town] and Lubbock [the location of her college alma mater]. . . . Because they're both small towns and Sheryl Swoopes is a local hero. Now what? I hope it doesn't change. It's important to me." Swoopes is perhaps the highest-profile active team-sport athlete to come out as a lesbian and the third WNBA player to do so. Sue Wicks of the New York Liberty, who came out shortly before her retirement in 2002, was the first active WNBA player to come out publicly about her sexual orientation.[39]

Does your opinion of celebrities change when they reveal they are gay or lesbian? How much discrimination or distress do you think a gay or lesbian celebrity experiences because of negative public attitudes about homosexuality?

Assess Yourself

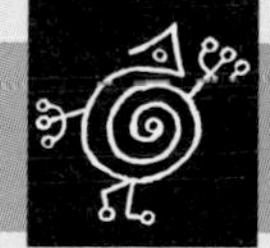

Gay and Lesbian Rights

Circle A for agree and D for disagree for each of the following items.

A D 1. It should *not* be legal to fire a gay or lesbian person from a job based solely on his or her sexual orientation.

A D 2. A gay or lesbian individual should *not* be denied custody of his or her children solely on the basis of sexual orientation.

A D 3. A gay or lesbian person should be allowed to designate his or her relationship partner as a recipient of spousal benefits on insurance benefit plans.

A D 4. A gay or lesbian couple should *not* be allowed to file joint income tax returns.

A D 5. A gay or lesbian couple should *not* be allowed to legally marry.

A D 6. A lesbian or gay person should *not* be allowed to adopt a child.

A D 7. A lesbian should *not* be allowed to use a sperm bank for insemination in order to get pregnant.

A D 8. Major television networks should *not* be able to show programs that depict lesbian or gay persons during prime-time hours (such as 7 to 9 P.M.).

A D 9. Grade school libraries and/or curriculum should include some books that depict families with gay members, such as gay parents.

A D 10. High school libraries and/or curriculum should *not* include some books about lesbians and gay persons.

A D 11. A person who claims to be gay should be encouraged to seek mental health therapy to change her or his orientation to become less gay and, thus, more heterosexual.

A D 12. A parent should *not* have the right to refuse his or her child, who is 17 years old or younger, room and board because the child is gay or lesbian.

A D 13. A parent should have the right to require a gay child, who is 17 years old or younger, to seek mental health therapy to become less gay and, thus, more heterosexual.

A D 14. Lesbian and gay persons should be allowed to serve in the military without having to hide their sexual orientation.

A D 15. Multicultural awareness programs and courses designed to fight discrimination and bigotry should include information on gays and lesbians in the same way that they present information on other minority groups.

Scoring

If you answered the items in the following designated direction, then give yourself one point for each: (1) A; (2) A; (3) A; (4) D; (5) D; (6) D; (7) D; (8) D; (9) A; (10) D; (11) D; (12) A; (13) D; (14) A; and (15) A.

Interpretation

If your score was 8 or higher, then you are considered to have an attitude more in favor of gay and lesbian rights. The higher your score, the more in favor of gay and lesbian rights you are. If your score was 7 or less, then you are considered to be less in favor of gay and lesbian rights. The lower your score, the less in favor of gay and lesbian rights you are. The maximum score is 15 and the minimum score is 0.

sexual orientation, extend benefits to same-sex partners, allow civil marriage for same-sex couples, and allow foreign partners of its homosexual citizenry to receive residency permits. Spain has a national gay rights law (established in 2005) that bans some antigay discrimination, including for housing, employment, and public and professional services. Spain provides homosexual couples with health care benefits, access to state widower's pensions, and alimony in the event of a separation. Spain allows same-sex couples the right to marry, adopt children, and inherit each other's property, making their legal status the same as that of heterosexual couples. Gay rights are more widely accepted in Europe than on any other continent. As of December 2006, three out of five countries that have legalized same-sex marriage are in Europe (Belgium, Netherlands, and Spain) and seventeen European countries have legalized same-sex civil unions.

ETHNIC, CLASS, AND GENDER BIAS IN HEALTH RESEARCH

The United States is a nation of diverse needs. The U.S. Census Bureau, Census 2000 reported the total population was 281,421,906 with 143,505,720 women (or 50.99 percent). The approximate ethnic characteristics of the total population of those reporting only one race were white 211.4 million; black or African American 34.6 million; Asian 10.2 million; American Indian and Alaska Native 2.4 million; Native Hawaiian and Other Pacific Islander over 398,000; and some other race over 15.3 million. Those reporting two or more races were 6.8 million. The statistics for Hispanic or Latino (of any race) are kept separately and integrated into the other race figures. The population for Hispanic or Latino (of any race) was 35.3 million, which breaks down into these

Viewpoint

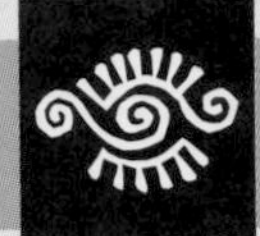

State Laws That Discriminate Against Homosexuals

Listed below are the states that, as of November 2005, have laws that discriminate against homosexuals. Where do you stand on these issues? Is it right to deny rights to citizens based on a demographic characteristic such as sexual orientation? How is discrimination based on sexual orientation different from (or the same as) discrimination based on gender, race, age, disability, or religion?

a. Has a law that prevents recognition of out-of-state same-sex marriage license.
b. Has a law that prohibits benefits for a state employee's unmarried partner.
c. Has amended the state constitution to ban same-sex marriage.
d. Has a law that prohibits homosexuals from adopting children.

State	Discriminatory Law
Alabama	a
Alaska	a, c
Arizona	a
Arkansas*	a, b, c, d
California	a
Colorado	a
Delaware	a
Florida	a,d
Georgia	a, b, c
Hawaii	a, c
Idaho	a
Illinois	a
Indiana	a
Iowa	a
Kansas	a, b, c
Kentucky	a, b, c
Louisiana	a, c
Mainea	
Michigan	a, b, c
Minnesota	a
Mississippi	a, c, d
Missouri	a, c
Montana	a, c
Nebraska	a, b, c
Nevada	a, c
New Hampshire	a
North Carolina	a
North Dakota	a, b, c
Ohio a, b, c	
Oklahoma	a, b, c
Oregon	c
Pennsylvania	a
South Carolina	a
South Dakota	a
Tennessee	a
Texas a, c	
Utah a, b, c, d	
Virginia	a
Washington	a
West Virginia	a

* On December 12, 2004, Arkansas Circuit Court Judge Timothy Fox ruled that children are not harmed by living with gay or lesbian parents and struck down an Arkansas state regulation that prevented a homosexual from adopting a child. The ruling is currently on appeal by the Arkansas Department of Human Services; thus, it is left on the list pending a final ruling.

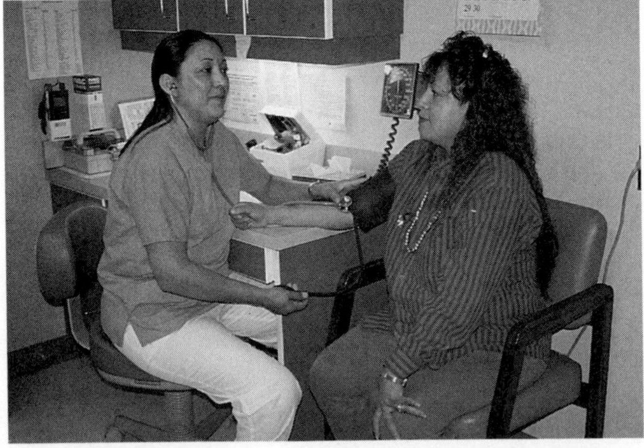

Flora Archuletta, a nurse at the Indian Health Center, has a special interest in Native American women's health issues.

groups: Mexican 20.6 million; Puerto Rican 3.4 million; Cuban 1.2 million; and other Hispanic or Latino 10 million. The age characteristics are reported in Table 1.1. Note how the percentage of women to the total population rises with age.

Historically, a majority of human health studies have been performed only with white, middle-class, young to middle-aged male subjects. Applications of research outcomes to individuals not represented in a study remain purely hypothetical. A case in point: The National Institutes of Health (NIH) was placed under congressional investigation in 1990 for failing to include female subjects in health studies that dictated diagnostic and prescriptive guidelines for both men *and* women. "The NIH excuse for not using females in such studies—that additional costs and complications are incurred with

TABLE 1.1 U.S. Age Population Characteristics for the Year 2000 (in millions)

	TOTAL	WOMEN	PERCENTAGE OF TOTAL
Under 5 years	19.1	9.3	48.7
5–9 years	20.6	10.1	49.0
10–14 years	20.6	10.0	48.5
15–19 years	19.9	9.7	48.7
20–24 years	19.0	9.3	48.7
25–29 years	19.2	9.5	49.5
30–34 years	20.4	10.1	49.5
35–39 years	23.1	11.6	50.2
40–44 years	22.8	11.5	50.4
45–49 years	20.2	10.3	50.9
50–54 years	17.4	8.9	51.1
55–59 years	13.4	6.9	51.5
60–64 years	10.8	5.7	52.7
65–69 years	9.6	5.1	53.1
70–74 years	8.9	4.9	55.0
75–79 years	7.3	4.3	58.9
80–84 years	4.9	3.1	63.2
85–89 years	2.7	1.9	70.3
90 years and over	1.4	1.0	71.4

women subjects because of their numerous physiological differences in comparison with men—is the very reason women should have been included."[41]

Gender bias is common in health research. Some medications prescribed for women have not been tested on women, and some diagnostic and treatment guidelines for women are based on studies performed strictly with male samples.

Ethnic bias is also very present in health research. Studies that do incorporate women as subjects typically limit the subject pool to white, middle-class, young to middle-aged females. Ethnic minorities remain significantly underrepresented in health research.

Socioeconomic bias is prevalent in the health field. The provision of continuous, high-quality health care is often limited to the middle and upper class—that is, to those who have plenty of money or can afford health insurance. Social programs for the underprivileged, such as Social Security, Welfare, Medicaid, and Medicare are limited and frequently targeted by politicians for budget cuts. The poor are often deprived of adequate health care, the middle class can usually manage to at least maintain good health care, and the wealthy can take the greatest advantage of the most up-to-date health information and medical treatment. In addition, even when health care is available, educational efforts about certain health risks or the availability of medical treatment are usually targeted toward the upper and middle class via restricted avenues such as a doctor's office or specialized magazines. Lower-income families may never know that a health service or a health risk exists unless special efforts are made to reach out to this population.

Another cultural issue of concern is geographic differences. The majority of inner-city families are poor, and they are often not aware of health services or cannot afford them. Rural families frequently do not have quick access to hospitals or specialists, and thus adequate health care may not be available when needed. Or the family may have to drive a long distance to receive emergency health care or special services. Urban and suburban families are the most fortunate regarding the availability and affordability of quality health care.

WOMEN'S HEALTH RESEARCH

Historically, women's health research focused on diseases affecting fertility and reproduction—a focus reflective of the value society placed on women, that of primarily being a reproductive organism. Other disease research has focused disproportionately on men. Despite this imbalance, new drug therapies tested on men, once approved, were prescribed to women without comparable trials of clinical safety or efficacy. For example, a 1994 study suggested that aspirin could help prevent heart attacks in men. Women were not included in this study even though heart disease was the number-one killer of U.S. women. Yet aspirin was now recommended to both men and women as a preventive measure for heart attacks. Women have been excluded from medical research for at least two reasons: (1) concerns about pregnancy during a trial and (2) concerns that women's changing hormone levels during menstrual cycles might skew test results. We now know that there are no significant reasons to exclude women in medical research. In most cases, both sexes respond similarly to many therapies; however, there may be exceptions. For example, women may need lower dosages, or therapies may need to be specific to women.

The first comprehensive effort to clinically study health issues for women was the Nurses' Health Study. The Nurses' Health Study began in 1976, enrolling about 121,000 nurses. In 1989 a second group of 116,000 was enrolled in the Nurses' Health Study II. The groups, designated NHS I and NHS II, were followed by means of a biennial mail questionnaire that inquired about lifestyle and health problems.

In response to public criticism of the lack of involvement of women subjects in its medical research, the National Institutes of Health in 1990 established the Office of Research on Women's Health (ORWH). The earliest undertakings of the ORWH included development of a research agenda to identify and address gaps in the biomedical community's knowledge of women's health, and strengthening and revitalizing already-existing NIH guidelines and policies for the inclusion of women and minorities in clinical studies.

The ORWH launched the Women's Health Initiative (WHI) in 1991. The WHI was transferred in October 1997 to the NIH division, the National Heart, Lung, and Blood Institute (NHLBI), where it is conducted as a consortium effort in cooperation with the National Cancer Institute and the National Institute of Arthritis and Musculoskeletal and Skin Diseases.

The WHI is a long-term, national study that focuses on strategies for preventing heart disease, breast and colorectal cancer, and osteoporosis in women, especially postmenopausal women. The WHI is one of the largest studies of its kind ever undertaken in the United States and involves more than forty centers nationwide and 162,000 American women ages 50 to 79, about 18 percent from minority groups. Enrollment in the study began in 1993 and ended in 1998. Some of the first results for the WHI were released in 2005. The WHI is conducting three primary clinical studies: hormone replacement therapy, dietary modification, and calcium and vitamin D supplements. Studies and reports can be located at the ORWH Web site (http://orwh.od.nih.gov).

In 1990 the U.S. Department of Health and Human Services released *Healthy People 2000: National Health Promotion and Disease Prevention Objectives.* This document outlined the strategic plan for improving the health of the public and paid special attention to women's health issues. The three primary goals for the nation were (1) to increase the span of healthy life for Americans, (2) to reduce health disparities among Americans, and (3) to achieve access to preventive services for all Americans. An important follow-up document was published in 1996 titled *Healthy People 2000: Midcourse Review and 1995 Revisions.* The latest revision, *Healthy People 2010,* has two primary goals: (1) to increase quality and years of healthy life and (2) to eliminate health disparities. *Healthy People 2010* "challenges individuals, communities, and professionals—indeed all of us—to take specific steps to ensure that good health, as well as long life, are enjoyed by all." It is available from the U.S. Department of Health and Human Services (see the Web site: www.health.gov/healthypeople/document/html).

CONCLUSION

Women have health needs and concerns that are unique to their gender. Thus, it is important to have a health text dedicated specifically to women. The culture of women has evolved, like all cultures do. Who women are today and the issues they face have developed over time as a result of both positive and negative events throughout history. This text addresses the importance of women's health issues within the context of social, political, and medical arenas.

We hope you enjoy using this text as much as we enjoyed writing it. The topic of women's health is vast and we do not suppose that we have covered everything. We do hope that we addressed most of the major issues. We now leave it to you to continue the journey and advocate for greater awareness and attention to the field of women's health.

Chapter Summary

- There are three common types of health action: proactive care, health care maintenance, and reactive care.
- Holistic health care incorporates all that we know about health and utilizes this information to keep the body, mind, and spirit healthy.
- Sexual discrimination affects women in the workplace, in the pharmacy, and in personal lifestyle choices.
- A major cultural bias is the absence of adequate representation of women and ethnic minorities in medical research.
- Women around the globe share many of the same health concerns. However, cultural differences significantly impact the type and severity of these concerns.
- The status of women's health must be examined from cultural, political, and social perspectives.

Review Questions

1. Why do we need a text specific to women's health issues?
2. Can you name and describe three common types of health action?
3. How would you describe holistic health care?
4. Why is cultural sensitivity necessary in health care?
5. Can you name the various types of cultural bias in health care?
6. What are some health issues that are shared by women around the globe?
7. What are some major contributions to the U.S. women's health movement of the 1960s and 1970s?
8. What are some major social and political events in the history of the U.S. women's movement?
9. What is the Nurses' Health Study?
10. What is the Women's Health Initiative?

Resources

Web Sites

Black Women's Health
www.blackwomenshealth.com
Centers for Disease Control, Women's Health
www.cdc.gov/women
Feminist Majority Foundation
www.feminist.org
Healthy People 2010
www.health.gov/healthypeople/document/html
Middle East and Islamic Studies Collection, Cornell University Library: Women and Gender Issues
www.library.cornell.edu/colldev/mideast/women.htm
Mujer (Hispanic women's organization)
www.mujerinc.net
National Asian Women's Health Organization
www.nawho.org
National Center for Health Statistics
www.cdc.gov/nchs
National Institutes of Health
www.nih.gov
National Organization for Women
www.now.org
National Women's Health Information Center
www.4woman.gov
National Women's Health Network
www.nwhn.org
Native American Women's Health Education Resource Center
www.nativeshop.org
Native Web
www.nativeweb.org
Office of Research on Women's Health, National Institutes of Health
http://orwh.od.nih.gov
Office of Women's Health, Food and Drug Administration
www.fda.gov/womens
U.S. Department of Health and Human Services
www.os.dhhs.gov
United Nations
www.un.org
United Nations Development Fund for Women (UNIFEM)
www.unifem.undp.org
Women's Human Rights Net
www.whrnet.org
World Health Organization
www.who.int/en
Women in the Middle East—Columbia University Libraries, Middle East and Jewish Studies
www.columbia.edu/cu/lweb/indiv/mideast/cuvlm/women.html

Videotape/DVD

Burns, K., and P. Barnes. 1999. *Not for Ourselves Alone: The Story of Elizabeth Cady Stanton and Susan B. Anthony.* Public Broadcasting System (PBS) Home Video.

References

1. *Columbia encyclopedia*. 6th ed. 2003. www.encyclopedia.com (retrieved September 22, 2006).
2. Ibid.
3. Ibid.
4. Ibid.
5. National Women's Hall of Fame. 2003. *Great women.* www.greatwomen.org (retrieved September 22, 2006).
6. Ibid.
7. Ibid.
8. Ibid.
9. *Columbia encyclopedia.*
10. United States Department of Interior, National Register of Historic Places. 2000. *History of frontier nursing.* www.frontiernursing.org/history_of_fsn.htm (retrieved March 17, 2004).
11. Shaw, S., and J. Lee. 2007. *Women's voices, feminist visions.* 3rd. ed. New York: McGraw-Hill.
12. Ibid.
13. Ruth, S. 2001. *Issues in feminism.* 5th ed. Mountain View, CA: Mayfield.
14. Shaw and Lee, *Women's voices.*
15. Kirk, G., and M. Okazawa-Rey. 2007. *Women's lives: Multicultural perspectives.* 4th ed. New York: McGraw-Hill.
16. Shaw and Lee, *Women's voices.*
17. Downs, M. 2001. Women's salaries in life sciences one-third less. *Women's eNews.* October 12. www.womensenews.org/article.cfm/dyn/aid/683 (retrieved February 14, 2006).
18. Townsend, B. 2002. WNBA players upset with pay: Female athletes know they face uphill climb to balance wage scale. *Dallas Morning News*, August 11.
19. About Women's Issues. 2006. Gender pay gap—women make less money. *New York Times.* http://womensissues.about.com/od/genderdiscrimination/i/isgendergap.htm (retrieved February 14, 2006).
20. Associated Press. 2001. Women file class action suit against MetLife. *USA Today.com*, March 13. www.usatoday.com/money/general/2001-03-13-metlife.htm (retrieved September 22, 2006).
21. Costco Class Web site. 2004. http://genderclassactionagainstcostco.com (retrieved February 13, 2006).
22. Associated Press. 2004. Judge certifies Wal-Mart class action lawsuit. *Business with CNBC*, June 22. http://msnbc.msn.com/id/5269131 (retrieved September 22, 2006).
23. National Organization for Women. Action alert: Oppose the Unfair Class Action "Fairness" Act. 2003. April 9. www.now.org/lists/now-action-list/msg00098.html (retrieved February 16, 2006).
24. National Organization for Women. Action alert: Support the Access to Legal Pharmaceuticals Act. 2005. June 23. www.now.org (retrieved February 16, 2006).

25. Jacobson, S., and G. C. Kovach. 2004. Birth-control battleground? *Denton Record-Chronicle*, April 1, p. 3A (originally printed in the *Dallas Morning News*).
26. About Women's Issues. 2006. Sexual harassment statistics in the workplace and in education. *New York Times*. http://womensissues.about.com/cs/sexdiscrimination/a/sexharassstats.htm (retrieved February 14, 2006).
27. Kinzie, S. 2006. Sexual harassment routine, college students in poll say. *Washington Post*, January 25, p. A02. www.washingtonpost.com (retrieved February 25, 2006).
28. Miller, Y. 2006. Survey: Students face sexual harassment in high school. *The Boston Bay–State Banner*. www.baystatebanner.com (retrieved February 25, 2006).
29. Bingham, C., and L. L. Gansler. 2005. *Class action: The landmark case that changed sexual harassment law*. New York: Anchor, p. 70.
30. Ibid., p. 70.
31. Ibid., p. 70.
32. Ibid., p. 71.
33. Ibid., pp. 71–72.
34. Ibid., p. 72.
35. Ibid., p. 72.
36. Equal Employment Opportunity Commission. 2003. Guidelines on discrimination because of sex. 1604.11 Sexual harassment. July 1, p. 186.
37. Bingham and Gansler, p. 382.
38. United States federal and state information. 2006. *Gay rights info*. www.actwin.com/eatonohio/gay/GAY.htm (retrieved February 14, 2006).
39. Associated Press. 2005. WNBA star Swoopes says she's lesbian. *MSNBC.com*. http://msnbc.msn.com/id/9823452 (retrieved September 22, 2006).
40. United States federal and state information, *Gay rights info*.
41. Chandler, C. 1991. The psychology of women: Approaching the twenty-first century. *Individual Psychology* 47 (4): 487.

Chapter Two

Becoming a Wise Consumer

CHAPTER OBJECTIVES

When you complete this chapter, you will be able to do the following:

- Define consumerism and identify the various components of consumer health
- Describe the benefits and practices of intelligent consumer choices
- Identify characteristics of effectual and qualified health care providers
- Differentiate between quackery and effective alternative healing and treatment methods
- Compare and contrast generic and brand-name prescription drugs
- Identify the types of information written on drug labels
- Identify medicinal drugs prescribed for common disorders such as weight control, depression, and anxiety
- Explain the difference between prescription and over-the-counter drugs and provide examples of both
- Evaluate beauty-enhancing products that claim to be safe and beneficial
- Analyze the benefits and risks of beauty-enhancing procedures
- Explain the influence that advertising has on the images of and attitudes toward women
- Explain the impact of advertising on the financial, emotional, and social aspects of consumer practices
- Describe the appropriate actions necessary to become a wise and effective health consumer

CONSUMERISM: WHAT IS IT?

Being a wise consumer takes time and energy. The lack of effective consumer skills and practices can cost you money. Do you have more time or money? If you are like most people, there are precious little of both. If you develop wise consumer skills and know where to seek assistance, would you not save both time and money? Yes! This chapter will help you to achieve this.

HOW WE CONSUME

Is there a "trick" to wise use of health-enhancement dollars? Perhaps the only trick is to become informed about the varied, and sometimes complex, health-related costs. We are deluged with consumer information every day from an array of sources, some of which are reliable and others that are not. Included among these are news releases, public service media campaigns, publications for

FYI

Consumer Bill of Rights[1]

I. Information Disclosure
Consumers have the right to receive accurate, easily understood information and some require assistance in making informed health care decisions about their health plans, professionals, and facilities.

II. Choice of Providers and Plans
Consumers have the right to a choice of health care providers that is sufficient to ensure access to appropriate high-quality health care.
Access to Qualified Specialists for Women's Health Services: Women should be able to choose a qualified provider offered by a plan—such as gynecologists, certified nurse midwives, and other qualified health care providers—for the provision of covered care necessary to provide routine and preventative women's health care services.

III. Access to Emergency Services
Consumers have the right to access emergency health care services when and where the need arises. Health plans should provide payment when a consumer presents to an emergency department with acute symptoms of sufficient severity—including severe pain—such that a "prudent layperson" could reasonably expect the absence of medical attention to result in placing that consumer's health in serious jeopardy, serious impairment to bodily functions, or serious dysfunction of any bodily organ or part.

IV. Participation in Treatment Decisions
Consumers have the right and responsibility to fully participate in all decisions related to their health care. Consumers who are unable to fully participate in treatment decisions have the right to be represented by parents, guardians, family members, or other conservators.

V. Respect and Nondiscrimination
Consumers have the right to considerate, respectful care from all members of the health care system at all times and under all circumstances. An environment of mutual respect is essential to maintain a quality health care system.

VI. Confidentiality of Health Information
Consumers have the right to communicate with health care providers in confidence and to have the confidentiality of their individually identifiable health care information protected. Consumers also have the right to review and copy their own medical records and request amendments to their records.

VII. Complaints and Appeals
All consumers have the right to a fair and efficient process for resolving differences with their health plans, health care providers, and the institutions that serve them, including a rigorous system of internal review and an independent system of external review.

VIII. Consumer Responsibilities
In a health care system that protects consumers' rights, it is reasonable to expect and encourage consumers to assume reasonable responsibilities. Greater individual involvement by consumers in their care increases the likelihood of achieving the best outcomes and helps support a quality improvement, cost-conscious environment.

women, their families, and their health care providers, toll-free hotlines, governmental clearinghouse services, and of course, advertisements via various mediums. Consumer information from these varied sources can increase awareness and knowledge, influence attitudes and choices, and promote demands for better consumer services. They have to be credible and proven sources of information; otherwise, the information is of little value.

Public access to both health information and health misinformation abounds. Americans spend billions of dollars on unproven, worthless, and sometimes dangerous health remedies, with more money spent on "disease-curing" quackery than on research to prevent or cure these same diseases. As women, we often want to attain the body and beauty promised via weight loss gimmicks, miracle potions, or unnecessary elective surgeries. Knowledge about health products and health care personnel, procedures, and facilities is valuable. You can protect both your money and your health by developing and using wise consumer skills. (See *FYI:* "Consumer Bill of Rights.").

As of April 14, 2003, health care providers were required to comply with the requirements of the Health Insurance Portability and Accountability Act of 1996, also known as **HIPAA.**

Establishing standards for the privacy of individuals, HIPAA created national standards related to the delivery of health care, health fraud and abuse, insurance portability, and simplification of electronic transmission of claims and privacy of medical records. The Privacy Rule requires (1) that patients receive information about their privacy rights, (2) that privacy procedures are adopted in hospitals and practices, (3) that employees are trained to understand the privacy procedures, (4) that a designated individual be in charge of privacy procedures, and (5) that patient records be secured.

Health Tips

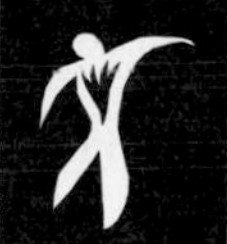

Selecting Your Health Care Provider

Upon entering the university, Elizabeth wants to search for a quality health care provider of the same caliber as her family-selected health care providers that she had for a number of years. She has two objectives: to locate two or three reputable physicians and then to determine which one best meets her health care needs. To do this, she will do the following:

To locate a provider

- Ask local friends and relatives for their recommendations.
- Check with the local medical society for suggestions specific to providers' specialty, sex, and age.
- Call local and/or regional women's health groups or organizations for suggestions.
- Call local hospitals to ask professional personnel about specific physicians.
- Check with the state medical society or licensing board to determine whether any complaints have been registered about a particular provider.

Once located, to select a provider

- Discuss his or her general health care practices; is he or she a single provider or a member of a group?
- What are the office location, the hours, fees, insurance requirements, and waiting period for appointments?
- Ask about the use of local health care facilities and interaction with other physicians.
- Is the physician an HMO member or in another health care group?
- Request a preliminary interview to determine rapport, mutual respect, treatment approaches, and referrals to specialists.

CHOOSING A HEALTH CARE PROVIDER

Selecting your health care providers is an important consumer skill. You will be sharing some of the most intimate concerns of your life with these persons. Qualifications, training, reputation, availability, and patient relation skills of health care providers are important. See *Health Tips:* "Selecting Your Health Care Provider" for suggestions about how to find the right provider for you.

Once you have visited the health care provider, consider the following questions: Do I like this provider? Do I feel respected? Does she or he take the time to answer my questions patiently? Was I able to understand the physician's information and instructions? Would this provider consider my health concerns and opinion as a part of a satisfactory treatment plan?

Health Care Providers

Health care providers include a variety of medical practitioners who have completed training in an accredited medical school and passed a medical examination. They can be divided into three groups:[2]

1. Independent practitioners who have been trained and licensed for all types of medical practices. There are medical and osteopathic physicians.
2. Independent practitioners with restricted practices such as podiatrists, dentists, psychologists, and optometrists.
3. Ancillary practitioners who practice only under the supervision of a medical practitioner. These include nurses, physical therapists, physician assistants, pharmacists, nurse practitioners, occupational therapists, and X-ray and laboratory technicians.

The following information gives a thumbnail sketch of health care providers with differing educational levels, skills, abilities, and responsibilities.

Physician The process of becoming a medical doctor, or MD, requires a minimum of 3 years of premedical college work for admission to medical school. However, 97 percent of premed students have a baccalaureate degree prior to admission.[3] Of those medical school students admitted in 2002, approximately 49.1 percent were women.[4] Students then spend 4 years in medical school, which should be accredited by a joint committee representing the American Medical Association (AMA) Council on Medical Education and the Association of American Medical Colleges. Following graduation, students must pass state or national board examinations to become licensed practitioners. (See *Women Making a Difference* to learn about a female physician who became surgeon general.)

Ever-changing research outcomes, improved technology, and new medicines create the need for developing medical specialties. Becoming a specialist such as a pediatrician, neurologist, or psychiatrist requires 3 or more years of additional training. Following the course work, the physician engages in additional clinical hours,

Women Making a Difference

Antonia C. Novello: Surgeon General of the United States, 1990–1993

Antonia C. Novello was born and educated in Puerto Rico, receiving an MD degree from the University of Puerto Rico School of Medicine at San Juan in 1970. Following a fellowship in the Department of Pediatrics at Georgetown University, she was in private practice until 1978. Dr. Novello then held various positions in public health service at the National Institutes of Health (NIH), rising to the position of Deputy Director of the National Institute of Child Health and Human Development in 1986. During her years at NIH, Dr. Novello earned an MPH degree from Johns Hopkins and made major contributions to the drafting and enactment of the Organ Transplantation Procurement Act of 1984, while assigned to the Senate Committee on Labor and Human Resources.

Antonia Novello was appointed surgeon general by President George H. W. Bush in 1990; she was the first Hispanic woman to hold this position. Dr. Novello focused on the health of women, children, and minorities as well as underage drinking, smoking, and AIDS. She helped to launch the Healthy Children Ready to Learn Initiative, and she worked with groups to promote immunization of children and childhood injury prevention. After her tenure as surgeon general, Dr. Novello served as the United Nations Children's Fund (UNICEF) Special Representative for Health and Nutrition from 1993 to 1996. Dr. Novello became commissioner of health for the State of New York in 1999. Antonia Novello has made a world of difference in the lives of women, children, and youth in her various health-related roles at the national level.

FYI

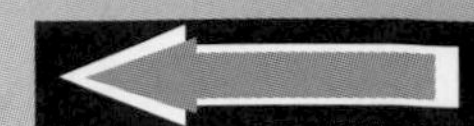

Periodic Checkups and Screening Tests[5]

Your doctor should ask about your . . .

- Family history, personal medical history, and any current medications, if any, that you take
- Dietary habits with special attention to fat, calories, fiber, iron, and calcium
- Exercise habits
- Use of any drugs, including alcohol and tobacco
- Safety practices (seat belt, safety equipment)
- Sexual practices related to disease prevention
- Birth control method (if any)
- What concerns you have about your health

Screening tests for generally healthy women include

- Blood pressure measurement: checked at least once or twice per year and during every doctor visit
- Clinical breast exam: yearly for all women aged 40 and over; every 3 years for women 20 to 40 years
- Mammography: yearly for women over 40; depending on family history of breast cancer, a physician may adjust these recommendations
- Pap smear: every 1 to 3 years beginning at age of first intercourse, or age 18
- Colorectal cancer: annual fecal occult blood test for age 50 and over and flexible sigmoidoscopy every 5 years
- Cholesterol screening: check every 5 years beginning at age 18, and more frequently as age increases or risks become prevalent
- Skin examination: every 3 years between 20 and 40 years of age, and every year for age 40 and over

obtains board certification, which means that the doctor has additional training, and passes a national examination in his or her specialty.

A doctor of osteopathy, a DO, is legally equivalent to a medical doctor and is licensed to practice in all states. Prior to admission to an osteopathy school, the student must have 3 years of college work related to the profession. During the 4 years of osteopathic college, the candidate will have over 5,000 hours of training, followed by a 1-year rotating internship at an approved hospital. If the DO decides to specialize, which about one-half do, a 2- to 6-year residency follows, depending on the chosen specialty.[6] Osteopathic doctors specialize in such areas as obstetrics, neurology, psychiatry, and anesthesiology. There is very little difference in the training of DOs and MDs. The difference is more in the philosophy of treatment. The American Osteopathic Association states that osteopathic medicine must closely follow the Hippocratic approach to medicine in that the body's musculoskeletal system is central to a person's well-being. Osteopathic medicine, because of its hands-on approach to diagnoses, can provide an alternative to surgery and/or drugs. The profession maintains its independence in order to provide a unique and comprehensive approach to health care.

Ordering a wide range of tests and X rays, taking blood, poking, prodding, and peering often compose the medical checkup. However, a more comprehensive look at an individual's lifestyle can often provide better quantity and quality of health information. A preventive health exam tailored to the age, risk factors, and lifestyle

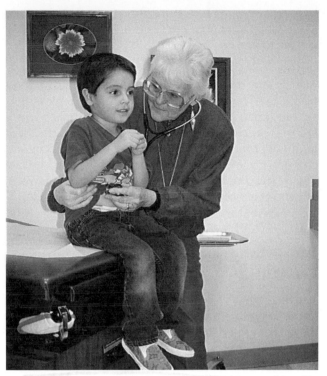

Bev Teagle, a nurse practitioner, examines 4-year-old Antonio.

of the patient can promote an enhanced quality of life and is more predictive of potential disease development. So, what constitutes a good periodic exam? See *FYI:* "Periodic Checkups and Screening Tests."

Physician Assistant A physician assistant (PA) works in the primary care medical setting under the supervision of a physician. He or she can give physical exams, prescribe drugs or therapies, and offer health counseling. Universities and medical schools that prepare PAs require varying entrance requirements and offer a curriculum that usually takes about 30 months to complete, including clinical training. Students may earn a Master of Physician Assistant Studies and then be a certified physician's assistant by passing an exam from the National Commission on the Certification of Physician Assistants. Because PAs are paid much less than physicians, health care programs often use them to help reduce the cost of health care. Physician assistants can work in private doctors' offices, hospitals, clinics, and other health care settings.

Nurse Practitioner A nurse practitioner can function as a primary care provider but often performs under a physician's supervision. Training includes additional nursing education, usually at the master's level, beyond the requirements needed to become a registered nurse (RN). Licensed by the state, registered nurses assess patients' physical and emotional needs and assist physicians and patients in prevention and treatment practices. Nurse practitioners are certified through the American Nurses Credentialing Center (ANCC) for work in geriatric, pediatric, and family health care, as well as in elementary and secondary school nursing. Nurse practitioners may also specialize in women's health and work in settings that treat health concerns of women.

Midwife Midwives are usually RNs who have received additional training and are certified to perform specific health care activities. One to 2 years of additional training is required from an approved school of midwifery. They can also earn nurse-midwife certification, CNM, which allows them to practice in almost every state by passing an exam from the American College of Nurse-Midwives.[7] Responsibilities include caring for pregnant women, managing labor and delivery, and caring for mother and baby after childbirth. A midwife may also be a vital part of the obstetrical team in physicians' offices, clinics, and hospitals. Midwives often are certified in CPR as well as neonatal resuscitation. In some states, midwives are required to obtain continuing education credits to maintain current knowledge in the field.

In the past, using midwives for childbirth and afterbirth care was disparaged by traditional health care, but recently, trained and qualified midwives have been found to offer effective, lower-cost, and patient-friendly health care. Currently, between 6 and 10 percent of all births in this country are attended by midwives, and some foremost medical schools in the United States offer certified midwife training programs.[8]

Mental Health Therapists Mental health professionals treat a variety of conditions related to one's mental and emotional well-being. Treatment can range from occasional outpatient counseling with single or group meetings to inpatient confinement using medication and electroshock. Seeking professional counseling and locating a competent and highly trained therapist are essential when you are concerned about your mental or emotional health.

Determining that you may need professional assistance with a mental or emotional health problem, what type of therapist should you seek? A wide range of mental health professionals have special training to work with a variety of issues. *FYI:* "Therapists for Mental and Emotional Health" explains the meaning of the letters following the therapists' names and the significance of each in helping you to select the best therapist.

Therapists should be trustworthy, nonjudgmental, empathetic, respectful, sincere, and well trained in their area of therapy. Consider the following criteria when determining the merits of a potential therapist:

- What are the credentials of the therapist?
- Is she or he a licensed therapist?

FYI

Therapists for Mental and Emotional Health[9]

Academic Degrees

Psychiatry *Doctorate in Medicine: MD*
Has completed medical training and has specialized residency in psychiatry. May also have additional training in psychoanalysis or psychodynamic training. Psychiatrists are the only therapists who can prescribe drugs.

Psychology

Doctorate in Psychology: PsyD
Has 6 to 7 years of graduate work and training with an emphasis on practical clinical course work rather than research.

Doctorate in Philosophy: PhD
Has 6 to 7 years of graduate work with training in research methodology and had a pychotherapy internship. Can administer psychological testing.

Doctorate in Education: EdD
Training similar to that received by a PhD. However, this degree is issued through graduate schools of education rather than science or psychology.

Therapy

Master of Science: MS
Has completed a 2-year program in clinical psychology after receiving a baccalaureate degree. Usually has training in psychotherapy techniques but not psychological assessmentor work.

Master of Social Work: MSW
Has completed a 2- to 3-year graduate program that emphasizes training in psychotherapy and social work.

Licensures by State Professional Boards*

Licensed Clinical Social Worker: LCSW
Licensed Marriage and Family Child Counselor: LMFCC
Licensed Professional Counselor: LPC
Licensed Marriage and Family Therapist: LMFT

*Note that these designations are licensures awarded by state professional boards. They do *not* refer to academic degrees. Licensure related to a professional specialty should be obtained. Otherwise, the "professional" may not truly be qualified.

- Will your insurance cover the costs of this therapy?
- What type of treatment does the therapist use?
- Will he or she prescribe medication?
- How long and how often should you expect to be in treatment?
- Do you know anyone who this therapist has treated for a similar problem? Was the treatment successful?
- Are any complaints about this therapist filed with local medical personnel or professional licensing boards?

There are always "professionals" who will take our money and provide poor quality and even harmful health care. In some states, it is legal to use such titles as "therapists," "counselors," and "sex therapists" without any specific or certified credentials. Be smart! Check for the appropriate credentials before investing time and money with a mental health professional. Locate trusted physicians, and check with family, friends, or coworkers who can recommend competent and qualified professionals to work with you.

Reporting Unprofessional Treatment

Knowing what to do if you have received inadequate, unprofessional, or unethical health care treatment is important. Taking action immediately by contacting proper authorities and providing written statements and any supporting documentation will aid you and other potential patients to avoid unnecessary, painful, incorrect, or even fatal treatment at the hands of a health care provider. To report this concern, write a letter to the hospital or doctor involved and send a copy to any or all of the following: a referring doctor, the administrator or director of the hospital or clinic, the local medical society, the state licensing board, your insurance carrier, and any local health consumer or women's health group. A doctor–patient relationship should be one of equality and mutual respect with you and your doctor making responsible and health-enhancing decisions together. An online complaint form is found at www.ftc.gov/ftc/consumer.htm.

HEALTH CARE DELIVERY

The socioeconomic circumstances and roles of women continue to evolve and change as they relate to parenting, employment, and relationships. Today, the health care needs of women vary significantly from the time when the "typical" female was a stay-at-home wife and mother and sheltered under her partner's health care plan and the long-time family physician. Meeting the changing needs of women's health care is the responsibility of the health care system, health-related institutions, and women themselves. How do we meet this challenge? There is a need to *improve* health care delivery for women and to *provide* for health needs whether women live in the inner city, rural America, or the "burbs." This could be accomplished by having health care clinics near public transport or in inner-city neighborhoods. An awareness of the differing health needs of women could be developed via better training in medical and nursing schools and by fostering an understanding attitude toward the special health needs of women.

Removing barriers to quality health care services is essential if women are to garner the necessary examinations, treatment, and rehabilitation. Barriers may include too little money for health care, lack of insurance, no transportation to and from health facilities, distant travel to health care providers, job-related demands, and no sick leave or time allotted away from the job. (Health insurance concerns are discussed later in this chapter.)

Solutions to effective health care delivery specific to the needs of women must include experts in medical, community, and government factions. All of these factions must identify the problems related to health care for women, determine the various alternatives and the positives and negatives of each, assess the possible solutions, and then act accordingly. A health care delivery system that addresses all women must be accessible, culturally relevant, affordable, and available.

HOME HEALTH TESTS

At-home methods to determine the status of one's health have come a long way from only using scales, thermometers, and taking your pulse. Over-the-counter home health test kits have expanded our access to faster results and vital information related to numerous health concerns. Well over $1 billion is spent annually in markets or online to monitor health conditions in the privacy of one's home. Home health tests can mean lower medical costs, better monitoring of chronic conditions, and earlier detection of health problems. Additionally, home health tests can be an easy-to-use method for providing private information in a brief amount of time. However, overreliance on these various tests (e.g., used as an indicator of diagnosis or cure) or misinterpretation of the results can be dangerous; a wise consumer will not make medical decisions without consulting with a medical professional. The FDA offers suggestions for purchasing home diagnostic tests and general precautions to consider.[10]

There are basically three types of home tests: (1) diagnostic tests (for sexually transmitted infections, ovulation, pregnancy, urinary tract infections), (2) continuous monitoring tests (for blood glucose, blood pressure) that are often recommended by one's physician to assist in overseeing an existing disease, and (3) screening tests to determine if a disease is present even though symptoms are not present, such as cholesterol testing or hepatitis screening. The best known are pregnancy tests, whereas the biggest sellers are blood glucose monitors and test strips used by individuals with diabetes. (See *FYI:* "Common Home Health Tests.") Together they account for 90 percent of home health test kits sold nationally.

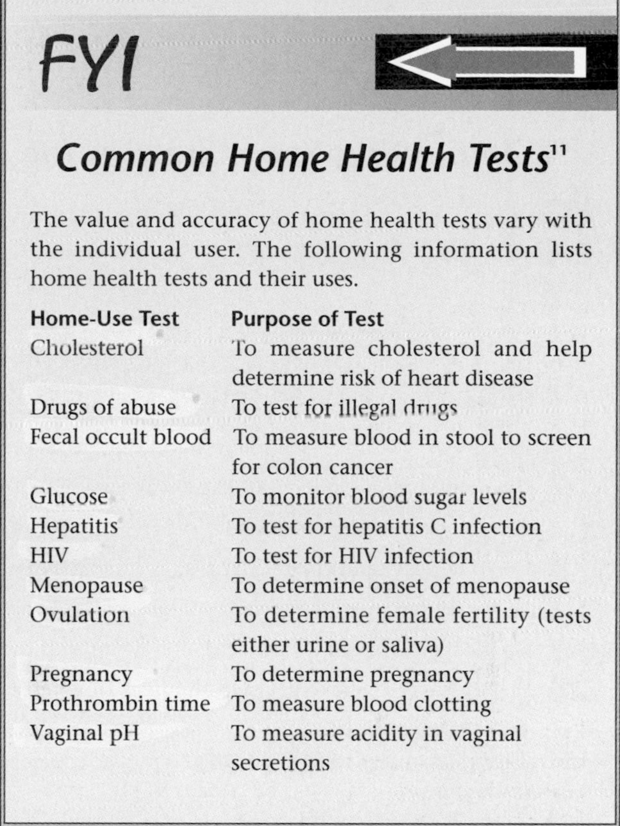

FYI

Common Home Health Tests[11]

The value and accuracy of home health tests vary with the individual user. The following information lists home health tests and their uses.

Home-Use Test	Purpose of Test
Cholesterol	To measure cholesterol and help determine risk of heart disease
Drugs of abuse	To test for illegal drugs
Fecal occult blood	To measure blood in stool to screen for colon cancer
Glucose	To monitor blood sugar levels
Hepatitis	To test for hepatitis C infection
HIV	To test for HIV infection
Menopause	To determine onset of menopause
Ovulation	To determine female fertility (tests either urine or saliva)
Pregnancy	To determine pregnancy
Prothrombin time	To measure blood clotting
Vaginal pH	To measure acidity in vaginal secretions

It has been estimated that one in seven medical tests, including those administered by health professionals, results in false findings. Certainly, the margin for error associated with the general consumer administering a test at home can be even greater. However, many of the use-at-home test kits, when used properly, can provide accurate and cost-effective results. Complete *Assess Yourself:* "Improving Your Chances for Accurate Home Health Test Results" to help improve the effectiveness of your test results.

COMPLEMENTARY AND ALTERNATIVE MEDICINE

Complementary and alternative medicine (CAM), such as herbs, acupuncture, chiropractic care, and massage therapy, increasingly are recognized as having the potential for relief, treatment, and cure of certain diseases. **Complementary medicine** is used *with* conventional medicine, and **alternative medicine** is used *in place of* conventional medicine. CAM has been defined as a group of diverse medical and health care systems, practices, and products that are not presently considered part of conventional Western medicine.[12] However, this is changing as the federal Committee on the Use of Complementary and Alternative Medicine by the American People recommends that health profession

Assess Yourself

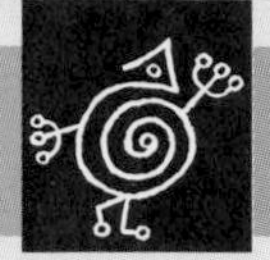

Improving Your Chances for Accurate Home Health Test Results

If you have purchased a home health test kit, answer the following questions. This information will assist you in obtaining accurate test results.

Question	Yes	No
1. Has the expiration date expired?	_____	_____
2. Has the kit been exposed to extreme heat or cold?	_____	_____
3. Are the directions for using the kit and chemicals clear to you?	_____	_____
4. Have you read and do you understand the special precautions, if any?	_____	_____
5. Did you follow the directions exactly as stated?	_____	_____
6. Did you time the test accurately and precisely as instructed?	_____	_____
7. Do you understand what the test kit is intended to find?	_____	_____
8. Do you know what to do when you obtain the results, whether they are positive or negative?	_____	_____
9. Do you know whom to contact to follow up with the results of the test?	_____	_____
10. Do you know where to get help administering the test if you are unsure about the directions?	_____	_____

If you answered eight or more of the questions with a positive response, your health kit test results should be accurate. If you answered less than eight with a positive response, you need to read directions more accurately and discuss the procedures with a medical professional.

schools, such as schools of medicine and nursing, incorporate sufficient information about CAM into the standard curriculum at the undergraduate, graduate, and postgraduate levels so that licensed professional can advise their patients about CAM in a competent manner.[13] Currently, 42 percent of U.S. citizens report that they have used at least one CAM therapy, and the number of visits to CAM providers exceeds the number of visits to all primary care physicians. The American public is currently spending over $27 billion a year on various CAM practices.[14] Women, with higher education levels overall, are more likely than men to use CAM therapies, and patterns of use vary among ethnic groups.

The National Institutes of Health now has a National Center for Complementary and Alternative Medicine (NCCAM), which investigates nontraditional healing regimens (see Chapter 5 for a more detailed description of the NCCAM and the use of mind–body medicine to heal and manage stress). Numerous medical schools, such as Georgetown University, University of Louisville, and University of Massachusetts in Worcester, offer courses and lectures on CAM medical therapies.[15]

Why has interest in alternative therapies experienced such phenomenal growth? Although we have seen amazing progress in high-tech medical practices, these procedures are often painful, expensive, and even dehumanizing. People began to seek therapies that would take healing a step beyond "treatment." Milestones in the women's movement toward alternative therapy began in the early 1960s with publication of books such as *The Feminine Mystique* by Betty Friedan, which enlightened many women and led to new heights of competence and empowerment. Near this time, yoga, meditation, and macrobiotic diets emerged as the idea of a mind–body connection in illness and wellness found its practitioners and patients. *Our Bodies, Ourselves,* initially published in 1973, created the desire in many women to take charge of their own well-being through increased knowledge about their own bodies and better education. Women desired a redefinition of the doctor–female patient relationship in which a partnership was formed that enabled them to become part of the decision-making healing process. Books such as *Type A Behavior and Your Heart* (Friedman and Rosenman, 1974), *The Relaxation Response* (Benson, 1975), *Anatomy of an Illness* (Cousins, 1979), and *Psychoneuroimmunology* (Ader, 1981) discussed the connection among our mind, our emotions, and our health. This literature led us to believe that, with effective training, we could become partners in our own level of health. Visiting a bookstore today, you will find an uncanny array of books related to alternative health–related practices. An important next step is for women to find the "right" type of alternative approach and the "right" practitioner, so the ability to control pain, reduce stress, and improve well-being is ours!

Unfortunately, in some instances the results have not been positive. Women were/are too often the victims of scam artists or quacks; our money is taken, but the results are less than desirable, even worse, harmful or deadly. However, there are certainly reputable alternative practitioners, medicines, and methodologies that offer, in some instances, more favorable results than conventional medicine. Let us look at a number of alternative therapies and find out what they are, how they "work," and possible risks and benefits of each.

Herbalism

Herbs could be called alternative "drugs" that promote the premise that many disorders or injuries can be treated with a plant or parts of a plant. Herbal medicine was practiced in ancient Rome, Greece, and Babylon and is still used throughout the world, especially in less developed countries. Historically, plants such as myrrh, oil of cloves, peppermint, and caraway were used to treat a range of disorders including sexually transmitted diseases, inflammation, and heart disease. Patent medicines (nonprescription drugs, protected by a trademark) contained a variety of plants such as ginger root, castor oil, juniper bush, and alfalfa. Herbalists found that drinks made of herbs soothe the nerves, aloe can soothe the skin, and leaves from foxglove contain digitalis, and so on.

It only takes a visit to a "health food" market to realize that herbs and products containing herbs are widely available. In fact, in the quest for a more "natural" approach to healing, Americans spend billions of dollars each year on herbal medicines, bulk herbs, and other herbal products. Brochures, books, and pamphlets espouse the benefits of available herbal "medicines," yet researchers state that we need to be wary of some of these medicines. Concerns about herbal medicines include lack of scientific "proof" that they indeed treat and heal health problems; most reports of herbal healing abilities are based on unfounded claims from folklore and some outdated reports. Herbs can be dangerous, even deadly in fact, and some herbs have been banned from sale, whereas others carry a warning on their labels. Herbs contain many hundreds of chemicals, and their reaction in the body can be unknown: perhaps helpful, but perhaps harmful. An excellent resource for herbal information is the Natural Medicines Comprehensive Database, which is available online.[16] Herbal medicines are not controlled by the **Food and Drug Administration** (FDA) and certain strengths of the herb can vary from product to product. Safe and effective medicines are available to treat conditions for which they are known to work (see FYI: "Herbs and Their Uses"). Purchasing and using unproven and potentially dangerous herbal medicines is not wise. It appears that it would be advantageous for Western researchers to continue to research and examine the benefits and risks of herbs.

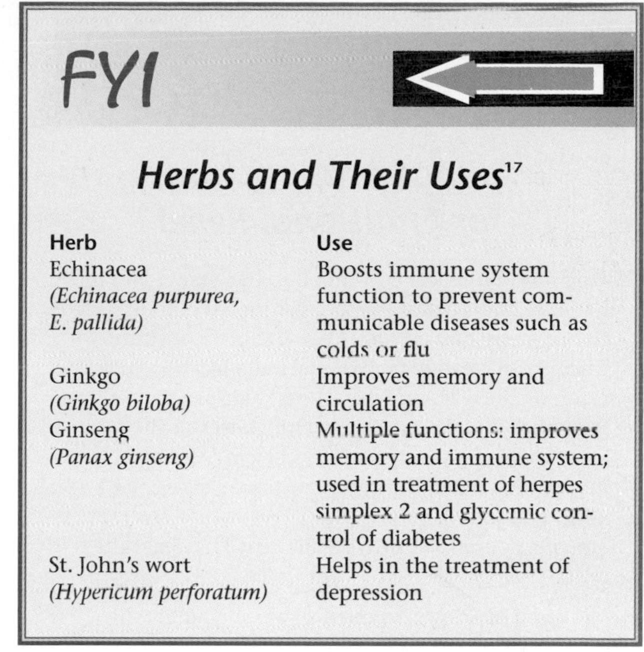

FYI

Herbs and Their Uses[17]

Herb	Use
Echinacea *(Echinacea purpurea, E. pallida)*	Boosts immune system function to prevent communicable diseases such as colds or flu
Ginkgo *(Ginkgo biloba)*	Improves memory and circulation
Ginseng *(Panax ginseng)*	Multiple functions: improves memory and immune system; used in treatment of herpes simplex 2 and glycemic control of diabetes
St. John's wort *(Hypericum perforatum)*	Helps in the treatment of depression

Acupuncture

In its 5,000-year history, acupuncture has been used by more people than any other form of alternative medicine. Acupuncture claims to restore balance (Qi) to promote healing and functioning through inserting needles at precise points on the body. Heat may be applied to the acupuncture point to promote the healing process. The premise is that meridians, channels of energy, run like energy throughout the body. When blockage in one part of a channel occurs, it impedes the flow to others. Acupuncture claims to remove the blockage and allow the usual flow through the meridians, restoring Qi and aiding the bodily organs with imbalances. The World Health Organization acknowledges acupuncture treatment for digestive and respiratory disorders, neurological and muscular ailments, and urinary, menstrual, and reproductive problems. It appears to be especially helpful for physical difficulties related to stress and tension.

Data from the Department of Health and Human Services 2004 survey found that 4 percent of the American public had tried acupuncture and that it is a more popular complementary medicine than homeopathy, naturopathy, and ayurveda.[18] The National Commission for the Certification of Acupuncturists is the certifying agency in this country. Acupuncturists have submitted scientific evidence to the FDA that

Her Story

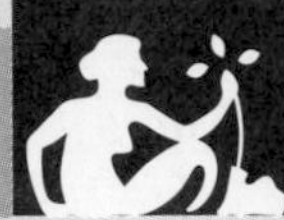

Ping: Acupuncture for Emotional Relief

Ping found that she continued to have more and more frequent bouts of anxiety and emotional outbursts close to her menstrual period. After she had consulted with three physicians and tried several tranquilizers, a coworker recommended acupuncture. Ping was open to, but skeptical of, the suggested treatment. However, she located a reputable acupuncturist and began a series of treatments with needles inserted at points along her back, arms, and legs. After 6 weeks of treatments, she was less anxious not only during premenstrual days but the rest of the time as well.

- Based on Ping's experience, would you be willing to try acupuncture yourself?
- What are the advantages of acupuncture? The disadvantages?
- How can you find a certified acupuncturist?

Health Tips

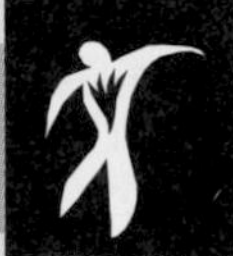

Acupuncture: Use Caution[20]

Consider the following when contemplating the use of acupuncture as alternative therapy:

- Although complications from acupuncture are few, serious complications can occur because it is an invasive procedure.
- No scientific data exist that prove acupuncture is successful in treating or reducing the risks of organic diseases.
- Acupuncture most often is used for pain relief, but the relief, if there is any, is usually brief.
- Training for acupuncture practitioners is often inadequate or unsupervised, and practitioners may use unscientific methods that are, at the least, not beneficial, or at most, harmful.

shows that the needles used in acupuncture do have the ability to heal. If the FDA decides to recognize the tools of acupuncture as bona fide medical instruments, then certain acupuncture treatments could be reimbursed by Medicare, Medicaid, and private insurers.

Women find relief with acupuncture for a variety of ailments: menstrual cramps, headaches, nausea, backaches, and depression. (See *Her Story:* "Ping: Acupuncture for Emotional Relief" and *Health Tips:* "Acupuncture: Use Caution.") Pain relief is the most common and well-documented use of acupuncture. With a certified acupuncturist using sterile equipment, this form of therapy has almost no side effects or risk of complication. However, it is important to remember that using acupuncture does not preclude seeing a physician and using medicinal drugs in conjunction with this type of alternative medicine.

Chiropractic Care

Reports of spinal manipulation appear in written records of ancient China and Greece. Indians in early America had family members walk on and maneuver their backbones to reduce problems with their spine. Another form of spinal manipulation, chiropractic, was founded around 1895 by Daniel David Palmer, a grocer and "magnetic healer" in Iowa.[19] After a number of battles with the AMA and other medical and political groups, chiropractic medicine became recognized as a method to treat disorders, with some degree of success, which chiropractors attribute to spinal manipulation.

There are over 50,000 licensed chiropractors in this country, and they make up the third largest group of health care practitioners, after physicians and dentists.[21] Chiropractors must complete 4,200 hours of study over a 4-year period and take both national and state board examinations to be a licensed practitioner. Although chiropractic is practiced in all 50 states, a chiropractor must pass the state board exam to be able to treat patients in certain states.[22] In many instances, chiropractice services are reimbursed through private as well as state and federal insurance providers.

Chiropractic medicine is nonscientific medical practices based on the belief that good health depends on the proper functioning of nerve impulse transmission through the nervous system. Therefore, when nerve impulse transmission encounters any type of interference, such as an ill-aligned spine, the person develops an illness. Chiropractic medicine claims that restoring the flow of nerve impulses through proper spinal manipulation can return the person to good health.

The medical science community is concerned about the claims of chiropractors because the claim that interference of nerve impulses is a cause of disease has not been proven scientifically. Additionally, the anatomical structure of the body does not lend itself to the healing and pain relief claims made by chiropractors. However, there does seem to be evidence that chiropractic medicine can be helpful in treating certain musculoskeletal ailments and relieving menstrual pain, which has a back-related component. There are also claims that manipulating and stretching muscles in the

Health Tips

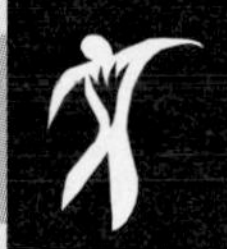

When to See a Chiropractor[23]

1. See your physician to determine the reason for your condition.
2. Select a chiropractor who is referred by the National Association for Chiropractic Medicine (www.chiromed.org).
3. Call first to find out about the kind of treatment offered:
   - Does the chiropractor primarily treat musculoskeletal problems?
   - Will he or she cooperate with your medical doctor to reach the best treatment for you?
   - How long and how often should you expect to be in treatment?
   - What are the charges and financial expectations?
   - To which professional associations does the chiropractor belong?
   - Can the chiropractor be reimbursed by your insurance company?

FYI

Assessing the Chiropractor[25]

Avoid the chiropractor who engages in the following practices:

- Takes repeated or full-spine X rays
- Does not attempt to assess the nature of the problem in a professional manner
- Claims that benefits to organ systems, immune function, or even a cure will result
- Offers vitamins or nutritional and/or homeopathic treatment
- Asks you to sign a contract for long-term care
- States that you will be kept healthy by regular checkups and manipulations
- Solicits other family members from you for treatment

back of the head can be beneficial for migraine and tension headaches.

Concerns arise about chiropractic care when chiropractors use treatment modalities for which they have no specific training such as physical therapy, "sports chiropractic," acupuncture, and sometimes nutritional and homeopathic medicine. Conventional medical practitioners worry that spinal manipulation may do more harm than good, especially if the pain has been long lasting or if a tumor or fracture is present. Additionally, some unethical chiropractors keep patients returning for unnecessary treatments and X rays.

There is movement in chiropractic medicine to focus on a scientific approach to musculoskeletal problems and eliminate procedures for which chiropractors have little or no training. Should you and your physician determine that you have a condition for which chiropractic medicine may be beneficial, such as low-back pain, refer to *Health Tips:* "When to See a Chiropractor" and *FYI:* "Assessing the Chiropractor."

Massage

Massage, in addition to feeling good, appears to offer healthful benefits for the promotion of healing of disease and injuries. Recent research confirms that massage therapy is an effective treatment for low back pain, helps breast cancer survivors both emotionally and physically, helps to ease pain after surgery, and boosts the immune system functions.[24] The same research found that children receiving a nightly massage also experience less anxiety and depression and have lower stress hormone levels. Researchers believe that massage helps to counteract the body's stress response, thereby reducing the ill effects stress hormones can have on the body.

Many active women, such as athletes, have experienced some relief from soreness, injury, and pain due to the use of massage therapy. This approach may eliminate the use of drugs and/or surgery to realize these benefits.

Trigger-point massage promotes the healing of muscle sprains, chronic tendonitis, and chronic muscle spasms, and **cross-fiber friction massage** assists in breaking up adhesions and stretches and realigns scar tissues with healthy muscle fiber.[26] Massages can also help to reduce fatigue and soreness in muscles by promoting muscle relaxation, increasing blood flow to muscles, and reducing inflammation and swelling.

Thirty-three states offer massage licenses, and the requirements to receive a license vary according to the state in which it is issued. Other states allow massage certification of individuals who acquire training and pass written and practical exams; these criteria vary according to state requirements. Either ask someone who has had a positive outcome using a masseur, or contact the American Massage Therapy Association at www.amtamassage.com for the name of the nearest licensed masseur. Time of massage sessions may be anywhere from 15 to 60 minutes and range in cost from $20 to $80 or more. Be sure the masseur you choose treats you in a respectful and professional manner. If not, as with any other practitioner, she or he should be reported to their professional association as well as to local authorities. Using massage, or any other alternative

Viewpoint 

Holistic Medicine Practices

Here are some characteristics of holistic medicine practices. Which ones do you consider to be worthwhile, and which ones lend themselves to questionable practices? Explain your position for each one.

- Uses nonscientific approaches to diagnose and treat medical problems
- Uses laypeople and other professionals in the treatment process
- Examines the lifestyle of the individual: nutrition, exercise practices, environment, emotions, use of chemicals, social interactions, and/or spirituality
- Encourages the woman's participation in all aspects of diagnosis and treatment
- Views illness as a means to evaluate and change one's lifestyle
- Emphasizes health as promotion of a healthy lifestyle rather than the absence of disease
- Emphasizes self-care rather than treatment and dependence on medical personnel
- Desires to reduce dependence on medicines, surgery, and treatment
- Promotes healing through meeting the needs of mind, body, and spirit of the individual

healing method, in lieu of determining the exact cause of the injury or pain through scientifically proven tests is not being a wise consumer.

Holistic Medicine

Holistic, or wholistic, medicine had its origin in ancient times and is derived from the Greek term *holo,* which means "whole." The whole person, which includes the physical, mental, emotional, social, and spiritual dimensions, is considered in the treatment and healing process. Although certain components of holistic medicine can be beneficial, other components embraced by holistic healers lend themselves to questionable medical practices.

Of the major concerns related to holistic medicine, the potential for use of nonscientific medical practices and for practitioners to provide useless, harmful, or even deadly care (for a large fee) is of greatest concern. Two long-time professionals who concerned themselves with the holistic healing movement believed it to be "a pabulum of common sense and nonsense offered by cranks and quacks and failed pedants who share an attachment to magic and an animosity to reason."[27] (See *Viewpoint:* "Holistic Medicine Practices.")

There is promise of effective treatment in many holistic health care practices, but until more funding is available for research to determine scientific proof of positive results, this concept of alternative health care will continue to be just that—an alternative.

Other Types of Alternative Health Care

Consider the following brief descriptions of various other alternative health care practices and you will see why the consumer needs information and guidelines to make wise choices.

Naturopathic medicine promotes the concept of the body's own natural healing ability through use of herbal medicine, nutrition, relaxation exercises, and acupuncture. *Reflexologists* use foot massage as a means to stimulate peak functioning of body systems. Massaging certain areas of the body to promote healing or pain reduction is the major premise of *craniosacral therapy*—skull, spine, and sacrum areas; *myofascial* and *Rolfing* massage connective tissue for pain relief and to promote structural integration; *myotherapists* manipulate trigger points in elbows, knuckles, and fingers to relieve pain and tension. *Yoga* attempts to integrate body, mind, and spirit with the universe through movement, relaxation, breathing techniques, and music. *Aromatherapy* is a practice in which aromatic oils are used in warm baths, massage oils, and other products. They can also be massaged into the body or inhaled for treatment of common disorders and to influence mind and emotions. Aromas may be used in a birthing environment to promote tranquility during the birthing process.

Using the best of Western medicine (orthodox health care) and the best of alternative health care practices may be a wise approach to obtaining the best health care possible. Although surgery, medicine, and physical therapy are essential treatments for the injured or critically ill woman, preventing major disease, promoting well-being, and providing the opportunity for partnership in health care have an important place. Medication and diagnostic tools for acute health problems combined with healing touch, needles, and herbs for tension, pain, and relaxation can be effective.

Health Quackery

In the search for "hope" when no other was offered or a "quick and painless fix" to any ailment or problem from wrinkle reduction cream to weight loss plans, U.S. citizens spend over $15 billion annually on a variety of products that purport to address these concerns.[28] When there is a health-related concern, there will often be some gimmick, potion, or practitioner available—for a price—to remedy the concern. These products promise

Assess Yourself

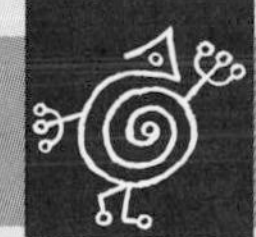

Assessing Alternative Health Care Claims and Products[29]

Does the practitioner or promoter exhibit these characteristics?	Yes	No
1. Promises quick, painless, drugless treatment or cure	_____	_____
2. Uses anecdotes or testimonials to support claim	_____	_____
3. Displays questionable credentials/titles	_____	_____
4. Uses pseudoscientific terminology	_____	_____
5. Claims that a single treatment can cure a wide range of illnesses	_____	_____
6. Claims persecution by organized medicine	_____	_____
7. Claims that many illnesses can be treated by nutrition	_____	_____
8. Advises use of vitamins/health foods for everyone	_____	_____
9. States surgery/X rays/drugs do more harm than good	_____	_____
10. Espouses "freedom of choice" to use unproven approaches	_____	_____
11. Claims to have a cure that is secret or known only in foreign countries	_____	_____

Any positive response should be regarded as suspicious!

that we can eat all we want and still lose weight, build a bigger bustline, melt away cellulite, or increase our libido. The FDA defines health **quackery** as the promotion of a medical remedy that doesn't work and is known to be false or unproven.[30]

Protecting Yourself

To protect yourself from loss of time, money, and possibly your health, complete *Assess Yourself:* "Assessing Alternative Health Care Claims and Products" to determine if the product and person are promoting quackery.

PRESCRIPTION DRUGS

Currently, the Food and Drug Administration (FDA) has approved more than 2,500 prescription drugs, all of which are intended to prevent, treat, or cure various types of illnesses. Prescription drugs are made of natural and/or synthetic chemicals and can be obtained only with a physician's written authorization.

Prescription drugs are potent, but when used as directed, they can produce positive results for treatment and healing. The FDA regulates prescription drugs for form, strength, safety, purity, effectiveness, and method of administration. More than 2.3 billion prescriptions are filled each year, including 1.02 billion refills and 1.29 billion new prescriptions.[31]

Prescription drugs have three names: the generic name, the chemical name, and the brand name. **Generic names** pertain to the kind of drug and also describe the drug, such as penicillin. Although generic drugs are identical in their chemical compounds with the same brand-name drug, generic drugs may *not* be equivalent in therapeutic effect. Legally, drugs are identified by their generic names and are listed by that name in the **United States Pharmacopoeia (USP).** The USP is responsible for conferring the official standards of identity, purity, and effectiveness for all prescription drugs. In laboratories, drugs are called by their **chemical name,** which usually refers to the chemicals from which the drugs have been developed. The **brand name,** under the control of the FDA, is patented by the pharmaceutical company, which develops, manufactures, and distributes the drug to pharmacies. The company that develops and tests the drug has exclusive rights to produce it for 17 years. Once the patent expires, other pharmaceutical companies are then permitted to manufacture the drug under another brand name or under its generic name. Table 2.1 provides a few examples of brand and generic names of commonly prescribed drugs.

Pharmacists can dispense generic drugs instead of brand-name products with a doctor's approval in almost all states. Brand-name drugs can be 30–50 percent more expensive than their generic counterparts, and approximately 400 different generic drugs can presently be substituted for brand-name drugs.[32] The equivalent effectiveness of generic and brand-name drugs is determined by scientists who measure the time it takes the generic drug to reach the bloodstream. The rate of absorption, called **bioavailability,** is then compared to the rate for the brand-name drug. If it is found that the generic and brand-name versions deliver the same amount of active ingredients into a patient's bloodstream with equal absorption rates, the two drugs are considered to be equivalent. The FDA ensures the equivalency of generic and brand-name drugs. However, even if drugs are therapeutically equivalent, they may not produce the same effects in all women.

Understanding Drug Labels

Carefully following the directions on a prescription label enables the consumer to receive the most effective results when taking a drug. A prescription label provides the patient's name and the physician's name as well as the name, address, and phone number of the pharmacy dispensing the drug. Drug-related information includes the name of the drug, the dosage form (liquid, capsule, tablet), and the strength of the drug, in either milligrams (mg) or ounces. How much, how often, and when to take the drug are indicated along with any special instructions and refill information. Essential information regarding warnings about drug–drug or food–drug interactions is also provided.[33] (See Figure 2.1.)

TABLE 2.1 Generic and Brand Names of Commonly Prescribed Drugs*

BRAND NAME	GENERIC NAME
Zovirax	acyclovir
Xanax	alprazolam
Valium	diazepam
Tylenol	acetaminophen

*Brand names are Capitalized; generic names are lowercased.

Almost half of all prescription drugs will fail to produce the desired effects because of incorrect use. Patients do such things as take too much or too little of a drug, take it too often or not often enough, skip doses, take it with food when directions say without food, drink alcohol when they're taking the drug, or use expired drugs. A woman needs to ask her physician and/or pharmacist critical questions and seek information that will permit her to use the medication safely and effectively. She should tell her physician about any previous allergic reactions to foods or medicines, any medication (including over-the-counter) being taken on a regular basis, any physical conditions for which she is being treated by other physicians, and if she is pregnant or breast-feeding.

Health Tips: "Questions to Ask When Taking Prescription Medicine" lists questions women should ask their physicians about prescription drug use. For practice, complete *Journal Activity:* "Questions to Ask When Purchasing Medications."

Commonly Prescribed Drugs

Two-thirds of the women who visit a doctor's office will have a written prescription in their hands when

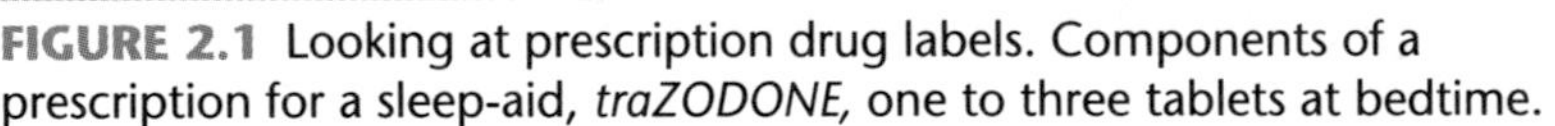

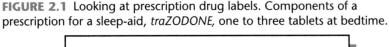

FIGURE 2.1 Looking at prescription drug labels. Components of a prescription for a sleep-aid, *traZODONE,* one to three tablets at bedtime.

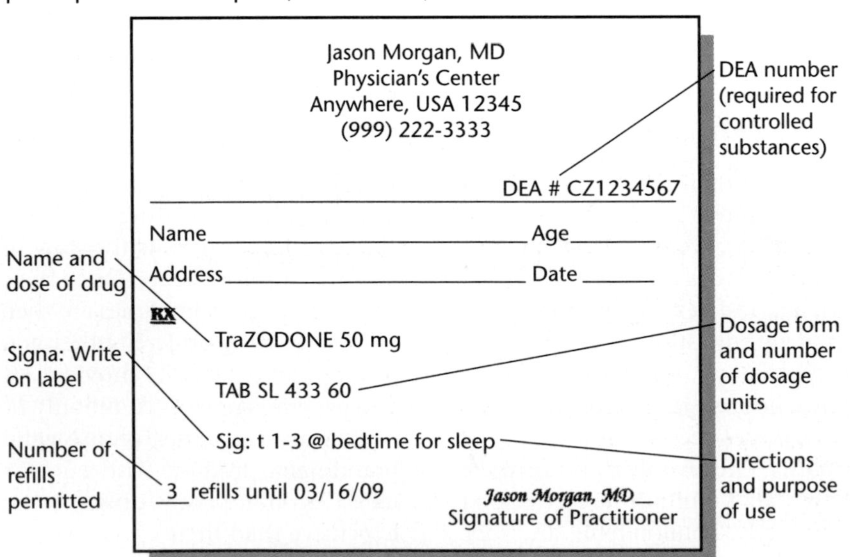

they leave the office. Between 1994 and 2005, the number of prescriptions have increased 71 percent, from 2.1 billion to 3.6 billion.[34] Substances that assist in weight management are among the most commonly prescribed drugs for women. Antidepressants, sedative hypnotics, and hormone regulation substances are also among the most commonly prescribed drugs for women.

Weight Control Substances Media sources portray the ideal and desirable woman as one who is tall, thin, well toned, and usually has long, blond hair. Although we cannot change our height, we can, if we choose, become blond and, in some instances, thin. This may not be everyone's "ideal," nor should we be expected to conform to the media's image. Yet we seem to think that this is the image we must have. Trying to create this image, a woman may use various drugs to find this thin, ideal person she believes can be uncovered if she could just lose those extra pounds. (See *FYI:* "The Ideal versus Reality.")

To aid in weight management and reduction, weight control substances can be obtained with a doctor's prescription or purchased as an over-the-counter product. Drugs prescribed to help manage weight often help in achieving short-term weight loss. However, unless an appetite suppressant drug is combined with a behavior modification program, once the drug is stopped, a woman will probably regain any weight she has lost. It should be remembered the most effective weight loss programs include a low fat diet, regular exercise, and perseverance. Morbidly obese women may turn to their

Health Tips

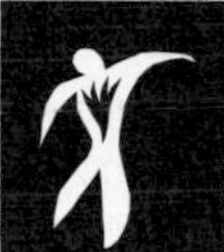

Questions to Ask When Taking Prescription Medicine

Asking basic questions and seeking information from your physician or pharmacist can assist you in receiving the proper medication for your health, as well as result in the most effective use of your consumer dollars.

- What is the purpose of this medicine?
- What are the possible side effects?
- What foods, beverages, or other medication should I avoid while taking this medicine?
- Exactly when and how do I take the medication?
- What should I do if I experience side effects?
- How long should I take this medication?

FYI

The Ideal versus Reality[35]

It is no wonder that medications to control weight are some of the most prevalent medicines used today. Consider the following:

- In the late 1960s, fashion models were 8 percent thinner than the average-sized woman; today, models are 23 percent thinner!
- Today, the average fashion model is 5'10" and weighs 110–115 pounds; the average American woman is actually 5'4" and weighs 140–145 pounds.
- If Barbie were a "real" woman, she would be 5'9" and have measurements of 36-18-33.
- One-third of American women wear size 16 or larger.
- The diet industry brings in revenue of approximately $33 billion annually.
- The estimated cost of obesity and obesity-related diseases is $70 billion annually.

Journal Activity

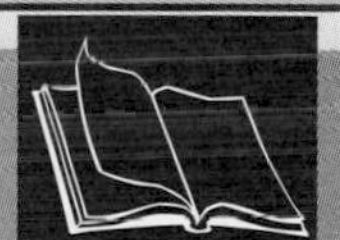

Questions to Ask When Purchasing Medications

Try this activity the next time you visit a pharmacy: Ask the pharmacist the questions in *Health Tips:* "Questions to Ask When Taking Prescription Medicine." You can do this activity when obtaining prescription medicine or purchasing an over-the-counter medication. Consider the following:

- Did the pharmacist answer your questions in language that you could understand?
- If you were unsure of the information, did you ask the pharmacist to provide additional information?
- Did the pharmacist treat you with respect and consideration?
- Did you feel comfortable with your interaction with this health professional?
- How was this activity beneficial to you regarding your own health care?

physician for help with weight reduction and weight maintenance. The physician may suggest prescription diet drugs, which are intended for initial efforts toward weight reduction and only for short-term assistance. Research studies demonstrate that diet drugs are only slightly effective, typically working only 10 percent better than programs that do not include diet drugs and losing their effect after about 6 months.

Previous diet drugs included phentermine drugs (Adipex-P), nicknamed *phen,* which was often prescribed with fenfluramine (Pondimin) or dexfenfluramine (Redux), nicknamed *fen*. Together they were known as *fenphen*. In 1997 the FDA asked drug companies to withdraw Pondimin and Redux due to research revealing that these drugs damaged the heart's mitral valve. Currently the *phen* drugs are still on the market, but the *fen* medications are no longer available.[36]

Xenical (generic name: orlistat) blocks the dietary fat in the bloodstream by almost one-third, which reduces the number of calories that are absorbed from a meal. However, as a result, Xenical also decreases the absorption of fat-soluble vitamins and beta-carotene; therefore, a multivitamin with vitamins A, D, E, and K needs to be taken 2 hours before or after a meal. This prescription drug is taken during each main meal, or up to 1 hour following the meal. However, if a woman misses a meal or the meal does not contain fat, Xenical should not be taken. Resume Xenical during the next meal at the usual dosage. Weight loss usually begins within 2 weeks and may last from 6 to 12 months. Side effects may include abdominal or back pain, diarrhea, dizziness, earache, fatigue, and gas with fecal discharge, headache, and other concerns. Of course, if any of these occur, contact your physician. This drug is not recommended for pregnant women as this new drug has not been adequately tested for use during pregnancy.

Meridia (generic name: sibutramine hydrochloride) works by boosting the level of particular chemicals in the central nervous system, which include dopamine, norepinephrine, and serotonin. This diet drug is recommended for women who have health problems such as high blood pressure (unless it is *not* being controlled by medication), diabetes, or high cholesterol in addition to a weight problem. It can be taken with or without food, and if a dose is missed, it can be taken as soon as remembered. Possible side effects can include abdominal or back pain, anxiety, constipation, dizziness, dry mouth, and others. Women who have uncontrolled high blood pressure or have had a stroke or suffer from heart disease should not use this drug. As with many other prescription drugs, Meridia may interact with a wide variety of other prescription and over-the-counter drugs. During pregnancy, this drug should be avoided; it is not known if Meridia appears in breast milk.

Fastin (generic: phentermine hydrochloride) is an appetite suppressant intended for short-term use as part of a comprehensive weight reduction plan. Fastin should not be taken for more than a few weeks because of possible side effects and decreased effectiveness as an appetite suppressant. Side effects can include constipation, dizziness, dry mouth, mood swings, loss of sex drive, and the inability to fall or stay asleep, among other effects. Fastin can create psychological dependency. Abrupt discontinuance can cause extreme fatigue, depression, and/or sleeping disorders.

Another often prescribed weight control substance is *Tenuate* (generic: diethylpropion hydrochloride). Similar to Fastin, it is also a short-term diet suppressant. However, it comes in two forms: immediate-release tablets and controlled-release tablets. It is essential that Tenuate be taken as prescribed because of its habit-forming and addicting qualities. Side effects such as blood pressure elevation, abdominal discomfort, mood swings, or sleep disruptions among others are possible. As with any other prescription drug, any changes or special concerns and situations should be discussed immediately with your physician.

Antidepressants Feelings of sadness, disappointment or helplessness, collectively known as depression, affect about 15 percent of the population at any given time. Women are twice as likely as men to be clinically depressed, and depression is the most common emotional disorder in women. A detailed discussion concerning depression in women is found in Chapter 4. Relief from depression often comes in the form of a prescription drug, and physicians consider age, symptoms, general health status, and side effects when deciding which antidepressant drug to prescribe.

Antidepressant drugs are intended to alleviate serious depression and are often used in combination with other types of therapy such as counseling and lifestyle changes. Instant relief from depression does not occur with antidepressant drugs; it usually takes 1 to 4 weeks to feel positive effects. It is important to consistently take the medication during this time so that essential chemical levels are reached in the blood. General side effects include blurred vision, light-headedness, dry mouth, and other effects. Antidepressant drugs are divided into four main classes: tricyclics (or heterocyclics), selective serotonin reuptake inhibitors, monoamine oxidase inhibitors, and the bipolar medication lithium.[37]

Tricyclic antidepressants have little effect on psychotic symptoms; however, they were found to elevate the mood of persons experiencing depression. Examples of tricyclics include *Norpramin, Sinequan,* and *Tofranil*. It may take several weeks before the medication becomes fully effective, and there are a number of side effects to each of these drugs, including dry mouth, constipation, and blurred vision. A woman should not abruptly stop taking these drugs if she feels she no longer needs them but, instead, decrease their use under the direction of a physician. If undergoing a medical procedure, such as surgery or dental work, if is important to report use of tricyclic antidepressants prior to procedures.

Selective Serotonin Reuptake Inhibitors (SSRIs) are among the most prescribed and greatest money-making drugs on the antidepressant market. SSRIs work by increasing the levels of serotonin and sometimes norepinephrine in the brain. Examples of SSRIs include Zoloft and Prozac, and a discussion of these drugs follows.

Zoloft (generic: sertraline) is prescribed for major depression including symptoms such as lack of interest in activities, disturbed sleep, reduced appetite, and feelings of worthlessness. It is thought that Zoloft alters part of the brain chemistry to balance its natural chemical messengers. Avoid Zoloft if you have taken any MAO inhibitors within the past 2 weeks. (See the discussion on MAOIs below.) Side effects may include dry mouth, constipation, dizziness, or headaches. Check with your physician if any of these or other side effects occur. You may initially lose 1 to 2 pounds, and it may take a few days or weeks to see any improvement with the depression. Do not drink alcohol while using this medication.

Prozac (generic: fluoxetine hydrochloride) is prescribed for continuing depression that can interfere with daily functioning. Prozac, another SSRI, increases the level of serotonin but not norepinephrine. Because SSRIs have fewer side effects than the tricyclic antidepressants, they are becoming the most frequently prescribed antidepressants in the United States. There are no negative cardiovascular side effects, sedative effects, or weight gain effects associated with SSRIs. Keep in mind, however, as with most medications, there are some potential unpleasant effects from using these drugs. Common side effects include diarrhea, increased or decreased appetite, nervousness, and abnormal dreams. Some evidence suggests that Prozac inhibits female orgasm. A word of caution: Do not take SSRIs with MAO inhibitors, which are other types of antidepressant drugs.

Monoamine oxidase inhibitors (MAOIs) increase the levels of numerous neurotransmitters in the body. These antidepressants, for example, *Nardil* and *Parnate,* are prescribed when no other antidepressant is effective and for individuals who have manic-depressive conditions. Studies indicate that MAOIs are somewhat more dangerous than other antidepressants because of the different neurotransmitters they affect. A long list of foods, such as aged cheese, smoked fish, or chianti wine, as well as other drugs cannot be taken with MAOIs. Physicians must be alerted to any and all medications a woman is taking prior to prescribing these antidepressants.

Lithium is prescribed for women suffering from the very serious disorder called bipolar illness, or manic-depression. When a woman is taking this drug, the symptoms of the manic phase—restlessness, little sleep, excessive energy—usually disappear within 5 to 14 days, and depressive symptoms are reduced. Drinking 10 to 12 glasses of water per day is essential while taking this medication to reduce dehydration. Side effects can include weight gain, nausea, tremor, and sometimes confusion and slurred speech.

Sedative Hypnotics

Anxiety is a feeling of unrest, excessive alertness, and hypervigilance. It may be caused by a chemical or hormonal imbalance or by emotional trauma. Anxiety can be debilitating and interfere with everyday happiness and responsibilities. Anxiety disorders, discussed more fully in Chapter 4, are divided into six categories: generalized anxiety disorder, simple phobias, agoraphobia, panic disorders, obsessive-compulsive disorder, and posttraumatic stress disorder. In addition to treating these disorders through behavioral modification and therapy, medication is often prescribed in the form of sedative hypnotics.

A group of sedative hypnotics called *benzodiazepines* have proven to be effective and safe when used to treat anxiety disorders, but they must be used as directed. These medications produce less drowsiness and a larger margin for safety than barbiturates. One of the best-known benzodiazepines is *Valium* (generic: diazepam), which was the largest selling prescription drug in the 1970s. *Xanax* (generic: alprazolam) is widely prescribed to treat anxiety disorders. Xanax is used for short-term relief of symptoms associated with anxiety or panic and, though it is most effective, it can lead to tolerance and dependency. *Ativan* is also used to treat anxiety disorders and has the potential for dependency. A number of common side effects may occur following benzodiazepine use, including agitation, confusion, constipation, drowsiness, dry mouth, and fluid retention.

Hormone Therapy

Hormone therapy is the process by which a woman increases the level of estrogen in her body. Decreased estrogen levels result from either natural or surgically induced menopause. Estrogen replacement therapy (ERT) raises levels of estrogen in the body, but produces some unpleasant side effects. An alternative to ERT is hormone replacement therapy (HRT), which provides both estrogen and progestin in the body. Many of the serious side effects resulting from ERT are greatly reduced by prescribing the combination of estrogen and progestin. Hormone therapy continues to be controversial among physicians who prescribe it and women who receive it. Physicians and women find weighing the health benefits against possible health risks both confusing and stressful. In Chapter 8, you will find an extensive discussion regarding hormone replacement therapy.

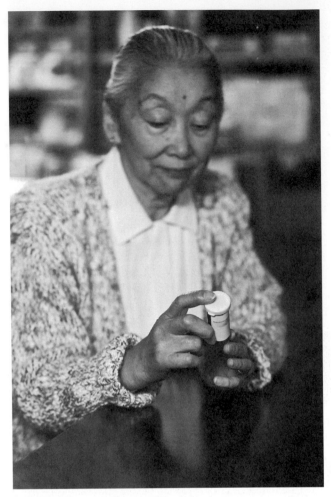

Reading prescription labels carefully is important for being a healthy and informed consumer.

Using Prescription Drugs Safely

Our bodies are chemical-laden machines. When we add chemicals such as prescription drugs, we may be brewing a chemical mix in our bodies that could result in undesirable, uncomfortable, and in some instances, unsafe **side effects.** Side effects often result from using the drug incorrectly, such as skipping a dose, taking too much, taking it at the wrong time, taking it with beverages other than water, or taking it with or without food when directions suggest differently. However, most side effects can be reduced or, even better, eliminated. Weight, age, gender, health status, and/or diet can affect how drugs react when used by women.

Health Tips: "Guidelines When Taking Medications" provides guidelines to follow when taking medications. Getting the most out of the medication you have been prescribed is as important as taking it correctly. *Assess Yourself:* "Safety Tips When Taking Medications" is a checklist to determine it you are using medicines safely.

Health Tips

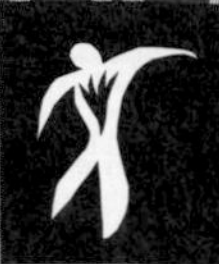

Guidelines When Taking Medications

Following safe guidelines can help enhance drug effectiveness and safety:

- Take the prescribed dosage; do not take more or less than instructed.
- Follow the directions on the label; modify only as your physician specifies.
- Ask the pharmacist or physician about directions if you are unsure about using the medication properly.
- Finish the prescription even after you are feeling better; women often relapse when they fail to finish all their medication.
- Seek a second opinion if you are concerned about taking the drug.
- Notify your physician immediately if you have any unusual or serious side effects.

Assess Yourself

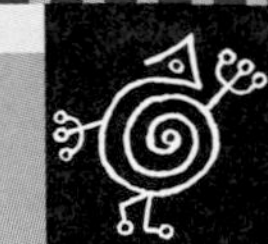

Safety Tips When Taking Medications

Do you	Yes	No
Alert all your physicians to all medications you are currently taking?	___	___
Refuse to share your medications with friends and family?	___	___
Store medication properly and away from light, heat, and moisture?	___	___
Use nonmedical treatment for occasional illnesses?	___	___
Review with your physician any medications used on a long-term basis?	___	___
Dispose of any medications that are expired or that you are no longer using?	___	___

The benefits resulting from using drugs that prevent, treat, and heal diseases correctly outweigh any risks one might encounter. Although medicines are powerful drugs, wise and careful use does eliminate most complications. (See *Health Tips:* "Caution: Watch for Tampering.")

Health Tips

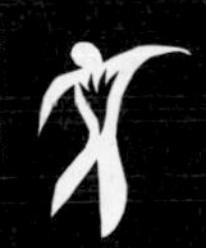

Caution: Watch for Tampering

Although prescription and over-the-counter drugs are considered to be packaged safely in the United States, manufacturers cannot make a *tamper-proof* package. It is important to know how to protect yourself from possible tampering and contaminating of medicines. You can protect yourself by doing the following:

- Inspect the outer package for tears, cuts, or punctures.
- Inspect the medicine and look for discoloration or damage.
- Look for tablets or capsules that appear to be different from others in the package.
- Never take medicine in the dark.
- Pay attention to the safety features provided by the manufacturer.
- Use time and care, and good common sense. It is your own best safety feature!

OVER-THE-COUNTER (OTC) DRUGS

More than 80 therapeutic categories with more than 100,000 drug products of over-the-counter (OTC) drugs are available without prescription in markets across the country today.[38] These include such categories as analgesics, antihistamines, stimulants, laxatives, topical analgesics, antacids, and others. Are these drugs safe and effective? The 1962 Kefauver-Harris Act required scientific evidence to prove that OTC drugs were safe and effective. A regulatory program was developed by the FDA in 1972 in which active ingredients of OTC drugs were assigned to one of three categories: *GRAS* (Generally Recognized as Safe), *GRAE* (Generally Recognized as Effective), and *GRAHL* (Generally Recognized as Honestly Labeled). These categories with their FDA-developed acronyms are used to effectively describe the safety of the ingredients found in OTC drugs. (See Table 2.2.)

In 1992 the U.S. General Accounting Office reported that the FDA is unable to determine the exact number of OTC products that are marketed each year, and that all of them may not be safe and effective. The Center for Drug Evaluation and Research (CDER) oversees OTC drugs, as well as prescription drugs, to ensure they are labeled properly and that the benefits outweigh the risks. OTC drugs usually have the following characteristics:

- Their benefits outweigh their risks.
- The potential for misuse and abuse is low.
- Consumers can use them for self-diagnosed conditions.
- They are properly labeled.
- Health practitioners are not needed for safe, effective use of the product.[39]

However, as more prescription drugs become OTC drugs, these OTC drugs are becoming safer and more effective. *FYI:* "How a Prescription Drug Becomes an OTC Drug" explains how this is done.

TABLE 2.2 FDA Categories for OTC Drug Ingredients

Category I	Ingredient is *GRAS* and *GRAE.*
Category II	Ingredient is either not *GRAS* and/or not *GRAE* and would be removed from stores within 6 months if the manufacturer did not prove its safety and effectiveness.
Category III	Insufficient data to determine the ingredient's safety and/or effectiveness. If the manufacturer cannot prove *GRAS* within one year, the drug becomes a Category II rather than a Category I drug.*

*Only drugs that have been proven safe and effective are now placed in the OTC market.

FYI

How a Prescription Drug Becomes an OTC Drug

Manufacturers who own a patent for a prescription drug must apply to the FDA for permission to reconstruct the formula for the drug to be sold as on OTC drug. Usually, the active ingredients are made less concentrated and safer to use without a doctor's prescription. Products do retain their prescription brand name. Once approval is given by the FDA, the former prescription drug can be marketed and sold as an OTC medicine. Examples of such products include Aleve for premenstrual discomfort, Monistat and Gyne-Lotrimin, which are creams to treat vaginal infection, and ibuprofen (Advil, Motrin, etc.) for headaches.

OTC Drugs Used by Women

Rising medical care costs are a major concern for those women who have little, if any, money for professional health care. Thus, self-diagnosis of illness is on the increase, which leads to frequent purchase of OTC drugs.

Hundreds of thousands of OTC drugs are purchased each year simply by consumer choice. Therefore, consumers must be informed about the advantages and the potential hazards of those medicines purchased without benefit of a physician's consultation or prescription.

To help reduce the misuse of OTC medicines, labeling and package inserts are provided with each drug and have become more reliable since the FDA assumed control over OTC medicines. FDA regulations mandate that labels on all OTC medication list information in the same order, arranged in a simple, eye-catching, consistent style, and use understandable terms. The following information is required on all OTC drug labels:[40]

- *Active ingredient:* the type of therapeutic substance and the amount of active ingredient per unit
- *Uses:* diseases, disorders, or symptoms the medication will treat or prevent
- *Warnings:* suggestions for safe use of the product, including when not to use, when to see a physician, possible interactions or side effects, use related to pregnancy or breast-feeding, keep out of reach of children
- *Inactive ingredients:* other substances in the product (colors, flavors)
- *Purpose:* product action or category (such as antacid, cough suppressant, painkiller)
- *Directions:* specific age categories, how to use, how much, how often, and how long to take the medication
- *Other information:* how to store properly and information about other ingredients

Other information found on labels includes the expiration date; the lot or batch number to help identify the product; the name and address of the manufacturer, packer, or distributor; the net quantity of contents; and what to do if an overdose occurs. By reading the information on each label, women should not have any problem in determining the purpose of the drug and the safe and effective way to take it.

Now let's look at some major categories of OTC drugs purchased by women.

OTC Weight Management Products Want to make a million dollars? Develop a diet pill that promises to remove unwanted fat without any physical exertion nor reduction in food intake and you will certainly be wealthy. Even though appetite suppressants are aids to weight loss or weight control, they simply cannot provide a healthy approach to quick weight loss.

Diet pills, creams, liquids, and supplements are available to suppress one's appetite, increase metabolism, and/or make a woman feel full and therefore less likely to eat large amounts of food. Some OTC weight management products have been removed from the marketplace because they either failed to meet their claims or were shown to be dangerous. Products that "burn fat," "dissolve cellulite," and provide a "natural" way to rid one's body of unsightly fat have failed to match their advertising claims and, in some cases, have created health problems for the user.

Are there any OTC weight management products that do work? If we mean that by taking them we can lose weight, then the answer is "yes." Diet products that can be purchased over the counter certainly do work—but only temporarily—and although body weight is lost, body fat remains. Diet pills "work" by decreasing the appetite due to stimulants in the products or by causing a quick loss of fluid due to the diuretic properties in the drug. Side effects from the use of diet pills can cause mild symptoms such as nausea, dry mouth, and dizziness, but more serious consequences such as stroke, seizures, and liver or kidney damage can also occur.

The chemical phenylpropanolamine (PPA) has been in numerous OTC diet pills and in cough and cold medications, acting as a decongestant. However, scientists at Yale University School of Medicine discovered that PPA increases the risk of hemorrhagic stroke (bleeding into the brain or into tissue surrounding the brain) in women. The FDA has removed all OTC and prescription drug products containing PPA from the market, and pharmaceutical companies have reformulated formulas to exclude PPA from their products. The FDA recommends that consumers read the labels of OTC drug products to determine if the product contains PPA and avoid these products.

As long as diet pills are ingested, a woman will lose weight, but when drug use is stopped, the lost weight usually returns. Why? Because eating patterns and exercise patterns have not changed! This is not a healthy weight loss method because women may not receive the nutrients needed when they are not eating healthy food. Although these pills can certainly reduce appetite and speed up metabolism, producing weight loss, there are better, healthier, and more permanent methods or combinations of methods available to reach your desired goal.

OTC Laxatives A laxative is a medicinal aid to help the body eliminate waste products, or "stool," from the body. OTC laxatives increase the bulk and water content of the bowel, thereby loosening it for better elimination. Laxatives are available in a number of different dosage forms: liquid, tablet, suppository, gum, powder, enema, and granule. Table 2.3 lists the different types of OTC laxatives available.

Although it is occasionally necessary to use a laxative product, frequent and continual use can lead to dependence and even the loss of muscular and neurological control of the bowels. Use of laxatives can lead

TABLE 2.3 Types of OTC Laxatives[41]

TYPE	ACTION	PRODUCTS
Stimulant	Agitates intestinal walls causing muscular contractions that expel fecal matter	Ex-Lax, Feen-a-Mint, Fletcher's Castoria, Modane
Lubricant	"Greases" stools, facilitating excretion	Agoral Plain, Fleet Mineral Oil Enema
Saline	Draws water into the bowel and allows for easier passage of stools	Milk of Magnesia, Citrate of Magnesia, Epsom Salts
Stool softener	Softens hard stools so that they can absorb more liquids and pass more easily	Colace, Dialose, Regutol, Surfak
Hyperosmotic	Draws water into the bowel to allow for easier passage of stool; less risk of salt depletion than with saline	OTC hyperosmotics like glycerin are only for rectal use; oral hyperosmotics require prescriptions
Carbon-dioxide-releasing agent	Produces carbon dioxide in bowels; gas pushes stool toward excretion	Ceo-Two (suppositories)
Bulk	Absorbs water into the intestine, swelling the stool into an easily passed soft mass; must be taken with 8 oz of water	TMetamucil, FiberCon, Serutan; and bran products such as found in cereals

Her Story

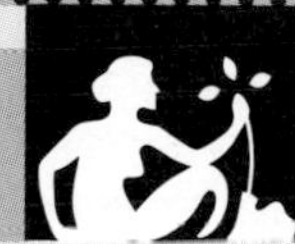

Aimee: Habitual Use of Laxatives

Aimee used a variety of laxative products to help her manage her weight. Even though she was aware of the possible consequences of habitual use of these products, Aimee relied on them to maintain the body image she felt she needed. Her roommate, Liz, began to see some negative effects on Aimee's physical appearance and demeanor. Usually an easygoing and even passive individual, Aimee became irritable, quick-tempered, fatigued, and developed a nasty-looking skin infection. It was not until Liz found Aimee vomiting and in severe abdominal pain that Aimee was willing to seek help for her habitual use of laxatives.

- What can Liz do to help Aimee find help for her problem?
- What resources are available for women in your college or community to assist with abuse of any type of drug?

to depletion of body fluids, salts, and essential nutrients. Another serious concern is that habitual use of OTC laxatives can inhibit the absorption and effectiveness of prescriptions and other OTC drugs. Depending on the type of laxative used, side effects such as belching, dizziness, fatigue, skin irritation, and irregular heartbeat may be experienced. (See *Her Story:* "Aimee: Habitual Use of Laxatives.")

The FDA has taken a number of measures to help regulate OTC products such as laxatives, as well as to remove products from the market that contain ingredients that cause serious side effects. Information about how the product works, how to use it properly, and the length of time needed to achieve the desired results can be found on packaging labels. Products with ingredients such as agar, guar gum, tartaric acid, ipomea, aloin, and ox bile have been removed from the marketplace until further research can prove them safe as well as effective.

Women can usually promote stool excretion regularity by making simple and healthful changes in diet and lifestyle. Increasing the intake of fiber-rich foods such as whole-grain breads; bran cereals; kidney, navy, and pinto beans; and fresh fruits and vegetables, while reducing foods such as cheeses, white bread, and meat are helpful ways to replace the need for laxatives. Irregularity can also be caused by stress, depression, an underactive thyroid gland, and even colorectal cancer. Seeing a physician to address these concerns can produce positive results. An increased exercise routine can promote regularity as can slowing down a fast-paced lifestyle to let nature take its course. If irregularity persists, or if the use of laxatives to achieve weight management continues, then a visit to a physician or psychotherapist is in order.

OTC Sleep Aids With the stress-filled lifestyles we all tend to live, getting a good night's sleep is sometimes difficult to achieve. If you do what millions of other women do, you probably visit the local pharmacy or discount store and select from a multitude of sleep aids that help promote sleep. Occasional use of some form of sleep aid is usually not harmful for temporary help.

However, for sleep difficulties or insomnia lasting longer than 3 weeks, one needs to consult a physician to receive a diagnostic evaluation.

The causes of sleep difficulties can be multiple and complex. Worries about school, relationships, or finances; overconsumption of products containing caffeine; too much activity or excitement before bedtime; or poor time management skills can all lead to sleep deprivation.

Among OTC products available for insomnia, most contain one of two types of an antihistamine: diphenhydramine (found in Compoz, Miles Nervine Caplets, and Nytol) or doxylamine succinate (found in Unisom, and Ultra Sleep). In some instances, products contain analgesics, or painkillers, for insomnia caused by pain. Examples of this type of product include Extra Strength Tylenol PM and Sominex Pain Relief.

Be aware of potential side effects and warnings related to the use of sleep aids. **Contraindications** are included for individuals with asthma, glaucoma, or prostate gland enlargements. Products should not be used without a physician's advice. Of course, sleep aids should not be taken when driving or operating power machinery, or when any task or responsibility calls for alertness. Pregnant or lactating women need to be cautious about the use of any sleep aid and should not use any OTC drugs containing doxylamine. Do not use sleep aids with alcohol or other sedatives and tranquilizers. Instead of using sleep aids, try the suggestions listed in *Health Tips:* "Natural Sleep Aids."

Prescription and OTC Drug Use during Pregnancy

Rubin and colleagues[42] analyzed the drug use of more than 2,700 pregnant females and found that 68 percent used at least one drug during their pregnancy. The average intake of drugs was 1.2 drugs per female while pregnant. Educated, married, white women with higher than average incomes were more likely to use legal drugs, especially OTC products, while pregnant.

Health Tips

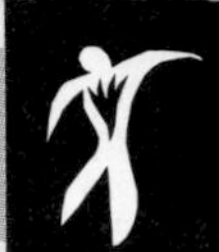

Natural Sleep Aids

Try these "natural" suggestions to help with sleep inducement before you go to bed:

- Engage in quiet and relaxing activities.
- Avoid any drinks containing caffeine.
- Have a bedtime routine such as a warm shower, a soothing lotion, cleaning your teeth, etc.
- Listen to quiet music and/or read for a while.
- Avoid exercise too close to bedtime.
- Avoid late meals.
- Sleep in clean, comfortable nightclothes and bedding.
- Try deep breathing and calming thoughts.

Journal Activity

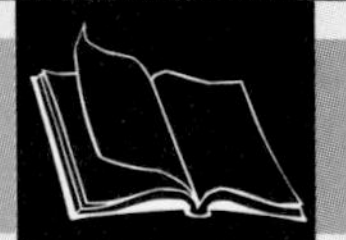

Recording the Medicines You Take

Find all the medications that you take on a regular basis. Divide them into prescription and OTC drugs, and use this chart to record essential information. This information can be useful when visiting your physician.

Date	Name of Medicine	Amount Taken	When Taken	Purpose	Refills
Example	Hurt-No-More Pain Pills	1–2 tabs 400 mg	3 times a day with meals	Headaches	2

Adapted from *Use medicine wisely.* Washington, DC: Food and Drug Administration.

The majority of these women gave birth to normal infants. However, women must be aware that each pregnancy is unique, and the best approach is to avoid exposing the fetus to unnecessary drugs. Therefore, it is strongly recommended that women avoid all medication, both prescription and OTC, if possible during pregnancy. Communication between pregnant women and their physicians, and strict adherence to the warnings about taking any drugs during pregnancy, *must* be a priority. (See *Journal Activity:* "Recording the Medicines You Take.")

BEAUTY-ENHANCING PRODUCTS AND PROCEDURES

Products

Women, and sometimes men, elect to use products to improve the way we look and feel about ourselves. Cosmetics of all descriptions, creams, lotions, hair products, and fragrances are developed and sold, for large profits, because there is a demand for them. As purchasers of these products, we need to be knowledgeable and aware in order to select products that meet our needs and desires.

Cosmetics Cosmetics as defined by the U.S. Food, Drug, and Cosmetic Act are "articles intended to be rubbed, poured, sprinkled, or sprayed on, introduced into, or otherwise applied to the human body . . . for cleansing, beautifying, promoting attractiveness, or altering the appearance."[43] Strangely enough, premarket approval is not required by the FDA for cosmetics. However, if a product proves to be harmful once it is on the market, the FDA can take legal action to obtain the manufacturer's safety data. Cosmetics are classified into thirteen categories: deodorants, eye makeup, skin care, fragrances, makeup other than eye (lipsticks, for example), hair coloring preparations, shampoos and other hair products, manicure products, shaving products, baby products, bath products, mouthwashes, and sunscreens.[44] Cosmetics containing poisonous or harmful substances may not, by law, be placed on the market. With the exception of color additives and a few prohibited ingredients, any ingredient or raw material may be used in the manufacture of cosmetics. See *Health Tips:* "Safety Tips for Beauty-Enhancing Products" for tips to protect yourself after you purchase cosmetics.

Cosmetic manufacturers must do the following to market their products: work in a sanitary environment and allow no filthy, putrid, or decomposed substances in the product; test for color additives and obtain FDA approval for their use in products; list ingredients on labels in descending order of predominance; and avoid the use of prohibited ingredients such as mercury compounds, chloroform, or vinyl chloride. If a manufacturer chooses to do so, it may register its manufacturing plant, cosmetic formulas, and report adverse reactions with the FDA. An increase in the demand for ethnic cosmetics has the manufacturers of products scrambling to meet this demand. An increase in the Latino and African American populations, as well as an increase in economic status of both groups, has been credited with this new market component. The youth of these particular groups appear to have boosted ethnic cosmetic sales.[45]

Skin Care Products Our skin continually renews itself by producing new cells deep within the skin layers and sloughing off dead cells on the skin's surface. Skin layers contain water and oil, but as we age less oil is produced within the skin and skin loses water faster, becomes dry, cracks, and develops fine wrinkles. When we attempt to replenish water and oil in our skin with moisturizers, we only moisturize the top layer of the skin. Because this is the skin layer that dries out, moisturizers need only to moisturize this layer. That can occur in two ways: use an occlusive type product that physically blocks moisture from leaving the skin (e.g., petroleum jelly) or use a "humectant" type product that attracts moisture from the skin and air and slows down the rate of water loss.[46]

Health Tips

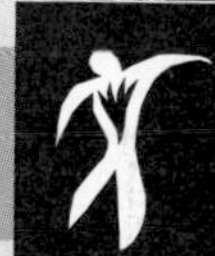

Safety Tips for Beauty-Enhancing Products

Protect yourself by following these guidelines to use cosmetics safely:

- When not in use, keep containers closed tightly.
- Store products, especially liquids, in a cool, dry place.
- Keep products away from sunlight as ingredients may degrade.
- Never moisten dry cosmetics or applicators with saliva.
- Toss out any cosmetics that smell strange, separate into layers, or have different colors or consistencies than when purchased.
- Do not share cosmetics or applicators or use in-store samples and applicators.
- Do not use cosmetics if you have an eye or skin infection.
- Be sure to wash cosmetic sponges and brushes with warm water and soap frequently; throw them away if they degrade or lose bristles.

Most skin care products have both types of ingredients as well as water. If a product is intended to be used for a drier type of skin, it will have more oil; for oily skin types, the product should have more or only humectants.

Ingredients in addition to oil and water add benefits, but may make the moisturizer more expensive. Ingredients found in today's moisturizers may include (1) sunscreen to reduce the damage caused by exposure to sun, (2) alpha-hydroxy acids which help rid the skin of dead cells, (3) tretinoin to help replace dead skin cells with new skin, and (4) petrolatum, which reduces scaling of skin and helps retain moisture.[47]

Moisturizers for the body and the face work similarly, but we tend to pay more attention to our face. Therefore, the advertiser more often promotes moisturizers for the face, and the consumer will find that face moisturizers are more expensive than those for the body. A comparison chart found on the *Consumer Search* Web site offers limited information about different type of moisturizers.[48]

Procedures

In attempting to obtain the image of women publicized by print and electronic media, women undergo intrusive and sometimes painful and disfiguring procedures. The demand for breast augmentation, face-lifts, chemical peels, tummy tucks, and liposuctions has increased. Why do women elect to go through these unpleasant and expensive procedures? (See *FYI:* "Reasons for Beauty-Enhancing Procedures.")

Cosmetic Surgery Cosmetic surgery is more prevalent than ever in our society, and we are more aware of the improved technology to achieve the image we desire. Television shows such as *Extreme Makeover* have brought the many possibilities of cosmetic surgery into almost every living room in America and created an awareness of beauty-enhancing procedures more than at any time in the past. **Cosmetic surgeons** now advertise their practice and provide "in-office" operating rooms and financing. What is the difference between a "cosmetic" and a "plastic" surgeon? A cosmetic surgeon specializes in procedures that enhance appearance such as face-lifts, breast reduction/augmentation, or "nose jobs." A **plastic surgeon** is trained in reconstructive surgery and performs procedures such as facial reconstruction, skin grafts, or hand surgery as well as cosmetic surgery. In selecting a cosmetic or plastic surgeon, look for the following: board certified in the area of surgical specialty; experience in the procedure you desire; recommendation from someone you trust who has had a procedure done by the surgeon; remains current with new procedures; communicates with you about the positives and negatives of the procedure and your motivation for having the surgical procedure; and has privileges at area hospitals.

> **FYI**
>
> ### Reasons for Beauty-Enhancing Procedures[49]
>
> - Anxiety over appearance based on a societal prejudice against aging females
> - To increase feelings of worthiness, often dependent upon childhood development situations
> - To maintain positive feelings about appearance
> - To fulfill a personal desire to achieve the best appearance possible
> - To attain an unconscious obligation to be a youthful and attractive member of society

Types of Cosmetic Procedures Many types of cosmetic procedures are available to accomplish a variety of desirable changes in one's appearance. The following list provides the common and medical procedural term and briefly explains the purpose of the procedures:

- Eyelid lift (*blepharoplasty*) corrects sagging or droopy lids above the eyes and/or bags below the eyes.
- Neck/face-lift (*rhytidectomy*) lifts the lower two-thirds of the face and improves sagging skin, jowls, double chin, and aging neck.
- Forehead or brow lift is accomplished with an ear-to-ear incision and removal of extra skin to reduce forehead and frown lines and to raise sagging eyebrows.
- Liposuction uses small tubes attached to a type of vacuum to remove pounds of fatty tissue from buttocks, upper arms, stomach, hips, or face.
- Chin (*mentoplasy*) or cheek (*malar*) augmentation provides for a more pleasing face contour by adding cheekbones and a stronger, more prominent chin line.
- Nose job (*rhinoplasty*) reshapes the nose by changing nostrils, building or removing the bridge, recontouring the tip, or cutting or adding bone or cartilage. This procedure may improve breathing (insurance may apply in this instance).
- Botulinum toxin injections (BOTOX) are biological toxins transformed into a therapeutic agent and are used to treat frown lines, crow's feet, and lines and wrinkles in many areas of the face, BOTOX smoothes wrinkles that contract during facial expressions. These injections are a temporary solution and last about 3 to 4 months, therefore requiring repeated treatments. Side effects such as facial numbness, swelling, or bruising may result from

this treatment. Women may feel a burning sensation during the injection.[50]

- Chemical peel (*phenol*) helps to remove, erase, or fade fine facial wrinkles, acne scars, or sun damage by use of certain types of acid such as phenol or trichloroacetic acid or use of certain types of laser.
- Dermabrasion scrapes top layers of the skin to help remove fine wrinkles and marred skin so that new and smoother skin will be produced.
- Collagen or fat injections help to fill out skin tissues to reduce wrinkling or scar tissue, "plump" up lips, or smooth the back of the hands.

Each of these procedures can have very positive benefits, but each can also be harmful and produce unexpected outcomes. The importance of utilizing a board-certified, experienced, and highly qualified surgeon is essential to avoid such side effects as infection, pooling of blood under the skin, nerve damage, numbness, scarring, or ill-positioned or hardening of implants. Side effects, such as bruising, swelling, redness, throbbing, numbness, tightness, and stiffness, can be expected, but they are usually temporary.

Breast Augmentation

Breast implants appeared on the market in 1962; in 2003 alone over 323,000 breast augmentation and reconstructive surgeries were performed.[51]

Prior to April 1995, **silicone gel–filled** and **saline implants** were available to any woman who could afford the procedure. However, continuing problems related to silicone gel–filled implants created a need for valid and reliable clinical research to determine the safety and long-term effects of these products. Hardening of the breast because of scar tissue shrinkage around the implant, possibility of negative effects on the immune system, risks of cancer development, and potential interference with mammogram readings all contributed to the investigation and eventual restrictions of silicone gel–filled implants. After being off the market for more than a decade, the FDA Advisory Committee has recommended that the restrictions on silicone breast implants be lifted. Multiple reasons are the foundation for this reversal, but the truth is that not much more is known about silicone implants than a decade ago.[52] However, in November 2006, the FDA stated that silicone implants from two manufacturers, Allergan and Mentor, are approved for breast augmentation in women aged 22 years and older and for breast reconstruction in women of any age.[53]

Of the women who get breast implants, the vast majority do so to increase the size of their breast, called **breast augmentation.** Saline pouches, filled with a saltwater solution, fill the inflatable implants and then are placed between breast tissue and the chest wall. These types of implants are presently available even though the safety of saline implants has not been proven. Concerns regarding saline implants relate to deflation due to leakage or rupture, which can require additional surgery to correct. Calcium deposits often develop, causing difficulty in reading and interpreting mammograms. Seepage of saline solution into the body may occur, creating a risk of developing an autoimmune disease.

Another breast augmentation procedure, called breast augmentation mammoplasty, is applied by injection (BAMBI). In this procedure, excess fat is suctioned from the buttocks, thighs, or abdomen and injected between the breast and the chest wall. The surgeon who developed this procedure, Dr. Gerald Johnson, claims that it can permanently increase the breast by one-half a cup size.[54] However, other cosmetic surgeons claim that the injected fat either breaks down and is absorbed into the body or develops a hard calcium mass that can mask or mimic breast cancer. Dr. Johnson, although no longer performing this procedure, claims that it is a safe and effective operation.[55] Perhaps with further study this procedure will be used again in future breast augmentation surgeries.

What do you think about breast augmentation? Answer the questions in *Viewpoint:* "Should Silicone Gel–Filled Breast Implants Be Available?" Women who have any type of breast implants are reminded to have regular checkups, especially if experiencing a change in size, shape, or consistency or feeling any discomfort. *Health Tips:* "Breast Augmentation Guidelines" provides guidelines that women should diligently follow.

Although information about different types of and precautions about cosmetic surgery is important if women choose to have any type of cosmetic surgical procedure, perhaps the more important questions are: Why are we seeing such an increase in the number of women who desire a "beauty-enhancing procedure" that carries so many risks? Shouldn't women be able to appreciate their "natural" qualities without feeling the need to undergo risky surgery, painful recovery, and undue expense for cosmetic procedures that may or may not yield positive results? Reading the next section about advertising and the media's portrayal of women may assist us in understanding the desire to enhance our physical being, even at the potential risk of experiencing negative health consequences.

EFFECTS OF ADVERTISING

We see the beautiful, slim bodies of attractive people having an exciting and fun time in a lovely environment many times every day through the magic of television or the turn of a page in a popular magazine. Everyone and

Viewpoint

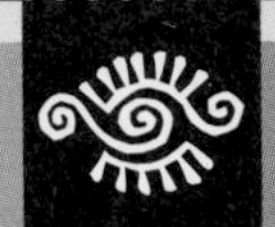

Should Silicone Gel–Filled Breast Implants Be Available?

The consequences of silicone gel–filled implants are not totally known, but it has been documented that implants should not be expected to last a lifetime; all implants leak silicone through their outer envelope; the health effects of this leakage are not truly clear; the percentage of silicone gel–filled implant ruptures is not known; the connection between silicone gel–filled breast implants and cancer, immune system disorders, and interference with mammogram readings, and the formation of calcium deposits is not clear. Because we do not have definitive answers to some of these possible health effects, should women still have the choice to have silicone gel–filled implants placed in their breasts if they so desire?

There appear to be some psychological benefits for women who elect to have their breasts enlarged. Women have reported feeling more attractive, more confident, and better about themselves. Do you think women who choose to take the unknown risks related to this surgery should be denied the right to make this choice? Why or why not?

Health Tips

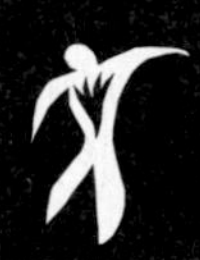

Breast Augmentation Guidelines

Follow these guidelines to prevent any potential danger from breast implants:

- Have regular breast exams by a qualified physician.
- Perform monthly breast self-exams.
- Have screening mammograms at intervals prescribed for your age group.
- Stay in contact with your regular physician as well as the cosmetic surgeon who performed the surgery.

everything appears to be just right! Whether it's wrinkle cream, beer, exercise equipment, or the latest weight control product, it's the advertiser's job to persuade people to buy products and services. Too often consumers must follow the concept of **caveat emptor**, a phrase that means "Let the buyer beware." In other words, it is the consumer's problem to determine if the advertisement is misleading, and she must make the decision to purchase at her own discretion or risk. Not fair! Consumers should be able to trust that the information presented by advertisements is accurate and truthful.

There have been strides toward truth in advertising and the products that are promoted. The Federal Trade Commission (FTC) was established in 1914 to protect citizens from unfair business practices. Congress expanded the responsibilities of the FTC with the 1938 Wheeler-Lea Amendment, which protects consumers against individuals or companies engaged in false advertisements of cosmetics, foods, drugs, and devices. The Fair Packing and Labeling Act of 1966 requires the labels on products involving foods, drugs, cosmetics, and medical devices to honestly inform consumers what they are buying and how it is to be used effectively.

Even with protective laws and agencies, consumers must still be aware, informed, and conscientious in regard to purchasing health-related products promoted by advertisers. The advertiser's objective is to sell a product; our objective is to purchase a product that is safe and effective for our needs. We hope the following information will be beneficial in assisting you, the female consumer, in selecting products that meet your needs and do not adversely affect your pocketbook.

Types of Advertising Techniques

Strategies for promoting health-related products (as well as other types of products) range from humorous and glitzy to sophisticated and ethereal. When purchasing a product to meet your needs, keep in mind a number of questions that will aid in your decision: How does it compare to other products? What is the evidence that the product works? Can any product really do what this product claims to do? Am I buying the product or trying to purchase the image that is portrayed by the advertisement?

Advertisers do an outstanding job of product promotion. Some advertisements are beneficial in helping us make a decision; other products are almost camouflaged as to their real purpose due to the hype (music, lighting, gorgeous people, celebrities, good times) used to promote the product. Awareness plays a significant part in making an informed decision about consumer issues. *FYI:* "Advertising Techniques for Health-Related Products" lists the techniques used by advertisers to sell their products. Which do you recognize in products you have purchased? Have any of these techniques persuaded you to purchase a cosmetic, drug, or device?

Through beautiful people, funny phrases, setting a mood, and testimonials, we are exposed to claims about products that are appealing and believable. Complete *Journal Activity:* "Analyzing Advertisements" to help you

FYI

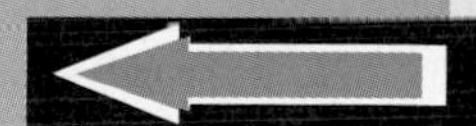

Advertising Techniques for Health-Related Products[56]

Technique	What You Hear	What You Can Ask
Bandwagon	Used by majority of hospitals/doctors; people rely on . . .	Does everyone use this? If so how do other companies stay in business?
Testimonials	By celebrities (sports, actors), by medical personnel	Do they know more than others? How much are they being paid to promote this product? Do they use the product?
Nonverbal/visuals	Music, colors, beautiful scenes and people, animation	What does this have to do with the effectiveness of products?
Humor, slogans	Jokes, silly costumes, phrases, songs, comedians	Helps to sell, but what does it mean? Is a product better because its ad is funny?
Power words	Works wonders, famous, revolutionary natural, amazing	What is the truth? What makes this product amazing or revolutionary or natural?
Scientific evidence	Studies say; doctors recommend; clinical trials indicate; scientists say . . .	What test, research, or clinical trials? What doctors? Which scientists?
Superiority	Leading brand, more effective, stronger, no other, best	Are differences significant? Who says it's more effective?
Emotions and attitudes	Relieves tension, improves mood; you'll feel sexier, feel better about self, feel good all over	How was this determined? Where is the evidence?

Journal Activity

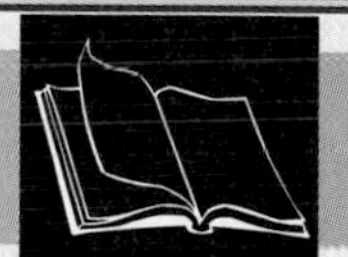

Analyzing Advertisements

Select advertisements from television and women's journals and answer the following questions related to the techniques presented in the FYI box on advertising techniques.

1. Does the person (celebrity or otherwise) have the credentials to know about the product he or she is promoting?
2. Can the product, in reality, do all the things it claims it can do?
3. Where is the scientific evidence that this product can produce the results for my well-being that it claims?
4. How do I know that the clinical trials produced the outcomes that the advertisement claims occurred?
5. Does the scenery or music or imagery in this advertisement make this product a better product than another in a less-appealing advertisement? As a result of this type of advertisement, will the cost of the product be higher than that of similar products?
6. Does the product claim to be painless, miraculous, fast and effective, FDA-approved, or guaranteed?
7. Does the product claim to work while you sleep, cure serious disease, retard aging, reduce fat without exercise, or improve your sex life?
8. Does the product claim that it can improve your social life, make you popular, or make you more appealing to other people?
9. Does the product claim to be an effective foreign product?
10. Is the cost of this product in accord with other brands of this type?

"see" beyond the image and glitz to find the real message, if there is one, about the product. Then determine if the product meets your needs.

Unrealistic Portrayals of Women

When advertisers promote products to women, the message is often that the product is necessary for us to be thinner, more attractive, or more youthful, or that it will improve our lifestyle. Promoting products in this manner sends the message that women are not thin, attractive, or young enough and that our situation in life can be improved by purchasing and using a particular product. Dissatisfaction with one's physique contributes to being vulnerable to advertisements that feature thin, young women who represent the "norm" of feminine beauty. Often the heart of female-directed advertisements plays to the lack of belief in one's self-worth or attractiveness. Women of today are programmed to believe they should be able to do and have it all—challenging careers, children and partners, and attractive, thin, and fit bodies. Therefore, if we don't achieve this "ideal," we often feel deficient and unworthy. Thus, advertisements often portray women who use certain products as attractive and successful in all areas of their lives. Examples of these include a young, thin, fit mother riding a bike with her son; a beautiful young woman with thick, blond hair sitting on the beach promoting shampoo; a woman displaying devices that can be worn to provide a face-lift effect without surgery; a gorgeous, young woman with long, thick dark hair promoting a hair conditioner; a beautiful, young Oriental woman with no wrinkles selling moisturizer; and a thin, young woman draped only in soft, see-through fabric and floating in a carefree position promoting a "soothing" line of hair products.

What about women who are of average to overaverage weight, are over 40 years of age, and may not have wrinkle-free complexions—are there no products for this group? Do only beautiful, thin, young, energetic women purchase products? No! Do these advertisements mean that we, of average looks and bodies, are not worthy of health-promoting and lifestyle-enhancing products? Is there some place for reality in advertising?

Advertisements also portray women as frivolous and preoccupied with self. In 1992, Quebec's Council for the Status of Women studied women in advertisements in 3,000 prime-time television shows reviewed over a 7-week period. The study determined that women were depicted as frivolous, superficial, ignorant, and incapable of doing difficult tasks.[57] Magazine advertisements directed at female consumers, unfortunately, depicted women in a similar manner. A Canadian writer reported that upon reviewing women's magazines, she observed an inordinate amount of information about dressing, eating, loving, shampooing, or exercising.[58] It can be disconcerting to be the gender viewed as superficial and perceived as having only a decorative contribution to make to society.

Is the mental and physical health of women negatively impacted when only thin and attractive models, implied as the cultural norm, are used in advertisements, or when women are portrayed as self-absorbed and frivolous? Advertisements that stereotype gender have been a major concern of feminist leaders. Has the image of women portrayed in the media been partially responsible for creating and maintaining limited social roles for women? In an analysis of research studies about women in advertisements from the 1950s through the 1980s, Bushy and Leichty[59] found that although there were not as many advertisements showing women in home or family settings, an increased number of advertisements showed women as decorative or in "alluring" roles in the ads.

Realistic Portrayals of Women

How about another view? A number of advertisements are beginning to portray women as decision makers who are financially independent. A phone company owned and operated by women, an automobile advertisement with a woman making the purchase decision, and a mortgage company showing a woman in the role of home buyer are examples of an enlightened and inclusive advertisement model. Another new approach finds advertisers seeking to find a neutral position; the trend is away from either-or images but, instead, seeks an image balanced between career and home.[60] Advertisers must place more emphasis on portraying women as capable, confident, and caring—as individuals who want factual information about products and services, not as individuals preoccupied by looks and images. An accurate and representative portrayal of women in advertisements can only be "healthful" for women, especially for women who are searching for their physical and psychological identities. (See *Journal Activity:* "Forming Your Own Opinion.")

As women continue to have a major financial impact on the marketplace, we will see advertisers present a more realistic image of women—one of an intelligent, pragmatic, attentive, concerned, and financially stable individual—because it is justified. (See *FYI:* "What Is Direct-to-Consumer Advertising?")

FINANCIAL CONSIDERATIONS

Health Insurance

All aspects of health care, ranging from prevention to treatment to cure, are essential to the health and well-being of all people. The continuing exponential growth

Journal Activity

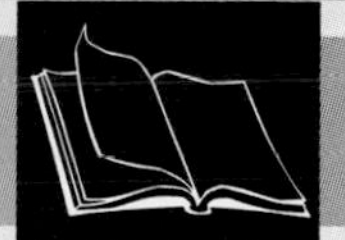

Forming Your Own Opinion

Complete the following activity to help you form your own opinion and develop perceptions about the portrayal of women in advertising. Monitor the media (television, radio, magazines, etc.) for their portrayal of women. Then answer these questions:

- Do you find evidence of traditional roles for women in the media?
- Is there evidence of sexism?
- Do you find advertisements in which women are portrayed as capable decision makers?
- Do you find women portrayed with a "Barbie doll" image?
- In advertisements including men and women, what is the implicit message about women?
- Do advertisers have a responsibility to portray both sexes in a manner that promotes the well-being of the individual?

FYI

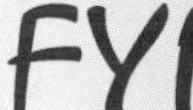

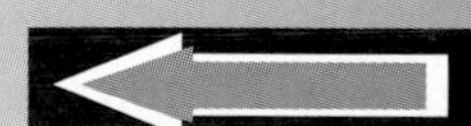

What Is Direct-to-Consumer Advertising?[61]

For decades, physicians or pharmacists have been expected to provide and interpret information, provided by pharmaceutical companies, about medications to their patients. However, as an increasing number of patients have become more involved in making their own health care decisions, some manufacturers have begun to create medical-related ads direct to consumers. In the past 20 years, direct-to-consumer (DTC) advertising has become increasingly popular.

These advertisements fall under the jurisdiction of the FDA, which helps to ensure that prescription drug information provided by drug firms is truthful, balanced, and accurately communicated. By surveying physicians and consumers, the FDA can determine if advertising rules need to be altered to help consumers better understand the benefits and risks of various medications.

of health care costs too often leaves individuals without the benefit of this vital care, especially the uninsured. Health insurance is a contract between an individual and/or a group and an insurance company, and it can assist individuals in meeting the demands and needs of paying for their health care. What types of health insurance plans are available, and how do we select one that meets our health needs and financial ability? See *FYI:* "The Three Basic Health Insurance Plans."

Health insurance plans vary according to the types of services offered and the price for coverage. *Basic health insurance* covers hospital, surgical, and medical expenses, and individual health plans differ according to the company and the contract. *Major medical insurance* (or catastrophic coverage) assists with any major and/or long-term illness, such as heart disease or cancer, and is usually a supplement to basic health insurance. *Comprehensive major medical insurance* combines basic health and major medical insurance plans to provide for the majority of health care needs. There is usually a deductible, often of $500 or more, which must be paid by the insuree before the insurance company is required to pay anything.

Not only do too many people not have health insurance, but people continue to lose the coverage they have—tens of thousands lose their health insurance each month, and more than 46 million Americans do not have any health insurance.[62]

Women and children are disproportionately represented among all uninsured individuals, with more than 23 million U.S. women uninsured. In addition, millions of women who are insured have difficulty accessing health care due to health coverage gaps, including noncoverage of essential services (medical screenings, dental care) and high deductibles or co-pays.[63] Uninsured women often postpone necessary health care, have limited access to preventive screenings such as a Pap test or cancer screenings, have delayed diagnoses of serious illness, often at incurable stages, receive less therapeutic care, and die at an earlier age or earlier in the disease process.[64] Uninsured or underinsured women usually have no regular doctor, do not fill needed prescriptions, and often use emergency rooms as their health care facility, which is more expensive and often less effective. Disparities exist between

FYI

The Three Basic Health Insurance Plans

The type of health insurance plan a woman has will determine the type of medical services, procedures, and practitioners she will be able to use. Here is a brief look at three basic types of plans.

- *Private, fee-for-service plan:* The individual or employer pays a certain amount each month that ensures a woman can receive health care on a fee-for-service basis. A deductible, paid by the patient, must be met and then the insurance pays a major portion, usually 80 percent, after the deductible is met. To lower costs of insurance, **preferred provider organizations (PPOs),** which are composed of private medical practitioners, provide services at a lower rate to a particular insurance company. Use of the PPO physicians produces lower health care fees; use of non-PPO physicians costs more.
- *Prepaid group insurance:* **Health maintenance organizations (HMOs)** are composed of various medical personnel who provide a wide range of medical services (e.g., specialists, lab work) for a prepaid amount that is usually deducted from each paycheck. There is often a co-pay (usually a minimal amount such as $15–$20) each time an HMO service is used. The HMO is usually associated with a hospital and provides care from a limited group of medical practitioners.
- *Government-financed insurance:* For women of certain ages and socioeconomic levels, the local, state, and/or federal government provides health care insurance under various types of plans. Briefly, two types of government insurance plans are (1) Medicare, which is paid from Social Security benefits for people 65 and older and for individuals with specific health concerns, and (2) Medicaid, which provides some health care coverage for individuals who meet certain financial criteria. These two types of coverage are discussed in greater detail in the text.

women of color and white women: Hispanic and African American women are two to three times more likely to be uninsured than are white women.

A comprehensive health insurance plan that meets the specific needs of women, especially low-income women, should (1) provide universal access—especially for women who work part-time or are seasonal, or who move in and out of the workforce; (2) be affordable—especially because women have average earnings that are 25 percent less than men's; (3) allow reimbursement for a range of providers—midwives, nurse practitioners, and other medical personnel who are effective but less expensive than physicians; (4) be nondiscriminatory; (5) have equal rating factors—adopt a community rating and prohibit the insurance industry from using gender as a rating factor; (6) require a minimum benefits package with preventive care, reproductive care (family planning, abortion, infertility), mental health benefits, drug abuse care, long-term health care, HIV AIDS treatment, and care for battered women. When considering health care insurance, assess the quality of the provisions by comparing these components to the policy components.

Medicare and Medicaid

Medicare, provided by the federal government Social Security Act, is a government health insurance program that provides health care benefits for individuals 65 years of age and older. Disabled women under 65 may also be eligible for Medicare. Medicare consists of two parts: *Part A* is the Hospital Insurance and *Part B* is Supplementary Medical Insurance. Part A helps to pay for inpatient care while in a hospital, or a skilled nursing facility, for home health care, and for hospice care. Medicare is a mandatory hospital insurance plan financed by federal Social Security taxes, but paid for by employers paying into Social Security on their employees' behalf and by self-employed persons. Part B helps to pay for physician services, outpatient care, lab tests, and other medical services and supplies. Monthly premiums paid by enrollees and from federal general revenues finance Part B Medicare. To enroll for Medicare, contact the Social Security Administration office found in the government section of your local phone book.[65]

Medicaid is a medical assistance program jointly financed by state and federal governments to help provide health care for low-income women with no health care. Eligible recipients include low-income women and those who cannot work; blind, elderly, and/or disabled individuals; low-income families with dependent children; and others with special circumstances. In 2004, 12.8 percent of the non-elderly population had health coverage through the use of Medicaid.[66] Of the Medicaid population recipients, women make up nearly 70 percent over the age of 15; women are twice as likely as men to qualify for Medicaid.[67] Even though states have expanded Medicaid coverage, 17.7 percent of women between the ages of 18 and 64 still do not have health insurance.[68] Federally mandated Medicaid services of significance to women include inpatient and outpatient hospital, physician, midwife, and certified nurse practitioner; laboratory and X ray; nursing home and home health care; rural health clinics; family planning; and early and periodic screening, diagnosis, and treatment for children under age 21. States have varying eligibility requirements, and the services are administered out of the county or state Human Servces office. Women can contact this office for assistance.

Social Security

Social Security (SS) is a protective program that provides benefits to workers and their families who have financial and health care needs. The program began in 1935 as a way to assist retired workers, most of whom were men, and the families of deceased workers. In the 1930s only a very small percentage of women worked in jobs outside the home; however, today about 60 percent of all women are employed outside the home and earn credit toward their retirement.[69] Women earn SS protection for themselves and their children, but also earn assistance if they become disabled and cannot work, and survivor benefits if they should die. Married women who choose not to work outside the home, or who enter the workforce for only a few years, may have Social Security benefits if their spouse retires, becomes disabled, or dies.

Retirement Benefits Retirement benefits vary according to age of the retiree. A woman can be eligible for benefits by age 62, but the payments will be permanently reduced because she will be receiving payments for a longer period of time than if she had waited until age 65. A woman will be eligible for full retirement benefits if she waits until she is 65 years of age to retire. In the future, the age in which full benefits are payable will be gradually increased—by the year 2027, a woman will need to be 67 years old to receive full retirement benefits.

If you are married, you can receive retirement payments on your husband's as well as your own employment record. There are often special circumstances related to SS retirement benefits, including age, former and current marital status, and the work history of both partners.

Special situations such as never being employed, self-employment, household worker, or service in the military have some unique aspects. Information related to these and other considerations can be obtained from the Social Security Administration office at www.ssa.org or from the local SS office. Social Security benefits related to remarriage, being widowed, and being divorced are multifaceted and sometimes complex.

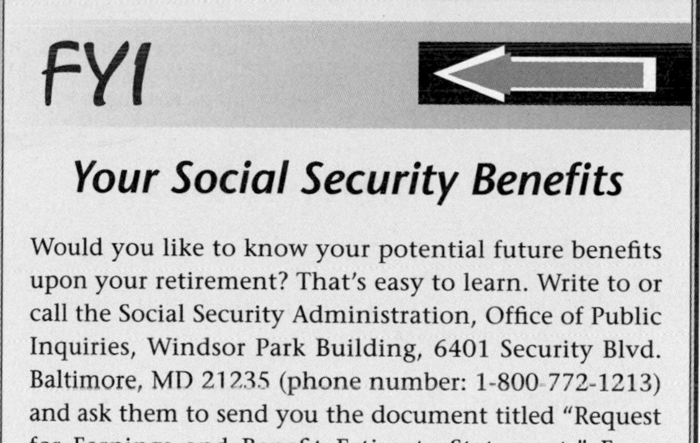

FYI

Your Social Security Benefits

Would you like to know your potential future benefits upon your retirement? That's easy to learn. Write to or call the Social Security Administration, Office of Public Inquiries, Windsor Park Building, 6401 Security Blvd. Baltimore, MD 21235 (phone number: 1-800-772-1213) and ask them to send you the document titled "Request for Earnings and Benefit Estimate Statement," Form #SSA-7004-SM OP-7, or go to the Web site www.ssa.gov to learn about Social Security.

Contact a representative from the local, state, or national Social Security office. (See *FYI:* "Your Social Security Benefits.")

TAKING ACTION AS A CONSUMER

Agencies

The Food and Drug Administration (FDA) has the responsibility to regulate the following products (with examples): foods (labeling, safety), drugs (approval, advertising), cosmetics (safety, purity), biological products (blood banks, human vaccines), medical devices (registration, approval), radiological devices (microwave, X-ray equipment), and veterinary products (pet foods, vet drugs) sold in interstate commerce. States enforce regulations on products that do not cross state lines. The states are also responsible for licensing health professionals such as dentists, physicians, and pharmacists as well as inspection and regulation of restaurants and health clubs.

The FDA offers a variety of services to assist the consumer with questions or concerns related to any product under its regulatory control. Consumer Affairs Officers (COAs) are located throughout the United States to answer questions and provide informational literature, either by print or through media. These officers (often referred to as public affairs specialists) will also speak to groups on specific topics related to drugs, fraud, safety, and many other topics of interest to consumers. Your local COA can be found under the Food and Drug Administration in the federal government section of the local phone book. The Consumer Inquiries Staff, located

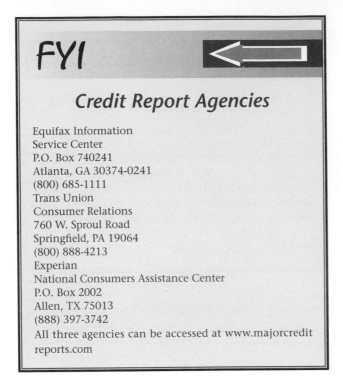

FYI

Credit Report Agencies

Equifax Information
Service Center
P.O. Box 740241
Atlanta, GA 30374-0241
(800) 685-1111
Trans Union
Consumer Relations
760 W. Sproul Road
Springfield, PA 19064
(800) 888-4213
Experian
National Consumers Assistance Center
P.O. Box 2002
Allen, TX 75013
(888) 397-3742
All three agencies can be accessed at www.majorcreditreports.com

in Washington, D.C., has the responsibility of answering consumers' questions of any type. This staff has the ability to utilize the expertise of a variety of federal agencies to find the answer to inquiries, about 2,500 each month. See the Resources at the end of this chapter for additional consumer resources.

Credit Reports

Reports of your credit history may be requested when you seek to purchase items such as an automobile, a home, or a large appliance. Credit bureaus collect and maintain great volumes of information on an individual's financial activities, including your buying and paying history. If a company wants to assess your creditworthiness, it can obtain a copy of your credit report from a number of credit agencies. Because of the increase in identity theft, it is essential to check your credit report regularly to determine if someone else is using any of your credit cards or bank accounts without your knowledge. You can obtain a copy of your credit report by contacting one of three national credit report agencies: Equifax, Trans Union, and Experian. (Addresses are provided in *FYI:* "Credit Report Agencies.") Each year, you can order one free credit report from one of these agencies. Check carefully to see if there are any inaccuracies or questionable listings of debts.

Knowing what to do if inaccuracies appear in your credit report is an important consumer skill. If you find inaccuracies, write to the credit bureau that issued the report and tell it report which credit listing is inaccurate. The credit report agency must, by law, reverify the information within a reasonable amount of time (usually 30–35 days) or the credit listing must be removed from your file. Information that is inaccurate or cannot be verified must be corrected or removed from your report. If you have some negative information on your report that is accurate, you may elect to write a brief explanation (about 100 words) to the credit bureaus and explain why the negative credit incident occurred. This may be helpful in obtaining credit even though the negative report usually must stay in your file for 7 years. Bankruptcy information is kept for 10 years. If this information appeared on one credit bureau report, it may appear on others. Therefore, it is a good idea to review all three major credit report agencies. Be sure to establish credit for yourself and not rely on your partner's credit line. There may be situations in which you will need to have established a credit rating for yourself.

Righting a Wrong

Even if we are wise consumers, there are times when we may be taken advantage of by an individual or a company or we may have purchased a faulty product. Knowing what to do and how to rectify this situation can be helpful and save time and money. Purchase-related paperwork of a product that is intended to last for a period of time should be saved in an organized file with other product-related information. If a problem occurs, contact the business (or person) that sold you the product and describe the problem and how you would like for it to be resolved. For example, do you want the product repaired or your money back? Keep a record of calls and/or letters to and from the company and include when and with whom you spoke. If the problem has not been resolved within a reasonable amount of time, then it is time to contact the company headquarters. Look on the packaging for a toll-free 800 number or call the toll-free 800 operator at 800-555-1212 to locate the number of the company. Most local libraries have a directory of 800 numbers, or you can get this information online (http://inter800.com or www.anywho.com.tt.html).

Many companies require a complaint to be in writing; therefore, knowing where to write and what to say can be valuable information. Look for the address of the product manufacturer on the packaging of the product. If it is not there, or you do not have the packaging, go to the reference section in your local library and search for the company address in one of the following books: *Standard & Poor's Register of Corporations, Directors and Executives;* the

FIGURE 2.2 Sample complaint letter.[70]

Your street address
Your city, state, zip code
Date

(Name of contact person if available)
(Title, if available)
(Company name)
(Consumer complaint division, if you have no contact person)
(Street address)
(City, state, zip code)

Dear (contact person):

Re: (account number, if applicable)

On (date), I (bought, leased, rented, or had repaired) a (name of product with serial or model number or service performed) at (location, date, and other important details of the transaction).

Unfortunately, your product (or service) has not performed well (or service was inadequate) because (state the problem). I am disappointed because (explain the problem: for example, the product does not work properly, the service was not performed correctly, I was billed the wrong amount, something was not disclosed clearly or was misrepresented, etc.).

To resolve the problem, I would appreciate your (state the specific action you want—money back, charge card credit, repair, exchange, etc.). Enclosed are copies (do not send originals) of my records (include receipts, guarantees, warranties, canceled checks, contracts, model and serial numbers, and any other documentation).

I look forward to your reply and a resolution to my problem, and will wait until (set a time limit) before seeking help from consumer protection or the Better Business Bureau. Please contact me at the above address or by phone at (home or other number with area code).

Sincerely,

(Your name)

Enclosure(s)

cc: (who you are sending a copy of this letter, if anyone)

Standard Directory of Advertisers; the *Trade Names Directory;* or the *Dun & Bradstreet Directory.* The *Thomas Register of American Manufacturers* can provide you with a list of manufacturers of thousands of products. After locating the address of the company, it is important to write a concise and reasonable, but not threatening, letter explaining what is wrong with their product and how you have attempted to resolve the problem. (See Figure 2.2.) Include your name, address, work or home phone numbers, and your company account number, if you have one. Provide the company with place and date of product purchase, and serial or model number of the product, and include copies, not originals, of all documentation. If, after a reasonable time, usually 2 to 4 weeks, you have not received satisfaction, file a complaint, along with a copy of your letter, with the local or state consumer protection agency that pertains to the nature of your concern. Addresses and phone numbers for agencies that govern banking, hospitals, insurance, products, and utilities can usually be found in the government pages of the telephone directory. Addresses for more specific agencies and companies are found in the *Consumer Action Handbook.*[71]

Chapter Summary

- Effective consumer skills include having an awareness and knowledge of health products and services, making informed choices, and knowing how to obtain better consumer services.
- There are important guidelines that can be utilized when locating and selecting a health care provider.
- A variety of health care practitioners provide special and specific services that can be beneficial to women's health.
- Alternative health care offers options to conventional medicine but as a rule is not taught in U.S. medical schools. Many of these alternative practices have not been scientifically proven to be medically beneficial.
- Fraudulent health care costs American citizens more than $10 billion annually; therefore, it is essential to recognize and report acts of fraudulent behavior.
- Prescription and over-the-counter (OTC) drugs can cause physical and psychological addiction as well as tolerance and withdrawal symptoms.
- Prescription drugs are legal drugs used to treat and/or cure diseases and may be obtained in generic or brand-name forms.
- Disorders such as obesity, depression, anxiety, and hormonal imbalances can be treated with a variety of prescription drugs.
- OTC drugs are purchased without a physician's prescription and can be used to treat various common ailments.
- Reading labels, following instructions, and consulting a physician as needed are important precautions to remember when taking OTC drugs.
- The physician's instructions should be strictly followed by pregnant women who use prescriptions and OTC drugs.
- Unrealistic portrayal of women has been created in order to promote the perception that certain types of products need to be purchased.
- Cosmetics, skin-care products, and facial and body cosmetic surgery are all products/procedures that can be expensive and risky; women can learn important guidelines for better selection of these products and procedures.
- Advertising is a major influence in the purchase of health-related products, and the media use a variety of techniques to sell these commodities.
- Women have specific needs in health insurance coverage yet are too often without important insurance coverage for themselves and their children.
- Information regarding health insurance, Social Security benefits, and retirement plans is needed by women in order to make health- and life-enhancing financial decisions.
- Medicare and Medicaid are government health insurance programs that provide health care benefits for women and children who meet specific criteria.
- Government and citizen consumer protection agencies provide avenues by which women can learn how to report problems with products/people/procedures and find assistance in correcting the problems.

Review Questions

1. What is the Consumer Bill of Rights, and what is its purpose?
2. What are the processes for locating and selecting a health care provider?
3. What are the advantages and disadvantages of using home health tests? Which are designed specifically for women?
4. Why are more women turning to alternative health care? What are some of the advantages and disadvantages of alternative health care?
5. How can you protect yourself from health care fraud?
6. What is the difference between brand-name and generic drugs?
7. What information is available on prescription and OTC drug labels, and what are the benefits of knowing this information?
8. What are three types of weight control prescription drugs and the pharmacological function of each?
9. What three federal laws were passed to help protect the consumer from poor-quality health products and inadequate health care?
10. Why are antidepressant drugs prescribed more for women than for men, and what precautions should be taken while using these drugs?
11. How can women use medicinal drugs safely?
12. What are the pros and cons of purchasing an OTC drug? Which are purchased specifically by women?
13. What are the various types of laxative products that are currently on the market?
14. What precautions should be taken when using OTC sleep aids?
15. What are some safety measures that women can take when selecting and purchasing cosmetics?
16. What are some of the concerns about cosmetic surgery? Why do many women elect to have these beauty-enhancing procedures?
17. What criteria should a woman use when selecting a cosmetic surgeon?
18. What is the purpose of the various advertising techniques used by companies to sell their products?
19. What techniques do advertisers use in promoting their products? Provide an example of a product for each of these techniques.
20. Why should women be concerned about how they are portrayed in advertisements?
21. What is the difference between basic, major medical, and comprehensive major medical insurance coverage?
22. Why are women and their children disproportionately uninsured in this country?
23. What health care benefits are provided by Medicare and Medicaid?
24. What elements should be included when writing a letter of complaint about a product, a professional, an agency, or a facility?

Resources

Web Sites

Agency for Healthcare Research and Quality
www.ahcpr.gov/consumer
American Society of Plastic Surgeons
www.plasticsurgery.org
Better Business Bureau
www.bbb.org
Consumer Health Sourcebook
www.chsourcebook.com
ConsumerLab.com
www.consumerlab.com
FDA Office of Women's Health
www.fda.gov/womens
Federal Citizen Information Center
www.pueblo.gsa.gov
Federal Trade Commission
www.ftc.gov/ftc/consumer.htm
FirstGov for Consumers
www.consumer.gov/index.htm
Food and Drug Administration
www.fda.gov
Medline Plus
www.medlineplus.gov
National Association for Chiropractic Medicine
www.chiromed.org
National Center for Complementary and Alternative Medicine
www.nccam.nih.gov
National Council Against Health Fraud
www.ncahf.org
National Women's Law Center
capwiz.com/nwlc/home
Natural Medicines Comprehensive Database
www.naturaldatabase.com
Quackwatch
www.quackwatch.com
Social Security Online
www.ssa.gov
U.S. Consumer Product Safety Commission
www.cpsc.gov

Suggested Readings

Block, S. B. and, G. A. Hirt. 2008. *Foundations of Financial Management.* 12th ed. New York: McGraw-Hill.

Blum, V. L. 2003. *Flesh Wounds: The Culture of Cosmetic Surgery.* Berkeley: University of California Press.

Brody, J. E., and D. Grady. 2001. *The New York Times Guide to Alternative Health.* New York: Henry Holt.

Coddington, D. C., E. A. Fischer, K. D. Moore, and R. L. Clarke. 2000. *Beyond Managed Care: How Consumers and Technology Are Changing the Future of Health Care.* San Francisco: Jossey-Bass.

Colvin, R. 2002. *Prescription Drug Addiction: The Hidden Epidemic.* Omaha, NE: Addicus Books.

Crister, G. 2005. *Generation Rx: How Prescription Drugs Are Altering American Lives, Minds and Bodies.* New York: Houghton Mifflin.

Ernst, E., M. H. Pittler, and B. Wider, 2006. *Complementary & Alternative Medicine: An Evidence-Based Approach.* St. Louis, MO: Mosby.

Griffith, H. W. 2005. *Complete Guide to Prescription and Nonprescription Drugs 2006.* New York: Berkley Publishing Co.

Institute of Medicine. 2001. *Crossing the Quality Chasm: A New Health System for the 21st Century.* Washington, DC: National Academy Press.

Kotler, R. 2005. *The Essential Cosmetic Surgery Companion: Don't Consult a Cosmetic Surgeon Without This Book.* Beverly Hills, CA: Ernest Mitchell Publishers.

Lewis, D., G. Eysenbach, R. Kikafka, P. Z. Stavri, and H. Jimison. 2005. *Consumer Health Informatics: Informing Consumers and Improving Health Care.* Traverse City, MI: Spring Publishers.

Lieberman, T., ed. 2000. *Consumer Reports Complete Guide to Health Services for Seniors: What Your Family Needs to Know about Finding and Financing, Medicare, Assisted Living, Nursing Homes, Home Care, Adult Day Care.* Three Rivers, MI: Three Rivers Press.

Rees, A. M. 2003. *Consumer Health Information Source Book.* 7th ed. Phoenix, AZ: Onyx Press.

Rybacki, J. 2003. *Essential Guide to Prescription Drugs.* 7th ed. New York: HarperCollins.

References

1. Consumer Advisory Commission on Consumer Protection and Quality in the Health Care Industry. 1997. *Final report, consumer bill of rights & responsibilities.* www.hcqualitycommission.gov/cborr (retrieved September 15, 2006).
2. Barrett, S., W. London, R. Baratz, and M. Kroger. 2007. *Consumer health: A guide to intelligent decisions.* 8th ed. New York: McGraw-Hill.
3. Ibid.
4. Barzansky, B., and S. I. Etzel. 2003. Education programs in US medical schools, 2002–2003. *Journal of the American Medical Association* 290:1190–96.
5. Smith, M. 2002. The screening test you need. *WebMD Medical News.* http://aolsvc.health.webmd.aol.com/content/article/54/65232.htm (retrieved September 15, 2006).
6. Barrett et al., *Consumer health.*
7. American College of Nurse-Midwives. *A career in midwifery.* www.midwife.org (retrieved September 15, 2006).
8. Payne, H., D. B. Hahn, and E. Lucus. 2007. *Understanding your health.* 9th ed. New York: McGraw-Hill.
9. 4therapy.com. 2000. *Understanding therapists' professional degrees.* www.4therapy.com/consumer/about_therapy/item.php?uniqueId=4936&categoryid=102& (retrieved September 15, 2006).
10. U.S. Food and Drug Administration. 2003. *Buying diagnostic tests from the Internet: Buyer beware.* www.fda.gov/cdrh/consumer/buyerbeware.html (retrieved September 15, 2006).
11. U.S. Food and Drug Administration: Office of In Vitro Diagnostic Device and Evaluation and Safety. *Home-use tests.* www.fda.gov/cdrh/oivd.consumer-homeuse.html (retrieved January 12, 2006).

12. National Institutes of Health: National Center for Complementary and Alternative Medicine. 2002. *What is complementary and alternative medicine (CAM)?* http://nccam.nih.gov/health/whatiscam (retrieved September 15, 2006).
13. Institute of Medicine, Committee on the Use of Complementary and Alternative Medicine by the American Public. 2005. *Complementary and alternative medicine in the United States.* Washington, DC: National Academies Press.
14. Ibid.
15. Barasch, D. S. 1994. The mainstreaming of alternative medicine. *Good Health* (October 4): 6–9, 36, 38.
16. Natural Medicine Comprehensive Database. 2003. www.naturaldatabase.com (retrieved September 15, 2006).
17. Common herbs. 2006. www.herbalgram.org/default.asp?c=common_herbs (retrieved September 15, 2006).
18. National Center for Complementary and Alternative Medicine. *Get the facts: Acupuncture.* http://nccam.nih.gov/health/acupuncture/(retrieved September 15, 2006).
19. Chiropractors. 1994. *Consumer Reports* 59 (6): 383–90.
20. Barrett et al., *Consumer health.*
21. Ibid.
22. American Chiropractic Association. 2003. *What is chiropractic?* www.amerchiro.org/level2_css.cfm?T1ID=13&T2ID=61 (retrieved September 15, 2006).
23. Chiropractors. *Consumer Reports.*
24. American Massage Therapists Association. 2005 *Research confirms massage therapy enhances health.* www.amtamassage.org/news/enhancehealth.html (retrieved on January 10, 2006).
25. Chiropractors. *Consumer Reports.*
26. Witherell, M. 1995. Massage: De-stress in minutes. *American Health* (September): 70.
27. Stalker, D., and O. Glymour. 1983. Engineers, cranks, physicians, magicians. *New England Journal of Medicine* 308:60–64.
28. Barrett et al. *Consumer health,* p. 37.
29. Ibid.
30. Ibid.
31. Carroll, C. R. 2000. *Drugs in modern society.* 5th ed. New York: McGraw-Hill, p. 280.
32. Barrett, et al., *Consumer health,* p. 410.
33. Food and Drug Administration. 2000. Requirements on content and format of labeling for human prescription drugs and biologics: Requirements for prescription drug product labels; proposed rule. *Federal Register* 65: 81081–131.
34. Prescription Kaiser Family Foundation. 2006. *Prescription drug trends.* www.kff.org/rxdrugs/upload/13057-05.pdf (retrieved May 1, 2007).
35. Kapusniak, L. 1997. Women's bodies should figure into standards. *Bryan-College Station* (Texas) *Eagle,* May 28.
36. PDR Health. 2003. *Battling anorexia, bulimia . . . and obesity.* http://consumer.pdr.net (retrieved September 16, 2006).
37. PDR Health. 2003. *Depression: How to recognize; what to do about it.* http://consumer.pdr.net (retrieved September 16, 2006).
38. Food and Drug Administration: Center for Drug Evaluation and Research. (2003). *Nonprescription products: What we do.* www.fda.gov/cder/Offices/OTC/whatwedo.htm. (retrieved September 16, 2006).
39. Center for Drug Evaluation and Research. 2003. *Nonprescription products.* www.fda.gov/cder/Offices/OTC/default.htm (retrieved September 16, 2006).
40. Center for Drug Education and Research. 2002. *The new over-the-counter medicine label: Take a look.* www.fda.gov/cder/Offices/OTC/default.htm (retrieved September 16, 2006).
41. Cummings, M. 1991. Overuse hazardous: Laxatives rarely needed. *FDA Consumer: DHHS Publication* (April), DHHS No. 92-1182.
42. Rubin, J. P., C. Ferencz, and C. Loffredo. 1993. Use of prescription & non-prescription drugs in pregnancy. *Clinical Epidemiology* 46 (6): 581–89.
43. U.S. Food and Drug Administration. 2002. *Is it a cosmetic, a drug or both? (or soap)?* www.cfsan.fda.gov/~dms/cos-218.html (retrieved September 16, 2006).
44. Ibid.
45. Cavanaugh, T. 1995. Ethics expand. *Chemical Marketing Reporter* 2 (17): SR 21–22.
46. Moisturizers. 1994. *Consumer Reports* 59 (9): 577–81.
47. Columbia University: Go Ask Alice. 2003. *Moisturizers.* www.goaskalice.columbia.edu/2408.html (retrieved September 15, 2006).
48. Consumer Search. 2004. *Moisturizer comparison chart.* www.consumersearch.com/www/family/facial_moisturizers/comparisonchart.html (retrieved September 16, 2006).
49. Goodman, M. 1994. Social, psychological & developmental factors in women's receptivity to cosmetic surgery. *Journal of Aging Studies* 8 (4): 375–96.
50. The American Society for Aesthetic Plastic Surgery. 2003. *Botulinum toxin injections.* www.surgery.org/public/procedures-injectables.php. (retrieved September 15, 2006).
51. U.S. Food and Drug Administration. 2004. *Making an informed decision about breast implants.* www.fda.gov/fdac/features/2004/504_implants.html (retriered May 1, 2007).
52. Jacobson, N. 2003. No clearer than it was before. *Washington Post,* October 26.
53. Food and Drug Administration. 2006. *Breast implants.* www.fda.gov/cdrh/breastimplants/qa2006.html#s1 (retrieved March 3, 2007).
54. Margolis, D. 1993. Fat chance: Rearrange the unwanted mass. *American Health* (March): 12, 18.
55. Ibid.
56. Barrett et al. *Consumer health.*
57. Shier, M. 1995. On being a boy toy. *Canada and the World Backgrounder* 60 (4): 8–10.
58. Ibid.
59. Bushy, J., and G. Leichty. 1993. Feminism & advertising in traditional and nontraditional women's magazine, 1950s–1980s. *Journalism Quarterly* 70 (2): 247–64.
60. Kanner, B. 1995. Advertisers take aim at women at home. *New York Times.*
61. Lewis, C. 2003. The impact of direct-to-consumer advertising. *FDA Consumer Magazine* online. (March/April). www.fda.gov/fdac/features/2003/203_dtc.html (retrieved September 16, 2006).

62. National Coalition on Health Care. 2004. *Health insurance coverage*. www.nchc.org/facts/coverage.shtml (retrieved March 3, 2007).
63. National Women's Law Center. 2005. *Women and health insurance*. www.nwlc.org/details.cfm?id=2186§ion=health (retrieved March 3, 2007).
64. Ibid.
65. *Medicare*. 2007. The Official U.S. Government Site for People with Medicare. www.medicare.gov/Coverage/Home.asp (retrieved May 1, 2007).
66. Employee Benefit Research Institute. 2004. *Sources of health insurance and characteristics of the uninsured, analysis of the March 2004 Current Population Survey*. Issue brief #276.
67. National Women's Law Center. 2004. *Women and Medicaid*. http://nwlc.org/WomenMedicaidUpdate.June2004.pdf (retrieved January 27, 2006).
68. Ibid.
69. Social Security Administration. 2003. *Social Security . . . what every woman should know*. SSA Publication No. 05-10127, ICN 480067. www.ssa.gov/pubs/10127.html#part6 (retrieved September 16, 2006).
70. Consumer Action Webpage. 2007. *2007 Consumer action handbook*. http//www.consumeraction.gov/pdfs/2007revisedCAH.pdf (retrieved May 1, 2007).
71. *Consumer Action Handbook*. 2003. Washington, DC: U.S. Office of Consumer Affairs. www.consumeraction.gov (retrieved September 16, 2006). You can also request this handbook by calling the federal Consumer Information Center at 1-800-878-3256.

Chapter Three

Developing a Healthy Lifestyle

CHAPTER OBJECTIVES

When you complete this chapter, you will be able to do the following:

- Define the dimensions of wellness in regard to the whole person concept
- Describe the health continuum, from wellness to illness, and appropriate intervention strategies
- Describe theories of learning and models of behavior change
- Plan a lifestyle change using the following: behavioral assessment, goal setting, behavioral contracting, initiation of behavior change, and periodic evaluation of progress

WHAT IS HEALTHY?

Do you consider yourself to be healthy? What do you compare yourself with to decide that you are healthy? How old do you feel? How long do you expect to live? These are not easy questions to answer primarily because living is a very complex process. Your health is dependent upon your personal lifestyle choices as well as upon uncontrollable elements, such as genetics, environmental conditions, the technological development of your country, your gender, your ethnicity, cultural issues, age-specific risks, and the potential for accidents.

This whole book serves as a guide for lifestyle assessment and enhancement for women. The ideas introduced in this chapter are meant to prepare you for the material presented in later chapters. And although much of the information in this chapter may be applied to anyone, you can use this information to help you understand how you, personally, make lifestyle choices. Think of this chapter as a presentation of the basic philosophies of health and behavior change.

Some people live to be over 100 years old and some die in infancy. Many factors must be considered in determining just how long you will actually live. Life expectancy figures are important in that they provide researchers with overall, statistical averages for tracking health concerns, but statistical averages do not consider the individual. The most important consideration for you is what you are doing to achieve a lifestyle that is enjoyable for you and that will prolong your enjoyment as much as possible.

This chapter presents average life expectancy figures and describes established models for healthy living. These health models serve as a basis for you to understand your own personal life concerns and can aid in the design of a lifestyle that suits you best.

Life Expectancy

According to the U.S. Census Population Clock, on March 9, 2006, the U.S. population was 298,266,107 and the world population was 6,502,389,908 (for the latest numbers, go to the U.S. Census Web site at www.census/gov). During the year 2003 an estimated 2,448,288 deaths occurred in the United States, and according to the National Center for Health Statistics, average life expectancy for a person living in the U.S. was 77.5 years from the time of birth. In the year 2003, the life expectancy for women was 80.1 years, an average of 5.3 years more than for men. The life expectancy for white women was 80.5 years, and for black women it was 76.1 years.

Women outlive men in almost every country and, on average, are expected to live 4 years longer than men. In 2005 the United Nations reported that the life expectancy of women in the world was 67.8 years and for men it was 63.7 years. Life expectancy refers to the number of years we are expected to live from birth. Although there is no way to predict how long each person is going to live at the time they are born, we can take an average of how long people have lived, which provides an indication of how long a certain cross section of a population might live. Life expectancy seems to be directly tied to income. The countries with the largest increase in life expectancy were also among the countries with the most rapid increase in their income per capita. There are big differences between regions. Africa has the lowest life expectancy with 55.7 years for women (52.7 for men). The HIV/AIDS epidemic is rampant in Africa. North America has the highest life expectancy with 80.2 years for women (73.5 for men). Among the obvious life-threatening health problems specific to women around the world is maternal mortality. The United Nations estimated in 2005 that each year about 600,000 women die of complications related to childbirth. With better maternal health care and education, this figure could change dramatically. Other factors that dramatically affect life expectancy are prolonged periods of war, civil strife, and genocide in a country or region. Table 3.1 provides a comparison of life

TABLE 3.1 Years of Life Expectancy at Birth for Women of the World

Country	Years
Africa	
Algeria	72
Angola	42
Benin	55
Botswana	37
Burkina Faso	48
Burundi	44
Cameroon	47
Cape Verde	73
Central African Republic	40
Chad	45
Comoros	65
Congo	53
Congo, Democratic Republic of Circumflex	44
Côte d'Ivoire	47
Djibouti	54
Egypt	72
Equatorial Guinea	44
Eritrea	55
Ethiopia	49
Gabon	55
Gambia	57
Ghana	57
Guinea	54
Guinea-Bissau	46
Kenya	46
Lesotho	38
Liberia	44
Libyan Arab Jamahiriya	76
Madagascar	57
Malawi	40
Mali	48
Mauritania	54
Mauritius	76
Morocco	72
Mozambique	43
Namibia	49
Niger	44
Nigeria	44
Réunion	80
Rwanda	45
São Tomé and Principe	64
Senegal	57
Sierra Leone	42
Somalia	47
South Africa	51
Sudan	58
Swaziland	33
Togo	56
Tunisia	75
Uganda	47
United Republic of Tanzania	46
Zambia	37
Zimbabwe	37
America, North	
Bahamas	73
Barbados	78
Belize	75
Canada	82
Costa Rica	81
Cuba	79
Dominican Republic	71
El Salvador	74
Guadeloupe	82
Guatemala	71
Haiti	52
Honduras	70
Jamaica	73
Martinique	82
Mexico	77
Netherlands Antilles	79
Nicaragua	72
Panama	77
Puerto Rico	80
Saint Lucia	74
Saint Vincent and the Grenadines	74
Trinidad and Tobago	73
United States of America	80
America, South	
Argentina	78
Bolivia	66
Brazil	74

(continued)

TABLE 3.1 ***(continued)***

Chile	81
Colombia	75
Ecuador	77
French Guiana	78
Guyana	66
Paraguay	73
Peru	72
Suriname	73
Uruguay	79
Venezuela	76
Asia	
Afghanistan	46
Armenia	75
Azerbaijan	70
Bahrain	76
Bangladesh	63
Bhutan	64
Brunei Darussalam	79
Cambodia	60
China	73
Hong Kong SAR	85
Macao SAR	82
Cyprus	81
Georgia	74
India	65
Indonesia	69
Iran	72
Iraq	60
Israel	82
Japan	85
Jordan	73
Kazakhstan	69
Korea, Dem. People's Rep. (North)	66
Korea, Republic of (South)	80
Kyrgyzstan	71
Lao People's Democratic Rep.	56
Lebanon	74
Malaysia	75
Maldives	66
Mongolia	66
Myanmar	63
Nepal	62
Occupied Palestinian Territory	74
Oman	76
Pakistan	63
Philippines	72
Qatar	76
Saudi Arabia	74
Singapore	81
Sri Lanka	77
Syrian Arab Republic	75
Tajikistan	66
Thailand	74
Timor-Leste	56
Turkey	71
Turkmenistan	67
United Arab Emirates	81
Uzbekistan	70
Vietnam	72
Yemen	62
Europe	
Albania	77
Austria	82
Belarus	74
Belgium	82
Bosnia and Herzegovina	77
Bulgaria	76
Croatia	78
Czech Republic	79
Denmark	79
Estonia	77
Finland	82
France	83
Germany	81
Greece	81
Hungary	77
Iceland	83
Ireland	80
Italy	83
Latvia	77
Lithuania	78
Luxembourg	81
Macedonia, The FYR of	76
Malta	81
Moldova, Republic of	71
Netherlands	81
Norway	82
Poland	78
Portugal	81
Romania	75
Russian Federation	72
Serbia and Montenegro	76
Slovakia	78
Slovenia	80
Spain	83
Sweden	82
Switzerland	83
Ukraine	72
United Kingdom	81
Oceania	
Australia	83
Fiji	70
French Polynesia	76
Guam	77
Kiribati	67
Marshall Islands	69
Micronesia	68
New Caledonia	78
New Zealand	81
Palau	75
Papua New Guinea	56
Samoa	73
Solomon Islands	63
Tonga	73
Tuvalu	65
Vanuatu	70

Reported by the United Nations for the Years 2000–2005.

Women Making a Difference

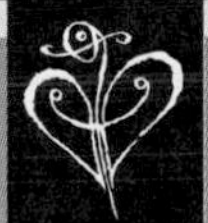

Maggie Kuhn: Senior Activist[1]

Maggie Kuhn was one of the founders of the Gray Panthers. She led a full and interesting life. She was born in Buffalo, New York, on August 31, 1905, in her grandmother's front bedroom; grew up in Cleveland; and graduated with honors from high school in 1922 and from college in 1926. She was sexually active with her boyfriend and utilized a diaphragm to prevent pregnancy. After college, she worked at the YWCA in Cleveland, Philadelphia, and later in New York, where she organized programs for working women, started classes on marriage and human sexuality, and provided programming for women workers assisting in the World War II effort. In 1950 she went to work for the Presbyterian Church for which she traveled extensively to teach social justice issues to clergy and laity; however, her salary was thousands less than that of men who had equal or lesser jobs. By age 41, she had two mastectomies. In 1958 she secured a mortgage and bought her own home in Philadelphia during a time when single women were not readily given loans because they were considered to be "undesirable risks." She commuted to work in New York City. In the 1960s, she developed a special interest in the problems of the elderly. During this period, the Presbyterian Church enforced its mandatory retirement policy upon her when she was 65 years old even though she did not yet desire retirement.

In 1970 Kuhn and five other active professional women who were facing retirement, founded the Gray Panthers to protest the Vietnam War and later to address numerous social issues specific to the elderly. These issues included minority discrimination by the Social Security system, discrimination of lending policies by banks, nursing home reform, health care policies and concerns, home health care advocacy, and combating the myths and stereotypes of old age. In 1976 she was diagnosed with uterine cancer and had a radical hysterectomy. In 1977 she was attacked by a man in a hotel corridor and forced into her hotel room where she was physically assaulted and robbed. She refused to let the mugging incident keep her from her work or her travels, but she never walked down a hotel corridor alone again. She had a number of romances, but chose to never marry or have children. She remained sexually active through her senior years and promoted the premise of sexual activity for the elderly. She remained active in social causes until she died in 1995.

- How well do you know the seniors in your life?
- Are you missing out on some really good life stories, and perhaps life lessons, by not taking more time to listen to the elder persons in your life?

expectancies for women around the world. After examining the table, research what might be contributing to a high or low life expectancy for women in various countries. For example, the countries of North and South Korea are geographically similar and located next to one another, but North Korean women have a life expectancy of 66 years while South Korean women have a life expectancy of 80 years. This is a tremendous gap in years of life expectancy. Consider how different political and social climates in each of these countries might impact life expectancy.

Japan has the greatest overall life expectancy for women at 85 years. Several factors go into making Japan number one in the rankings, including a low rate of heart disease, which is associated with their traditional low fat and high soy and fish diet, and, until recently, limited use of tobacco.

More and more people are living longer, healthier lives. In the United States it is estimated that 76 million baby boomers will start retiring in the year 2010. The nation is about to experience a great demographic shock. Between 2010 and 2030 the over-65 population is expected to rise more than 70 percent while the population paying payroll taxes to support the elderly will rise less than 4 percent. While seniors can place a financial burden on a country, they can also serve as an incredible resource of knowledge and wisdom giving much to enrich a community. Take, for example, the case of Maggie Kuhn who at the age of 65 organized senior citizens to protest the Vietnam War in 1970. The group was named the Gray Panthers. Kuhn and the Gray Panthers successfully addressed numerous issues in the community, especially those that stereotyped or discriminated against the elderly. (See *Women Making a Difference:* "Maggie Kuhn: Senior Activist.")

People living to be over 100 years old fascinate most of us. Those reaching 100 years or more are called centenarians. The United Nations World Population Revision released in 2000 included for the first time the numbers of octogenarians (ages 80–89), nonagenarians (ages 90–99), and centenarians (ages 100 and older). In 1998 around 135,000 persons in the world were estimated to be aged 100 years or older. The number of centenarians is projected to increase sixteen-fold by the year 2050 to reach 2.2 million. (See *Her Story:* "Jeanne Calment: Portrait of a Centenarian.")

Her Story

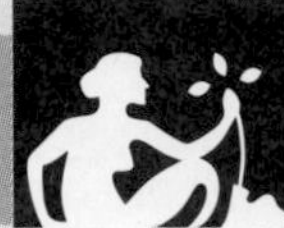

Jeanne Calment: Portrait of a Centenarian[2]

Jeanne Calment died in 1997 at the age of 122. She was born in France in 1875, before the Eiffel Tower was built. She remembered when a Dutch painter named Vincent van Gogh visited her hometown, Arles, in the south of France in 1888. She recalled that he was "very ugly, ungracious, impolite, crazy. I forgive him. They called him 'the Nut.'" Now both she and van Gogh are very famous people.

- Do you know any centenarians?
- Have you asked them to recall events in history from their point of view?

Leading Causes of Death

The U.S. Centers for Disease Control reported the leading cause of death for the U.S. population in 2002 was heart disease followed by stroke (cerebrovascular diseases), chronic lower respiratory diseases, accidents (unintentional injuries), diabetes, influenza/pneumonia, Alzheimer's disease, kidney diseases (nephritis, nephritic syndrome, and nephrosis), and septicemia (blood poisoning). Cultural factors such as gender, age, and race may influence trends, and it is often necessary to look at data more closely in order to have an accurate perspective (see Table 3.2).

For example, in examining the 2002 data reported by the Centers for Disease Control for females in the United States, HIV disease was the fifth leading cause of death for black females aged 15 to 24 years, the number-one cause of death for black females aged 25 to 34, and the third leading cause of death for black females aged 35 to 44. In contrast, HIV disease as a cause of death for white women was fourteenth for ages 15 to 24, eighth for ages 25 to 34, and ninth for ages 35 to 44. Thus, HIV disease was a much more prevalent cause of death for black females than for white females. A very different profile is demonstrated for suicide as a cause of death for females. As a cause of death for white females, suicide was sixth for ages 5 to 14 years, third for ages 15 to 24, third for ages 25 to 34, and fourth for ages 35 to 44. In contrast, as a cause of death for black females, suicide was fourteenth for ages 5 to 14 years, sixth for ages 15 to 24, tenth for ages 25 to 34, and thirteenth for ages 35 to 44. Thus, suicide was a much more prevalent cause of death in the year 2002 for white females than for black females.

The leading causes of death for people in economically advanced countries may be very different from those for people in impoverished, developing countries. Lack of education, income, nutrition, and access to adequate health care are major contributors to diseases and deaths in poor countries. According to the United Nations Statistics Division, in 2001, 21 percent of the population in the developing world was extremely poor with 530 million working men and women living on less than $1 a day. In 2002 an estimated 815 million people in developing countries had too little to eat to meet their daily energy needs. The lack of food can be most perilous for young children since it retards their physical and mental development. Food crises are a result of several contributing factors including declining agricultural productivity, drought, growing populations, economic failures and conflicts. In 2004, of the thirty-five countries requiring emergency assistance—the majority of them in Africa—most were in conflict or postconflict situations. Overcoming hunger is possible as demonstrated by the United Nations report that more than thirty countries reduced hunger by at least 25 percent during the last decade; fourteen of these countries were in sub-Saharan Africa.

The United Nations reported in 2005 that each year almost 11 million children worldwide die before the age of 5 (or 30,000 children per day), and most of these children live in developing countries. Most of these deaths are from diseases that are easily preventable with vaccines or conditions that can be successfully treated with proper attention and medication. Five diseases, including AIDS, account for half of all deaths in children under the age of 5. Among diseases that can be eradicated through immunization, measles is the leading cause of death for children. Measles strikes 30 million children a year, killing 540,000 and leaving many others blind or deaf.

The United Nations reports that complications during pregnancy and childbirth are a leading cause of death and disability among women of reproductive age in developing countries. More than half a million women die each year from such complications, and twenty times that many suffer serious injuries or disabilities that can cause lifelong pain. There were an estimated 529,000 maternal deaths worldwide in 2000 with 445,000 of these reported to be from sub-Saharan Africa and southern Asia.

According to the United Nations, HIV/AIDS is the fourth leading cause of death for both women and men worldwide. More than 20 million people around the world have died of AIDS since the epidemic began. The United Nations Statistics Division reported that in 2004 an estimated 39.4 million people were living with HIV, which is the highest number on record. Nearly two-thirds of HIV-infected persons live in sub-Saharan Africa, where the prevalence rate among adults has reached 7.2 percent. Slowing the spread of HIV/AIDS is a major goal of the United Nations. Globally, the epidemic

TABLE 3.2 Leading Causes of Death for Females

This table is a list of the top five leading causes of death in the year 2002 for U.S. females by age and race with percent of total deaths as reported by the Centers for Disease Control, National Center for Health Statistics.

All races, all ages	%	*White, all ages*	%	*Black, all ages,*	%	*Asian/Pacific Is., all ages*	%	*American Indian, all ages*	%
Diseases of heart	28.6	Diseases of heart	28.8	Diseases of heart	28.3	Malignant neoplasms	26.9	Malignant neoplasms	19.3
Malignant neoplasms	21.6	Malignant neoplasms	21.6	Malignant neoplasms	20.9	Diseases of heart	25.0	Diseases of heart	18.6
Cerebrovascular diseases	8.0	Cerebrovascular diseases	8.1	Cerebrovascular diseases	7.7	Cerebrovascular diseases	10.8	Accidents	8.6
Respiratory diseases	5.2	Respiratory diseases	5.6	Diabetes mellitus	5.2	Diabetes mellitus	4.0	Diabetes mellitus	7.2
Alzheimer's disease	3.4	Alzheimer's disease	3.6	Kidney diseases	2.8	Accidents	3.9	Cerebrovascular diseases	5.8
All races, 1–4 yrs.	%	*White, 1–4 yrs.*	%	*Black, 1–4 yrs.*	%	*Asian/Pacific Is., 1–4 yrs.*	%	*American Indian, 1–4 yrs.*	%
Accidents	30.1	Accidents	32.0	Accidents	24.3	Accidents	29.0	Accidents	34.1
Congenital defects	12.1	Congenital defects	12.7	Assault (homicide)	14.0	Malignant neoplasms	10.1	Assault (homicide)	17.1
Assault (homicide)	9.2	Malignant neoplasms	9.5	Congenital defects	11.1	Assault (homicide)	10.1	Diseases of heart	9.8
Malignant neoplasms	9.1	Assault (homicide)	7.3	Malignant neoplasms	8.1	Congenital defects	8.7	Congenital defects	7.3
Diseases of heart	3.8	Diseases of heart	3.5	Diseases of heart	4.5	Diseases of heart	2.9	In situ/benign neoplasms	4.9
All races, 5–14 yrs.	%	*White, 5–14 yrs.*	%	*Black, 5–14 yrs.*	%	*Asian/Pacific Is., 5–14 yrs.*	%	*American Indian, 5–14 yrs.*	%
Accidents	34.0	Accidents	34.0	Accidents	33.1	Accidents	33.3	Accidents	47.5
Malignant neoplasms	16.0	Malignant neoplasms	18.1	Malignant neoplasms	9.9	Malignant neoplasms	15.6	Assault (homicide)	13.1
Congenital defects	6.8	Congenital defects	7.6	Assault (homicide)	7.3	Assault (homicide)	5.6	Malignant neoplasms	8.2
Assault (homicide)	5.4	Assault (homicide)	4.5	Respiratory diseases	5.2	Diseases of heart	4.4	Congenital defects	4.9
Diseases of heart	3.9	Diseases of heart	3.6	Congenital defects	5.2	Septicemia (blood poison)	3.3	Cerebrovascular diseases	3.3
All races, 15–24 yrs.	%	*White, 15–24 yrs.*	%	*Black, 15–24 yrs.*	%	*Asian/Pacific Is., 15–24 yrs.*	%	*American Indian, 15–24 yrs.*	%
Accidents	46.0	Accidents	51.4	Accidents	25.5	Accidents	39.9	Accidents	52.7
Assault (homicide)	8.6	Malignant neoplasms	8.7	Assault (homicide)	18.9	Malignant neoplasms	11.2	Suicide	12.0
Malignant neoplasms	8.3	Suicide	7.4	Diseases of heart	6.8	Assault (homicide)	9.0	Assault (homicide)	9.6
Suicide	6.7	Assault (homicide)	6.0	Malignant neoplasms	6.5	Suicide	8.5	Malignant neoplasms	6.0
Diseases of heart	3.9	Diseases of heart	3.2	HIV disease	3.8	Diseases of heart	4.0	Diseases of heart	1.8
All races, 25–34 yrs.	%	*White, 25–34 yrs.*	%	*Black, 25–34 yrs.*	%	*Asian/Pacific Is., 25–34 yrs.*	%	*American Indian, 25–34 yrs.*	%
Accidents	23.3	Accidents	27.3	HIV disease	14.7	Malignant neoplasms	24.1	Accidents	34.9
Malignant neoplasms	15.9	Malignant neoplasms	17.4	Accidents	12.1	Accidents	22.0	Malignant neoplasms	10.8
Diseases of heart	8.2	Suicide	9.2	Diseases of heart	11.6	Suicide	12.5	Liver disease/cirrhosis	10.3
Suicide	7.2	Diseases of heart	7.1	Malignant neoplasms	11.4	Assault (homicide)	10.1	Assault (homicide)	8.7
Assault (homicide)	6.5	Assault (homicide)	4.9	Assault (homicide)	10.2	Diseases of heart	6.1	Suicide	5.1
All races, 35–44 yrs.	%	*White, 35–44 yrs.*	%	*Black, 35–44 yrs.*	%	*Asian/Pacific Is., 35–44 yrs.*	%	*American Indian, 35–44 yrs.*	%
Malignant neoplasms	26.9	Malignant neoplasms	28.9	Malignant neoplasms	20.6	Malignant neoplasms	43.8	Accidents	25.0

(continued)

TABLE 3.2 *(continued)*

Accidents	14.0	Accidents	16.0	Diseases of heart	15.5	Accidents	9.3	Liver disease/cirrhosis	14.3
Diseases of heart	12.1	Diseases of heart	11.1	HIV disease	12.5	Diseases of heart	8.3	Malignant neoplasms	13.3
Suicide	4.6	Suicide	5.8	Accidents	8.1	Cerebrovascular diseases	7.0	Diseases of heart	6.0
HIV disease	4.5	Liver disease/cirrhosis	3.6	Cerebrovascular diseases	4.9	Suicide	6.0	Cerebrovascular diseases	4.5
All races, 45–54 yrs.	%	*White, 45–54 yrs.*	%	*Black, 45–54 yrs.*	%	*Asian/Pacific Is., 45–54 yrs.*	%	*American Indian, 45–54 yrs.*	%
Malignant neoplasms	37.8	Malignant neoplasms	40.2	Malignant neoplasms	29.0	Malignant neoplasms	52.5	Malignant neoplasms	24.8
Diseases of heart	16.0	Diseases of heart	14.5	Diseases of heart	21.6	Diseases of heart	11.0	Accidents	10.6
Accidents	6.5	Accidents	7.1	Cerebrovascular diseases	6.2	Cerebrovascular diseases	8.4	Diseases of heart	9.1
Cerebrovascular diseases	4.3	Cerebrovascular diseases	3.6	HIV disease	4.7	Accidents	6.2	Liver disease/cirrhosis	9.1
Diabetes mellitus	3.5	Diabetes mellitus	3.2	Diabetes mellitus	4.5	Suicide	2.5	Diabetes mellitus	7.5
All races, 55–64 yrs.	%	*White, 55–64 yrs.*	%	*Black, 55–64 yrs.*	%	*Asian/Pacific Is., 55–64 yrs.*	%	*American Indian, 55–64 yrs.*	%
Malignant neoplasms	41.5	Malignant neoplasms	43.4	Malignant neoplasms	32.5	Malignant neoplasms	46.0	Malignant neoplasms	27.1
Diseases of heart	19.9	Diseases of heart	18.7	Diseases of heart	26.4	Diseases of heart	16.6	Diseases of heart	16.6
Respiratory diseases	5.4	Respiratory diseases	6.1	Diabetes mellitus	6.4	Cerebrovascular diseases	8.6	Diabetes mellitus	10.1
Cerebrovascular diseases	4.4	Cerebrovascular diseases	3.9	Cerebrovascular diseases	5.9	Diabetes mellitus	4.0	Liver disease/cirrhosis	5.8
Diabetes mellitus	4.3	Diabetes mellitus	3.7	Kidney diseases	2.9	Accidents	3.1	Accidents	4.9
All races, 65–74 yrs.	%	*White, 65–74 yrs.*	%	*Black, 65–74 yrs.*	%	*Asian/Pacific Is., 65–74 yrs.*	%	*American Indian, 65–74 yrs.*	%
Malignant neoplasms	34.8	Malignant neoplasms	35.7	Malignant neoplasms	29.1	Malignant neoplasms	34.9	Malignant neoplasms	25.9
Diseases of heart	23.6	Diseases of heart	22.8	Diseases of heart	28.8	Diseases of heart	23.4	Diseases of heart	20.0
Respiratory diseases	7.8	Respiratory diseases	8.6	Diabetes mellitus	7.3	Cerebrovascular diseases	11.0	Diabetes mellitus	11.7
Cerebrovascular diseases	5.8	Cerebrovascular diseases	5.5	Cerebrovascular diseases	7.1	Diabetes mellitus	5.2	Respiratory diseases	6.5
Diabetes mellitus	4.5	Diabetes mellitus	3.9	Kidney diseases	3.5	Accidents	2.5	Cerebrovascular diseases	6.1
All races, 75–84 yrs.	%	*White, 75–84 yrs.*	%	*Black, 75–84 yrs.*	%	*Asian/Pacific Is., 75–84 yrs.*	%	*American Indian, 75–84 yrs.*	%
Diseases of heart	29.2	Diseases of heart	28.9	Diseases of heart	32.6	Diseases of heart	29.4	Diseases of heart	27.3
Malignant neoplasms	22.0	Malignant neoplasms	22.2	Malignant neoplasms	20.1	Malignant neoplasms	22.3	Malignant neoplasms	19.2
Cerebrovascular diseases	8.9	Cerebrovascular diseases	8.7	Cerebrovascular diseases	9.5	Cerebrovascular diseases	12.2	Diabetes mellitus	9.0
Respiratory diseases	6.8	Respiratory diseases	7.3	Diabetes mellitus	6.1	Diabetes mellitus	5.5	Cerebrovascular diseases	8.3
Diabetes mellitus	3.6	Alzheimer's disease	3.7	Kidney diseases	3.3	Influenza/pneumonia	3.7	Respiratory diseases	5.3
All races, 85+ yrs.	%	*White, 85+ yrs.*	%	*Black, 85+ yrs.*	%	*Asian/Pacific Is., 85+ yrs.*	%	*American Indian, 85+ yrs.*	%
Diseases of heart	29.2	Diseases of heart	37.2	Diseases of heart	37.2	Diseases of heart	36.5	Diseases of heart	30.2
Malignant neoplasms	22.0	Cerebrovascular diseases	10.5	Malignant neoplasms	10.7	Cerebrovascular diseases	13.7	Malignant neoplasms	12.7
Cerebrovascular diseases	8.9	Malignant neoplasms	9.7	Cerebrovascular diseases	10.4	Malignant neoplasms	10.8	Cerebrovascular diseases	8.8
Respiratory diseases	6.8	Alzheimer's disease	6.0	Alzheimer's disease	4.3	Influenza/pneumonia	5.8	Influenza/pneumonia	6.7
Diabetes mellitus	3.6	Influenza/pneumonia	4.6	Diabetes mellitus	4.3	Diabetes mellitus	3.2	Alzheimer's disease	4.7

shows no signs of slowing with an estimated 4.9 million people becoming infected with HIV in the year 2004 and 3.1 million deaths due to AIDS this same year (500,000 of these deaths among children under 15 years of age). Nearly half of all people living with HIV are females, and as the epidemic worsens, the share of infected women and girls is growing. In sub-Saharan Africa, 57 percent of those infected with HIV are female.

We live in a global society and it is important to consider the health of women not only in the country in which we live but in other countries as well. Worldwide poverty and disease place a strain on the global economy. Economic and social services from countries that are relatively better off are sent as assistance to countries that lack the resources to combat poverty and disease. When certain countries are in despair, in some ways the whole world is impacted by the pain and suffering. We must remain ever diligent in our pursuit of health and wellness for women worldwide.

WHOLE PERSON CONCEPT

Your health status is not limited to the physical realm because you also have emotions, thoughts, and spirit. These all work together to bring about your state of well-being. Each of these interacts with the other, so, if you are affected in one area, the other areas will also be impacted. When examining your lifestyle, it is important to look at the whole picture of your health.

Mind, Body, and Spirit

One comprehensive conceptual model of individual health involves all three of the following elements: psyche, soma, and spirit (mind, body, and spirit).[3] The psyche involves your emotional, attitudinal, and mental state. Soma, or body, refers to your physical status. Spiritual health is your philosophy about living for yourself and living with others. Have you thought about yourself in these three different ways?

Two major categories of factors influence your status as a whole person: endogenous factors and exogenous factors. **Endogenous factors** are those events that occur within you. Examples are the presence or absence of illness, a positive or negative attitude, ability to have intimacy, and so on. **Exogenous factors** are external events that influence you, such as the type of personal relationships you have, the weather, stressful events, and so on. Endogenous and exogenous events interact to create an impact on your whole person. Can you think of some things occurring within and around you that impact your health? (To assess you current health habits, see *Assess Yourself:* "Personal Health Inventory.")

Dimensions of Wellness

Wellness has been described as consisting of six major dimensions: physical, emotional, social, occupational, intellectual, and spiritual.[5] Do you think it is possible to pay attention to all six dimensions in your life? Some

Assess Yourself

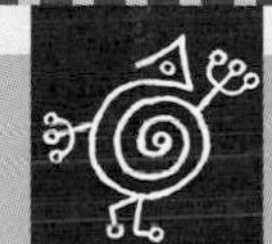

Personal Health Inventory[4]

Circle the number for each item that best describes you.

CIGARETTE SMOKING

Note: If you never smoke, enter a score of 10 for this section and go to the next section on Alcohol and Drugs.

	Almost Always	Sometimes	Almost Never
1. I avoid smoking cigarettes.	1	0	
2. I smoke only low tar and nicotine cigarettes or I smoke a pipe or cigars.	2	1	0
Cigarette Smoking Score: 10			

ALCOHOL AND DRUGS

	Almost Always	Sometimes	Almost Never
1. I avoid drinking alcoholic beverages or I drink no more than 1 or 2 drinks a day.	4	1	0
2. I avoid using alcohol or other drugs (especially illegal drugs) as a way of handling stressful situations or the problems in my life.	2	1	0
3. I am careful not to drink alcohol when taking certain medicines (for example, medicine for sleeping, pain, colds, and allergies) or when pregnant.	2	1	0
4. I read and follow the label directions when using prescribed and over-the-counter drugs.	2	1	0
Alcohol and Drug Score: 10			

(continued)

Assess Yourself (continued)

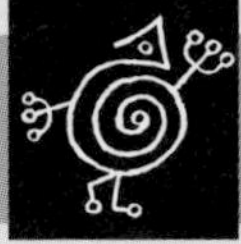

	Almost Always	Sometimes	Almost Never
EATING HABITS			
1. I eat a variety of food each day, such as fruits and vegetables, whole-grain breads and cereals, lean meats, dairy products, dry peas and beans, and nuts and seeds.	4	1	0
2. I limit the amount of fat, saturated fat, and cholesterol I eat (including fat on meats, eggs, butter, cream, shortenings, and organ meats such as liver).	2	1	0
3. I limit the amount of salt I eat by cooking with only small amounts, not adding salt at the table, and avoiding salty snacks.	2	1	0
4. I avoid eating too much sugar (especially frequent snacks of sticky candy or soft drinks).	2	1	0
Eating Habits Score: 4			
EXERCISE/FITNESS			
1. I maintain a desired weight, avoid being overweight or underweight.	3	1	0
2. I do vigorous exercise for 15–30 minutes at least 3 times a week (examples include running, swimming, brisk walking).	3	1	0
3. I do exercises that enhance my muscle tone for 15–30 minutes at least 3 times a week (examples include yoga and calisthenics).	2	1	0
4. I use part of my leisure time participating in individual, family, or team activities that increase my level of fitness (such as gardening, bowling, golf, and baseball).	2	1	0
Exercise/Fitness Score: 3			
STRESS CONTROL			
1. I have a job or do other work that I enjoy.	2	1	0
2. I find it easy to relax and express my feelings freely.	2	1	0
3. I recognize early, and prepare for, events or situations likely to be stressful for me.	2	1	0
4. I have close friends, relatives, or others to whom I can talk about personal matters and call on for help when needed.	2	1	0
5. I participate in group activities (such as church and community organizations) or hobbies that I enjoy.	2	1	0
Stress Control Score: 10			
SAFETY			
1. I wear a seat belt while riding in a car.	2	1	0
2. I avoid driving while under the influence of alcohol and other drugs.	2	1	0
3. I obey traffic rules and the speed limit when driving.	2	1	0
4. I am careful when using potentially harmful products or substances (such as household cleaners, poisons, and electrical devices).	2	1	0
5. I avoid smoking in bed.	2	1	0
Safety Score: 10			

Interpretation: There is no total score for this inventory. Compare your individual scores for each topic with the scales below.

9–10 Excellent! Your answers show that you are aware of the importance of this area to your health.

6–8 Your health practices in this area are good, but there is room for improvement.

3–5 Your health risks are showing! You should seek out information on changing your behaviors in this area.

0–2 Your answers show that you may be taking serious and unnecessary risks with your health in this area. It is definitely time to take the steps to change your behaviors. Seek out information and assistance about behavior change.

feel that this may be one ultimate goal of wellness. You may not be able to pay attention to all six at once, but you can take turns on each one at different times in your life, depending on which is most important to you at the time. (See *FYI:* "Descriptions of Wellness.")

Holistic Wellness Model

Another way to conceptualize health is as five primary dimensions of wellness—physical, emotional, social, occupational, and intellectual—and two basic components within each dimension, a personal component and a spiritual component.[6] (See Figure 3.1.) The personal component is striving for the satisfaction of your own personal needs, such as nutrition, exercise, shelter, income, relaxation, recreation, education, and personal achievement. The spiritual component is striving for a relationship or connection with other persons and things, such as family, friends, community, country, world, and higher power. This includes enhanced awareness, knowledge,

FYI

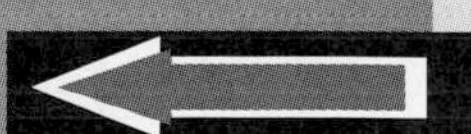

Descriptions of Wellness[7]

- *Physical wellness* is the willingness to take time each week to pursue activities that increase physical flexibility and endurance. A physically well person understands and employs the relationship between nutrition and body functioning.
- *Emotional wellness* is an awareness and acceptance of a wide range of feelings for oneself and others. It includes an ability to freely express and manage feelings effectively. An emotionally well person functions autono-mously, yet is aware of personal limitations and the value of seeking interpersonal support and assistance.
- *Social wellness* is the willingness to actively participate in and contribute to efforts that promote the common welfare of one's community. A socially well person lives in harmony with fellow human beings, seeks positive interdependent relationships with others, develops healthy sexual behaviors, and works for mutual respect and cooperation among community members.
- *Occupational wellness* is the personal satisfaction and enrichment one experiences through work. The occupationally well person has integrated a commitment to work into a total lifestyle and seeks to express personal values through involvement in paid and unpaid activities that are rewarding to the individual and valuable to the community.
- *Intellectual wellness* is self-directed behavior that includes continuous acquisition, development, creative application and articulation of critical thinking, expressive and intuitive skills, and abilities toward the achievement of a more satisfying existence.
- *Spiritual wellness* is the willingness to seek meaning and purpose in human existence, to question everything, and to appreciate the intangibles that cannot be explained or understood readily. A spiritually well person seeks harmony between that which lies within the individual and the forces that come from outside the individual.

FIGURE 3.1 Holistic wellness model. The spiritual component starts from deep within ourselves (center dark circle) and extends outward (dark lines), influencing our personal component (outer white circle) and connecting us with our community.

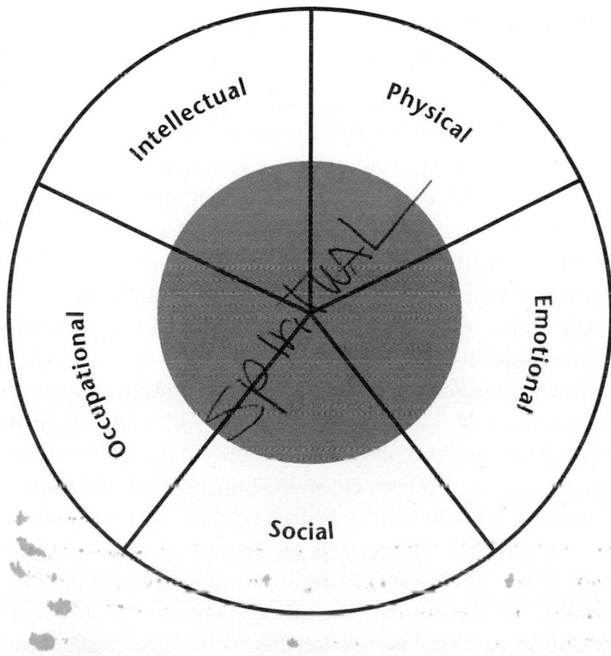

and love of others. Sometimes an issue or event is not clearly in one area but rather may coexist in more than one wellness dimension and in more than one component, spiritual or personal, at a time.

Developing a healthy lifestyle is a process. It is a goal worth working toward, but it can often be a life goal. Total attention to all wellness dimensions at the same time is very difficult to achieve. Thus, the holistic wellness model is not a mandate, but it is a guide for living.

ACHIEVING OPTIMUM WELLNESS

You must decide for yourself how you want to design your lifestyle. Life events and demands may pull you in one direction or another, and balance may not be possible until the events and demands are worked through. As a woman, your style of living is going to look different from that of a man. In fact, everyone's lifestyle is different. Wellness models can be used to assess your lifestyle based on an ideal. However, it is ultimately up to you to decide how you want your life to be the same or to be different. (See *Journal Activity:* "Your Personal Wellness Guide" and then complete *Assess Yourself:* "Rate Your Wellness.")

Even if you currently have an illness or disorder, you can still achieve the optimum level of wellness

Journal Activity

Your Personal Wellness Guide

Use the following guide to become more aware of your own personal wellness. Read the questions and record your ideas. A few examples have been provided to get you started. Some of the dimensions and components may overlap. You may want to include behaviors for both a personal component (a focus more on yourself) and a spiritual component (a focus more on other). See Figure 3.1 as a guide.

- How do you participate in physical wellness?
  Examples:

Personal Component	*Spiritual Component*
nutrition, vitamins	volunteer at a food bank
regular exercise	charity walk-a-thon
get a massage	support a sick friend

- How do you participate in emotional wellness?
  Examples:

Personal Component	*Spiritual Component*
have a positive attitude	avoid blaming others
seek personal therapy	listen and be supportive
express your needs	respect needs of others

- How do you participate in social wellness?
  Examples:

Personal Component	*Spiritual Component*
ask to be included	invite others along
ask for honesty and respect	be honest and respectful
receive community assistance	be a community volunteer

- How do you participate in occupational wellness?
  Examples:

Personal Component	*Spiritual Component*
be in a job you like	help others get a job
develop your skills further	teach job skills to others
invest your money	recycle products

- How do you participate in intellectual wellness?
  Examples:

Personal Component	*Spiritual Component*
learn	teach
be creative or artistic	encourage creativity
broaden your experience	share your experience

Assess Yourself

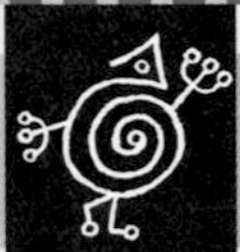

Rate Your Wellness

Refer to the holistic wellness model in Figure 3.1. Rate how well you believe you are attending to the personal (a focus more on self) component and spiritual (a focus more on others) component for each of the five dimensions of wellness as explained in the Journal Activity. You will have ten separate ratings, one for the personal component and one for the spiritual component in each of the five wellness dimensions. Use the following scale: 1 = not enough attention, 2 = enough attention, 3 = too much attention.

Now ask yourself the following questions:

- Is one wellness dimension attended to more than another? If so, why?
- Do you have balanced focus on both the personal and spiritual components of each wellness dimension? Or, is one component given more attention than the other? If so, why?
- What adjustments, if any, would you like to make in your spiritual or personal focus, or in each wellness dimension to be more balanced?
- Do you have any areas in conflict? If so, how can this conflict be resolved?
- Are you ready and/or able to make a commitment today to focus more on a particular area?

that is right for you. Design a lifestyle that maximizes your own health potential and contributes to your longevity.

WORLD WELLNESS

There are six primary environmental issues for world wellness: air, water, energy, food, toxins, and nature.[8] These are described further as air quality, water quality, sustainable energy and recycling, sustainable agriculture, hazardous material and waste management, and protection of wilderness areas and rain forests. The basic essentials of life include air, water, food, physical activity, and sexual activity. Because the earth sustains us, the world must be kept in good shape in order for humans to continue to survive.

In the area of environmental health, many questions remain to be answered. For example, should action be taken to reduce the possible risks of exposure to residential electric and magnetic fields? Should an alternative to water chlorination be found to reduce the chlorination by-product cancer risk in drinking water? Should policies be developed to reduce greenhouse gas emissions to prevent global warming? People who advocate precautionary measures believe we should act now. Those who adopt a more conservative approach prefer we wait until clear evidence supports the existence of

Her Story

Melissa: Contribution to World Wellness

Melissa Crabtree does her part to heal and preserve the environment. She is an active environmentalist. She teaches others to appreciate and love the environment by interacting with it on a very personal level. During the spring, she is a white-water river raft guide. In the winter, she is a cross-country ski guide and works on a ski patrol. In the summer she teaches canoeing and sea kayaking. Melissa is also a songwriter and performs her music about the environment across the country at women's music festivals and nightclubs.

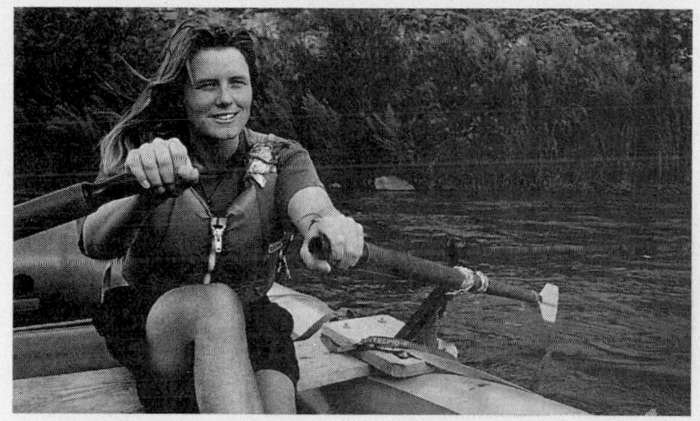

Health Tips

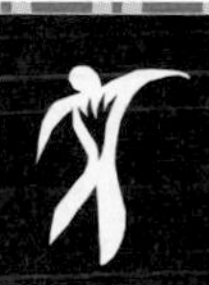

Enhancing World Wellness

It is very easy to participate in world wellness. You can do small things every day that can have a big impact. Here are some ideas to get you started.

- Turn out the lights in every room you are not using.
- Do not throw litter on the ground.
- Join a community litter cleanup group.
- Recycle newspaper, paper, plastic, bottles, and aluminum.
- Use biodegradable soaps and detergents; many of these are available in your local grocery store or health food store.
- Plant a garden and grow food.
- Plant and care for a tree.
- Drive environmentally safer vehicles having low exhaust output and safer air-conditioning systems.
- Share a ride or carpool.
- Take short showers, and don't fill the tub all the way when taking a bath.
- Fix water drips and leaks as soon as possible. Water is more precious than gold.
- Use less water in your toilet tank with each flush by setting the water level lower.
- Do not purchase products from companies that regularly violate environmental protection laws.

Journal Activity

Your World Wellness Guide

How are you contributing to world wellness in each of these six areas?

- Maintaining and/or improving air quality
- Maintaining and/or improving water quality
- Saving energy and/or recycling
- Growing and/or saving food
- Preventing and/or reducing toxins and pollutants
- Preserving and/or enhancing nature

the problem. There are many factors to consider in the environmental decision-making process.[9]

It is vital that we attend to the issues of world health in addition to individual health. What does world wellness have to do with women's health? Well, the world is often referred to as *Mother Earth,* and she does nurture our survival. The Mother Earth concept is perhaps the earliest and strongest female archetype that exists for women. (See *Her Story:* "Melissa: Contribution to World Wellness"; *Health Tips:* "Enhancing World Wellness"; and *Journal Activity:* "Your World Wellness Guide.")

The United Nations Fourth World Conference on Women, held in Beijing in 1995, made an important contribution to the global wellness of women. The Platform for Action for this conference was an agenda for women's empowerment and reaffirms the fundamental principle set forth in the World Health Organization's 1994 Vienna Declaration and Program of Action adopted by the World Conference on Human Rights: "[T]he human rights of women and of the girl child are an inalienable, integral and indivisible part of universal human rights."[10] Critical areas of concern for the Beijing conference were

- The burden of poverty on women
- Unequal access to education and training
- Unequal access to health care
- Violence against women
- The effects of armed or other kinds of conflict on women, including those living under foreign occupation
- Inequality in economic structures and policies
- Inequality in the sharing of power and decision making
- Insufficient mechanisms to promote the advancement of women
- Lack of respect for and inadequate promotion and protection of the human rights of women
- Stereotyping of women and inequality in women's access to and participation in all communication systems, especially in the media
- Gender inequalities in the management of natural resources and in safeguarding of the environment
- Persistent discrimination against and violation of the rights of the girl child

The twenty-third special session of the United Nations General Assembly on Women 2000: Gender Equality, Development and Peace for the Twenty-First Century took place in June 2000 and adopted a political declaration and outcome document titled "Further Actions and Initiatives to Implement the Beijing Declaration and Platform for Action." This special session of the General Assembly was convened to review current status in the implementation of the plans set forth at the Beijing Conference.[11] The progress of the Beijing Platform is monitored by the United Nations departments of the Division for the Advancement of Women and the Bureau on the Status of Women.

The fiftieth session of the United Nations Commission on the Status of Women was held in February–March 2006. The main themes of this session were (1) enhanced participation of women in development: to create an enabling environment for achieving gender equality and the advancement of women, taking into account the fields of education, health and work; and (2) equal participation of women and men in decision-making processes at all levels. Reports of the sessions of the United Nations Commission on the Status of Women are available from the United Nations Web site for the Division for the Advancement of Women (see *Resources:* "Web sites" in the Resources at the end of this chapter).

WELLNESS VERSUS ILLNESS

Health is viewed along a continuum of wellness to illness with a whole myriad of possibilities in between. **Health intervention** is defined as the act or fact of interfering so as to modify.[12] Health interventions fall into at least three categories: education, prevention, and treatment. (See Figure 3.2.)

Education

Health education involves research and study in the causes, prevention, and treatment of disorders and diseases. It also involves the publication and distribution of this information to the public. Paramount to education is the concept of health promotion. **Health promotion** efforts include

- Dissemination through literature and workshops of information regarding healthy lifestyles, enhancement of life quality, and illness prevention
- Provision of information about early warning signs of disorders and diseases
- Provision of information regarding community services for assessment, such as health checkups
- Assistance in the development of personal health programs in each of the wellness dimensions

The American Cancer Society has an extensive education program. They publish pamphlets about the warning signs of breast cancer, posters of women using breast self-examination, and even poems written by and about survivors of breast cancer.

Prevention

Preventive health action is defined as measures serving to avert the occurrence of illness or disease.[13] According to the public health service model for prevention,

FIGURE 3.2 Health interventions continuum.

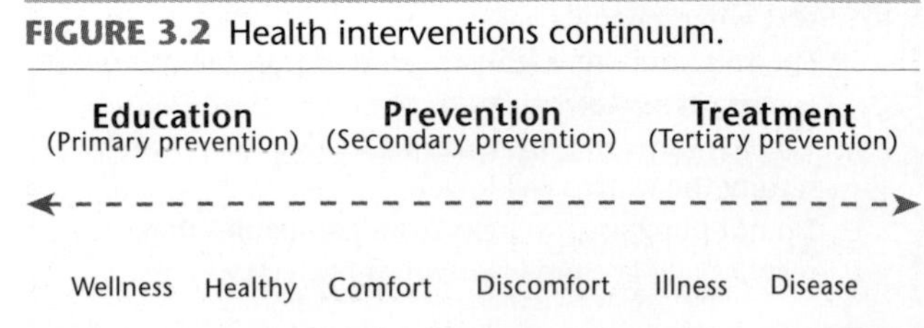

services may be directed toward the individual (host), toward the source (agent), and toward the environment that encourages and supports, or sustains, the source. This is referred to as the epidemiological model. **Epidemiology** is the study of the relationships of the various factors determining the frequency and distribution of diseases in a human community.[14] For example, let us consider three preventive measures regarding the health risks of drinking alcohol for pregnant women. First, an educational campaign is directed toward women explaining the increased risk to the woman and to her fetus from alcohol consumption while she is pregnant. This preventive action is directed at the individual or host. This educational campaign can take many forms, such as information provided by physicians or other health care providers, educational materials distributed at prenatal care clinics, and information articles in popular women's magazines or other publications. Second, a legislative bill requires that alcohol products manufacturers and distributors place a statement on their product containers warning that use of that product while pregnant may cause a health hazard. This preventive action is directed at the source or agent. Third, advertisers of these products are required to include on any printed advertisement of their product the warning of the health hazards of drinking alcohol while pregnant. This preventive measure is directed at an environment that may support alcohol consumption, in this case, the advertising industry.

Prevention efforts can be divided into three types: primary, secondary, and tertiary. **Primary prevention** is an extension of health education. Based on what we know, we can take steps to enhance the quality of life and prevent the development of illness. Primary interventions include efforts that assist with the prevention of most discomfort, disorders, diseases, and premature death. This prevention can be accomplished by sufficient attention to those things that keep us healthy—such as proper diet, regular exercise, a positive attitude, stress management and relaxation, fostering relationships, avoidance of toxins and pollutants, avoidance of the abuse of drugs and alcohol, avoidance of tobacco, and looking both ways before crossing the street. The bottom line is to live smart and be well.

In spite of your best efforts, you could possibly still experience some degree of discomfort, disorder, or disease in your life. **Secondary prevention** identifies persons who are in the early stages of "unhealth," which may lead to the development of disorders or illnesses. Secondary prevention attempts are interventions used to stop unhealthy behaviors and seek any necessary treatment.

Tertiary prevention is the application of an intervention to treat an existing disorder or illness. This is for the purpose of preventing the disorder or illness from getting worse. Tertiary prevention can also involve rehabilitation efforts, which attempt to facilitate recovery to the highest degree of health possible for an individual.

Treatment

Treatment interventions are applied to halt the progress of a discomfort, disorder, or disease and, if possible, move the individual away from discomfort and toward increased health. A woman who has entered menopause may experience extreme discomfort that accompanies this phase, such as hot flashes and mood swings. She may want to seek the assistance of a health provider for the purpose of considering hormone replacement therapy, or instead she may want to seek the advice of an herbologist for herbs that can reduce the discomforts of menopause.

Health treatment can involve intervention by a mental health provider, a physical health provider, or both. Examples of mental health providers include mental health counselors, social workers, psychologists, drug and alcohol counselors, marriage and family therapists, and psychiatrists. Examples of physical health providers include physicians, nurse practitioners, nurses, dentists, rehabilitation therapists, osteopaths, chiropractors, herbalists, massage therapists, and physical therapists.

It is up to you to decide from whom you would like to seek treatment and what type of treatment you wish to receive. It is best to act as an educated consumer and be as familiar as possible with the current and most effective treatment or treatments for your condition. It is also advisable to seek an opinion from more than one health professional, whenever appropriate, to explore additional possibilities regarding diagnosis and treatment.

LEARNING AND BEHAVIOR

In considering learning behavior you must understand the role of primary reinforcers: positive, negative, and punishment.[15] A **positive reinforcer** is rewarding. If your behavior is followed by something perceived by you as rewarding, then you will more likely repeat that behavior. If you exercise and feel better, then you may be more likely to exercise more. A **negative reinforcer** is the removal of something uncomfortable, and this too can be rewarding; thus, if your behavior is followed by the removal of something uncomfortable to you, then the likelihood that you will repeat that behavior increases. For example, if telling an individual to stop criticizing you unnecessarily results in a positive outcome, you are more likely to assert yourself again. **Punishment** involves the presentation of something uncomfortable. Thus, when your behavior is followed by punishment, the likelihood of that behavior being

Her Story

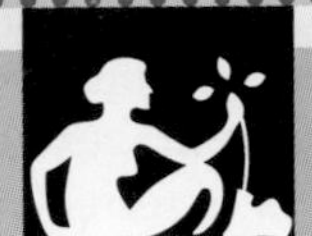

Danette: Resistance to Change

Danette came into therapy complaining of extreme stress in her life. She played a major role as a caretaker to her children, spouse, and peers. She left no time for herself. She had anxiety and extreme headaches. The counselor suggested that she reprioritize her life, learn and use assertiveness skills, and incorporate time and stress management techniques. These skills and techniques were recommended to her by the therapist because they are known to be documented, effective strategies for assisting with Danette's kind of problem. However, Danette persisted in her complaints without trying the techniques even though she seemed to understand that they would in fact help her situation. The counselor suspected that Danette might have less obvious motives contributing to her resistance to change (secondary reinforcers), motives that Danette herself might not be completely aware of. Through continued exploration of Danette's values and belief systems, the counselor discovered that Danette believed she was not a worthwhile person unless she sacrificed herself for others. It was further discovered that this was a very old belief that Danette learned as a child from her mother: "To be a good person you must always sacrifice yourself for others, otherwise you are a selfish person." This belief became integrated into Danette's lifestyle when she was rewarded with praise in childhood whenever she acted accordingly. When Danette realized that this old belief was creating difficulty for her, she decided to put it aside in certain situations so that she could make healthier choices in her life.

- How can Danette determine when the act of putting another's needs before her own is too much sacrifice?
- In what other ways can Danette be assured that the needs of others are being met without always having to be the one who meets the needs of these others?

repeated by you decreases. For example, if you drink too much alcohol and become very sick, you will be less likely to drink so much again.

The concept of learned behaviors is basically simple. However, how would you explain resistance to change even with the presentation of reinforcers? Resistance to change is often a result of the existence of secondary reinforcers. A **secondary reinforcer** is much less obvious but still has some influence over behavior. If you are experiencing difficulty in changing your behavior, then consider less obvious reasons that may be holding you back, such as an interfering belief or value. (See *Her Story:* "Danette: Resistance to Change.")

Hierarchy of Needs

The importance placed on a reinforcer is dependent upon the value that you give it. This can vary greatly from person to person. However, the "Hierarchy of Needs" is a way of exploring the motivating potential of a reinforcer.[16] At least five sets of goals, usually referred to as basic needs, are common to all persons: physiological, safety, love, esteem, and self-actualization. These needs contribute to motivating actions or behavior. Maslow summarizes the Hierarchy of Needs as shown in Figure 3.3.

FIGURE 3.3 Maslow's hierarchy of needs.

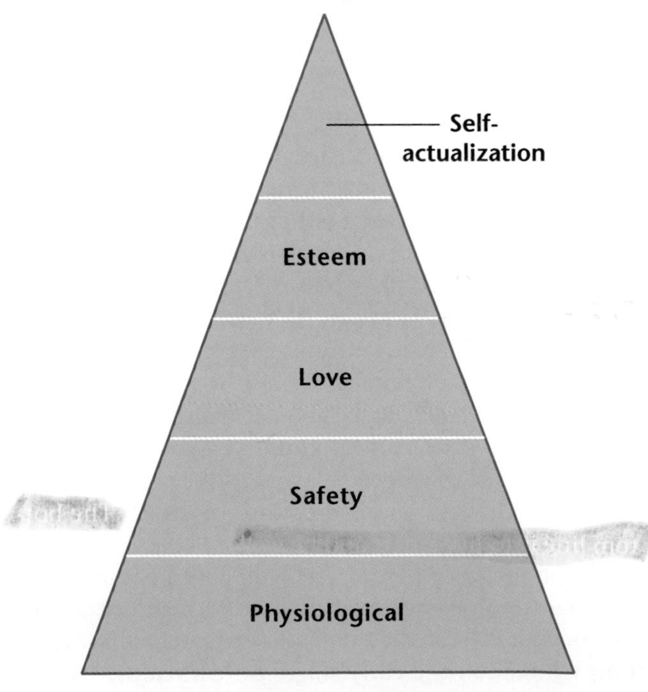

Physiological needs, the lowest level on the hierarchy, refer to such things as freedom from hunger, sufficient oxygen, adequate water, sufficient sleep, freedom of movement, and sexual activity. Safety needs refer to such things as protection from danger, nonisolation, sufficient trust to build relationships, freedom from fear, and freedom from deprivation. Love needs are composed of such things as love, affection, and belongingness. Esteem needs refer to such things as the desire for

Her Story

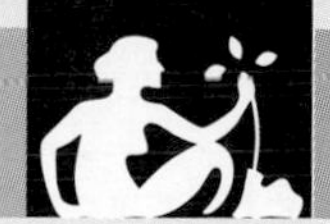

Charlene: Hierarchy of Needs

Charlene, an 18-year-old college student, was diagnosed with an eating disorder called anorexia nervosa. Charlene was a member of the gymnastics team, and she felt she needed to make her weight as low as possible to stay on the team. She was literally starving herself to death because of her belief that she was overweight and her fear that she would get kicked off the team. Her body weight became dangerously low and, starved for nutrition, it began to rob her muscles and organs of vital nutrients. Her situation had become life threatening. In this case, Charlene placed a higher priority on esteem needs than on physiological needs. Thus, she was motivated to behavior based on the area of her life in which she believed there was the greatest need. Charlene's belief was not well grounded in reality, because she was an anorexic who was willing to starve her body in an effort to feel better about herself.

- How can education and counseling about the concept of the hierarchy of needs be used to help Charlene?
- How can you relate each level in the hierarchy of needs to your own life and the decisions you have made about your health and well-being?

respect from others, self-respect, self-esteem, achievement, adequacy, confidence, and independence. Self-actualization needs, the highest level on the hierarchy, are the need or desire to become everything one is capable of becoming, to strive for ideals, and to strive for success or life satisfaction.

Typically, you do not move up the Hierarchy of Needs until your lower needs are met sufficiently. However, there may be instances when upper-level needs take precedence over lower-level needs. (See *Her Story:* "Charlene: Hierarchy of Needs.")

THEORIES AND MODELS OF BEHAVIOR CHANGE

There are many models and theories that suggest ways to change health behaviors. Some of these were developed many years ago but still present ideas that are very relevant today.

The Transtheoretical Model

The transtheoretical model of change, sometimes referred to as the multicomponent stage model, suggests that you will experience several stages as you attempt to change your health behavior over time.[17] The first stage is precontemplation, the time when you are not seriously thinking about changing during the next 6 months. The second stage is contemplation, when you are seriously thinking about behavior change during the next 6 months. The third stage is action, the 6-month period following an overt modification of a behavior. The fourth stage is maintenance, the period after action until the unwanted behavior is permanently modified or terminated. The final stage is termination, when you are no longer tempted by the unwanted behavior, and you feel confident in your ability to resist relapse.

Theories of Reasoned Action and Planned Action

The theory of reasoned action promotes three primary concepts that affect behavior change: your attitude toward performing the behavior, standard beliefs about what relevant others think you should do, and your motivation to comply with those others.[18] In other words, sometimes you may do certain things because other people who are important to you or have power over you think that you should do them. This concept is often referred to as the subjective norm. Doing things because others think you should can work in both positive and negative ways. For example, if Charlene's coach keeps encouraging her to lose more and more weight, then the coach may actually reinforce Charlene to be anorexic. However, if Charlene's coach encourages the athletes to maintain a proper, nutritious diet, then Charlene will be less likely to engage in unhealthy eating behavior. The theory of planned action is similar to the theory of reasoned action with one addition. The theory of planned action adds the concept of perceived behavioral control. The perceived ease or difficulty of performing the behavior is assumed to reflect past experience as well as anticipated obstacles and impediments. The more favorable the attitude and subjective norm with respect to behavior, and the greater the perceived behavioral control, the stronger should be the individual's intentions to perform the behavior under consideration.[19]

Self-Efficacy

The perception of potential benefits of action is related to the concept of self-efficacy. **Self-efficacy** is the conviction that one can successfully execute the behavior or behaviors required to produce desired outcomes.[20] Let's say that you were, in fact, significantly overweight. Your ability to design and stick to a plan of behavior change would depend on your belief that you could do it. Self-efficacy suggests that people's beliefs in their ability to perform specific behaviors influence the following:[21]

- Choice of behavior and the situations that will be avoided or attempted
- Effort expended in a specific task
- How long one will persist with a task even when facing difficulties
- Emotional reactions such as positive emotions with perceived success or negative emotions with perceived lack of success

A strong sense of self-efficacy is essential for the promotion of healthy behavior change.

Now that you have reviewed the various models and theories that suggest how behavior is changed, it is time to consider how you can develop your own individualized plan of action.

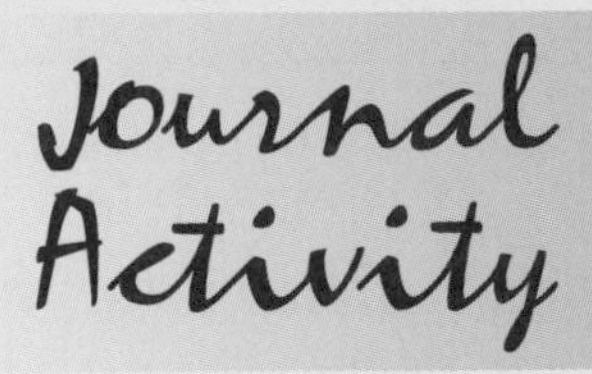

Your Personal Health Behavior Inventory

Make a list of your existing health-promoting behaviors. Now make a list of your existing health-inhibiting behaviors. Consider two questions at this point: (1) Which behaviors present the greatest threat to your health, and (2) which behaviors do you need to target first?

PLANNING YOUR LIFESTYLE CHANGE

You can manage many lifestyle changes through a self-help plan of action. This involves three primary steps: take a personal inventory, maintain a helpful attitude, and develop a plan of action. The plan should be realistic and developed with an attitude of appreciation for even the smallest of movements toward the goal. Patience is also a major key when persevering a lifestyle change.

Personal Inventory

The first step in a self-help plan is to take a personal inventory. This involves an evaluation of personal health habits and practices. (See *Journal Activity:* "Your Personal Health Behavior Inventory.")

Helpful Attitude

A realistic and positive attitude is paramount to successful behavior change. It is important not to set goals too high nor expect outcomes too quickly. Both of these attitudes can lead to discouragement and even termination of effort. It is also important to view behavior change as a lifestyle change rather than just a temporary goal. Otherwise, success that is achieved may be short-lived. Avoid an attitude of denial or deprivation; these can result in preoccupations of thought or impulsive actions that worsen the targeted behavior. Instead, find healthy substitutes for the things that you are reducing or eliminating from your life.

Plan of Action

Essential principles of lifestyle management when structuring a plan of action include (1) assessing behavior, (2) setting specific and realistic goals, (3) formulating intervention strategies, and (4) evaluating progress.[22]

Assessment of current behaviors involves the process of counting, recording, measuring, observing, and describing. Assessment tools are usually daily logs, journals, and diaries. The assessment phase is completed when there is sufficient information to form a behavior profile, state specific goals, and customize a program that matches your unique circumstances and personality.

Goal setting involves establishing specific and realistic goals for behavior change. Specific goals are concrete, observable, and measurable. Realistic goals are reasonable and relate to personal circumstances. Goal setting should start off small to facilitate initial successes that will provide further motivation for continued participation in the personal lifestyle change program.

Intervention strategies should be personalized to fit your needs. Common intervention strategies include the use of stimulus control, healthy positive reinforcers, and positive behavior substitution and behavioral contracts. Stimulus control includes the reduction or elimination

FIGURE 3.4 Behavior change contract.

BEHAVIOR CHANGE CONTRACT

Name: ______________________ **Date of Contract:** __________

Identified health area for change: ______________________

____

Long-term goal: ______________________

____

Intermediate goals: ______________________

____

____

____

Estimated time to achieve each intermediate goal: ______________________

____

____

____

Rewards for achieving intermediate goals: ______________________

____

____

____

Support network (persons and facilities): ______________________

____

____

______________________ ______________________
Signature of Participant **Signature of Witness**

of the stimulus that encourages the original unhealthy behavior. For example, to help you stop smoking cigarettes, you might use nicotine patches that have gradually lower dosages of nicotine. The presentation of healthy positive reinforcers or rewards will increase the potential for healthy behaviors to be reported. For example, if you are attempting to overcome procrastination, you can reward yourself with an activity you enjoy, such as a bike ride, after you complete a chore. Positive behavior substitution is the incorporation of a healthy behavior that is incompatible with the unhealthy behavior, such as walking instead of watching television or chewing gum instead of smoking.

A **behavior change contract** is a written agreement in a behavior change program. Most contracts state long-range and intermediate goals, target dates for completion, rewards, intervention strategies, names of friends and resources to serve as a support network, and witnesses to the agreement who serve as sources for encouragement. (See Figure 3.4 for a sample behavior change contract, and then complete *Journal Activity:* "Behavior Change Contract.")

To evaluate your progress, you must regularly monitor goal-related activities. Consistent monitoring provides information necessary for determining progress toward your goal. Periodic monitoring (weekly or monthly) is

Journal Activity

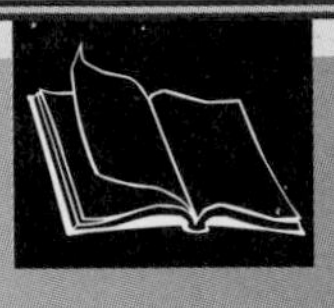

Behavior Change Contract

Write a behavior change contract in your journal. Keep a record in your journal of your activities related to the contract. Assess your progress periodically. Remember to reward yourself in healthy ways for demonstrating progress toward your goals. Don't forget to frequently seek out encouragement and guidance from your support system.

better than daily monitoring. Monitoring can be done in the form of charts, graphs, or lists or descriptions of behaviors and attitudes.

CONCLUSION

The information and activities in this chapter encourage you to understand and, if needed, change your lifestyle. The remaining chapters have additional information and activities to help you with your own personal health journey.

Chapter Summary

- Wellness encompasses the whole person concept including the following dimensions of health: physical, emotional, social, occupational, intellectual, and spiritual.
- The primary dimensions of world wellness are air, water, energy, food, toxins, and nature.
- The three primary health-related intervention strategies are education (primary prevention), prevention (secondary prevention), and treatment (tertiary prevention).
- The basic hierarchy of needs for humans are physiological, safety, love, esteem, and self-actualization.
- A self-help plan involves three primary steps: taking a personal inventory, having the right attitude, and developing a plan of action.
- A plan of action involves the following steps: assessment, goal setting, intervention strategies, and evaluating progress.

Review Questions

1. Can you name and describe the six dimensions of wellness?
2. What are the environmental issues for world wellness?
3. What are the three types of interventions utilized in the health services?
4. What are reinforcers?
5. Can you describe the hierarchy of needs?
6. Can you describe the transtheoretical model for change?
7. Can you describe the theory of reasoned action and the theory of planned action?
8. What is self-efficacy?
9. Can you devise a self-help plan for behavior change?

Resources

Web Sites

American Hospital Association
www.aha.org
American Medical Association
www.ama-assn.org
American Nurses Association
www.ana.org
Centers for Disease Control
www.cdc.gov
National Institute of Environmental Health Sciences
www.niehs.nih.gov
Natural Healers
www.naturalhealers.com
Office of Rural Health Policy
www.ruralhealth.hrsa.gov
United Nations, Division for the Advancement of Women
www.un.org/womenwatch/daw/index.html
United Nations, Statistics Division
http://unstats.un.org
U.S. Census Bureau
www.census.gov
U.S. Environmental Protection Agency
www.epa.gov

Videotape

Northrup, C. (1998). *Women's Bodies, Women's Minds.* Chicago: JWA Video. Web Site: www.jwavideo.com.

Suggested Readings

Borysenko, J. 1988. *Minding the Body, Mending the Mind.* Toronto: Bantam Books.

Chopra, D. 1991. *Perfect Health: The Complete Mind/Body Guide.* New York: Harmony Books.

Dossey, B. M., L. Keegan, L. G. Kolkmeier, and C. Guzzetta. 1989. *Holistic Health Promotion: A Guide for Practice.* Rockville, MD: Aspen.

Kabat-Zinn, J. 1990. *Full Catastrophe Living: Using the Wisdom of Your Body and Mind to Face Stress, Pain, and Illness.* New York: Delacorte Press.

Moyers, B. 1993. *Healing and the Mind.* New York: Doubleday. (Also available as a series of videotapes.)

Myss, C. 1996. *Anatomy of Spirit.* Westminster, MD: Random House.

Northrup, C. (1998). *Women's Bodies, Women's Wisdom.* New York: Bantam.

Siegel, B. 1992. *Love, Medicine and Miracles.* New York: Harper & Row.

References

1. Kuhn, M., C. Long, and L. Quinn. 1991. *No stone unturned: The life and times of Maggie Kuhn.* New York: Ballantine Books.
2. Wagner, C. 1999. The centarians are coming. *Futurist,* May, pp. 16–23.
3. Allen, R., and R. Yarian. 1981. The domain of health. *Health Education* 12 (4): 3–5.
4. Assessment adapted from *Health style: A self test.* U.S. Department of Health and Human Services (PHS) 81-50155.
5. Hettler, W. 1979. *Six dimensions of wellness.* Stevens Point, WI: National Wellness Institute, University of Wisconsin; Hettler, W. 1990. Six dimensions of wellness. *Guidepost: American Counseling Association* 33 (September): 1.
6. Chandler, C., J. Holden, and C. Kolander. 1992. Counseling for spiritual wellness: Theory and practice. *Journal of Counseling and Development* 71 (2): 168–75.
7. Opatz, J. 1986. Stevens Point: A long-standing program for students at a midwestern university. *American Journal of Health Promotion* 1 (1): 60–67.
8. Hettler, W. 1991. Environmental issues for world wellness. *Guidepost: American Counseling Association* 33 (17): 17.
9. Tong, S., and Y. Lu. (July, 1999). Major issues in the environmental health decision-making process. *Journal of Environmental Health* 62 (1): 33–35.
10. United Nations. (1995). Fourth World Conference on Women: Platform for action. www.un.org/womenwatch/daw/beijing/platform/plat1.htm (retrieved September 22, 2006).
11. United Nations. (2000). Beijing + 5: Process and beyond. www.un.org/womenwatch/daw/followup/bfbeyond.htm (retrieved September 22, 2006).
12. *Mosby's medical, nursing and allied health directory.* 4th ed. 1994. St. Louis: Mosby.
13. Ibid.
14. Ibid.
15. Skinner, B. F. 1953. *Science and human behavior.* New York: Macmillan.
16. Maslow, A. H. 1943. A theory of human motivation. *Psychological Review* 50 (July): 370–96.
17. Prochaska, J., and C. DiClemente. 1992. Stages of change in the modification of problem behaviors. *Progress in Behavior Modification* 28: 183–218.
18. Fishbein, M., and I. Ajzen. 1975. *Belief, attitude, intention and behavior: An introduction to theory and research.* Reading, MA: Addison-Wesley.
19. Ajzen, I. 1988. *Attitudes, personality and behavior.* Chicago: Dorsey Press.
20. Bandura, A. 1986. *Social foundations of thought and action.* Englewood Cliffs, NJ: Prentice-Hall.
21. Lyn, L., and K. R. McLeroy. 1986. Self-efficacy and health education. *Journal of School Health* 56 (2): 317–21; Schunck, D. H., and J. P. Carbonari. 1984. Self-efficacy models. In J. D. Malarazzo and others, *Behavioral health: A handbook of health enhancement and disease prevention,* pp. 230–47. New York: John Wiley & Sons.
22. Anspaugh, D. J., M. H. Hamrick, and F. D. Rosato. 2006. *Wellness: Concepts and applications.* 6th ed. New York: McGraw-Hill.

Mental and Emotional Wellness

CHAPTER FOUR

Enhancing Emotional Well-Being

CHAPTER FIVE

Managing the Stress of Life

Part Two

Enhancing Emotional Well-Being

Chapter Four

CHAPTER OBJECTIVES

When you complete this chapter, you will be able to do the following:

- Describe self-in-relation theory
- Demonstrate assertive communication and effective listening skills
- Delineate the steps for effective problem solving
- Describe activities for enhancing self-image and self-esteem
- Identify the types of eating disorders
- Describe the natural stages of the grief process
- Identify the types of depression

THE EMERGING SELF

How is it that you become the person that you are? How do you develop your values, beliefs, feelings, thoughts, and ideas about yourself, others, and the world around you? How does your personality emerge, and what contributes to the happiness and unhappiness in your life? How do you decide when it is time to change, and to think, feel, believe, or behave differently about something or someone? Whom do you decide to include in your social support system as persons who influence you and help you? These are important questions to consider as you explore your personal development and your emotional health.

THEORIES OF DEVELOPMENT

Until 1979 when psychologist Carol Gilligan began to challenge the views of earlier male psychologists,[1] the psychology profession generally supported the long-held societal belief that women were inferior to men. For example, in 1905, Sigmund Freud, who is considered to be the father of psychology, designed the theory of psychosexual development around the experiences of the male child, depicting women as envying that which they lacked, such as a penis, and being "driven" largely by a highly "irrational" and oftentimes "hysterical" portion of female anatomy, the uterus. From Freud's view, differences between men and women resulted from women's developmental failure to meet the male standard.[2] As a physician, Freud relied heavily on traditional medical training and terminology to describe the emotional conditions of his patients. Women who presented as emotionally distraught were referred to by physicians of this era as "hysterical." The origin of the word *hysteria* derived from the Greek *ustera* or *hustera*, meaning "of the womb." Thus, an emotionally distraught, or hysterical, woman was considered one whose behavior originated from the womb. Taking into consideration nineteenth-century medicine's general view of the inferior anatomy of women as compared to men's anatomy, a common cure for women's emotional distress in the late 1800s was a hysterectomy, that is, removal of the uterus. Many unnecessary hysterectomies were performed throughout the late 1800s and across much of the 1900s because of a biased view toward women and women's anatomy. Up until the women's rights movement in the 1960s and 1970s, little consideration was given, by the medical profession at large, to the possibility that much of nineteenth- and twentieth-century women's emotional distress could have been the result of the prevalent oppression of women who were forced into social and political positions inferior to men.

Jean Piaget did not acknowledge the value of the female pattern in his theory of cognitive development in 1932. Piaget equated normal child development with male development and considered females to be far less developed in capacities that would allow them to deal adequately with the realities of adult life. Piaget based his assumption on his observations of adolescent children playing games. Boys focused more on a resolution of conflicts by following established rules to the letter, whereas girls were more tolerant in their attitudes, more easily reconciled to innovative solutions, and more willing to make exceptions if the rules did not seem to result in fair outcomes relative to the situation. Piaget determined that the female pattern of conflict resolution lacked the necessary legal sense that was essential to moral development; thus, he determined that girls were inferior to boys.[3] Piaget failed to recognize that the approach that girls took to conflict resolution, although different from that of boys, was an equal or sometimes more favorable approach to resolving the conflict depending upon the circumstances of the particular situation.

Lawrence Kohlberg, in 1969, derived his theory of moral development without considering the potential benefits of gender differences.[4] Kohlberg explains that gender differences develop because girls play games that are less likely to involve strict rules, such as hopscotch and jump rope. And, he observed, when conflicts over rules do develop in girls' games, the games often end. Rather than elaborating a set of rules to settle the dispute, girls subordinate the continuation of the game in favor of the continuation of relationships. This type of solution to conflict resolution was considered inferior by Kohlberg. Thus, when Kohlberg developed a scale to measure moral development, he utilized an exclusively male subject group; so, when measured by Kohlberg's scale, women are consistently found to be deficient in moral development.

In 1968 another prominent psychologist, Erik Erikson, did recognize gender differences by noting that in males the ability to develop an identity precedes intimacy development, but the development of intimacy occurs along with identity development in females. This tendency for women to identify themselves through their relationships with others remains strong for most women throughout their life. Despite Erikson's observation of gender differences, his life-cycle stages consistently depicted the male pattern as the standard for healthy psychosocial development.[5]

As a response to gender bias within the psychology profession, Gilligan proposed to the profession that a new psychology for women be developed that was independent of comparisons to male standards and that encouraged women to trust their own judgments about themselves. The psychology profession gradually began to respond to Gilligan's suggestion, and sensitivity to women's issues continues to evolve within the field. In fact, the American Psychological Association has a subdivision dedicated entirely to the psychology of women.

Women's Relational Model of Development

Traditional male models of development emphasize the separation and individuation process as primary for psychological well-being, but women demonstrate a very different process. The self-concept of a woman, her identity and self-esteem, is strongly associated with her relationship to others. The ability to relate to others is a woman's strength, and it enhances her process of empathy. This tendency of girls and women to relate self to others, and to even sacrifice self-achievement in order to preserve a relationship, was observed by early psychologists, such as Piaget, Kohlberg, and Erikson, but they erroneously dismissed this demonstration as inferior to the male process. A woman tends to foster and encourage relationships as an integral part of her self-identity. This relational approach to psychological understanding was initially called "self-in-relation theory," and it was primarily developed by women psychologists and their associates working together at the Stone Center at Wellesley College in the late 1980s and early 1990s.[6]

What began as self-in-relation theory has emerged to be referred to as **gender-relations theory,** and it is a response to traditional Western psychology that emphasizes separation and individuation but neglects the intricacies of human interconnection. Men tend to identify themselves mostly through their work and competition; this is the model of normal human development espoused by Western psychology. Women tend to identify themselves mostly through persons and relationships; this is largely ignored by Western psychology. Gender-relations theory espouses that the primacy of responsive relationships is a powerful determinant of women's psychological reality—women mostly develop their sense of self through their connections with others, whereas men mostly develop their sense of self through separating from others. Maintaining a healthy sense of self, while in relation with others, is a key to self-worth and self-esteem for women. In many cases, the primary problem for a woman in therapy is "how to be the kind of self she wants to be, a being-in-relationship, now able to value the very valuable parts of herself, along with her own perceptions and desires—and to find others who will be with her in that way."[7] A woman's sense of self can be annihilated due to her tendency to give up self in order to maintain a relation with another. "Women tend to define power as having the strength to care for and give to others, which is very different from the way men have defined power."[8]

To encourage a woman to separate and individuate completely from another is asking her not to be a woman. Truly, some women become too enmeshed with others, as in the case of a woman who repeatedly returns to an abusive partner. When dysfunctional relationships occur, the goal is not to get a woman to stop her relational aspect of self but instead to channel it in a healthier way. A tendency women must watch out for is giving too much of themselves to others. A woman who spends all of her time fostering others and not enough time nurturing her own needs and desires can begin to feel lost and empty. The Stone Center relational model emphasizes the centrality of connection in women's lives. Understanding this is core in helping a woman find fulfillment.

Sociocultural Influences

Sociocultural influences (SCIs) may significantly impact your emotional health. Examples of SCIs include, but may not be limited to, family members, family history, family values, religious doctrine, media, school activities and personnel, community events, national events, world events, historical events, friends, famous persons, and significant others. These SCIs can affect you in many different ways. As you experience them in your life you will choose, either consciously or unconsciously, to integrate them into your self in some meaningful way. Once integrated, these SCIs can guide and direct your thinking, feeling, believing, and behaving. The influence of these SCIs in your life can lead to life satisfaction and the pursuit or achievement of wellness, or they can lead you to some points of dissatisfaction or dysfunction. In fact, some SCIs may have a positive impact early on in your life but will eventually lose their usefulness as you grow and change and thus may eventually begin to have negative consequences in your life. It is important to be

Her Story

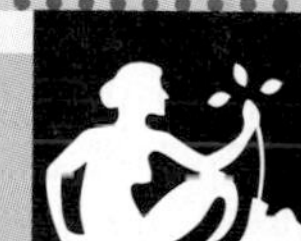

Ning: Sociocultural Influences

Ning was unhappy in her college major. She came to the student counseling center for advisement. The career tests that she took all suggested that she would be much happier in a different area, in this case, theater arts. She confirmed to the counselor that she had wanted to be a theater major since high school, at which she starred in several school stage plays. When the counselor began to suggest that Ning change her major from premedicine to theater arts, Ning became very uncomfortable and said she just could not do that. With further probing, she explained that her parents fully expected her to be a physician and that she dare not change out of her premed major or they would be very upset with her. She described that her parents' definition of a successful career included medicine, but not the theater. The influence that Ning's parents had on her was so strong that Ning felt like she could not choose her own profession for fear of alienating the love of her parents and demonstrating disrespect toward them.

Ning decided to stay in counseling to explore how she developed her beliefs and values and to determine how these may be serving her well or not serving her so well in her life. This process of mindful self-exploration assisted Ning in making new choices in her life that would result in greater happiness for her. One choice was to develop a style of assertive communication with her parents that would help Ning to express her needs and desires in a better way but would also, in her opinion, not demonstrate disrespect for her parents, which was very important to Ning. After talking to her parents and working through their differences of opinion, Ning chose to change her major to theater arts. She was much happier, and she felt that, although her parents were still somewhat disappointed in her choice, they now were more accepting of her desire to strive to do her best in a career for which she was more highly motivated to succeed.

- Have you ever had an internal conflict over something really important to you?
- How could mindful self-exploration help you to examine, understand, and potentially resolve this conflict?

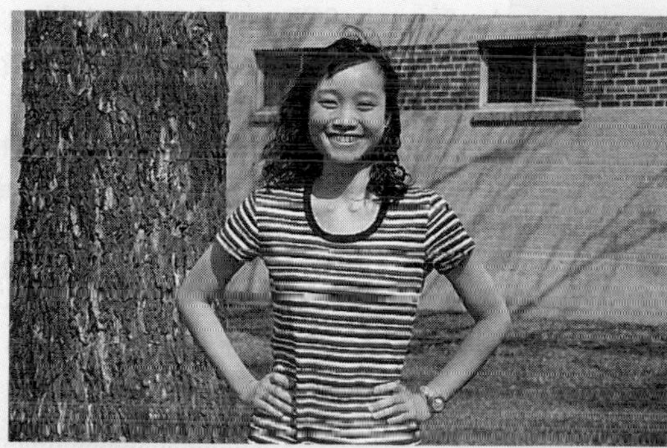

Ning resolved those issues that led to her life dissatisfaction through the process of a mindful self-exploration of the sociocultural influences upon her life.

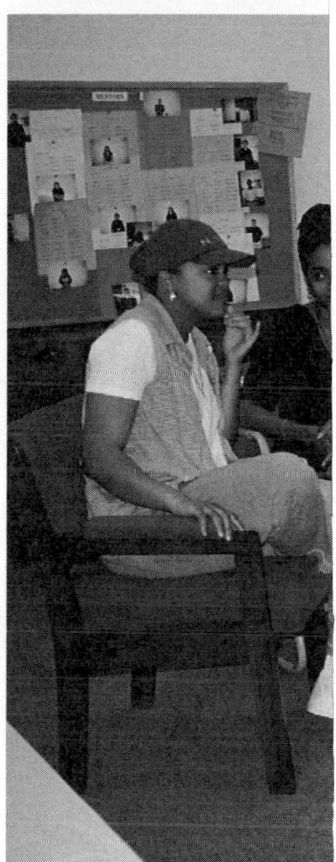

A personal growth group is

Journal Activity

Mindful Sel

Identify three things you
your life and write each
paper. Now do the same fo
about yourself or your life
three things you are unha
write down the sociocultu
have integrated into your
processes that may have c
happiness or unhappiness
parental messages you recei
"should" be from televisio
beliefs, modeling persons y
be included.) If you have t
try asking a friend for som

FYI

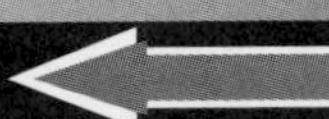

What Is Assertiveness?

Assertiveness, or assertion, is standing up for personal rights and expressing thoughts, feelings, and beliefs in direct, honest, and appropriate ways that do not violate another person's rights. Assertiveness involves the use of "I" messages, for example: "This is what *I* think." "This is what *I* feel." "This is how *I* see the situation." These types of messages express "who the person is" and are said without dominating, humiliating, or degrading the other person.

"Assertiveness involves respect—not deference. Deference is acting in a subservient manner as though the other person is right or better simply because the other person is older, more powerful, experienced, knowledgeable, or is of a different sex or race. Deference is present when people express themselves in ways that are self-effacing, appeasing, or overly apologetic."[9] With assertion, one must communicate respect for self and for others.

Health Tips

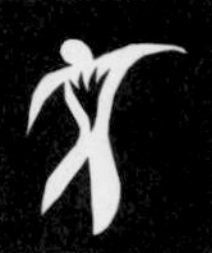

When Do You Need to Be Assertive?

Applying assertive behavior may be required in many situations in order to get your needs met in a healthy manner. Here are just a few examples in which you may need to be assertive:[12]

- Maintaining assertion in the face of someone's aggression and personal attack
- Being assertive with repair people who overcharge or do not properly do the work
- Giving supervisory criticism
- Presenting yourself at a task meeting where others ignore, discount, or put down your ideas
- Negotiating salary increases, and dealing with changes in job title or job function
- Being assertive with colleagues who make sexist, racist, or condescending remarks
- Expressing feelings of hurt, anger, and disappointment with people who are close to you

skills to individuals and groups. Assertiveness training teaches the differences between assertive, aggressive, and nonassertive behavior and increases experience in applying responsible assertive behavior. *FYI:* "What Is Assertiveness?" explains what assertiveness is.

A need for assertiveness training is more prevalent for women than for men because many messages from American society tend to encourage boys to be aggressive career professionals while encouraging girls to be passive caregivers and homemakers. Assertive behavior is more common in working women than in homemakers. In a study regarding women's views about leisure time, homemakers were less likely than working women to feel assertive, competent, or independent during their leisure. They felt more constrained by lack of skills and opportunity, poor self-image, fear, personal values, and the belief that some leisure activities are only for men.[10]

Adventure-based activities can have a positive influence on assertiveness enhancement for women. Ropes course training is one such activity. Women must overcome obstacles, usually constructed in an outdoor wilderness area, that include crossing rivers on rope ladders, scaling high walls, swinging across chasms on ropes, rock climbing, or rappelling down cliffs. Adventure-based courses have produced positive changes in women participants, such as increases in women's abilities to take risks, to practice assertive leadership, to solve problems effectively, and to feel more competent in general.[11] Participants in adventure-based courses for women report that feelings of power and achievement emerge in this setting.

In spite of the positive impact that assertiveness can have in your life, such as enhancing your success in a career and increasing your ability to meet your needs and the needs of significant others, there is some pressure exerted by society for women to not be assertive. For example, one study of 122 men between the ages of 17 and 25 years rated women described as independent and assertive as less physically attractive than women described as affectionate and compassionate.[13] What is especially significant about this study is that the two groups of women had been rated as equally physically attractive by a separate sample of men when no personality characteristics were described. It was only with the addition of the differentiating personality characteristics that men now found one group, the independent and assertive women, less physically attractive than the other group.

Sending assertive messages is an important step for getting your needs met. *Health Tips:* "When Do You Need to Be Assertive?" and *FYI:* "Types of Assertive Messages" provide examples of when and how to be assertive.

Being an effective communicator is also important in creating positive and productive interactions.

Effective Communication

The components of **effective listening** and **effective communication** are appropriate body language, encouraging responses, paraphrasing, clarification, and summarization.[14] Effective listening begins with

FYI 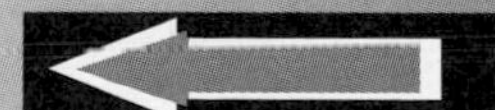

Types of Assertive Messages[15]

There are six basic types of assertive messages: *I want* statements help to clarify to both yourself and others what you really want. For example, "I want you to call when you are going to be late." *I feel* statements help express your feelings without attacking the other person. For example, "I feel embarrassed when you criticize my clothes in front of my friends." *Mixed feelings* statements name more than one feeling and explain where each is coming from. For example, "I enjoy going out and doing things with you, yet I feel it is unfair that you frequently do not bring enough money and ask me to pay for you." *Empathic assertion* presents some sensitive understanding about the other person and then expresses how you feel. For example, "I know you said that you are angry and do not want to talk about it. However, I feel we need to talk about it when you feel ready." *Confrontive assertion* is necessary when there are contradictions such as differences between what a person says and what she or he does. For example, "I know you said you would teach the newer students some of the beginning information as part of your internship, yet you consistently put them off or do not show up for appointments. I want you to be more responsible and follow through on the tasks that you agreed to do." *I language assertion* is useful for expressing difficult negative feelings. For example, "When you cancel a weekend event with me because you say you are busy working and then I find out you went out with someone else, I feel rejected and humiliated. I need for you to be honest with me about why you do things or it could damage our friendship."

Journal Activity 

Practice Assertive "I" Messages

Practice writing assertive *I messages* to someone you would like to communicate with assertively. Here is a template for writing I statements:

> I feel (emotion) when (behavior) and would like (behavioral request).

Now, let's look at some examples containing I messages:

> I feel (irritated) when (dirty clothes are left on the floor), and I would like (you to pick up your dirty clothes each day).
>
> I feel (glad) when (I see you have taken the trash out), and I would like (to thank you).

appropriate body language. When someone is talking, be attentive. Watch the person's his face and, when appropriate, make eye contact. From time to time, make brief encouraging responses (one to three words only) to let the person know you are listening, for example, "I see" or "I hear you." Sometimes a brief nod is appropriate. The purpose of encouraging responses is to let the individual know you are listening without implying agreement at this point. When the individual pauses, attempt to paraphrase what has been said; that is, in one or two sentences, restate in your own words what has been told to you.

Occasionally, effective listening involves a need for clarification if you are having difficulty understanding the person talking. Clarification can be achieved through brief exploratory statements and open-ended questions. An exploratory statement is an attempt to request further information without disrupting the flow of communication by the other person. An example exploratory statement would be, "Tell me more about your need for space." Another example of an exploratory statement would be, "Please give me more details about how you see our relationship evolving." An example of an open-ended question would be, "When you said my being late for meetings causes a disruption, could you tell me in what ways so that I might better understand your concern?" Open-ended questions usually ask what, when, where, or how.

When the individual stops talking, briefly summarize the main contents of what you think was communicated and then ask the person if he or she feels you understood. This effective listening process can then be followed by communication from you to the other person regarding your thoughts, ideas, or needs. Assertive communication can be useful at this point. The goal of effective listening is that each party be heard and understood. Then, via assertive communication, attempts can be made at caregiving, problem solving, conflict resolution, or negotiation and compromise. (Complete *Journal Activity:* "Practice Assertive 'I' Messages.")

Effective Problem Solving

Everyone appreciates the love, warmth, and potential companionship that can come from a relationship. Most people do not consider or adequately prepare for the disagreements or conflicts that will inevitably arise in any type of relationship, be it family, friends, relationship partner, or colleagues at work. Some individuals have misconceptions about conflict and disagreements that can impair adequate resolution. Many people incorrectly believe that a conflict must automatically be their fault, or that they must win a conflict, or that they should be able to handle a conflict so well that the problem never recurs.[16] Here are some other similar kinds of misconceptions to avoid: a compromise means losing and being less powerful than the other person; conflict should be avoided at any cost; your solution is the only worthwhile one; all conflicts must be resolved; and one party must be right and one must be wrong in any conflict.

Successful **problem solving** is a step-by-step approach of planning and negotiating and involves all parties to be affected. A common model for problem solving and negotiation involves six basic steps: defining the problem, generating possible solutions, evaluating the solutions, making the decision, determining how to implement the decision, and assessing the success of the solution.[17] After assessing success, some adjustments might have to be made, but it is important that all involved parties have a say in any adjustments to the original agreement.

Self-Esteem Enhancement

Self-esteem is based on the distance between the perceived self and the ideal self. The perceived self is how you currently see yourself. The ideal self is how you believe you "should" be. The greater the distance between the perceived self and the ideal self, the lower your self-esteem.

Self-esteem enhancement is the process of reducing the distance between the perceived self and the ideal self. In cases of low self-esteem, typically the ideal self is too unrealistic. Thus, the process here would be to bring the ideal self into reality, to make the view of the ideal self more realistic and less perfectionistic. Once the ideal self is more realistic, then you can have a healthier opinion about yourself and greater self-esteem. When you desire to make some changes, having good self-esteem is prerequisite to making healthier and more realistic decisions about change.

Individuals who have low self-esteem are often discouraged persons. Activities that help to instill a belief in oneself can raise self-esteem, bring the ideal self into a healthier perspective, and build success and confidence. Participation in adventure programs, sports, music and arts, and community service are just a few examples of activities that enhance self-esteem through the experience of success while having fun.

Low self-esteem can originate from discouraging messages we received from our parents. Parents serve as primary role models and message senders. For a woman, the most common primary role model is her mother. The presence of critical messages or the absence of encouraging messages from a woman's mother can create severe doubt in a woman's own judgment and ability throughout her life span.

If we feel trapped by unfulfilled needs that arose out of childhood experiences, we first need to understand them as best we can. In terms of the self-concept, it is helpful to understand how much of any belief about ourselves is an accurate reflection of us and how much is the product of circumstance or other people's misperceptions.[18]

At some point in their life women have to ask, "Whom are we to believe?" An integral part of moving on is learning to trust our own judgments as much as or more than our parents'.

Not only is it important to feel good about yourself, but it also may be important to let others know this. Characters who were boastful or positive about themselves were rated by undergraduate college students as being more competent than characters who made negative statements about themselves.[19] Thus, bragging about yourself may enhance the opinion that others have about you.

The process of maintaining or enhancing self-esteem in women may vary across cultures. Conditions that impact self-esteem were compared for young Asian, black, and white women in America.[20] The best predictors of good self-esteem among Asian women included having children, having nonconflicting social networks, and experiencing positive life events. For black women, the best predictors of good self-esteem included having educational opportunities and nonconflicting social networks. For white women, the best predictors of good self-esteem included the absence of negative life events, the presence of nonconflicting social networks, and a good income. (See *Health Tips:* "Understanding and Enhancing Self-Esteem in Women.")

Image Building

A positive image of self is central to feeling good and being successful. A key element to building and maintaining a positive self-image is to focus on being what you want to be—that is, building an image from the inside out instead of trying to be what others want you to be.

Society presents many messages about the supposed "ideal image." This is a myth; there is no such thing as the "ideal woman." Every woman has something unique to offer on an emotional, physical, mental, social, occupational, and spiritual level. It is the differences you present that help to make the world diverse and complete.

To enhance your self-image, start by loving yourself and accepting yourself as you are right now at this very moment. If you can do this, then any changes you want to make in yourself can be much more fun instead of seeming so difficult and laborious.

A preoccupation with body image can reach elevations significant enough to be considered clinical in nature. **Body dysmorphic disorder (BDD)** is the classification of body-image disturbance reserved for the non—eating

Health Tips

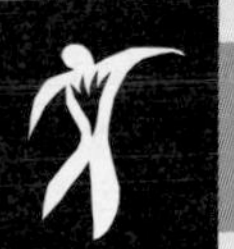

Understanding and Enhancing Self-Esteem in Women

IMPAIRED COMPETENCE DEVELOPMENT

- Self-esteem is based on competence, and competence means having a sense of control over our self and mastery of our environment.
- Acquiring self-competence is more difficult for female children (and female adults) because males are more highly valued in our society, females have more limits placed on them from childhood through adulthood, and females are more susceptible to discrimination and violence than males in childhood and adulthood.

HINDRANCES TO SELF-ESTEEM DEVELOPMENT AND MAINTENANCE

- Women are stereotyped to play the role of caretaker and servant: good mother, good wife, good woman, and the weaker sex—to sacrifice herself for others.
- Prominent health and mental health care models are designed and maintained mostly by men and thus are sorely lacking in a proper understanding of and attention to women's issues.
- There is a tendency to medicate a woman who is anxious and depressed instead of fostering a sense of her personal power through therapy.

TEN TIPS FOR SELF-ESTEEM ENHANCEMENT

- Identify and challenge negative feelings and thoughts you have about yourself and other women. Women with low self-esteem often are critical of other women, thereby contributing to the problem in a larger sense.
- Examine and challenge self-critical tapes (and the origins of these messages, most likely from a critical parent).
- Build up a large repertoire of positive feelings and thoughts about yourself and repeat them daily (even if you do not believe them yet).
- Practice assertive behavior.
- Learn to set limits and boundaries on what you will and will not do, what you will not tolerate from others, and what you expect from others.
- Enhance your ability to practice effective communication.
- Enhance your problem-solving and decision-making abilities.
- Learn to filter out or ignore stereotypical messages from other persons and the media about body-image preferences and gender-role expectations.
- Avoid the temptation to be a "martyr"; learn to delegate responsibility so that you have more time for yourself.
- Participate in activities that challenge you to grow and contribute to a sense of self-competency and personal power.

disorder population. BDD is a preoccupation with an imagined defect in appearance that results in distress in social or other important areas of life functioning.[21] Preliminary evidence suggests that BDD is diagnosed with approximately equal frequency in women and in men. BDD behaviors include frequent mirror checking or avoidance of mirrors, frequent comparisons to others, and excessive grooming behavior. Dysmorphophobia is the label the Europeans have assigned to BDD and the term used by the World Health Organization and the *International Classification of Diseases* diagnostic reference.

Image and the Media

Glamorous images projected in the media have contributed to harsh self-criticism by women regarding their own body image. Television, movies, and magazines present images of women that seem real but are, in fact, impossible to compete with. Many models and actresses have what is considered to be an ideal body image, but they also have all of the best clothes designers, hair dressers, and makeup staff. These professionals spend many hours sculpting a woman into a form that is, supposedly, "ideal" but that is pretty unrealistic most of the time. What they have created is an image of a woman that does not occur naturally in the world. One example is the glamorization of Barbara Stanwyck, a well-known actress in the United States in the mid-1940s, '50s, and '60s. Ms. Stanwyck had a "figure fault" by Hollywood standards; her hips were considered to be too low in the back and thought to look odd when she was walking. A famous designer in Hollywood at the time created a new design for Ms. Stanwyck to hide this "flaw." The design created by Edith Head was a dress with a high midriff, as opposed to a well-defined waistline that would accentuate the hips. This new design resulted in a taller, sleeker-looking Barbara. The dress design was incorporated into Ms. Stanwyck's wardrobe and was presented in the 1941 movie *The Lady Eve*. After this, Barbara Stanwyck had a career boost and played more glamorous roles. Edith Head's high midriff dress design, known as "The Lady Eve dress," was copied by many designers and purchased in abundance by women all over the country who wanted to camouflage their waistline or hips.[22] This type of camouflaging of a woman's natural image can be seen throughout history. More public efforts have been put into hiding a woman's natural image than in accepting the nature of a woman's uniqueness.

There have been instances where the media industry has been beneficial to the image of women. For example, the movie wardrobe of Marlene Dietrich, a famous actress of the 1930s, '40s, and '50s, made wearing pants more socially acceptable for women at a time when dresses had been socially demanded.[23] It is important to remember that in the movie and fashion industry, what is "in" one day may be "out" the next. This should add emphasis to the point that diversity and uniqueness enable us to be individuals and still fit in.

For the most part, the media have contributed more to the fictional "ideal woman" image than to the healthy "real woman" concept. In the 1990 movie *Pretty Woman,* Julia Roberts was portrayed as having a beautiful and desirable perfect body type. What the general public did not know was that several models were used as stand-ins. When Ms. Roberts's body was supposedly revealed, it was actually one of these body doubles that was being shown.[24] Thus, the "pretty woman" was not considered pretty enough for Hollywood standards. In fact, on the movie poster to advertise the film, Julia Roberts's head was superimposed on another woman's body. The unsuspecting public was led to believe that the woman on this poster was actually Julia Roberts. Another example of how the media promotes a fictionalized presentation of how women "should be" is the cover girl on a 1990s modeling magazine who was actually computer generated. Different parts of different women, including different facial features, were put together to create a whole new woman. An unsuspecting public can be easily misled by media magic tricks.

The **glamorization** of women, or basing the desirability of a woman on her body shape, mainly thinness in the arms, legs, face, and waist, and largeness of breasts and hips (the hourglass figure), is thought to have begun in the 1830s when the camera was invented.[25] This type of woman's figure was additionally popularized in the late 1800s by male artist Charles Gibson, who created the "Gibson girl" in a series of his paintings, which presented the supposed ideal woman.[26] Gibson's fictional depictions became very popular, and women strived to model after them.

Modern media technology is now reaching newly developing countries, and these societies are being exposed to fictionalized presentations of the ideal woman's body image. As this media technology is made more available in these countries, we have seen the instigation and rise of eating disorders and other emotional distresses that accompany striving to become the fictional ideal woman.[27]

There are ethnic differences in how women view body-image satisfaction. White women in the United States report greater levels of disordered eating and dieting behaviors and attitudes and greater body dissatisfaction than Asian Americans and African Americans.[28] Low self-esteem and high public self-consciousness are associated with greater levels of problematic eating behaviors and attitudes and body dissatisfaction.

There are some differences in how men and women view their own body. Women reportedly have lower body-image satisfaction than men, and self-esteem is linked to body-image attitudes more for women than for men.[29] These differences are evident as early as adolescence, in that adolescent males are found to feel more positive about their bodies than are adolescent females.[30]

Most women do not actually have unattractive and unacceptable bodies. It is more likely that society has been generating unfair messages to women about how they "should" and "should not" look so that most women feel that they may have unattractive bodies or features. The reality is that most women's sense of unattractiveness has been created by media bias. It is difficult to turn around a pattern of thinking that has endured for such a long time. Some progress has been made in countering the fictional images of a woman's body. However, society has a long way to go. In the meantime, the image of women will sustain harsh criticism as it continues to be based on biased and unrealistic thinking.

Eating Disorders

Poor body image has been identified as the central factor in the development of eating disorders. Ninety percent of people with an eating disorder are female.[31] Eating disorders include **anorexia nervosa, bulimia nervosa,** and **binge eating disorder.** Anorexia nervosa is starving oneself, sometimes even to death, because of a personal belief that one is unattractive or unlovable. Bulimia nervosa is eating and then vomiting soon afterward or using a laxative to get rid of the food in order to avoid weight gain. Binge eating disorder involves binge eating but not purging (vomiting and laxative abuse) afterward.

The National Institute of Diabetes and Digestive and Kidney Diseases reports that about 2 percent of all adults (as many as 4 million Americans) have binge eating disorder. About 10 to 15 percent of people who are mildly obese and who try to lose weight on their own or through commercial weight-loss programs have binge eating disorder. The disorder is even more common in people who are severely obese, and it occurs more frequently in adults than adolescents. (See *Women Making a Difference:* "Celebrities Support National Eating Disorders Association.")

Women Making a Difference

Celebrities Support National Eating Disorders Association

Country music superstar Sara Evans became an ambassador for the National Eating Disorders Association lending her voice during the 19th Annual Eating Disorders Awareness Week, February 26th–March 4th, 2006. Evans is best known for her hit songs "Born to Fly," "Perfect," "Suds in the Bucket," "Cheatin'," and "A Real Place to Start." Evans said, "I am so honored to announce my affiliation as an ambassador for NEDA. Thankfully, I have never suffered from an eating disorder, but am well aware of our society's obsession with body image. My passion for this cause is much more personal. I almost lost my best friend to anorexia. I am lending my voice as an entertainer, a mom and a friend because I want to bring great awareness to this cause." "[Sara] Evans joins NEDA Ambassadors Paula Abdul (*American Idol*); Jamie-Lynn Sigler (*The Sopranos*); Scarlett Pomers (*Reba*); actress Tracey Gold; model and producer Carfe Otis; and author, lecturer and actionist Jessica Weiner, who have all overcome eating disorders themselves and are using their spotlight to reach out to anyone who may be struggling with anorexia, bulimia, or other disordered eating. Also, reaching out as an ambassador on behalf of NEDA is model, TV host, author, lecturer and plus-sized clothing designer Emme, who has long promoted healthy body image."[32]

Bulimics are at risk for a number of serious health problems. The use of laxatives eventually creates a dependency upon them for normal bowel function. The constant vomiting causes teeth to erode and salivary glands to enlarge due to the effects of acidic stomach fluids that pass through the mouth.

Approximately 5 to 10 percent of persons with anorexia die as a result of either starvation or suicide.[33] Most of these deaths are sudden and are probably due to irregular heartbeats or coma induced by low blood sugar. Chances of death are highest in anorectic women who lose more than 30 percent of their original weight and in those who rely on purging to enhance their weight loss. Eating disorders have the highest mortality rate of all psychiatric disorders.

Approximately 0.5 to 1 percent of women between the ages of 15 and 30 have anorexia.[34] Onset is typically between the ages of 14 and 18 years with almost all cases starting between the ages of 11 and 22. Approximately 1 to 3 percent of adolescent and college-age women have bulimia.[35] In addition, persons who miss a diagnosis of anorexia or bulimia by only one criterion are diagnosed with the clinical condition **EDNOS (Eating Disorder Not Otherwise Specified).** The prevalence of EDNOS is twice that of anorexia and twice that of bulimia at 2 to 6 percent of the population.[36] Many therapists who treat eating disorders suggest the criteria for anorexia and bulimia are too restrictive because they exclude so many persons on the basis of just one criterion. For example, if a client exhibits all criteria required for anorexia except she still has her menstrual period or she has an inconsistent menstrual period, then she does not qualify for the diagnosis of anorexia because the required criterion is for her to have a complete absence of a menstrual period for three consecutive months, a criterion that is usually only present once the anorexia has progressed to a later, and potentially life-threatening, stage. Exclusion from an eating disorder category on the basis of one criterion is problematic in that one, it significantly dilutes the statistics for the number of persons struggling with a serious eating disorder (EDNOS is typically not reported by databases), and two, insurance companies are less likely to reimburse clients for EDNOS because of a mistaken belief that EDNOS is less serious, and three, significantly less research is performed on EDNOS even though it is much more prevalent than anorexia or bulimia. Also, it is important to note that women who do not quite meet the criteria for a clinical eating disorder may suffer from a number of subclinical eating disorders. For example, many women who diet obsessively use some similar techniques such as bingeing, vomiting, or abusing laxatives, diet pills, and diuretics to keep their weight under control.

It is more difficult for women to lose weight because women's bodies are designed to retain fat so that the population can survive during times of famine with women still able to breast-feed from fat stores. A healthy woman has as much as 20 to 30 percent body fat, whereas a healthy man has only about 10 to 15 percent.

Results of a survey of teenage girls reported that 90 percent of white girls were dissatisfied with their bodies and that 62 percent had dieted within the past year.[37] This contrasted sharply with results among black teenage girls: 70 percent were satisfied with their bodies, and 64 percent said that it was better to be a little overweight than underweight.

The Centers for Disease Control reports that eating disorders are a serious problem among adolescents, particularly among girls in their teenage years. In 1999, 36.4 percent of female high school students perceived themselves to be overweight. Although some of these students may truly be overweight, many are not. More than 12 percent of the students reported not eating in the 24 hours preceding the CDC survey to lose weight or to avoid gaining weight; 7.6 percent reported taking diet pills, powders, or liquids without a doctor's advice

FYI

Treatment for Eating Disorders[39]

Common issues for persons with an eating disorder include

- Perfectionism.
- Dichotomous thinking.
- Diminished awareness of internal standards.
- Overreliance on external reinforcement.
- Desire to please and caretake others.
- Sense of helplessness and being out of control.
- Avoidance of emotions.

The most common approach to the treatment of an eating disorder is

- Appropriate assessment and diagnosis.
- Treatment focused on having a realistic body image and resolving personal issues that impair one's ability to do this.
- Multidisciplinary approach involving a mental health therapist, a physician, and a nutritionist.
- Medication: none for anorexia; some antidepressants are helpful with bulimia (such as fluoxetine, known as Prozac) in combination with mental health therapy.

Family therapy is the treatment of choice for anorexia. Cognitive-behavioral therapy is the treatment of choice for bulimia. A combination of individual and group treatment can be effective for both anorexia and bulimia. Inpatient hospitalization may be necessary for anorexics whose body weight causes medical complications or drops dangerously low. Inpatient hospitalization may be required for bulimics who are unresponsive to psychological treatment. Day treatment programs for eating disorders are rapidly rising in popularity because insurance companies are more often choosing not to reimburse for hospital treatment.

to lose weight or to avoid gaining weight; and 4.8 percent reported having vomited or taken laxatives to lose weight or to avoid gaining weight. These behaviors were consistently more prevalent among females.

Women who suffer from an eating disorder frequently have a poor self-concept. The treatment for eating disorders requires a combination of personal mental health counseling and nutritional guidance. (See *FYI:* "Treatment for Eating Disorders.")

Resolving Grief over Loss

During your life, you will lose someone or something very important to you. This will probably happen many times in your lifetime. Losing someone or something meaningful is very painful. Understanding the grief resolution process is an important life skill for coping with the pain accompanied by loss.

Grief is the emotional experience of loss, whereas **mourning** is the actual expression of loss, those behaviors that take place as a result of the grief experience.[38] An actual loss or some memory of a previous loss can serve as a trigger to experience the emotions of grief. These emotions then result in behaviors to mourn the loss. It is important to mourn the loss to reconcile the emotions of grief. Unreconciled or poorly reconciled grief experiences can lead to unhealthy behaviors.

Grief is a normal response to loss. It does not matter what or who has been lost. The more meaningful the thing or person that is lost, the more intense will be the sense of loss. People grieve in various ways. Some seek support, and others grieve silently and alone. Some recover quickly whereas others are bereaved for a very long time. There is no one right way to grieve. However, the grief process must not consume your life to the degree that you become dysfunctional and risk losing additional things that are important and necessary, such as relationships and employment.

The support of close friends and family is helpful during bereavement. Sometimes it may become necessary to seek the assistance of a mental health professional experienced in facilitating the grief recovery process. Grief support groups are common. Individuals who participate in a community grief support group or professional grief counseling often recover more quickly from their bereavement. People tend to work through loss in healthier ways and integrate loss more effectively when assistance from others and a variety of resources are readily available. Resources form the basis of a **support network** consisting of three systems that focus on (1) clarifying how you derive meaning from life through your beliefs and values, (2) how you access support from those around you, and (3) how you draw upon your own personal strengths and abilities.[40]

Recovering from loss does not necessarily mean that you will no longer experience any pain from the memory of the loss. It does mean that you will regain a sense of being okay and going on with your life. Recovery means that you are no longer consumed by the loss and can incorporate new beginnings and new ways of thinking into your life. The first 6 months after a loss are usually the most difficult. The formal bereavement or grieving process typically takes about 2 years, although the sense of pain usually subsides gradually over this 2-year period. Even after the 2-year period, you may find certain dates related to the loss just as difficult, for example, the birthday of a deceased child or the anniversary of the death of a spouse or relationship partner.

Some commonalities have been discovered in the **grief process.** One grief process model describes grief from the loss of a loved one as having three phases, each with its own set of characteristics, challenges, and choices: early mourning, mid-mourning, and late mourning.[41] The early mourning phase lasts from the time you first hear about the loss to the final disposition of the body and personal belongings of the deceased. This phase can last as long as 3 to 6 weeks after the funeral. Challenges to face include getting through the funeral, dealing with funeral details, notifying family and friends, settling estate arrangements, and preparing for the transitions to come.

Mid-mourning is the phase of having to face the harsh reality of the loss. As others begin to get on with their lives, you will find it difficult to do so. You may suffer deep separation feelings, pain, or anxiety. You may have difficulty distinguishing fact from fantasy, and physical symptoms may develop such as sleep disturbance, reduced appetite, anxiety attacks, headaches, stomachaches, and shortness of breath. Your health may be fragile during this phase, and it is extremely important, difficult as it may be, to exercise and eat a nutritious diet. During this phase there can be a flood of emotions, intense sadness, and loneliness as well as feelings of guilt, depression, powerlessness, abandonment, anger and rage, fear, and panic. You may choose to be alone in order to grieve completely. However, it is also important to seek out and maintain a support system during this vulnerable time.

The late mourning phase focuses on getting on with your life. Your feelings will focus less on grief, although anger and sadness may still be prevalent, and more on attitudes and perceptions as they relate to moving on with your life. An attitude of acceptance has gradually evolved, and an integration of the loss into your life scheme has occurred.

Another grief process model involves **five stages of grief:** denial, anger, sorrow/despair/depression, bargaining, and acceptance.[42] These stages can be experienced in any order and more than once in the grieving process.

Denial is often the initial reaction, although it can be experienced again at any time. Denial is a buffer of protection against the shock and trauma of the loss. It allows us time to adjust to the event. This stage is accompanied by a feeling of numbness and disbelief. As is the case with each of these stages, it is important to work through the denial. From there, one must regain and maintain a presence of mind as soon as possible so that one can function in the world realistically. Seeking and receiving support and understanding from others is very important during this time.

When you have lost someone or something important to you, you can become very angry. You may want to lash out and hurt others with your words and deeds. It is important to remember that what you are angry about is the loss, and you should not become destructive toward yourself or others as a result. Anger can be worked through by talking with others. Anger is a natural part of the grief process, and it needs to be expressed, but in a healthy manner.

Sorrow, despair, and depression are natural and healthy ways to express sadness from a loss. Crying is useful for releasing the sadness. Ritualistic ceremonies, such as funerals, wakes, and memorial services, are often held to facilitate opportunities for expressing sadness with others who are also feeling the loss or wish to support you in your loss. These ceremonies can assist with the transitions that are necessary from one stage to another in the grieving process.

Bargaining is a desperate attempt to stay in control. This stage is accompanied by our attempts to second-guess the situation or try to reverse the loss. We might say things like "If only I had done this or that, then this would not have happened" or "If I promise this thing or that thing, everything will be okay again." Although the bargaining stage does not necessarily have many healthy aspects, it is still a very common experience during bereavement. The persistent and gentle assurance and reassurance by those close to you that "there is nothing you could have done" or "there is nothing you can do now" will help you through this potentially destructive stage.

Acceptance is the final stage of grief, although it is possible to recycle through the previous stages again. Acceptance is the final goal of the grief process. In this stage, we come to accept the loss that has occurred. We come to terms with reality. We understand that our life will always be different having been impacted by the loss, but that we can and will go on. We can let go of our doubts and anger and lift our sadness. We can go on and live our lives fully again.

DEPRESSION

A common emotional health concern for women is the presence of symptoms associated with depression. **Depression** is an emotional state of persistent dejection that may range from mild discouragement to feelings of extreme despair. These feelings are usually accompanied by loss of motivation, loss of energy, insomnia, loss of appetite, and difficulty in concentrating and making decisions.[43] Persons who have had a stressful or traumatic event often experience depression afterwards. (See *FYI:* "Prevalence of Depression.") A chemical imbalance in the brain, primarily that of the neurotransmitter serotonin, is thought to be a precursor to depression. The causes of this imbalance may include the experience of stress or trauma or a genetic predisposition toward depression.

The World Health Organization ranks depression as the world's fourth most devastating illness, measured in total years of healthy life stolen by death or disability. According to WHO projections, depression will have climbed to second place by 2020, exceeded only by heart disease.

Prevalence of Depression

The National Institute of Mental Health estimates that between 17 and 20 million Americans develop depression each year. One of every five adults may experience depression at some time in their lives, but less than half of the people suffering from depression receive treatment. Twice as many women as men suffer from depression, although everybody, including children, can develop the illness. Have you ever been depressed or known anyone who was depressed? If so, what resources did you find most helpful with managing or treating the depression?

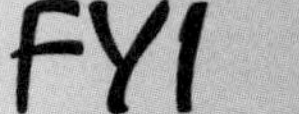

Common Types of Clinical Depression[49]

Major depressive episode involves the presence of at least five of the following symptoms for most of the day for at least a 2-week period:

- Feelings of sadness or emptiness
- Diminished interest or pleasure
- Weight loss
- Insomnia
- Feelings of worthlessness or inappropriate guilt
- Diminished ability to think or concentrate
- Recurrent thoughts of death or suicide

Dysthymic disorder involves the presence of at least two of the following symptoms for most of the day for at least 2 years (1 year for adolescents and children):

- Poor appetite or overeating
- Insomnia
- Low energy or fatigue
- Low self-esteem
- Poor concentration or difficulty making decisions
- Feelings of hopelessness

Major depressive disorder is typically the reccurrence of a major depressive episode (two or more within two consecutive months).

Bipolar disorder is a mixture of major depressive episodes and manic episodes. Manic episodes are a distinct period of persistently elevated, expansive, or irritable mood lasting at least 4 days, and that is clearly different from the usual non-depressed mood. If numerous periods of depressive symptoms and numerous periods of manic symptoms occur, the individual may be diagnosed as having **cyclothymic disorder** (a chronic fluctuating mood disturbance involving numerous periods of mania and depression).

Types of Depression

Individuals may have just a few characteristics associated with depression, or they may have more severe symptoms indicative of a clinical depression. Women are twice as likely as men to be diagnosed with a clinical depression, and thus the cost of depression is borne disproportionately by women.[44,45] Most research suggests that women are at greater risk for depression because of interplay between environmental factors (such as social stressors), biological factors (such as hormones), and genetic factors (such as family history).[46]

Clinical depression usually requires intervention by a trained mental health professional. The most common types of clinical depression are major depressive episode, dysthymic disorder, major depressive disorder, and bipolar disorder (commonly referred to as manic depression; see *FYI:* "Common Types of Clinical Depression"). In any given community, it is estimated that between 10 and 25 percent of women will develop a major depressive disorder sometime in their lifetime.[47] These prevalence rates for major depressive disorder seem to be unrelated to ethnicity, education, income, or marital status.

Psychosocial Stressors and Depression

Some researchers believe that the higher incidence of depression in women is because they respond to depressing life events differently than men. Men tend to cut off the depression before it has serious consequences, whereas women tend to remain focused on their depressed mood in ways that prolong its duration and intensify its effects (this is referred to as rumination).[48] (See *Viewpoint:* "Women Have Better Emotional Memories.")

Researchers believe that women have higher incidences of depression than men because they experience more stress and discrimination. Women are subject to unique psychosocial stressors that can initiate depression and impede recovery. Examples include conflict between domestic and job demands, gender discrimination in financial and political venues, and pressure by society to maintain a prescribed body image. Body-image dissatisfaction has been linked to low self-esteem and higher rates of depression.[50]

Perceived lower social support for women as compared to men is linked with higher rates of depression for women.[51] Also, significantly more women than men are living in poverty, and poor women have more frequent and uncontrollable adverse life events (danger, violence, crime, etc.) than men.[52] (See *Viewpoint:* "Why Are Women More Susceptible to Depression?")

Viewpoint

Women Have Better Emotional Memories

Women have better emotional memories than men. In a study appearing in the *Proceedings of the National Academy of Sciences* in July 2002, researchers utilized brain MRI (magnetic resonance imaging) to track the activity of the brain while recalling emotional stimuli. Women's brains seem to be wired both to feel and recall emotions more keenly. Turhan Canli, professor of psychology at the State University of New York, Stony Brook, points out that a risk factor for depression is rumination, or dwelling on a memory and reviewing it time after time. This study illuminates a possible biological basis for rumination and suggests another reason depression is more prevalent in women. Do you agree that women can recall emotional events better than men? Do you agree with the possibility that women have a higher prevalence for depression because they have a better emotional memory than men?

Viewpoint

Why Are Women More Susceptible to Depression?

There are many theories about why depression is more prevalent in women than in men. Do women experience more psychosocial stressors that lead to depression? Or do women tend to focus on depressing life events more than men so that depression lingers and is more severe in women? Are women socialized to reveal their feelings more often so they are more willing to report that they are depressed, or are they more willing to seek assistance for their depression? Does the physiology of women and the influence of hormones lead to increased incidences of depression? What is your theory about why women have a higher incidence of depression than men?

Research links depression in women with the experience of a higher number of life stressors and negative life events as compared to men.[53,54] Negative life events include serious illness or injury of self or a close family member, relationship discord or divorce, loss of a job, loss of a parent, and death of a family member. Severe adverse life events over which women feel little to no sense of control has been determined to be a major risk factor for women.[55] In one study, a depressive episode in response to adverse life events was found to be three times more likely in women than in men.[56] In another study, women who developed depression following a severely threatening event were more likely to reflect feelings of humiliation and being trapped as compared to women who had not developed depression following such an event.[57]

Women's higher rates of traumatic stressors are shown to be significant contributors to gender differences in major depression. Traumatic stressors such as sexual assault, sexual harassment, relationship partner violence, and childhood sexual abuse have all been linked to depression in women.[58,59,60]

The interpersonal and psychological functioning of women can be significantly impaired from the experience of childhood trauma. Childhood physical abuse, incest, and parental alcoholism have each been associated with higher rates of depression, higher sexual assault rates, lower self-esteem, and greater involvement with a chemically dependent partner.[61]

Women who had experienced childhood abuse and/or adult abuse were studied over 8 years by researchers who discovered that childhood and adult abuse were both independently related to chronic or recurrent depression in these women.[62] Women college undergraduates who reported exposure to abuse between their parents (parental partner abuse) during their childhood were described as having depression and low self-esteem.[63]

The Reproductive System and Depression

Research on the influence of biological factors on depression is somewhat inconclusive. Fluctuations in female hormones and other biochemicals may influence the frequency of depression in women. It is known that gonadal and adrenal steroids affect neurotransmitters, which play a role in regulating mood and behavior and neuroendocrine physiology.[64] The hormones of progesterone and estrogen both affect the neuroendocrine, neurotransmitter, and circadian systems, which affect the synthesis and release of both serotonin and norepinephrine, which in turn influence the development of depression.[65,66] However, most research does not support a definitive relationship between depression and normal fluctuations in ovarian hormones except for the few women who may have had some underlying emotional or social vulnerability during the hormonal fluctuation or who have a family history of depression.[67,68] Further research is needed to clarify the impact and role that endocrinology plays in the onset of depression.

Menstruation and Depression Severe premenstrual mood changes have been associated with a lifetime history of major depression. Premenstrual symptoms appear

Assess Yourself

Premenstrual Dysphoric Disorder (PMDD)

The most severe type of menstruation-related mood distress is **premenstrual dysphoric disorder (PMDD).** The criterion for diagnosing this condition is that for most of the menstrual periods over the past year the woman must have experienced at least five or more of the following eleven categories of symptoms:

1. Depressed mood or self-deprecating thoughts
2. Anxiety or tension
3. Sudden feelings of sadness or tearfulness
4. Persistent anger, irritability, or interpersonal conflicts
5. Decreased interest in usual activities (work, school, and so forth)
6. Difficulty concentrating
7. Lethargy or easy to fatigue
8. Marked change in appetite, overeating, or food cravings
9. Hypersomnia or insomnia
10. Feeling of being overwhelmed or out of control
11. Other physical symptoms, such as breast tenderness or swelling, headaches, joint or muscle pain, a sensation of bloating or weight gain.[69]

to have their highest prevalence in women in their late 20s and 30s. Approximately 80 percent of women report mild to minimal mood or somatic (physical) changes premenstrually, and an estimated 5 percent of women experience severe premenstrual symptoms.[70] Common premenstrual symptoms include depressed mood; irritability; hostility; anxiety; changes in sleep, appetite, energy, and libido; and somatic symptoms. (See *Assess Yourself:* "Premenstrual Dysphoric Disorder (PMDD).")

Depression Related to Pregnancy and Childbirth

Many women experience some negative emotions after childbirth.[71] Between 50 and 80 percent of women experience a mild postpartum dysphoria, or "the blues." This typically occurs the third or fourth day after delivery and lasts 1 to 2 weeks. Women giving birth to their first child are more susceptible to postpartum dysphoria and may experience it up to 8 weeks postpartum. The more severe condition of postpartum depression occurs in 10 percent of all women after delivery, and it has a greater duration. The onset may occur from 6 weeks to 4 months after delivery and last from 6 months to a year. These women may have any of the following complications: depression, mania, delirium, or psychosis. Postpartum psychosis is a rare condition and is often dangerous. Approximately 2 out of 1,000 new mothers (about 3,500 women each year in the United States) develop postpartum psychosis.[72] (See *Her Story:* "Andrea Yates: Postpartum Depression and Psychosis.")

Typically, pregnancy is associated with a low incidence of psychiatric disorders. But for women with a history of even mild emotional problems, pregnancy and childbirth can result in worsened or new psychiatric disorders, sometimes severe enough to endanger a woman's

Her Story

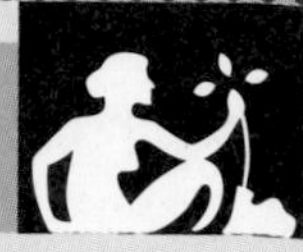

Andrea Yates: Postpartum Depression and Psychosis

On June 20, 2001, 36-year-old Andrea Yates, a Texas mother of five, methodically drowned all of her children, ages 6 months to 7 years. Andrea Yates had been treated for postpartum depression since the birth of her 2-year-old. She had been on medication and had attempted to kill herself in 1999 shortly after childbirth. She cited her reason for attempted suicide as being afraid she would hurt someone. Her depression was compounded by episodes of dissociative thought and psychosis. Even with this emotional instability, her husband insisted she continue to home-school all of the children. Andrea Yates was indicted for murder and pleaded "not guilty by reason of insanity." She was found guilty of murder and sentenced to life in prison. She most likely avoided the death penalty because of her emotional condition.

On January 5, 2005, Yates's murder convictions were overturned because a key witness, who depicted her as knowing right from wrong, had given erroneous testimony. While she waited for her new trial, she stayed in the prison psychiatric ward where she continued to receive treatment. On July 26, 2006, Andrea Yates was found "not guilty by reason of insanity." The ruling was based on the determination that Yates had suffered from severe postpartum psychosis and, in a delusional state, believed Satan was inside her and that she killed her children because she was trying to save them from hell. She was committed to a mental health facility, and mental health experts say she may be there for the rest of her life. Each time she gets better with treatment, she realizes what she did and descends again into a state of severe emotional distress or psychosis.

- Do you think Andrea Yates should be held responsible for the deaths of her children?
- If Ms. Yates became pregnant again, would her future children be at risk?
- What responsibility did Andrea's husband bear for the safety and welfare of his wife and children?
- Should women be assessed for signs of postpartum depression when they receive their 6-week postpartum checkup? What is the role of the medical community in ensuring that women receive proper diagnosis and treatment of postpartum depression?

life or her baby's.[73] Mood changes in pregnancy most often occur in women who are predisposed to emotional problems; the rapidly changing hormonal levels during pregnancy exacerbate the condition. Major elevations of steroid hormones occur during pregnancy, yet in contrast to their effect on mood during the menstrual cycle, these steroid elevations usually do not contribute to severe mood changes during pregnancy. It is thought that a change in gonadal steroid receptors during pregnancy may modify the impact of elevated steroid levels,[74] but further research is required to substantiate this.

Antepartum (before labor) and postpartum (after delivery) depression can be made worse with the presence of major life stressors. Among financially impoverished inner-city women, antepartum depression was found among 27.6 percent and postpartum depression was found among 23.4 percent.[75] These rates were about double those found for middle-class women. African American and European American women did not differ in their rates of depression. The larger incidence of antepartum and postpartum depression in the impoverished inner-city women was most likely due to the stress of their financial plight.

Menopausal Depression The severe hormonal shifts associated with menopause may incite depression. A survey of working, postmenopausal women reported that at least 40 percent of those surveyed faced difficulties in the work environment due to menopausal symptoms, including weight gain, hot flashes, irritability, depression, bloating, and mood changes.[76]

Infertility and Depression Research on the relation of infertility to depression is based on clinical observations and the self-report of women. Infertility patients tend to report feeling damaged, defective, guilty, less attractive, less desirable, and lacking in capability. Almost half of all women seeking assistance at fertility clinics exhibit some symptoms of depression: 40 percent demonstrate moderate symptoms and 7 percent exhibit severe symptoms.[77] Depression in fertile women has been shown to increase when their partners are diagnosed as being infertile. Attempts to become pregnant can give rise to intense mood swings, anxiety, irritability, emotional liability, and depressive symptoms.

Abortion and Depression The emotional impact of abortion is not yet fully understood. Mediating social factors such as the woman's religious beliefs and her family value system may negatively or positively impact postabortion mood. Also, women who have a history of emotional vulnerability may be more susceptible to a melancholic postabortion mood.

The scientific literature does not support the idea that severe guilt and depression often follow from a legal abortion. In fact, the predominant response is one of relief. Guilt and depression, when reported, are typically mild and transitory and do not affect the ability of the woman to function socially. Most women report the greatest distress prior to the abortion. The positive psychological effects of abortion have not been fully assessed, but some studies indicate that women feel more self-directed and more independent and have greater self-efficacy after an abortion.[78]

Do not be fooled by something called "post abortion stress syndrome" (PASS). It sounds scientific, but it is a fictitious condition invented by conservative religious groups to frighten women. There is no clinical evidence to support the existence of PASS, and it is not recognized by any professional medical or mental health organization.

Depression and Genetic Liability

Normal hormonal changes may serve as triggers for psychiatric illness in genetically vulnerable women. Research with female twins determined that there is a genetic liability for the onset of major depression in women who experience stressful events.[79] Thus, the tendency to develop depression may be inherited. Major depressive disorder is 1.5 to 3 times more common among first-degree biological relatives of persons with this disorder than among the general population.

Medication for Depression and Anxiety

The most common medication for the treatment of depression is Prozac (fluoxetine). Similar drugs that are also prescribed for depression include Zoloft (sertraline), Paxil (paroxetine), and Effexor (venlafaxine). All of these drugs work by selectively raising serotonin levels in the brain, the neurotransmitter thought to be most responsible for regulating moods. These drugs are classified as SSRIs, or selective serotonin reuptake inhibitors. They allow serotonin to linger longer in the synaptic cleft (space between neurons) thereby increasing the amount of serotonin available for absorption by receiving neurons along the neuronal pathway. Some 5 million Americans have taken Prozac, and more than 900,000 prescriptions are written every month.[80]

Manic-Depression Manic-depressive disorder, referred to clinically as bipolar disorder, is a condition in which an individual cycles through episodes of mania and depression.[81] During manic episodes the person may exhibit euphoria, irritability, recklessness, and wild or belligerent behavior. During the depressive episodes the person is extremely sad with feelings of hopelessness. Between manic and depressive episodes, individuals can function normally. The disorder typically begins in adolescence or early adulthood and continues throughout a person's life. Manic-depression affects almost 2 million Americans and puts grave stress on a person, which can result in job loss, divorce, or even suicide. Manic-depression is equally common in both women and men (unlike major depressive disorder, which is more common in women). However, in men the first episode is most likely to be a manic episode, whereas in women the first episode is more likely to be a depressive episode.[82]

Manic-depression can be controlled through medication, the most common being lithium carbonate (Eskalith) or lithium citrate (Lithonate).[83] But long-term use can have some negative side effects, such as certain skin conditions (acne, psoriasis, swelling) and hypothyroidism. Hypothyroidism can be controlled by taking supplementary thyroid medications. Lithium use is not recommended during pregnancy as it may cause the child to have malformed heart and blood vessels. Persons who miss the manic-phase emotional rush may not be motivated to take the medication, which tends to flatten affect.

Anxiety Anxiety is the body's natural "fight-or-flight" response gone out of control. (See more about the fight-or-flight response in Chapter 5.) Several broad categories of anxiety disorders are recognized by the psychiatric profession, including generalized anxiety disorder, panic attacks, panic disorder, phobias, obsessive-compulsive disorder, and posttraumatic stress disorder.[84] Generalized anxiety affects about twice as many women as men.[85] About a third of all people who have it eventually recover, although men seem to have a slightly better recovery rate than women. Multiple symptoms may occur during anxiety, including heart palpations, trembling, shaking, sweating, shortness of breath, nervous stomach, tight throat, goose bumps, flushing, dry mouth, dizziness, tightness or pains in the chest, diarrhea, heartburn, and belching. Prolonged anxiety can lead to headaches, sleep problems, and chronic fatigue. Anxiety is treated with antianxiety drugs such as Xanax (alprazolam) and Valium (diazepam), one of the original antianxiety drugs, still prescribed today. Such drugs are most effective when used in conjunction with counseling.

A woman experiencing both anxiety and depression who is taking antianxiety drugs should consult a physician about switching to an antidepressant.[86] The antianxiety drugs are not effective in treating depression and, unlike antidepressants, they can be addictive. (See *Viewpoint:* "Are We Overmedicating but Undertreating Depression and Anxiety?")

Positive Experiences versus Depression

Women who have positive experiences can enhance their self-esteem and decrease depression. Studies confirm a negative relationship between depression and the sense of humor in that as humor increases, depression decreases.[87] Support has been found for a positive relationship between achieving the dream of life success and mental health for midlife women.[88] In addition, women who indicated low self-esteem and a negative evaluation of self showed marked improvements in esteem and self-evaluation over a 7-year period due to positive life changes such as increased quality of personal relationships and work status.[89]

Viewpoint

Are We Overmedicating but Undertreating Depression and Anxiety?

In our fast-paced society there is a tendency for depressed or anxious persons to ask for a quick fix from their physician who too often complies with a prescription for the client's condition without consultation with or referral to a mental health provider. While there exist many effective medications for depression and anxiety, medications treat only the resulting physical symptom and do not affect the initial cause of the depression or anxiety. In other words, much anxiety and depression is a result of experiencing pain and suffering from a negative or traumatic life event. Mental health counseling is the treatment of choice for resolving personal issues and healing emotional wounds created from life experience. Medication in combination with mental health therapy can be very helpful in the early stages of treatment because the medication may allow severely impaired individuals to receive greater benefits from the counseling. However, medication without mental health treatment can actually mask the lingering effects of a psychosocial stressor that needs to be attended and prolong the negative impact of the stressor. For example, a woman who is having anxiety attacks and who has a verbally abusive relationship partner needs mental health treatment, and medication alone will not resolve her discomfort. Or, a woman who feels depressed because her relationship partner cheated on her needs to attend to her feelings of anger and betrayal and resolve the impact of this event on her relationship and her self, and not just try to numb her pain by taking medication. Do you agree that many medications are prescribed for depression and anxiety without an accompanying recommendation for mental health therapy? Do you think that every initial prescription for anxiety and depression should be accompanied by a recommended referral to a mental health provider for at least an evaluation and possible counseling? Do you think there is a tendency to medicate a woman who is depressed or anxious instead of empowering her through mental health therapy?

Developmental Issues and Depression

There are no consistent gender differences in rates of depression among prepubescent children. However by midadolescence, ages 13 to 15, girls show significantly higher rates of depressive disorders and depressive symptoms than boys.[90] Major depressive disorder is twice as common in adolescent and adult females as in adolescent and adult males.[91] Although not overlooking the biological differences of males and females that become more prevalent during adolescence, additional possible explanations for the emerging differences in the rates of depression exist. First, girls enter early adolescence responding to frustration and distress with a style that is less effective and action-oriented than boys. Second, girls begin to face uncontrollable stressors in early adolescence to a greater extent than boys.[92] Data suggest that girls exhibit more passive and introspective coping styles, which are associated with longer and more severe depressive symptoms; girls undergo biological changes that are less favored by society, and girls and women face more negative life events and social conditions such as sexual abuse and stronger parental and peer expectations.

The most likely age for women to develop depression is in their 20s and 30s.[93] However, a woman in her mid-40s and 50s is also vulnerable to the onset of depression. It is not yet clear whether menopause in midlife by itself predisposes women to depression, but many major life events that occur around this time of life may contribute to depression. Facing the social stigma that devalues the worth and beauty of middle-aged and older women can also be demoralizing. Older women, in their 60s and beyond, face increased medical problems and concern over the limited number of years left in their life. Their physical condition may put limitations on their activity level, and many friends and family have died. These issues can contribute to feelings of depression for the older woman.

Family of Origin Issues and Depression

Many research studies demonstrate the influence of familial factors on depression, especially for persons who have experienced adverse or threatening life events. Chronic depression in women has been associated with family of origin experiences reflecting severe losses, including neglect, rejection, abandonment, and physical, sexual and emotional abuse.[94] Persons who came from a loving family but still developed depression have reported they lacked an empathic caretaker who could soothe emotional reactions to traumatic losses during critical periods of childhood.[95] Research suggests that "chronically depressed women have often adapted as best they could to an environment that discouraged appropriate mourning by assuming a cognitive-emotional mask, unconsciously defending themselves against expressing or even experiencing the painful emotions generated by their losses. As a result, unresolved mourning typically lies at the root of long-term depressive patterns, especially for women who adapted to their unfortunate childhood circumstances by using a placating approach to secure relationship with significant others."[96] In other words, many women who develop depression did not have the emotional support in childhood necessary to cope effectively with trauma and traumatic loss. Parents may have discouraged and suppressed emotional expression by family members and even encouraged masking and denial of negative emotions thereby leaving significant emotional wounds unattended. Motivations for parents to suppress emotional expression by family members range from a need to keep family "secrets" (such as incest, child abuse, domestic violence, alcoholism/drug abuse) to a simple desire to present the family image to the community in the most favorable light.

Multicultural Issues of Depression and Suicide

African American women may experience racism as an additional stressor that may contribute to depression. Female status, lower social class, and downward social mobility are all related to greater depression.[97] Racism itself can be a factor in whether a black woman is properly diagnosed with or treated for depression. Black female psychiatric patients were diagnosed with depression at a rate 42 percent higher than that of white women, and more black women were more likely to receive drug therapy than white women. It is unclear whether this reflects a discriminatory attitude or is an accurate reflection of the condition of these patients.

Hispanic women and Latinas in the United States may experience economic deprivation, migration, and political discrimination as risk factors for depression. Hispanic women who experienced discrimination, gender-role conflicts, and concern about starting a family in a preceding 3-month period had significantly higher rates of depression than Hispanic women who did not experience these circumstances.[98] Also, many migrant Hispanic women experience gender-role conflicts within their own traditionally male-dominated culture.

Some Asian women have an economic situation as favorable as that of white women in the United States, but immigrant women who had completed eight or fewer years of education were at a high risk for racial and social discrimination.[99] This was most common in immigrant women from Vietnam, China, Guam, the Philippines, Samoa, and Korea. Gender-related risk factors such as low self-esteem are significant problems for many Asian women and may contribute to depression.

Native American women (including Alaskan Natives) are among the least visible and least researched groups in the United States. Compared with other U.S. women, the death rate for Native American women is six times higher for alcoholism (ten times higher for ages 25–45), five times higher for cirrhosis and liver diseases, three times higher for homicide, three times higher for accidental death (for ages 15–54), and three times higher for motor vehicle accidents.[100] In addition, suicide is twice as high among Native American women than among the general U.S. population. Risk factors associated with depression for Native Americans include poverty, lack of education, and larger numbers of children.

Low parental support is a significant predictor for adolescent depression as is low self-esteem; low levels of attachment to either parents or peers, or both; underinvolved parents or authoritarian parents; and depressed parents.[101] An unstable family life was a major factor in 50 to 80 percent of all adolescent suicides. Rates of adolescent suicide have been on the rise and have tripled since the 1950s. Lesbian and gay youth are two to three times more likely to commit suicide than other youths, and 30 percent of all completed youth suicides are related to the issue of sexual identity.[102] The single largest predictor of mental health in this group was self-acceptance. A general sense of self-worth, with a positive view of their sexual orientation, appears to be critical for good mental health.

More men than women die by suicide with a ratio of 4:1 (males:females). More women than men report a history of attempted suicide, with a gender ratio of 3:1 (females:males). The strongest risk factors for attempted suicide in adults are depression, alcohol abuse, cocaine use, and separation or divorce. The strongest risk factors for attempted suicide in youth are depression, alcohol or other drug abuse, and aggressive or disruptive behaviors. (See Table 4.1.)

In the *World Health Report 2001,* the WHO examined suicide trends across the globe for the past 20 years. These rates vary considerably. For example, suicide rates are up in Mexico, India, Brazil, and Russia, but down in the United States, Japan, and China. It is very difficult, if not impossible, to find a common explanation for this variation. However, alcohol consumption and easy access to firearms seem to be positively correlated with suicide across all industrialized and developing countries. (See *FYI:* "International Approaches to Suicide Prevention.")

For women who are beaten or sexually assaulted, the emotional and physical strain can lead to suicide. The WHO research suggests that abused women endure enormous psychological suffering because of violence. Many are severely depressed and display symptoms of posttraumatic stress disorder. They may be chronically fatigued but unable to sleep; they may have nightmares and use alcohol and drugs to numb their pain; or they may become isolated and withdrawn. In one study in Leon, Nicaragua, researchers found that abused women were six times more likely to be diagnosed with mental distress than were nonabused women. Likewise, in the United States women battered by their partners have been found to be between four and five times more likely to be depressed than are nonabused women.

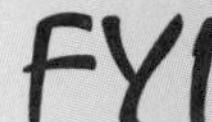

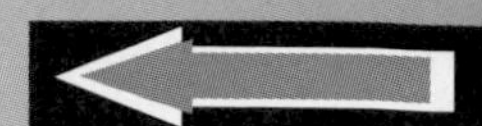

International Approaches to Suicide Prevention

In *World Health Report, 2001,* the WHO reports two different national approaches to suicide prevention.

Finland

Between 1950 and 1980, suicide rates in Finland increased by almost 50 percent among men and doubled among women. The government launched a comprehensive suicide prevention campaign in 1986 and, by 1996, had achieved an overall reduction in suicide rates of 17.5 percent. More than 100,000 health and mental health professionals participated in the national suicide prevention effort.

India

In 1997 more than 95,000 persons in India killed themselves (that is, one suicide every 6 minutes). One in every three was in the 15 to 29 year age group. India has no national policy or program for suicide prevention. In response to the growing suicide problem, a voluntary charitable organization was formed. Sneha is affiliated with Befrienders International, an organization that provides "listening therapy" with human contact and emotional support. Sneha has helped establish ten centers in various parts of India and is helping to set up the first survivor support groups in India.

THE COUNSELING OPTION

There might be times in your life when you or someone you know needs counseling to assist with a mental or emotional concern. A mental health counselor

TABLE 4.1 Suicide Rankings for U.S. Females in the Year 2002

This table is a list of the rankings for suicide as a leading cause of death for females by age and race with a percent of total deaths that suicide accounts for as reported by the U.S. Centers for Disease Control, National Center for Health Statistics.

ALL RACES		WHITE		BLACK		ASIAN/PACIFIC ISLANDER		AMERICAN INDIAN	
All ages	%	All ages	%	All ages	%	All ages	%	All ages	%
Not in top 15	—	Not in top 15	—	Not in top 15	—	Twelfth	1.1	Thirteenth	1.2
1–4 yrs	%	1–4 yrs.	%	1–4 yrs.	%	1–4 yrs.	%	1–4 yrs.	%
Not in top 15	—	Not in top 15	—	Not in top 15	—	Not in top 15	—	Not in top 15	—
5–14 yrs.	%	5–14 yrs.	%	5–14 yrs.	%	5–14 yrs.	%	5–14 yrs.	%
Sixth	2.2	Sixth	2.6	Fourteenth	0.9	Sixth (tied)	2.2	Fifth (tied)	3.3
15–24 yrs.	%	15–24 yrs.	%	15–24 yrs.	%	15–24 yrs.	%	15–24 yrs	%
Fourth	6.7	Third	7.4	Sixth	3.1	Fourth	8.5	Second	12.0
25–34 yrs.	%	25–34 yrs.	%	25–34 yrs.	%	25–34 yrs.	%	25–34 yrs.	%
Fourth	7.2	Third	9.2	Tenth	1.7	Third	12.5	Fifth	5.1
35–44 yrs.	%	35–44 yrs.	%	35–44 yrs.	%	35–44 yrs.	%	35–44 yrs.	%
Fourth	4.6	Fourth	5.8	Thirteenth	1.0	Fifth	6.0	Sixth	3.8
45–54 yrs.	%	45–54 yrs.	%	45–54 yrs.	%	45–54 yrs.	%	45–54 yrs.	%
Eighth	2.3	Seventh	2.9	Not in top 15	—	Fifth	2.5	Seventh	2.4
55–64 yrs.	%	55–64 yrs.	%	55–64 yrs.	%	55–64 yrs.	%	55–64 yrs.	%
Eleventh	0.8	Eleventh	0.9	Not in top 15	—	Tenth (tied)	1.0	Not in top 15	—
65–74 yrs.	%	65–74 yrs.	%	65–74 yrs.	%	65–74 yrs.	%	65–74 yrs.	%
Not in top 15	—	Not in top 15	—	Not in top 15	—	Fourteenth	0.6	Not in top 15	—
75–84 yrs.	%	75–84 yrs.	%	75–84 yrs.	%	75–84 yrs.	%	75–84 yrs.	%
Not in top 15	—	Not in top 15	—	Not in top 15	—	Not in top 15	—	Not in top 15	—
85+ yrs.	%	85+ yrs.	%	85+ yrs.	%	85+ yrs.	%	85+ yrs.	%
Not in top 15	—	Not in top 15	—	Not in top 15	—	Not in top 15	—	Not in top 15	—

can be very effective at facilitating the recovery process either through therapy or by recommending available resources.

The therapeutic orientation of the counselor may make no difference in how effective the counselor is with a client; however, one therapeutic orientation is designed specifically to assist women. **Feminist therapy,** also referred to as gender equity therapy, empowers women through an egalitarian (equity-based) relationship with the therapist. Women are so frequently abused, attacked, or discriminated against in society that their self-concept and sense of self-worth may be depleted. Feminist therapy assists in rebuilding and reinforcing a woman's inner strength and ability to survive, overcome, and succeed in the face of emotional burdens.

Feminist therapists often respond to a client's issues or problems by understanding the impact of societal gender-role expectations on the client. Feminist theory examines issues such as how men and women are similar and different in their moral decision making, the way they relate to others, and how they contribute to and confront abuse and violence.[103]

When looking for a mental health professional, it is wise to get a referral from someone who has knowledge about the capabilities and expertise of a particular counselor that might be helpful for you. This referral might come from a family member, a friend, a physician, a teacher, or a spiritual counselor. If a referral is not possible, the telephone yellow pages can suggest several possibilities, though the expertise and training of a counselor cannot be guaranteed this way.

In setting up your first appointment, feel free to interview the counselor before agreeing to enter into the therapeutic relationship. This is usually done over the telephone before meeting in person. Inquire about his or her educational background, professional training, experience, professional credentials, and approach to counseling. You have a right to know about the training, credentials, and counseling approach of any counselor that you are considering.

Mental health providers are required by most states to be licensed or certified by a health board in order to practice counseling. In addition, counselors who have been found guilty of a breach of ethics or illegal acts risk losing their license to practice. These controls and standards are in existence to help protect the consumer from abuse, neglect, and sexual or other exploitation by their therapist. Not all states require that counselors be licensed or certified by a state health board. Thus, it is especially important to explore the background and training of a counselor who is not credentialed by a state licensing or certification board.

EMOTIONS AND HEALTH

Sometimes people talk about good emotions and bad emotions, or healthy emotions and unhealthy emotions. However, it is not the emotion itself that is good or bad, nor is it necessarily the emotion that is healthy or unhealthy. Emotions are natural states that result from the perceived impact of an event or the memory of an event. Emotions serve as guideposts to help you understand just what kind of an impact something has on you. Emotions are designed to direct your behavior for life development and life survival. It is the choice of behavior that follows an emotion that can be judged as good or bad, appropriate or inappropriate, or healthy or unhealthy.

Keeping your emotions pinned up inside you can be very detrimental to your health. Suppressing your feelings can cause escalating tension in the body. Releasing your feelings and thoughts on a regular basis by talking to someone, laughing, or crying can help relieve the pressure that is building inside you. Without regular release, the pressure can rise to the point where you explode, and you say or do things that are harmful to yourself or to others.

Confiding in others appears to protect the body against damaging internal stresses and seems to have long-term health benefits.[104] Whenever possible, confide in friends or family members whom you trust. When this is not sufficient to get you through a stressful time, seek out the services of a professional mental health provider. What you feel and think is important, and sharing your feelings and thoughts with someone else in confidence can be good for you.

CONCLUSION

Life is a challenge and it helps to have guidance from significant others, teachers, and role models. It also helps to have life skills that help you to cope with the demands that life presents. The greater the personal support system you have and the more life skills you learn and practice, then the higher the likelihood that more of your emotions will be happy ones instead of sad ones, or that the sad ones that you do have will not linger as long. However, remember that emotional health is not determined by how many happy feelings you have versus how many sad feelings. Both happy and sad feelings are normal and natural responses to life's challenges. If you have a good support system and well-developed life skills, the many challenges that life presents can be more enjoyable and perhaps less harsh than they otherwise would be.

Chapter Summary

- Being aware of the various social influences that impact your development can enhance your potential life satisfaction.
- Assertiveness training is a life skill that can enhance self-confidence and result in improvements in relationships and performance.
- Effective listening is required to facilitate healthy communication.
- When conflicts or problems arise, effective problem solving is a useful tool to reach resolution. This involves a step-by-step process: defining the problem, generating solutions, evaluating solutions, making a decision, and implementing the decision.
- Building and maintaining a positive self-image is paramount to feeling good about yourself and achieving successes.
- Similar to self-image, self-esteem involves being realistic about who you think you should be, and loving and accepting who you already are.
- The journey through life will include the loss of loved ones along the way. The grief process is a normal response to loss.
- When life's challenges become too great, depression may arise. If you feel lost and alone, you need to reach out to others for support.
- Sometimes seeking out personal therapy is necessary to facilitate growth when you feel stuck in an uncomfortable emotional state.

Review Questions

1. Can you briefly describe the primary premise of self-in-relation theory, also known as gender-relations theory?
2. What are some of the social and cultural influences that can impact the development of the self?
3. What are some situations in which one may need to be assertive?
4. What are the six basic types of assertive messages? Give examples.
5. What are the basic components of effective listening? Give examples.
6. What are some misconceptions about conflict and problem solving?
7. What are the six basic steps to problem solving? Can you describe what is involved with each of these steps?
8. What is a key element to building and maintaining self-image?
9. What are three types of eating disorders?
10. Can you define self-esteem?
11. What is the process of self-esteem enhancement?
12. What are the three phases of mourning and the five stages of the grief process?
13. Can you name and describe the various types of depression?
14. What are some common predictors of suicide?
15. Can you describe the focus of feminist therapy?

Resources

Web Sites

American Association for Marriage and Family Therapy
www.aamft.org

American Counseling Association
www.counseling.org

American Psychiatric Association
www.psych.org

American Psychological Association
www.apa.org

Eating Disorders Resource Catalog
www.gurze.com

National Eating Disorders Association
www.nationaleatingdisorders.org

National Institute of Mental Health
www.nimh.nih.gov

Mental Health America
www.nmha.org

Screening for Mental Health
www.mentalhealthscreening.org

World Psychiatric Association
www.wpanet.org

Videotapes/DVDs

Anger Management for Parents (1995)
Facing Death (1995)
A Family in Grief (1995)
Learning to Manage Anger: The Rethink Workout for Teens (1995)
The Practical Parenting Series (1995)
Research Press, Champaign, IL, Phone: 217-352-3273.
The Brain: Inside Information: The Brain and How It Works
Exploring Your Brain: The Brain Body Connection
Films for the Humanities & Sciences, Box 2053, Princeton, NJ 08543-2053. Phone: 800-257-5126, Website: http://www.films.com

Killing Us Softly 3: Advertising's Image of Women
Recovering Bodies: Overcoming Eating Disorders
Sexual Harassment: Building Awareness on Campus
Slim Hopes: Advertising and the Obsession with Thinness
Media Education Foundation, 26 Center Street, Northampton, MA 01060. Phone: 800-897-0089, Website: www.mediaed.org

Suggested Readings

Ahrons, C. 1994. *The Good Divorce.* Philadelphia: Harp.

Alberti, R. 1994. *Making Yourself Heard: A Guide to Assertive Relationships.* Obispo, CA: Impact.

Anderson, P. 1991. *Affairs in Order: A Complete Resource Guide to Death and Dying.* New York: Macmillan.

Bass, E. and L. Davis, 1994. *The Courage to Heal: A Guide for Women Survivors of Child Sexual Abuse.* 3rd ed. New York: HarperCollins.

Benziger, K. 1992. *Overcoming Depression: A Self-Help Workbook.* Westminster, CA: KBA.

Burns, D. 1993. *Ten Days to Self-Esteem!* New York: Morrow.

Butler, P. 1992. *Self-Assertion for Women.* San Francisco: HarperCollins.

Cash, T. F. 1997. *The Body Image Workbook: An 8-Step Program for Learning to Like Your Looks.* Oakland, CA: New Harbinger.

Copeland, M. E. 2001. *The Depression Workbook: A Guide for Living with Depression and Manic Depression.* 2nd ed. Oakland, CA: New Harbinger.

Courtois, C. A. 1996 *Healing the Incest Wound: Adult Survivors' Therapy.* New York: W. W. Norton.

Deits, B. 1992. *Life after Loss: A Personal Guide Dealing with Death, Divorce, Job Change and Relocation.* Tuscon, AZ: Fisher Books.

DeSpelder, L. A. and A. L. Strickland. 2005. *The Last Dance: Encountering Death and Dying.* 7th ed. New York: McGraw-Hill.

Fay, A. 1994. *Prescription for a Quality Relationship.* Obispo, CA: Impact.

Fisher, B. 1992. *Rebuilding When Your Relationship Ends.* Obispo, CA: Impact.

Freeman, S. J. 2005. *Grief and Loss: Understanding the Journey.* Belmont, CA: Wordsworth.

Hecker, L., and S. Deacon. 1998. *The Therapist Notebook: Homework, Handouts, and Activities for Use in Psychotherapy.* New York: Haworth Press.

Hundley, M. 1993. *Awaken to Good Mourning.* Arlington, TX: Crocker Associates.

James, M., and D. Jongeward, 1996. *Born to Win.* Cambridge, MA: Da Capo Press.

Lazarus, A., C. Lazarus, and A. Fay. 1993. *Don't Believe It for a Minute: Forty Toxic Ideas That Are Driving You Crazy.* Obispo, CA: Impact.

Ledray, L. E. 1994. *Recovering from Rape.* New York: Henry Holt.

Matsakis, A. 2003. *The Rape Recovery Handbook: Step-by-Step Help for Survivors of Sexual Assault.* Oakland, CA: New Harbinger.

McKay, G., and D. Dinkmeyer. 1994. *How You Feel Is Up to You: The Power of Emotional Choice.* Obispo, CA: Impact.

Neeld, E. 1990. *Seven Choices: Taking the Steps to New Life after Losing Someone You Love.* New York: Clarkson N. Potter.

Newman, L. 1991. *Somebody to Love: A Guide to Loving the Body You Have.* Chicago: Third Side Press.

Palmer, P. 1994. *I Wish I Could Hold Your Hand: A Child's Guide to Grief and Loss.* Obispo, CA: Impact.

Preston, J. 1989. *You Can Beat Depression: A Guide to Recovery.* Obispo, CA: Impact.

Preston, J. 1993. *Growing beyond Emotional Pain: Action Plans for Healing.* Obispo, CA: Impact.

Smead, R. 2000. *Skills for Living: Group Counseling Activities for Young Adolescents.* Champaign, IL: Research Press.

Zerbe, K. 1995. *The Body Betrayed: A Deeper Understanding of Women, Eating Disorders, and Treatment.* Carlsbad, CA: Gurze Books.

References

1. Gilligan, C. 1979. Women's place in man's life cycle *Harvard Educational Review* 49 (4): 431–46
2. Gilligan, C. 1982. *In a different voice: Psychological theory and women's development.* Cambridge, MA: Harvard University Press.
3. Ibid.
4. Ibid.
5. Ibid.
6. Jordan, J. (Ed.) 1977. *Women's growth in diversity,* New York: Guilford.
7. Ibid., pp. 24–30.
8. Ibid., pp. 24–30.
9. Lange, J., and P. Jakubowski. 1976. *Responsible assertive behavior.* Champaign, IL: Research Press, pp. 7, 218–20.
10. Harrington, M. 1995. Who has it best? Women's labor force participation, perceptions of leisure and constraints to enjoyment of leisure. *Journal of Leisure Research* 27 (1): 4–24.
11. Hart, L., and L. Silka. 1994. Building self-efficacy through women-centered ropes course experiences. Special issue: Wilderness therapy for women: The power of adventure. *Women and Therapy* 15 (3–4): 111–27; Aubrey, A., and M. MacLeod. 1994. So . . . What does rock climbing have to do with career planning? Special Issue: Wilderness therapy for women: The power of adventure. *Women and Therapy* 15 (3–4): 205–16.
12. Lange and Jakubowski, *Responsible assertive behavior.*
13. Keisling, B., and M. Gynther. 1993. Male perceptions of female attractiveness: The effects of targets' personal attributes and subjects' degree of masculinity. *Journal of Clinical Psychology* 49 (2): 190–95.
14. Dillard, J., and R. Reilly. 1988. *Systematic interviewing: Communication skills for professional effectiveness.* Columbus, OH: Merrill.
15. Jakubowski, P., and A. Lange. 1978. *The assertive option.* Champaign, IL: Research Press, pp. 157–69.
16. Jakubowski and Lange, *The assertive option.*
17. Gordon, J. 1974. *Teacher effectiveness training.* New York: Wyden Books.
18. Sanford, L., and M. Donovan. 1988. *Women and self-esteem: Understanding and improving the way we think and feel about ourselves.* New York: Penguin, pp. 97, 101.
19. Miller, L., L. Cooke, J. Tsang, and F. Morgan. 1992. Should I brag? Nature and impact of positive and boastful disclosures for women and men. *Human Communication Research* 18 (3): 364–99.

20. Woods, N., M. Lentz, E. Mitchell, and L. Oakley. 1994. Depressed mood and self-esteem in young Asian, black, and white women in America. *Health Care for Women International* 15 (3): 243–62.
21. American Psychiatric Association. 2000. *Diagnostic and statistical manual of mental disorders.* 4th ed. text revision *(DSM-IV-TR).* Washington, DC: APA.
22. American Movie Channel (AMC). *The Hollywood fashion machine.* AMC television broadcast March 2, 1996.
23. Ibid.
24. Kilborne, J. 1995. *Slim hopes: Advertising and obsession with thinness.* Video. Northampton, MA: Media Education Foundation.
25. Cohen, B. 1986. *The snowhite syndrome.* New York: Macmillan; Wolf, N. 1991. *The beauty myth.* New York: Anchor/Doubleday; Fallon, A. 1990. Culture in the mirror: Sociocultural determinants of body image. In T. Cash and T. Pruzinsky, *Body images: Development, deviance and change.* New York: Guilford.
26. Zimmerman, J. 1997. An image to heal. *Humanist* 57 (January/February) (1): 20.
27. Lee, A., and S. Lee. 1996. Disordered eating and its psychosocial correlates among Chinese adolescent females in Hong Kong. *International Journal of Eating Disorders* 20 (2): 177–83; Ben-Tovim, D. 1996. Is big still beautiful in Polynesia? *Lancet* 348: 1047–48.
28. Akan, G., and C. Gril. 1995. Sociocultural influences on eating attitudes and behaviors, body image, and psychological functioning: A comparison of African-American, Asian-American, and Caucasian college women. *International Journal of Eating Disorders* 18 (2): 181–87.
29. Furnham, A., and N. Greaves. 1994. Gender and locus of control correlates of body image dissatisfaction. *European Journal of Personality* 8 (3): 183–200.
30. Koff, E., J. Rierdan, and M. Stubbs. 1990. Gender, body image, and self-concept in early adolescence. *Journal of Early Adolescence* 10 (1): 56–68.
31. Probst, M., W. Vandereycken, H. Van Coppenolle, and G. Pieter. 1995. Body size estimation in eating disorder patients: Testing the video distortion method on a life-size screen. *Behaviour Therapy and Research* 33 (8): 985–90.
32. National Eating Disorders Association. 2006. 19th Annual National Eating Disorders Awareness Week, 2006. www.nationaleatingdisorders.org (retrieved March 15, 2006).
33. Carlson, K. J., S. A. Eisenstat, and T. Ziporyn. 1997. *The women's concise guide to emotional well-being.* Cambridge, MA: Harvard University Press.
34. Ibid.
35. Ibid.
36. Ibid.
37. Ibid.
38. Wolfelt, A. D. 1997. *The journey through grief: Reflections on healing.* Fort Collins, CO: Center for Loss and Life Transition.
39. Kalodner, C. R., and J. L. Delucia-Waack, 2003. Theory and research on eating disorders and disturbances in women. In M. Kopala and M. Keitel (eds.), *Handbook of counseling women,* pp. 506–32. Thousand Oaks, CA: Sage.
40. Hundley, M. 1993. *Awaken to good mourning.* Arlington, TX: Crocker Associates, p. 83.
41. Ibid.
42. Kübler-Ross, E. 1969. *On death and dying.* New York: Macmillan.
43. APA, *Diagnostic and statistical manual of mental disorders.*
44. Korenstein, S. G., and B. A. Wojcik, 2002. Depression. In S. G. Kornstein and A. H. Clayton (eds.), *Women's mental health: A comprehensive textbook,* pp. 147–165. New York: Guilford.
45. Wells, M., C. J. Brack, and P. J. McMichen, 2003. Women and depressive disorders. In M. Kopala and M. Keitel (eds.), *Handbook of counseling women,* pp. 429–457. Thousand Oaks, CA: Sage.
46. Gotlib, I. H., and C. L. Hammen, eds. 2002. *Handbook of depression.* New York: Guilford.
47. APA, *Diagnostic and statistical manual of mental disorders.*
48. Nolen-Hoeksema, S. 1990. *Sex differences in depression.* Stanford, CA: Stanford University Press.
49. APA, *Diagnostic and statistical manual of mental disorders.*
50. Furnham, A., and N. Greaves. 1994. Gender and locus of control correlates of body image dissatisfaction. *European Journal of Personality* 8 (3): 183–200.
51. Downey, G. and J. C. Coyne. 1990. Children of depressed parents: An investigative review. *Psychological Bulletin,* 108: 50–76.
52. Brown, G. W., and P. M. Moran. 1997. Single mothers, poverty, and depression. *Psychological Medicine,* 27: 21–33.
53. Goodman, S. H. 2002. Depression and early adverse experiences. In I. H. Gotlib and C. L. Hammen (eds.), *Handbook of depression,* pp. 245–67. New York: Guilford.
54. Kendler, K. S., R. C. Kessler, M. C. Neale, A. C. Heath, et al. 1993. The prediction of major depression in women: Toward an integrated etiologic model. *American Journal of Psychiatry* 150: 1139–48.
55. Mazure, C. M., M. L. Bruce, P. K. Maciejewski, and S. C. Jacobs. 2000. Adverse life events and cognitive-personality characteristics in the prediction of major depression and antidepressant response. *American Journal of Psychiatry* 157: 896–903.
56. Maciejewski, P. K., H. G. Prigerson, and C. M. Mazure. 2001. Sex differences in event-related risk for major depression. *Psychological Medicine* 31: 593–604.
57. Brown, G., T. Harris, and C. Hepworth. 1995. Loss, humiliation and entrapment among women developing depression: A patient and non-patient comparison. *Psychological Medicine* 25 (1): 7–21.
58. Golding, J. M. 1999. Intimate partner violence as risk factor for mental disorders: A meta-analysis. *Journal of Family Violence* 14: 99–132.
59. Nolen-Hoeksema, S. 2000. The role of rumination in depressive disorders and mixed anxiety/depressive symptoms. *Journal of Abnormal Psychology* 109: 504–11.
60. Weiss, E. L., J. G. Longhurst, and C. M. Mazure. 1999. Childhood sexual abuse as a risk factor for depression in women: Psychosocial and neurobiological correlates. *American Journal of Psychiatry* 156: 816–28.
61. Fox, K., and B. Gilbert. 1994. The interpersonal and psychological functioning of women who experienced

childhood physical abuse, incest, and parental alcoholism. *Child Abuse and Neglect* 18 (10): 849–58.
62. Andrews, B. 1995. Bodily shame as a mediator between abusive experiences and depression. *Journal of Abnormal Psychology* 104 (2): 277–85.
63. Silvern, L., J. Karyl, L. Waelde, and W. Hodges. 1995. Retrospective reports of parental partner abuse: Relationships to depression, trauma symptoms and self-esteem among college students. *Journal of Family Violence* 10 (2): 177–202.
64. McGrath, E., G. P. Keita, B. R. Strickland, and N. F. Russo. (Eds.). 1993. *Women and depression: Risk factors and treatment issues.* Washington, DC: American Psychological Association.
65. Parry, B. L. 2000. Hormonal basis of mood disorders in women. In E. Frank (ed.), *Gender and its effects on psychopathology,* pp. 61–84. Washington, DC: American Psychiatric Press.
66. Young, E. A., A. Korszun, and M. Altemus. 2002. Sex differences in neuroendocrine and neurotransmitter systems. In S. G. Kornstein and A. H. Clayton (eds.), *Women's mental health: A comprehensive textbook*, pp. 3–30. New York: Guilford.
67. Nolen-Hoeksema, S. 2002. Gender differences in depression. In I. H. Gotlib and C. L. Hammen (eds.), *Handbook of depression,* 492–509. New York: Guilford.
68. Burt, V. K., and K. Stein, 2002. Epidemiology of depression throughout the female life cycle. *Journal of Clinical Psychiatry* 63, 9–15.
69. APA, *Diagnostic and statistical manual of mental disorders.*
70. McGrath et al., *Women and depression.*
71. Ibid.
72. Carlson et al., *The women's concise guide to emotional well-being.*
73. Ibid.
74. McGrath et al., *Women and depression.*
75. Hobfoll, M., C. Ritter, J. Lavin, M. Hulsizer, et al. 1995. Depression prevalence and incidence among inner-city pregnant and postpartum women. *Journal of Consulting and Clinical Psychology* 63 (3): 445–53.
76. High, R., and P. Marcellino. 1994. Menopausal women and the work environment. *Social Behavior and Personality* 22 (4): 347–53.
77. McGrath et al., *Women and depression.*
78. Ibid.
79. Kendler, K., R. Kessler, E. Walters, and C. MacLean. 1995. Stressful life events, genetic liability, and onset of an episode of major depression in women. *American Journal of Psychiatry* 152 (6): 833–42.
80. Carlson et al. *The women's concise guide to emotional well-being.*
81. Ibid.
82. APA, *The diagnostic and statistical manual of mental disorders.*
83. Carlson et al., *The women's concise guide to emotional well-being.*
84. APA, *The diagnostic and statistical manual of mental disorders.*
85. Carlson et al., *The women's concise guide to emotional well-being.*
86. Ibid.
87. Thorson, J., and F. Powell. 1994. Depression and sense of humor. *Psychological Reports* 73 (3): 1473–74.
88. Drebing, C., W. Gooden, S. Drebing, and H. Van de Kemp. 1995. The dream in mid-life women: Its impact on mental health. *International Journal of Aging and Human Development* 40 (1): 73–87.
89. Andrews, B., and G. Brown. 1995. Stability and change in low self-esteem: The role of psychosocial factors. *Psychological Medicine* 25 (1): 23–31.
90. Nolen-Hoeksema, S. 1994. An interactive model for the emergence of gender differences in depression in adolescence. *Journal of Research on Adolescence* 4 (4): 519–34.
91. APA, *Diagnostic and statistical manual of mental disorders.*
92. Nolen-Hoeksema, An interactive model for the emergence of gender differences in depression in adolescence.
93. Carlson et al., *The women's concise guide to emotional well-being.*
94. Wells, Brack, and McMichen. *Women and depressive disorders.*
95. McWilliams, N. 1994. *Psychoanalytic diagnosis: Understanding personality structure in the clinical process.* New York: Guilford.
96. Wells, Brack, and McMichen, *Women and depressive disorders,* pp. 433–434.
97. McGrath et al., *Women and depression.*
98. Ibid.
99. Ibid.
100. Ibid.
101. Ibid.
102. Gibson, P. 1989. Gay male and lesbian youth suicide. In *Prevention and intervention in youth suicide* (Report to the Secretary's Task Force on Youth Suicide), M. Feinleib, ed. (vol. 3, pp. 110–42). Washington, DC: U.S. Department of Health and Human Services.
103. Sharf, R. S. 2006. Feminist therapy. In *Theories of psychotherapy and counseling,* 3rd ed. Albany, NY: Brooks/Cole.
104. Pennebaker, J. 1990. *Opening up: The healing power of confiding in others.* New York: William Morrow.

Chapter five

Managing the Stress of Life

CHAPTER OBJECTIVES

When you complete this chapter, you will be able to do the following:

- Describe the anatomy and physiology of stress
- Identify the warning signs of too much stress
- Summarize the different types of life stressors
- Describe the impact of stress on women
- Demonstrate effective coping strategies for stress management

CONCEPTS OF STRESS

You, like most people, have a lifestyle that, in one way or another, and at some time or another, can create stress in your life. **Stress** is the body's response to demands. A **stressor** is the demand itself. Such demands can include everyday life events such as getting up, going to work or school, being at work or school, rushing home to fix dinner, dashing off to play a quick game of tennis, spending time with the family in the evening, and catching up on work at home before going to bed at night. Stress is not something you can ever completely get away from; however, it is something you can learn to understand and to manage. Figure 5.1 identifies the types of stressors we encounter.

Stress and Perception

The way in which you might respond to an event depends greatly on how you may perceive that event. Perceptions can vary greatly from person to person. Perceptions can be impacted by immediate potential consequences and by a cumulation of life experiences. For example, students who must take a final exam may each have different stress responses to the event depending on their own expectations of self and/or the value of the event.

Where do the expectations you place on yourself and on others come from? Many psychologists believe that expectations come from your social environment—the messages you receive from your family, friends, and society that you integrate into your own belief and value system. These expectations can be less than, equal to, or exceed the demand of a particular situation. If your expectations of yourself are at a certain criterion for performance and you do not meet that criterion, then you will probably be greatly bothered by this failure. The level at which you set the criteria for success is going to affect how much stress you experience in trying to meet or surpass that goal. Having realistic expectations of yourself is important in managing your stress level.

Look outside of yourself and beyond family members by examining the goals and ambitions of your peers and healthy role models. This will help you determine what

FIGURE 5.1 Types of stressors.[1]

Stressors can be grouped into five categories

- Social stressors—noise, crowding, etc.
- Psychological stressors—anxiety, worry, etc.
- Psychosocial stressors—loss of a job, death of a family member, spouse, or friend, etc.
- Biochemical stressors—heat, cold, injury, pollutants, poor nutrition, etc.
- Philosophical stressors—value system conflict, lack of purpose, lack of direction, etc.

is realistic and what is not. This is not meant to imply that you should not strive toward excellence; instead, you should choose specific areas to excel in. Trying to excel in every area of life is too stressful and exhausting.

In some situations, some amount of stress is necessary to motivate you to perform and strive to do your best. Too little stress, as well as too much stress, can impede performance. A moderate amount of stress can drive you to try harder and to improve your current abilities. If you want to win the sports tournament or a grand prize at the state fair, then you have to work hard. Hard work involves stress.

The same kind of sensitivity to being realistic and self-aware may direct you to adjust the demands of a situation to your preferred stress level. Imagine that you were asked to perform the following tasks within the next week: write a professional paper, prepare a major presentation, have ten appointments, attend a wedding, and play in an all-weekend tennis tournament. How are you going to accomplish all of these tasks and still find time to do daily home chores, exercise, eat nutritionally, and find time to relax, much less sleep? It would be difficult to maintain this kind of schedule and expect to stay healthy for very long. In addition, you may not enjoy this high of a demand level; it may create much more stress in your life than you prefer. You might need to prioritize events and exercise assertiveness by saying "no" to some demands or by renegotiating completion dates. In addition, you might recruit some assistance for those tasks that you cannot complete alone within a realistic time span. We examine stress and time management strategies later in the chapter.

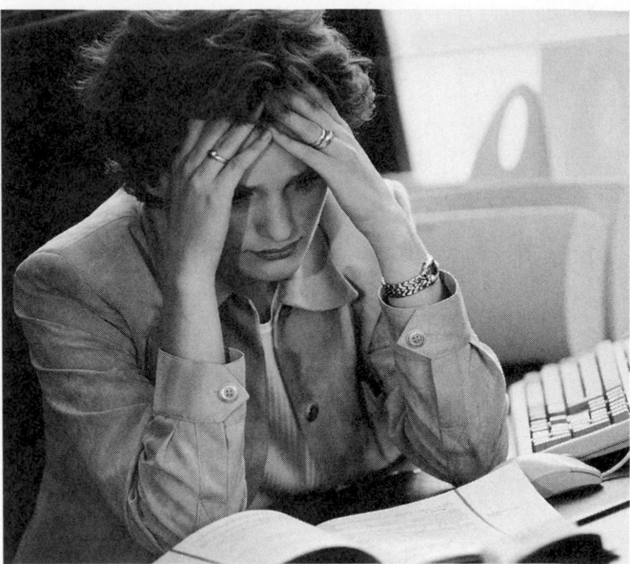

Too much to do and too little time to do it.

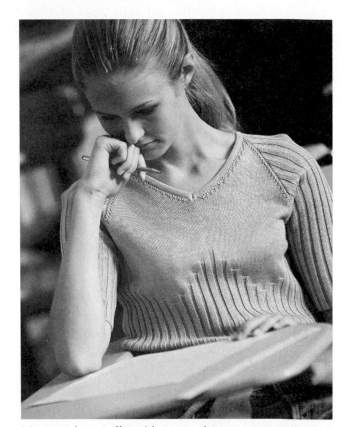

Many students suffer with test anxiety.

Positive versus Negative Stress

Not all stress is bad. There is constructive stress and destructive stress. Whereas debilitating or excessive stress is often referred to as **distress,** constructive stress is called **eustress** (prefix *eu* from Greek meaning "good").[2] Stress arousal can be a positive motivating force that improves the quality of life. Initially, as stress increases, so do health, performance, and general well-being. However, as stress continues to increase, an *optimal stress* level is obtained, and if stress continues beyond this point to *maximum stress,* performance quickly declines and health begins to erode. Complete *Journal Activity:* "How Do You Handle Stress?" to determine how you handle stress.

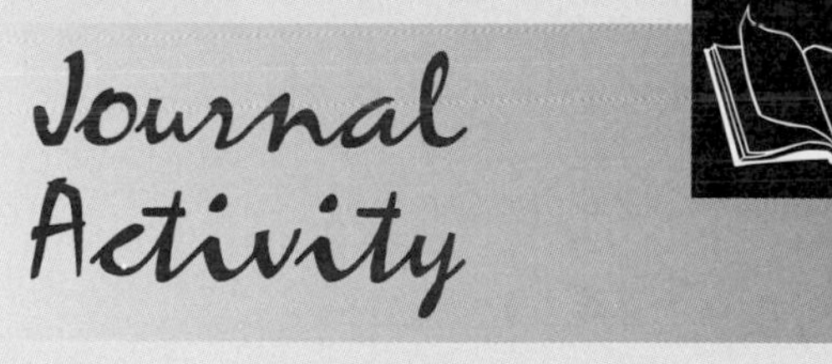

Journal Activity

How Do You Handle Stress?

Think of some times in your life when you experienced stress from events in each of the five categories of stressors (see Figure 5.1). Write about each experience and suggest ways to alter or manage those stressors. Altering a stressor is finding a way to change the event to be less stressful by extending deadlines, getting assistance, and so on. Managing the stressor is finding a way to experience less stress during the stressor by practicing relaxation exercises, eating healthy foods, and so on.

THE STRESS RESPONSE

Fight-or-Flight Response

The **fight-or-flight response** is your body's natural response to a perceived danger.[3] The body goes on alert, and various physiological changes occur that will allow you to survive the threat. For instance, imagine that you are walking through a beautiful mountain forest with luscious pine trees, and a fresh breeze is blowing your hair. You are relaxed and allowing your mind to wander and enjoy the experience. You hear the sound of thunder overhead. You look up and suddenly you realize that the thunder is actually the sound of a large boulder falling down from the cliff above and heading for your path. Instantly your body begins to respond to the threat. Blood vessels constrict, forcing more blood toward your heart and lungs. Your heart begins to pound, sending blood to vital organs. Your lungs open up and your breathing gets faster. Your pupils dilate so that you can see better. Adrenalin is sent into your system to give you a burst of strength. With all of this added metabolic help you are able to leap away from the boulder as it explodes past you. In this particular instance, you chose the "flight" response—and a wise choice it was because you might not have been able to defeat the large boulder in a fight. When the perceived threat is past, your body will begin to return to its prearousal condition. It takes longer for your body's systems to return to a state of relaxation than it does to become aroused. So you may be a little shaky for several minutes or so, depending on how often you replay the experience in your mind.

The stress response created by a life-threatening event is easy to recognize. However, your body has the ability to respond to stressors in varying degrees according to how important an event is perceived or imagined to be by you. Just getting out of bed and rushing to work or school can elevate the stress response, although to a degree much less noticeable than when running from an avalanche of rock. The stress response helps you to maximize your performance and to survive danger. However, if your stress response is not turned off periodically, it can create wear and tear on your body's systems. (See general adaptation syndrome, described below). Your body will begin to break down and illness can set in. New research suggests that women and men respond differently to stress at the hormonal level. (See "Female Researchers Discover That Women Respond Differently to Stress than Men Do.")

General Adaptation Syndrome

The **general adaptation syndrome (GAS)** is a specific pattern of responses that your body experiences as a reaction to continuous life demands or threats.[4] The GAS has three stages: (1) alarm reaction (which is the same as the fight-or-flight response just described), (2) stress resistance, and (3) stress exhaustion. In the alarm reaction stage, hormones are released that create the arousal response in your body necessary to respond to the demand being placed upon it from the environment. The stress resistance stage is when your body tries to return to a state of internal balance that existed before the onset of the stress; this state is referred to as **homeostasis.** The persistent presentation of stressors throughout the day results in cumulative stress. As stressors continue to be presented and the stress response occurs followed by the body working to return to balance, your body eventually becomes exhausted. This is the stress exhaustion stage when parts of your body begin to break down.

You can learn to voluntarily control the stress response. Then you can give yourself the added burst when you need it, but also monitor the use of the stress response and turn it way down or even totally off frequently. You can conserve your stress response in the same way that you conserve electricity in your home: the less you use, the less you have to pay for later. To control your stress levels, learn to use some of the relaxation exercises described later in the chapter.

Anatomy and Physiology of Stress

An event in your life begins the journey to becoming a perceived stressor as a message to your cerebral cortex, the higher centers of the brain. (See Figure 5.2.) The thalamus,

Women Making a Difference

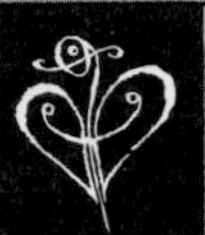

Female Researchers Discover That Women Respond Differently to Stress than Men Do

Shelley Taylor of the University of California at Los Angeles (UCLA) and her colleague Laura Cousino Klein are researchers in the area of stress. One day they were discussing how men and women seem to respond differently to life stress. Men tend to respond to stress by aggressing toward the stressor in either an overt (open) or covert (secretive) fashion. Overt aggression might be to complain, to argue, or to quit their job; or, covertly, men may use drugs or alcohol to numb the effects of the stressor or exercise vigorously to release the stressor.[5] In contrast, women respond to stress much differently than men do.[6] When women are stressed they tend to seek support from other women (to befriend) and talk about their stress. Professional women and especially working professional mothers deal with their stress by redirecting energy to care for their homes and children (to tend). After discussing it at length, Taylor and Klein set out to discover the possible physiological source for the behavior difference between women and men in responding to stress.

Taylor and Klein discovered that the hormone oxytocin is released as part of the stress response in women. This hormone buffers the fight-or-flight responses and encourages women to tend to their children and to gather with other women. When women actually engage in this tending and befriending behavior, more oxytocin is released, which further counters stress and produces a calming effect. This finding may explain why men and women respond differently to stress and why women live longer than men. Men produce high levels of testosterone when under stress, which reduces the calming effects of oxytocin.

This tendency for men to aggress in response to a stressor (either overtly—"fight," or covertly—"flight"), and for women to tend and befriend in response to a stressor is a part of human primal survival instinct. According to Taylor, survival of the species meant that females had to learn to protect their young from danger, and, as there is strength in numbers, gathering with other females was an effective strategy for protecting the young and each other from predators and for finding support for coping with a variety of other types of stressors as well.[7] Thus, using Taylor's speculations as a basis for argument it seems reasonable and long overdue to reconsider the generally accepted concept of the fight-or-flight response. The traditional survival response to stress referred to in the stress literature for many years as the fight-or-flight response should be differentiated, one for men—the fight-or-flight response—and one for women—the tend-and-befriend response. This differentiation could explain why women tend to seek out professional counseling services at a significantly higher rate than do men: under stress women seek out someone to talk to whereas men tend to isolate. These different primal tendencies in response to stress may also explain some gender differences in relationship communication patterns—women like to talk about a stressor at length whereas most men do not.

the part of the brain that serves as the main relay center for sensory impulses to the cerebral cortex, sorts the information, makes a decision that the event is indeed of a stressful nature and, thus, a stressor is perceived. Next, another part of the brain, the **hypothalamus,** is stimulated. Once the hypothalamus is stimulated, two major response pathways are activated in the body: the endocrine system and the autonomic nervous system.

Endocrine System

The **endocrine system** is activated by the anterior section of your hypothalamus. The anterior portion of the hypothalamus gland releases a hormone called the corticotropin-releasing factor (CRF). CRF stimulates the **pituitary gland** of the brain, and it releases **adrenocorticotropic hormone (ACTH).** ACTH is continuously released into the body via the bloodstream in small amounts during the day. However, a mental or physical demand can cause up to twenty times this amount to be secreted within seconds. ACTH stimulates the adrenal cortex of the **adrenal glands,** located on top of the kidney, which secrete **corticoids.** The adrenal glands secrete mostly glucocorticoids, primarily cortisol, and mineralocorticoids, primarily aldosterone.

Aldosterone, transported by the blood, acts on the kidney to increase sodium absorption. This creates an increase in osmotic pressure that forces extracellular fluid into the blood, causing an increase in blood volume and an increase in blood pressure. Cortisol creates metabolic alterations in the body, increasing the **metabolic rate** in response to stress and decreasing the metabolic rate when stress is no longer perceived. The body attempts to get as much glucose into circulation as possible. Glucose is the body's most basic source of energy. If the stress response is maintained, glucose may become depleted and the body will then begin to draw off of the remaining energy reserves, fat deposits,

FIGURE 5.2 The stress response: physiological reactions to a stressor.

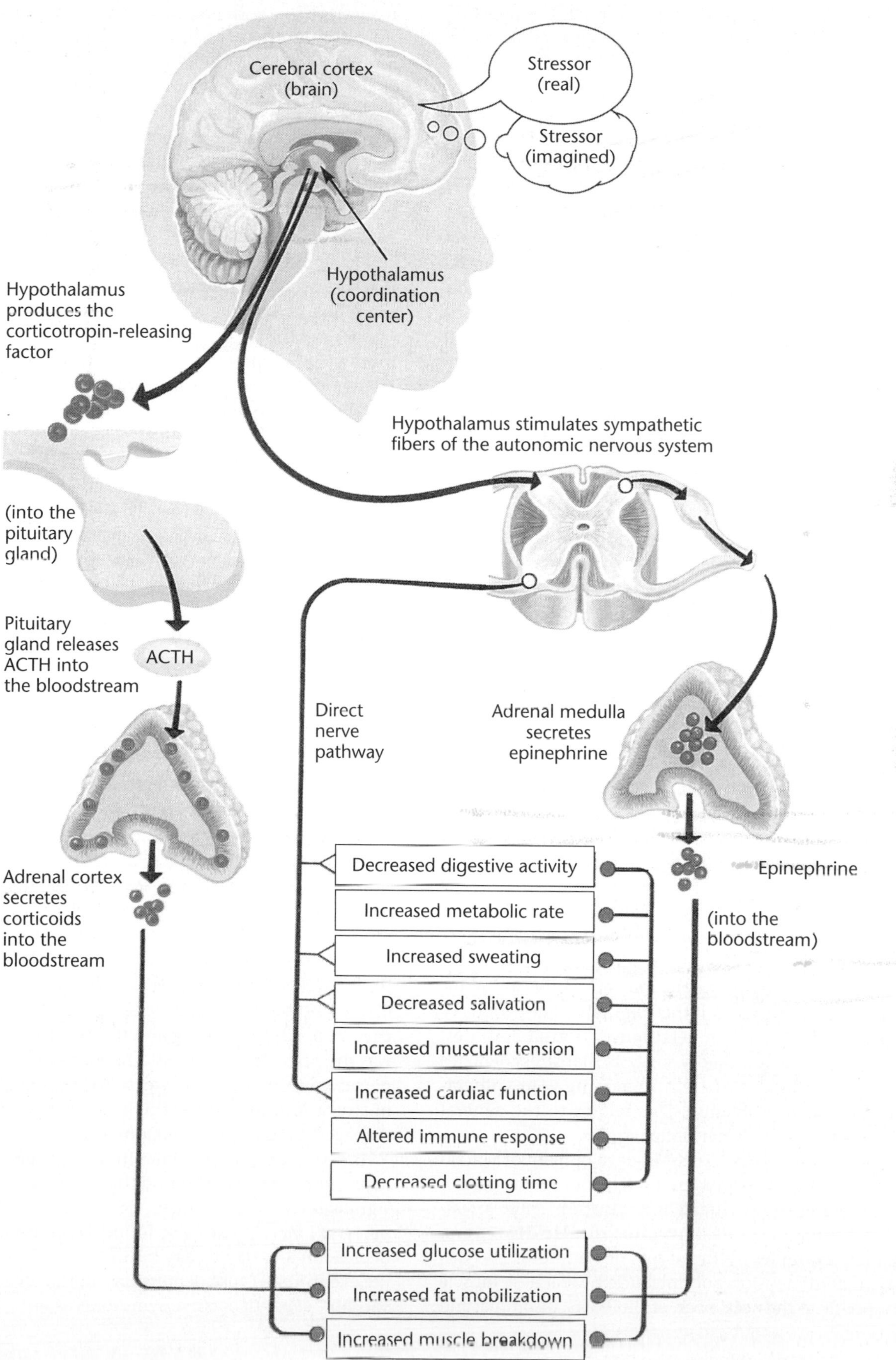

and muscle tissue. As the body meets the demands and relief begins to occur, excess cortisol levels will act to shut down the production of CRF in the hypothalamus and the physiological stress response will begin to stop.

Autonomic Nervous System

The **autonomic nervous system (ANS)** is activated by the posterior section of your hypothalamus. The autonomic nervous system excites and inhibits various bodily functions. It stimulates motor functions, blood sugar production, and inhibitory functions. The ANS stimulates the adrenal medulla of the adrenal glands, which then secretes the catecholamines **epinephrine** (adrenalin) and **norepinephrine** (adrenalin-like substances). Norepinephrine increases blood pressure and the strength and frequency of the heartbeat. Epinephrine increases oxygen consumption, relaxes smooth muscles of the digestive system, increases carbohydrate metabolism, dilates arterials in the heart and skeletal muscles, accelerates heart rate, increases the volume of the blood, and decreases blood clotting time.

The shutdown of the digestive system during stress reduces the production of saliva, a fluid that contains digestive enzymes, and may result in a dry mouth. Also, decreased digestive activity can contribute to indigestion and stomachaches from poorly digested food.

DISTRESS AND THE BODY

Stress and "Dis-ease"

Prolonged stress can put your body at "dis-ease." The longer the body is under a strain, the more likely this disease will lead to uncomfortable and sometimes disabling symptoms or disorders. Your body is not capable of maintaining high levels of stress or arousal for prolonged periods of time without its systems beginning to break down. The stress response in humans is better designed for short bursts of energy and strength to survive immediate and short-lived challenges or dangers. Your body can maintain greater health status if there are sufficient periods of nonarousal between the heightened arousal episodes. The stress-adaptation theory suggests that stress depletes your reserve capacity, thereby increasing your vulnerability to health problems.[8] This relates to the general adaptation syndrome mentioned earlier.

Prolonged stress can lead to the development of a broad range of stress-related disorders, from the somewhat painful and annoying to life-threatening diseases. These stress-related disorders are called **psychosomatic disorders.** Just a few examples of these types of symptoms and disorders include tension and migraine headaches; muscle pain specific to the neck, back, or shoulders; insomnia; and anxiety. Chronic stress may contribute to serious conditions such as depression, digestive disorders (ulcers, colitis, and irritable bowel syndrome), cardiovascular disorders (high blood pressure, heart arrhythmias), and pancreatic disorders (diabetes). Your immune system is most vulnerable to the effects of prolonged stress. Hormones released during the stress response, specifically adrenal hormones, can have a destructive effect on important immune system cells. Under prolonged periods of stress, your immune system will become less capable of fighting off illness and disease, thus making you more prone to colds, flu, or bacterial infections.

Research has demonstrated on three different stress measures that participants reporting high stress were more likely than those reporting low stress to develop upper respiratory infections.[9] Conversely, persons with more social support networks have been shown to have greater resistance to upper respiratory illness.[10] It is likely that the social support diminished the effects of stress.

One of the largest studies on heart disease, with 5,115 participants aged 18 to 30 years from four different states in the United States, showed a relationship between increased job strain and increased high blood pressure. Job strain is defined as "a demanding and stressful work environment with little latitude, flexibility or option for coping with these demands."[11]

Stressful major life events have been associated with a higher frequency of cutaneous symptoms (skin sensations such as burning, crawling, tingling, pricking, pins and needles, pain, tenderness, numbness, itching, and easy bruising).[12] The most frequently reported body region affected was the scalp (59.9 percent) and the most frequently reported symptom was itching (69.3 percent).

A landmark study determined that stress kills off telomeres, part of the cellular structure (the caps at the end of chromosomes).[13] This destructive process leads to premature aging. This research is the first evidence-based link between stress and aging. In this study, researchers examined thirty-nine women aged 20 to 50 who had been caring for a child with a serious chronic illness. They found that every time the cell structure divided in these women, the telomeres got shorter until they stopped functioning and the cell died. A key factor was the perception of stress. The more stresses a woman perceived in her life, the worse she scored on the level of stress. And the higher the level of stress, the greater damage was found to the telomeres.[14]

Investigating a possible link between stress and depression, researchers found that depressed women had significantly higher levels of perceived stress than depressed men.[15] They also found a connection between depression and day-to-day hassles in that not just major life events may cause depression but that everyday stressors may cause depressive symptoms as well.

Stress has been linked to eating disorders. After completing a baseline measure of restraint, forty-six binge-eating college women kept daily diaries assessing depressed affect, stress, coping, and binge eating for 30 days.[16] Regardless of depressed mood, higher stress was associated with increased risk of same-day binge eating; distraction coping was associated with increased risk of future binge eating; and social support was associated with decreased risk of same-day binge eating. In addition, vulnerability to binge eating in women who differ in terms of dietary restraint level was related to their coping responses to stress.

Stress has been related to problems with sleeping. A study investigated workplace characteristics and nocturnal sleep in 709 men and women employees.[17] Gender-stratified analyses revealed that high overcommitment was associated with poor sleep in men, while in women poor sleep was related to the amount of overcommitment in combination with perceived job reward. Thus, for men the amount of work effort is a significant determinant of disturbed sleep, and for women, the amount of work effort–reward balance is a significant determinant of disturbed sleep.

The National Institute of Mental Health reports in 2003 that stress slows the body's healing and recovery process by lowering levels of key immune system chemicals; thus, cuts and bruises take longer to heal. Stress hormones can also contribute to osteoporosis in women by interfering with calcium absorption. The hormones secreted into your system during stressful events help you to survive in an emergency situation, but these hormones can also contribute to brittle bones, infections, and even cancer. If these hormones are being triggered daily due to stress, with little relief, they may lead to disease. (See *FYI*: "Stress and Wound Healing.")

Stress and Wound Healing

Clinical observation has suggested that negative mood or stress is associated with slow wound healing. Basic mind–body research is now confirming this observation. Matrix metalloproteinases (MMPs) and the tissue inhibitors of metalloproteinases (TIMPs) play a role in wound healing. Using a blister chamber wound model on human forearm skin exposed to ultraviolet light, researchers have demonstrated that stress or change in mood is sufficient to modulate MMP and TIMP expression and, presumably, wound healing. Activation of the hypothalamic-pituitary-adrenal (HPA) and sympathetic-adrenal medullary (SAM) systems can modulate levels of MMPs, providing a physiological link among mood, stress, hormones, and wound healing. This research suggests that activation of the HPA and SAM systems, even in individuals with the normal range of depressive symptoms, could alter MMP levels and change the course of wound healing in blister wounds.

Source: National Institutes of Health, National Center for Complementary and Alternative Medicine, August 2005, Mind-body medicine: An overview. Web site: http://nccam.nih.gov/health/backgrounds/mindbody.htm (retrieved March 26, 2006).

Stress Amenorrhea **Stress amenorrhea** is specific to women. Stress amenorrhea is when menstruation stops because of physical or mental stress.[18] Stress can also cause irregularity in the menstrual cycle; that is, time between periods can vary significantly and so can flow rates. Fasting, irregular eating habits, or too much exercise can also place enough stress on the body to cause menstrual irregularity or cessation. If you experience menstrual cessation or irregularity, consult with your health care provider as you would with any other conditions of concern.

Migraine The National Institute of Neurological Disorders and Stroke (NINDS) reports that migraine headaches affect 28 million Americans, of whom 75 percent are women. The migraine prevalence in the United States is 17.6 percent for females and 6 percent for males. The International Headache Society reports that a similar high prevalence is found in Europe and most parts of the world. In the United States, white women report more migraines (20.4 percent) than do African Americans (16.2 percent), and Asian Americans have the lowest levels of migraine (9.2 percent). This may indicate a genetic or cultural component. About 70 percent of migraine sufferers relate a positive family history for migraine. Migraine symptoms peak during productive years of life, between the ages of 25 and 55. In children, both males and females have a fairly equal prevalence before the age of puberty, and some studies suggest that the prevalence of migraine may be increasing in the United States.

Migraine symptoms occur in various combinations and include pain, extreme sensitivity to light and sound, nausea, and vomiting. Migraine is often described as an intense pulsing or throbbing pain in one area of the head. Some individuals can predict the onset of a migraine due to visual disturbances called the migraine aura.

Female sufferers often report that migraine has affected their ability to be in control of their life. It can affect confidence or ability to cope. Many describe feeling frustrated, angry, resentful of their condition, guilty for having the condition, or embarrassed by the condition. Many women do not realize how common this

FYI 

Migraine Sufferers

Women need to understand that migraine is a legitimate biological condition that can be quite disabling. Far too many women feel embarrassed by this condition. A telephone survey of 284 female migraine sufferers revealed that one-third felt that migraines have affected their ability to be in control of their life.[19] Twenty-one percent responded that it has affected their confidence or their ability to cope with life. These women reported feeling frustrated (80 percent), angry (52 percent), resentful (41 percent), guilty (33 percent), and embarrassed (20 percent). Some 14 percent reported that their self-esteem has been negatively affected by others' perception of migraine. The impact of migraine on family life is higher in women because of their child care and other family and general household responsibilities. Of all the women surveyed, 32 percent reported that migraine has had a negative impact on their relationship with their children, with the majority of these mothers reporting that they cannot engage in activities with their children during a migraine attack.

Health Tips 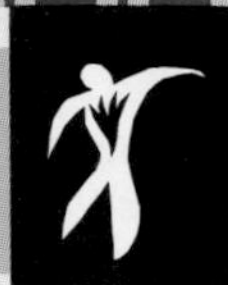

Migraine, Medicine, and Food

Medicines to avoid that may bring on a migraine attack:

- Oral contraceptives
- Stimulants
- Diuretics
- Blood vessel dilators
- Decongestants
- Antidepressants
- Asthma medications
- Certain painkillers

Foods to avoid that may bring on a migraine attack:

- Caffeine, commonly found in coffee, tea, and colas
- Common food additives, such as monosodium glutamate (MSG), common in meat tenderizers and Chinese food
- Alcohol
- Foods that contain tyramine, such as chocolate or cocoa, aged cheeses, vinegar, liver and kidney or other organ meats, sour cream, lima beans, nuts, citrus fruits, bananas, avocados, yogurt, and yeast extracts
- Substances that contain nitrates, such as smoked fish, bologna, pepperoni, bacon, frankfurters, corned beef, pastrami, canned ham, and sausages
- Aspartame, an artificial sweetener sold under the trade names Nutrasweet and Equal

condition is and instead feel ashamed or weak because of it. (See *FYI:* "Migraine Sufferers.")

The cause of the migraine is not precisely known, but a strong genetic connection has been identified and specific abnormal genes may play a role in some forms of migraine. Traditional explanations of the cause of migraine headaches focused on the external environment or internal hormones that caused the blood vessels of the head to constrict and then dilate from built-up pressure causing inflammation. The NINDS reports that new research is beginning to challenge the simplicity of this explanation. The onset of migraine is much more complex than simple constriction and dilation of the blood vessels in the head. Investigators now believe that migraine is caused by inherited abnormalities in certain cell populations in the brain. Using new imaging technologies, scientists can see changes in the brain during migraine attacks. Scientists believe that there is a migraine pain center located in the brainstem, a region at the base of the brain. As neurons fire, surrounding blood vessels dilate and become inflamed, causing the characteristic pain of a migraine.

Various factors can trigger a migraine and, usually, it takes one or more of these together to cause an attack. Common migraine triggers include stress, the letdown after a period of stress, glare and eyestrain, changes in the weather, sleep irregularities, certain medicines, tobacco or tobacco smoke, grinding or clenching your teeth, allergies, eating irregularly, fasting, and dietary factors. *Health Tips:* "Migraine, Medicine, and Food" summarizes additional migraine triggers to watch for.

Both the frequency and the intensity of migraine headaches worsen at those times in a woman's life that are associated with hormonal fluctuation such as around menstrual periods and menopause. Researchers say that female sex hormones are related to migraine attacks. There are no consistent abnormalities found in patients who suffer from migraine, either chemical or hormonal, but it is suspected that changing levels of progesterone and estrogen, the main female hormones, are the trigger for menstrual migraine, and that it is mainly the withdrawal of estrogen which triggers the attack.[20] Menstrual migraine can be treated with the same protocol as nonmenstrual migraine. However, preventive therapy can be considered with nonsteroidal drugs or estrogen supplements.[21,22] Oral contraceptives may increase the frequency and severity of attacks in some women. A very small subgroup of women with migraine have an increased risk of stroke: those who suffer from migraine with aura (visual disturbances preceding the headache), who smoke, and who are taking combined oral contraception.[23]

A research study was conducted with 81 menstruating women with clinically diagnosed migraine in which the women kept a 98-day diary.[24] The results showed that an excess risk of headache occurred perimenstrually (around the menstrual period) and was highest on days 0 and 1 of the cycle (day 0 being the first day of menses). A significantly elevated risk on days 0 and 1 was observed for migraine without aura (visual disturbances that precede the headache) and for tension-type headache. Elevated risks were also observed in the 2 days before the onset of menses for migraine without aura. A significantly lower risk was observed around the time of ovulation for all kinds of headaches. Pain intensity was slightly greater for migraine headaches during the first 2 days of menses.

Another study was conducted with 1,943 female students randomly selected from a university school of medicine and pharmacy who completed a questionnaire about headaches and the menstrual cycle.[25] Both migraine and nonmigraine headaches were found to be worse during menstruation, and the women with migraine headaches experienced more frequent, more severe, and more complex headaches than those with nonmigraine headaches. The researchers also found that both menstrually related migraine and menstrually related nonmigraine began on approximately the first day of menstruation. This shows that menstrual migraine occurs during peak fluctuation in estrogen levels. Women with nonmigraine headache can also experience fluctuation of these hormones, although to a lesser degree than in women with migraine.[26]

Migraine significantly decreases during pregnancy, disappearing in 70 percent of women migraine sufferers.[27] About 40 percent of women suffer from headaches the first week after giving birth. Migraine at this time is more frequent in women who had migraine headaches prior to becoming pregnant.

In strict medical terms the menopause is actually the last menstrual period.[28] However, the term is often used for all the hormone fluctuations and resulting symptoms that women get both before and after the last menstrual period. Menopause is actually the failure of the ovaries to produce estrogen. The years leading up to menopause and shortly after are called the climacteric, or perimenopause. It is during perimenopause that many women find that migraine gets worse and those who previously had not noticed much of an association with their periods start having monthly migraine attacks. Hormone replacement therapy can help perimenopausal migraine.[29] You can read more about hormone replacement therapy in Chapter 8.

If you suffer from migraine headaches, it is a good idea to consult with your health care provider to get an accurate diagnosis. There are three basic ways to approach migraine treatment: prevention through health practices, prevention through medication, and reducing discomfort and restoring functioning with medication during an attack. Health prevention practices include watching what you eat and drink because some substances can trigger a migraine attack. Hormone therapy may help some women, and stress management strategies, such as exercise, relaxation, biofeedback and other therapies, may be helpful. In addition, medications to prevent a migraine may be taken on a daily basis. Some medications developed for epilepsy and depression may prove to be effective treatment options as well. Consult your health care professional to determine the treatment that is best for you. See *Her Story:* "Kathryn: Stress-Induced Migraine Headaches" for a personal look at someone who suffers from migraines.

To reduce discomfort and restore functioning during a migraine attack, the prescription drugs called *ergots* can be helpful.[30] Ergots are a family of migraine medications

Her Story

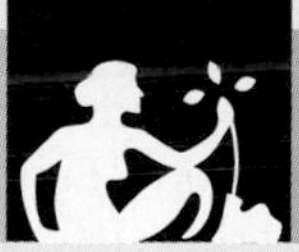

Kathryn: Stress-Induced Migraine Headaches

Kathryn had experienced migraine headaches most of her life. She was going to graduate at the top of her college class in about 2 months and get married a week later. She was very busy maintaining her academic standing in school and planning her wedding. Her migraines were really getting in her way of being able to function. After an assessment it was determined that Kathryn had stress-induced migraine headaches. One common symptom of migraines is cold hands, measured as an exterior finger temperature less than 90°. In Kathryn's case, her finger temperature was consistently in the seventies, even though it was warm outside and comfortable in the room. Following eight sessions of relaxation training that incorporated some biofeedback therapy (to be discussed later in this chapter), Kathryn learned to raise and maintain a finger temperature above 90° even outside of the therapy setting. Her migraines disappeared and she was able to go on with her life with much less pain and discomfort.

- Do you know someone who suffers with migraines? What is it like for them?
- Have they tried stress management and relaxation exercises to help them with their migraine headaches?

that originally derived from a fungus that grows on rye. They interact with receptors for the brain chemical serotonin, which regulates mood, pain awareness, and blood vessel tone. Ergot drugs reduce inflammation and have a powerful effect on blood vessels, causing them to constrict. This vasoconstrictive property helps relieve the throbbing pain of migraine, but these drugs are not recommended for people with high blood pressure, heart disease, or peripheral vascular disease. Ergotamine tartrate is available in several different brands. Combinations containing caffeine in addition to ergotamine are available in tablets (Wigraine) and suppository (Ercf). Ergomar is a tablet that dissolves under the tongue giving somewhat quicker results. Bellergal-S combines ergotamine with belladonna and phenobarbital. Ergotamine may produce nausea as a side effect; however, an antinausea drug taken beforehand can help with this. Dihydroergotamine is related to ergotamine but has a less powerful effect on blood vessel constriction, making it somewhat safer to use; it is also available in a fast-acting nasal spray (Migranal) or self-injection (DHE-45). Isometheptene (Midrin) is a migraine medication that contains acetaminophen and dichloralphenazone (a mild sedative) and is often chosen for migraine sufferers who cannot tolerate ergot drugs.

Another family of prescription medications designed to reduce discomfort and restore functioning during a migraine are triptans, which target specific groups of serotonin receptors that are known to play a role in migraine headaches.[31] Triptans have some negative side effects and are not suitable for all persons. However, triptans have fewer side effects than the ergot drug family. Triptans currently available in the United States include sumatriptan (Imitrex), naratriptan (Amerge), zolmitriptan (Zomig), rizatriptan (Maxalt), eletriptan (Relpax), frovatriptan (Frova), and almotriptan (Axert). Imitrex is currently the most frequently prescribed medication for migraine.

Simple over-the-counter analgesics can sometimes be helpful in reducing milder migraine pain.[32] Simple pain relievers include aspirin (Bufferin, Bayer), acetaminophen (Tylenol), ibuprofen (Advil, Motrin, Nuprin), ketoprofen (Orudis), and naproxen (Naprosyn, Aleve). These last three are nonsteroidal anti-inflammatory drugs (NSAIDs). Some NSAIDS are available in prescription strength or through injection at an emergency room, such as ketorolac (Toradol). Some over-the-counter pain relievers have drug combinations that contain caffeine; caffeine can constrict the blood vessels to reduce the inflammatory swelling (dilation) of the blood vessels. Extra Strength Excedrin and Excedrin for Migraine combine acetaminophen and aspirin with caffeine. Aspirin-Free Excedrin contains acetaminophen plus caffeine, and Anacin combines aspirin and caffeine. Over-the-counter analgesics can cause stomach irritation and are not recommended for people with ulcers. Frequent long-term use of some analgesics can cause liver damage.

STRESS AND PREGNANCY

Maternal stress, or stress during pregnancy, can be harmful for both expectant mothers and the babies they are carrying. The March of Dimes reported in 2007 that high levels of stress may increase the risk of preterm labor, infant low birth weight, labor and delivery complications, and miscarriage. Maternal stress hormones may influence fetal development directly or alter uteroplacental blood flow via maternal, placental, or fetal blood flow mechanisms. Catecholamines, produced by the adrenal glands during periods of stress, reduce uterine artery blood flow from 30 to 100 percent, resulting in fetal distress, low infant birth weight, and premature labor. Stress-induced blood vessel constriction (vasoconstriction) may reduce uteroplacental blood flow and exchange and contribute to intrauterine growth retardation. Finally, the immunosuppressive effects of hypothalamic-pituitary-adrenal axis activation that is typical with the stress response may result in maternal infection, which in turn is a risk factor for preterm labor.

Relaxation therapy including biofeedback can be very useful for pregnant women to learn to control and minimize the stress response. Biofeedback-assisted relaxation may also reduce labor and delivery time. Biofeedback therapy is discussed later in this chapter.

STRESS AND LIFESTYLE

Major Life Events

Major life events can create significant stress in your life. When you have a financial crisis, a death in the family, a break off of a relationship, or so on, the pain of such an event and the adaptation required to adjust to the consequences generated by the event can present huge challenges for you. Several attempts to describe and measure the impact of such major life events have been made. However, the degree of stress experienced is dependent on how each individual uniquely perceives the event.

College Stress

It is difficult to specify the sources of stress for college students because they represent many diverse backgrounds located at many different institutions. It has been reported that up to 50 percent of the college students who seek counseling complain of difficulty studying or anxiety, tension, and depression due to poor grades, and fear of doing poorly in courses.[33]

Some of the more common factors related to college student stress include adapting to a new environment, expectations of parents, meeting demands of faculty members, pressure to achieve good grades, rising costs of higher education, and pressure to find employment before and after graduation. For the first time in their lives, many college students must find their own way in structuring and managing time for coursework, jobs, socializing, recreation, and daily chores.

Undergraduate college women are more likely than men to report an unacceptable stress level.[34] To reduce stress, college women are more likely to indicate a need to limit commitments, exercise more, and worry less. Frequent reasons given by women in college for not reducing stress are lack of time and lack of self-discipline.

Freshmen are probably the most vulnerable college group. The freshman class has the highest dropout rate, and 30 percent of first-year students frequently feel "overwhelmed by all I have to do." Nearly twice as many female students report feeling overwhelmed, 39 percent to only 20 percent of males. Why do women report higher levels of stress than men?

In 2002, the Higher Education Research Institute at the University of California at Los Angeles conducted a study of attitudes and goals of first-year college students. The survey indicates women students spent more time working at goal-oriented tasks, and men students spent more time partying and playing. While women students' habits increased their stress, men students spent more time actively releasing stress. Women's high stress levels in college may be related to their plans while in college. For example, more women (44 percent) than men (33 percent) reported needing a job to pay for college, and women spent more time studying, volunteering, doing housework and child care, and joining student activities.

Most college students need assistance to adjust to the demands of college life. Among the most beneficial survival strategies are notetaking techniques, stress reduction tips, study skills tips, test-taking strategies, time management, writing skills tips, public speaking skills, financial management, and finding a supportive social group. Most college campuses have resources to help you in any of these areas.

College stress is very pronounced for the nontraditional student, one who is older, maybe married with children, and perhaps commuting long distances to campus. The nontraditional student may also be holding down a part-time or full-time job. Also, difficult choices frequently have to be made, for instance, studying for a college exam versus taking a child to soccer practice. For these students, priorities are difficult to establish and maintain, and a great deal of help and support is needed from friends and family if they are to succeed in college.

Daily Life Hassles

It is not just major life events that can affect your stress level. Those little daily life hassles can eat away at your composure and elevate your stress level by a significant amount. Hassles are irritants that can range from minor annoyances to fairly major difficulties. Contrary to hassles, some daily events can uplift your life by creating good feelings. Uplifting events can serve as sources of peace, joy, or satisfaction. Some hassles and uplifting events occur often, whereas others are relatively rare. It is often a combination of the presence or absence of hassles and uplifting events in your life that impacts your stress level and coping ability. Typical hassles are such things as misplacing or losing things, troublesome neighbors, the health problems of a family member, and having to wait in lines. Typical uplifting events are such things as being lucky, being rested, feeling healthy, and enjoying a hobby. Daily hassles prove to be a better predictor of the manifestations of stress symptoms than uplifting events, which are a deterrent to the manifestation of stress symptoms.[35] Thus, it seems that we may assign greater meaning to the hassles in life than we spend appreciating the uplifting events.

Complete *Assess Yourself:* "Stress Checklist" to help determine your stress level.

IMPACT OF MULTIPLE ROLES

The demands on today's woman are extreme. They often involve any combination of the following: maintain a household, care for a family, and work in or outside of the home. A woman is expected to play multiple roles in her life, such as daughter, sibling, spouse, mother, boss, employee, pet owner, friend, neighbor, social volunteer, and hobbyist. Dedication to each of these various roles can create a major strain. It is often difficult for a woman to find time for herself, much less find time to relax, because of all the demands placed upon her. Society often views the woman as the "giver" of assistance rather than the "receiver" of assistance. Women may experience different levels and types of stress depending on the particular role they play. In addition, high demands in combination with a sense of low control over how tasks are done makes a task more stressful.[36] Persons in nonprofessional positions, such as a secretary, have high demands placed on them, may find their jobs monotonous, and may experience boredom, frustration, and even a decline in self-esteem. Consequently, they have higher overall stress levels than persons in professional positions, such as a teacher. Furthermore, women seem to cope better with stress than men; however, women seem to have more stress to handle.

Stressors are different for employed women with children than they are for full-time homemakers with children. As a result, they require different kinds of support to enable them to cope effectively with their chosen

Assess Yourself

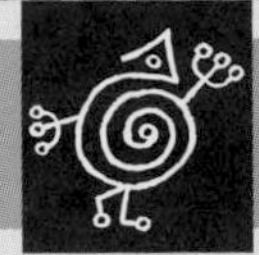

Stress Checklist

Check the following symptoms you have experienced in the past 3 months.

_____ 1. Worrying
_____ 2. Feeling anxious or uneasy
_____ 3. Going over the same thing in your mind
_____ 4. Feeling pushed
_____ 5. Unable to concentrate
_____ 6. Cold hands or feet occasionally
_____ 7. Tiredness at the end of the day
_____ 8. Sore or stiff neck
_____ 9. Occasional headaches (1 or 2 per month)
_____ 10. Irritable
_____ 11. Frequent headaches (more than 2 per month) or an occasional severe headache (at least 1 every 3 months)
_____ 12. Indigestion or stomach problems
_____ 13. Backaches
_____ 14. Irregular sleeping pattern (either sleeping too much or not sleeping)
_____ 15. Prolonged feelings of depression or anxiety (more than 1 week)

Interpretation: Items numbered 1 through 5 are typically associated with mild to moderate levels of stress. Items numbered 6 through 10 are typically associated with a moderate level of stress. Items numbered 11 through 15 are typically associated with a severe level of stress.

(Note: The Stress Checklist is not a thorough assessment instrument for stress. It is designed to be used for the purpose of a quick health screening. It is also important to consider additional possible causes for the symptoms listed other than stress. Stress symptoms can be evaluated for severity by trained professionals.)

- *Mild stress*—Changing your lifestyle or routine may help to reduce stress.
- *Moderate stress*—Although changing your lifestyle or routine may help to reduce stress, sometimes a more thorough assessment of the stress symptoms may be necessary. Direct intervention may be needed. This might include activities such as stress management instruction or biofeedback therapy to help prevent and/or alleviate symptoms.
- *Severe stress*—More thorough assessment and immediate intervention may be needed. The type of intervention will depend on the results of the more thorough assessment. Activities could include any or all of the following: a lifestyle modification to lessen the stress, stress management instruction, biofeedback therapy, physical and/or mental health counseling, or medication.

roles.[37] One example is the cost of child care for employed women, which is a huge financial stressor on most families. Employed women identify work, children, and household duties as the most frequent stressors, whereas nonemployed women identify children, finances, and self-concerns as stressors.

There are advantages and disadvantages to being either a woman not employed outside of the home or a woman employed outside of the home.[38] Each experiences stress, but in different ways. Women employed outside of the home and women not employed outside of the home experience, on average, similar levels of depressive symptoms. As compared to women employed outside of the home, full-time homemakers benefit from having less responsibility for things outside of their control. Women employed outside of their home appear to benefit from having less routine work than full-time homemakers.

A national longitudinal survey of a representative sample of 1,256 adults demonstrated that women's higher incidence of psychological distress than men's is associated with differences in men's and women's contributions to household labor.[39] Men performed on average 42.3 percent of the housework compared to 68.1 percent reported by women. Among married respondents, the gender differences in household labor were larger, with wives performing more than twice as many hours of household labor than husbands and doing over 70 percent of the housework as compared to 36.7 percent for men. The least distressed persons in the study were the ones who performed only about 50 percent of the housework. Those who did more than this or less than this had increasing levels of psychological distress. Thus, women are exceeding the amount of housework they should perform to receive maximum psychological benefits. And men, with an average of doing only 42.3 percent of housework, have room for increasing their contribution to housework without experiencing increased distress. This could benefit both genders.

Employment status moderates the effect of the division of household labor but not the effect of the amount of household labor. For those keeping house full-time, the least depressed perform almost 80 percent of housework, whereas for those employed full-time, the minimum level of depression occurs at performing 45.8 percent of housework.[40] Thus, persons with full-time employment and who performed more than or less than 45.8 percent of the housework had increasing levels of psychological distress.

The busy, stress-laden lifestyle of the modern woman has been described as "the hurried woman syndrome."[41] This is experienced primarily by women between the ages of 25 and 55 who have children living at home. The three major symptoms are fatigue or a low mood, weight gain, and low sex drive (libido). It is estimated that 50 million women suffer from these symptoms each year and reported that stress is probably the single most important factor that causes women to complain about hurried woman syndrome.

Women of middle age have a demanding multiple role position. As primary family caregivers, these women may be caring for their own children, their spouse, their grandchildren, and their elder parents. With the rising cost of child care, many young adults are turning to their parents to help take care of their kids. The middle-aged grandmother may be thrilled at the opportunity to spend time with her grandchildren, but it is a demanding task. In addition, the parents of the middle-aged woman may be experiencing a decline in health and require assistance with driving, cleaning house, preparing meals, and visits to a health care provider. These many roles that the middle-aged caregiver might fulfill can contribute to cumulative stress and have a negative impact on her emotional and physical health.

Researchers investigated autonomic and endocrine responses to acute stressors in twenty-seven women who were or are presently caring for a spouse with progressive dementia (high chronic stress group) and thirty-seven noncaregivers who were category matched for age and family income (low chronic stress group).[42] On measures prior to the presentation of the acute stressor, the caregivers reported greater stress, depression, and loneliness than the comparison group. The acute stressors were a math task and an evaluated speech task, each 6 minutes in length. Measures during and after the acute stressor reported that caregivers, compared to noncaregivers, exhibited a quicker response by stress hormones and higher blood pressure and heart rate. Progressive dementia is unpredictable, irreversible, and devastating to social relations. Many long-term caregivers for a spouse with progressive dementia live in strained relationships. Caregivers report more depressive symptoms than noncaregivers, and the impact of chronic psychological stress for caregivers carries physiological costs as well, making caregivers more vulnerable to the negative impact of acute stressors.

Researchers examined the relationship over time between women's paid work and their informal caregiving for aging or infirm relatives.[43] The sample was 293 white women who were wives and mothers born between 1905 and 1934. The results showed that women were equally likely to become caregivers regardless of whether they were employed. The investigation clarified the timing of women's caregiving and its association with their employment in several ways. First, caregiving was found to be an increasingly common role for U.S. women; over three-fifths of the women in this study were engaged in caregiving at some time in their lives and most typically in later midlife (ages 45–65). Second, the role of caregiver remains prominent as women age, even as they relinquish the role of paid worker. Third, while caregiving may be a major interruption in one's anticipated life experiences, researchers found that it does not necessarily interrupt women's labor force participation. Fourth, caregiving appears to be increasingly a role that is more, not less, characteristic of women's lives, as seen by the rising incidence of caregiving across succeeding birth cohorts. And fifth, position in social culture and level of education affect the likelihood of women working outside the home and caregiving at the same time. During the later years of adulthood, women with more education are more apt to be in the workforce than are women with less education, but the pattern is reversed for caregiving. It could be that women with only a high school education or less may not have the resources to pay for professional care or that women with a higher education tend to "invest" their time in paid work rather than in unpaid caregiving.

Women in middle adulthood are considered the **sandwich generation.** They are sandwiched between caring for their elderly parents while still providing for their children and sometimes even providing day care for their grandchildren. These multiple caregiver demands can put a severe financial and emotional strain on a woman.

Caregiving is the fastest growing unpaid profession in America. More than 22 million American households (1 in 4) are involved in caring for an older person. There exist many potential stressors for caregivers. These include

- Lack of knowledge of resources in a community.
- Lack of knowledge about alternative care facilities and their differences such as nursing homes, assisted living, and retirement homes.
- Lack of knowledge about Medicare/Medicaid.
- Lack of knowledge of home health aides or elder care services.
- Long-distance caregiving—caregiver living in a different city, state, or country than the person receiving care.
- Poorly coordinated community services for assisting the caregiver.
- Chronic care not receiving as much attention by the health community as acute care.

Chronic caregiving can be very stressful. Common signs of caregiver stress include anger, denial, insomnia, health problems, depression, exhaustion, loss of concentration, irritability, anxiety, and withdrawal.

In addition to caring for elderly parents, many middle-aged women provide a significant portion of daily/weekly care for their grandchildren and/or have older children who still live at home. This trend is on the rise and seems to be related to

- Higher divorce rates.
- Increases in the number of single-parent households.
- Cuts in federal funding for social services (especially child care).
- Increases in birthrates among teen-agers.
- Grandparents' being recruited by family and social services to care for a grandchild when a parent is no longer able to care for the child (because of substance abuse, emotional problems, unemployment, work-schedule conflicts, high cost of child care, incarceration, neglect, etc.).

Grandparents who provide significant care for grandchildren may feel out of control regarding the choices available; they may feel trapped by circumstances. They may feel uncertain about custodial rights and in their decision-making responsibility regarding the grandchild. While they have a responsibility to care for the child, they may not feel they have the legal right or power to exercise major decisions regarding him or her.

Stress can lead to violence. Women who experienced violence in their relationship described stress as a significant predictor of marital aggression within one year following their wedding.[44] In other words, the greater the stress level that was present in the lives of each of the partners, the more violence was present in the relationship.

Stress is a common problem among women. From a sample of 1,000 British women who completed a survey, 79 percent indicated that they felt overly stressed.[45] The main manifestation was identified as increased irritability, this being most pronounced among working mothers with children under 16 years of age. Twenty-five percent of all women aged 15 to 24 turned to smoking, and 23 percent of subjects aged 25 to 34 turned to alcohol as a means of relieving stress.

Stress, anxiety, and depression have been found to be among the most frequently reported health problems for women.[46] Significant factors contributing to these mental health problems include lower socioeconomic status, being an ethnic minority, being a member of a complex family structure, a lowered quality of family relationships, and intensity around participation in the labor market.

MULTICULTURAL ISSUES

Spiritual Beliefs

Cultural perspectives can impact health. Religious beliefs or, in the broader spectrum, spiritual beliefs can influence your frame of mind. Some beliefs emphasize a fatalistic philosophy—that one has no control over destiny. Other beliefs emphasize hope and a positive outlook on life—that one will reap positive rewards for efforts. Positive or hopeful attitudes seem to enhance health, whereas pessimistic or fearful attitudes can contribute to health deterioration.[47]

Ability to Acculturate

Degree of acculturation can impact health perspectives. Acculturation is how well an individual has adjusted to and become integrated into a community or country she or he has moved to. Being a newcomer in a foreign environment can be stressful just because you do not know very many people, have not built up a good support system yet, and cannot utilize new resources. For example, Mexican American women who are more acculturated to the "Westernized" culture (one with a prevalent biomedical basis for health and well-being) have less belief in and reliance on traditional folk healing than do Mexican American women with less acculturation. Thus, the acculturated women experience less stress as a result of feeling more in control over medical outcomes.[48] The less acculturated women expressed having a somewhat lower sense of control over their own health.

Racial Issues

Ethnicity can impact the degree of stressors or support an individual experiences. Race, for example, is a significant predictor of both levels of social support and occupational stress for women. African American women report lower levels of coworker support than do Caucasian women.[49] Women in Japan are suffering significant stress from that culture's current emphasis on overwork.[50] Putting in long hours to beat the competition can take its toll on the body and the emotions. Being a member of an ethnic minority group can be stressful as a result of the amount of bigotry and discrimination that still exists in the world today.

Age Factors

Research has identified differences in numbers and types of stressors and resulting health problems for women by age groups.[51] The presence of healthy personality traits that may help cope with stress was also examined. Young women (18–29 years) reported high stressors (second to middle-aged women), less-healthy personality traits, and significantly more physical and emotional symptoms of health problems than middle-aged or older women. Middle-aged women (30–45 years) had significantly more stressors than the other women, but their healthy personality traits may have contributed to their having fewer health problems than younger women. Older women (46–66 years) had the fewest stressors, highest healthy personality traits, and fewest symptoms of health problems compared to the other age groups.

According to this research, "In their roles and relationships as wives, mothers and employees, women experienced multiple stressors such as inadequate physical and emotional support from their spouse/partner, along with parenting and employee difficulties that contributed to their health problems. Young and middle-aged women were more stressed, juggling the multiple responsibilities and demands of their spouse, children, ageing parents, and their occupation, while trying to maintain their own 'inner balance.'"

Stressors can be more specific to certain age groups. Women in their twenties suffer from the syndrome referred to as the "type E woman"—being everything to everybody.[52] These women are divided among three competing goals in life: they want a career, a relationship, and a family. Retired women workers experience significant financial stress even in the early years after retirement.[53] This is even more significant for unmarried retired women workers. Women not only enter old age poorer than men but become poorer with age as a consequence of widowhood, higher health care expenditures, and pay and pension inequities.[54]

FINANCIAL STRESS

The ever-rising costs of living and unhealthy economic trends have placed a burden of financial stress on women. Many women are required to seek employment, and often work at more than one job, in order to pay all of the bills. The mobility of our society almost requires that women own their own mode of transportation or pay for public transportation. Paying rent or mortgage payments takes a huge bite out of women's income. The rising cost of food impacts pocketbooks daily. Clothes get more expensive all of the time, and women are expected to wear a variety of colors and designs. They are not supposed to wear just one or two types of suits or outfits to work whereas this is acceptable for men. Also, it is easy to accrue high-interest debts from using credit cards when cash is not available to purchase an attractive temptation of clothing or to put food on the dinner table. Also, women are more likely to shop as a means to relax than are men.[55] Accruing finance charges can stretch the limits of a paycheck and create additional stress in the lives of women.

The Impact of Technology

The advancement of technology has made it difficult to remain an active and informed participant in the community without a financial investment. If you are unavailable, people expect to be able to leave a message on an answering machine or with an answering service, or send you a letter via e-mail or fax. Access to television or radio programming is a vital link to staying informed about recent events so that you can understand what in the world everyone else is talking about. Employers or college professors may expect you to meet shorter deadlines because of the availability of desktop computers and the accessibility to computerized information networks and sophisticated software. Staying involved with a high-tech world is very expensive and very stressful.

The Workforce, Women, and Stress

Some women are not paid enough to make ends meet at the end of each month. Though some progress has been made over the years, the average wage earned by women is still significantly below that of men. The gender pay gap is universal. A 2000 study reported that women across the globe make significantly less than men: Japan 63.6 percent, Austria 69.2 percent, Canada 69.8 percent, Spain 71.1 percent, Switzerland 73.6 percent, United Kingdom 74.9 percent, Germany 75.5 percent, United States 76.3 percent, Finland 79.9 percent, New Zealand 81.4 percent, Italy 83.3 percent, Sweden 83.5 percent, Australia 86.8 percent, and France 89.9 percent.[56] Both Australia and Sweden have specific policies to help protect women from the gender gap; Australia has a comparable-worth policy so that incumbents receive equal pay for equal work, and Sweden has adopted a number of polices related to family leave and child care to equalize gender roles in the family. It remains unclear to researchers as to the reasons behind the more equitable gender pay ratios of France and Italy. Women employed full-time in the United States earn about two-thirds as much as men.[57] This is an economic disadvantage that may affect health.[58]

Women are more than twice as likely as men to work in part-time jobs. These types of positions are even more segregated than full-time work and offer less training, fewer promotional opportunities, and fewer employment benefits. Women executives are significantly outnumbered by men, and more than 90 percent report that a glass ceiling prevents women from reaching the top in any great numbers. More than half say they have been sexually harassed on the job, but their most likely response was to ignore the harassment. Women executives are likely to be married and have children and are likely to report feeling stressed and burned out, the result of juggling work and a disproportionate load of family obligations.[59]

Many women are expected to be primary caregivers to their children and have a difficult time earning a wage while caring for their dependents. Women who receive financial assistance through social service programs often are not able to provide for themselves and their dependents and find the resources to invest in an education, training, or employment opportunity. Thus, these women are often not able to break from the cycle that keeps them dependent on social services and limits their opportunities to engage in self-development or careers.

It is quite common that women in a relationship are likely to have a spouse or partner who is also working. However, this is often still not enough to eliminate or significantly reduce financial worries. When both partners are working, an added stress is placed on the relationship. It becomes difficult to find time to spend with family members, and the time that is spent often is not of high quality, such as during family crises or hurried activities.

EMPLOYMENT AND HEALTH

Many women work outside of their home because they want to. A career is often a way to discover additional personal significance and self-worth. Employed women are physically healthier than nonemployed women, and participation in the labor force improves health over time.[60] Accumulating evidence suggests that, when compared with not working for pay, employment improves health. Thus, we can expect that women's lower likelihood for employment will negatively affect their health.[61]

Working against Stereotypes

Due to current social trends and to antidiscrimination legislation that has opened opportunities in the workplace to women, more women are exercising their right to pursue careers. Some are even in fields that were once, and may still be, dominated by men. The pressure to perform and not fail is constant for many women in the workplace. The entrance into fields once dominated by men is still relatively new. Thus, women are heavily scrutinized by men and by other women to determine if they are truly capable of performing their duties on the job. The nature of this scrutiny is often unfair for women in that they must far exceed the expectations placed on men in the same job in order to demonstrate that they are capable.

The "equal pay for equal work" principle led to the passage of legislation that makes it illegal to pay any worker (usually a female or a minority group member) lower rates of pay than that paid to others (usually white males). Some employers still use evasion to avoid compliance by using a different title for positions held by women and ethnic minorities, despite only minor differences in assigned duties, to justify a lower rate of pay.[62]

Women who are competing with negative social stereotypes are often forced to become superachievers. High and persistent achievement-oriented individuals are often referred to as "Type A" persons. Type A persons find it difficult to slow down and relax, often equating relaxation with laziness. Type A persons are more prone to developing and maintaining stress symptoms. Type A women have greater frequency of illness and higher blood pressure than non–Type A women.[63] This could be a direct link to the rising numbers of cardiovascular illnesses reported among women.

Viewpoint

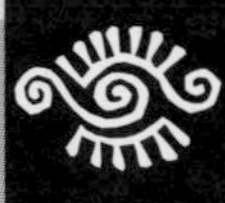

Tired or Toxic?

Research suggests that the environment has become so toxic that it is giving rise to new illnesses such as atypical immune system dysfunction and chronic fatigue syndrome. The medical community is slow to accept this proposition despite existing evidence. Many women with these disorders are considered hypochondriacs because of the hesitancy by some health providers to diagnose the toxic affects of pollution on the body. What do you think about pollutants in the environment possibly having toxic effects on the body?

ENVIRONMENTAL STRESS

Many elements in the environment can produce stress. Overcrowding in the home, in the neighborhood, or at work is a common cause of irritability and tension. Chemical toxins and pollutants can create stress on the body that affects physical and psychological well-being.[64] Even everyday items can be toxic to most people. Toxins that we come into contact with on a daily basis include insecticides, household cleansers, and personal toiletries including shampoos and cosmetics. Just the odor from any of these chemicals can cause severe negative reactions in the body. The "closed-building syndrome" refers to the escalation of airborne infectious illnesses and allergic reactions to pollutants because of recycled air. Closed-loop ventilation systems provide minimal access to fresh air and little opportunity for contaminated air to escape. Spending time in a high-rise office building, shopping mall, or commercial airplane could be risky because many of these facilities do not have sufficient circulation of fresh air. (See *Viewpoint:* "Tired or Toxic?")

Noise pollution is a common and frequent stressor. Women have been found to be more sensitive to high-pitched noises, like the continuous machine noise from a computer. This noise generates high levels of irritability and stress for women, whereas it does not seem to bother men.[65] (See *FYI:* "Ergonomics.")

Just as some noise can create stress, other sounds have a relaxing effect. Music with a soft, slow, flowing movement created by the piano, cello, harp, or violin can soothe and calm the body and mind. Soothing sounds also occur naturally in the environment: rustling leaves

FYI 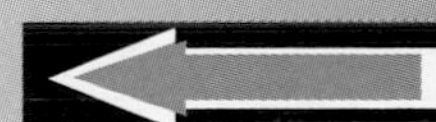

Ergonomics

Ergonomics is the science that seeks to adapt working conditions to suit the worker. A working environment that does not suit the worker can place stress and strain on the mind and the body. Let's look at the example of the computer station. Many people develop back or neck aches due to the strain of sitting in front of a computer for extended hours of work. Thus, through the study of postural positioning, new chairs were devised to help alleviate the strain on the body. These new "ergonomically correct" chairs range in design from an S-shaped chair that provides a padded knee rest to a giant rubber ball chair that provides complete leg and knee support; each of these designs straightens the back and pulls the shoulders back thus preventing back and neck strain. Typing at the computer keyboard for long periods of time can lead to the development of a very sore wrist, hand, or arm and can be serious enough to be diagnosed as carpal tunnel syndrome. This condition was alleviated with the design of ergonomically correct keyboards, which do not require such a wide reach to each key. Carpal tunnel syndrome can be treated via physical therapy or biofeedback therapy. Some people even have surgery for this condition, which is recommended only as a last resort.

Now, let's examine the computer screen. The brightness of this screen can cause eyestrain and severe headaches. To alleviate this problem some computers now have the ability to adjust the color and brightness of the screen. You can also purchase a tinted cover for your computer screen that will tone down the glare. Some computers can be very noisy, which can result in irritability and headaches for the user. Thus, computers are now designed to produce only minimal amounts of noise from the hard drive and the printer, so a quieter working atmosphere is created.

Take a look at your own working environment. Is there anything you can change that will make your work easier and more comfortable, and result in a happier and healthier place to work? How about your living environment? Can you make some adjustments in your home to create a safer and more pleasant place to live?

on a tree; distant sounds of crickets, frogs, or birds; and water moving in a stream or from a waterfall, or ocean waves rolling onto the shore.

The concept of "safe neighborhood" is vital to consider in relation to stress levels. It is very difficult to relax when your life is endangered. There are numerous instances for which a woman or her family and friends are at risk: from gunshots, bullets striking your home, or being hit by a stray bullet; the car breaking down on the side of the road; walking in an isolated area; and having to remember to lock yourself in at night and even during the day. The high incidence of rape and other violence against women is evidence that women are not safe in this world.

FYI 

Clinical Anxiety Disorders[66]

- Panic attack—sudden onset of intense apprehension, fearfulness, or terror often associated with the feeling of impending doom. Symptoms include shortness of breath, palpitations, chest pain or discomfort, choking or smothering sensations, and fear of "going crazy" or losing control.
- Agoraphobia—anxiety about, or avoidance of, places or situations from which escape might be difficult; the anxiety typically leads to an avoidance of a variety of situations such as being alone outside of the home, being in a crowd of people, traveling, and being in an elevator.
- Specific phobia—anxiety provoked by exposure to a specific object or situation.
- Social phobia—anxiety provoked by exposure to certain types of social or performance situations.
- Obsessive-compulsive disorder—characterized by obsessions that cause marked anxiety and/or by compulsions that serve to neutralize anxiety.
- Posttraumatic stress disorder (PTSD)—persons who are victims of assault frequently experience PTSD. An individual suffering from PTSD will reexperience the traumatic event through dreams, recurrent images, or flashbacks. The person may try to avoid anything or anyone that reminds her of the event and will have persistent symptoms of increased arousal, such as difficulty sleeping, difficulty concentrating, irritability or outbursts of anger, an exaggerated startle response, and hypervigilance (being overly alert).
- Acute stress disorder—symptoms similar to those of PSTD but these occur within the first month after the trauma and are short lived.
- Generalized anxiety disorder (GAD)—persistent and excessive anxiety and worry for at least 6 months; individuals with GAD often worry about routine life circumstances such as job, finances, family, and daily chores and schedules.

STRESS AND ANXIETY

There are a number of clinical anxiety disorders related to stress. (See *FYI*: "Clinical Anxiety Disorders" and *FYI*: "Prevalence Rates of Anxiety Disorders.") Specific phobia is the most common anxiety disorder and the second

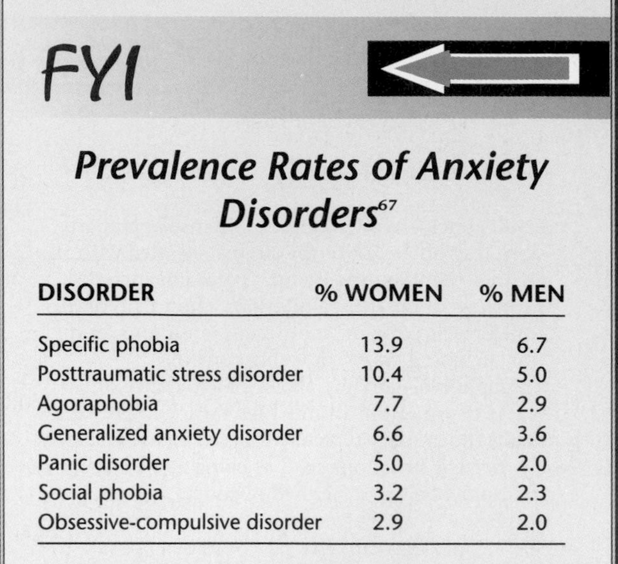

FYI

Prevalence Rates of Anxiety Disorders[67]

DISORDER	% WOMEN	% MEN
Specific phobia	13.9	6.7
Posttraumatic stress disorder	10.4	5.0
Agoraphobia	7.7	2.9
Generalized anxiety disorder	6.6	3.6
Panic disorder	5.0	2.0
Social phobia	3.2	2.3
Obsessive-compulsive disorder	2.9	2.0

most common of all psychiatric disorders occurring in about 14 percent of women (and 7 percent of men) in the United States.[68] The only two anxiety disorders for which women are not at significant increased risk (over men) are social phobia and obsessive-compulsive disorder. The most effective mental health treatment for anxiety disorders is cognitive behavioral therapy.[69] Cognitive behavioral therapy recognizes the role that thoughts and emotions play in shaping behavior and assists an individual in recognizing and changing irrational thoughts and exaggerated feelings that result in dysfunctional behavior. Hypnotherapy is often used as an adjunct with cognitive behavioral therapy for some anxiety disorders. Hypnosis creates a state of focused attention in which people can experience changes in perception, cognition, and emotion. Eye movement desensitization and reprocessing (EMDR) is also sometimes used in treating anxiety disorders. EMDR combines cognitive-behavioral and physiological interventions to reduce symptoms associated with posttraumatic stress disorder and other anxiety disorders. Relaxation training is incorporated into most treatment regimes for anxiety disorders, and biofeedback-assisted relaxation training is the most effective applied relaxation therapy. Medications for treating acute (short-term) anxiety are Xanax (alprazolam) and Valium (diazepam; one of the original antianxiety drugs still prescribed today), but both of these can be addictive. Medication for chronic (long-term) clinical anxiety is usually an antidepressant that is a selective serotonin reuptake inhibitor (SSRI), such as Prozac (fluoxetine), Zoloft (sertraline), or Paxil (paroxetine); or a selective serotonin-norepinephrine reuptake inhibitor (SSNRI), such as Effexor.[70] Very often a combination of mental health treatment and drug therapy can get the best results in the early stages of treatment. As mental health treatment progresses, one goal is to move the client to the point of no longer needing drug therapy.

Her Story

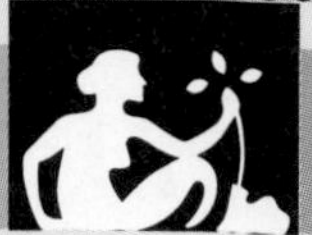

Linda: Posttraumatic Stress Disorder

Linda was assaulted by a stranger with a knife. She survived the attack. Along with some deep cuts on her hands, she experienced significant emotional trauma. She exhibited all of the symptoms relevant to posttraumatic stress disorder. She was afraid to be alone, found crowds to be extremely anxiety provoking, and was startled by the smallest events, such as someone walking too close to her. After mental health counseling to help Linda recover from PTSD, which also incorporated many relaxation techniques, Linda's symptoms were all either significantly reduced or eliminated.

- Do you know anyone who has ever had anxiety from experiencing a traumatic event?
- Were they able to overcome it completely?
- Did they seek assistance from a mental health provider?

STRESS AND TRAUMA

Individuals who become victims frequently experience severe stress. The stress reaction can be immediate or delayed. It can be brief, or it may last for years. The stress reaction from trauma experiences can take on a variety of manifestations including heightened startle and fear responses, anxiety and panic attacks, distancing from friends and family, and avoidance of strangers or crowded places. Mental health counseling can be effective in facilitating the healing process for trauma victims. (See *Her Story:* "Linda: Posttraumatic Stress Disorder.")

September 11, 2001, marked the single most disastrous terrorist event in U.S. history. Nineteen Islamic extremists hijacked four commercial airliners, crashing two into the World Trade Center towers in New York City, one into the Pentagon in Washington, D.C., and one in an open field in Pennsylvania. The victims of this tragedy included people of many different nationalities along with rescue personnel who were caught in the rubble when the twin towers collapsed. Many of the bodies from the disaster were never found. The trauma experienced after this act was global. Almost every country in the world sent condolences and many declared "national days of mourning." Reports of insomnia, anxiety, generalized fears, and depression were common. Fear of flying left passenger airliners empty, and the aftermath of the attacks created great financial turmoil around the world. Many survivors of the September 11 terrorist event suffered posttraumatic stress symptoms, and most U.S. citizens experienced a heightened level of anxiety.

Women in New York City were two times more likely than men to have posttraumatic stress disorder (PTSD) 5 to 8 weeks after the September 11, 2001, terrorist attacks.[71] Data from a telephone survey of randomly selected residents in Manhattan assessed demographic information, lifetime experience of traumatic events, life stressors, social support, event exposure variables, postevent concerns, perievent panic attacks (having a panic attack within the first few hours after the terrorist attacks occurred), and probable PTSD related to the attacks. The researchers concluded that specific behavioral and biographic factors explained most of the excess burden of probable PTSD among women after the terrorist attacks. The data suggested that the higher prevalence of PTSD in women after the attacks was largely explained by the effect of previous experience of unwanted sexual contact, the burden of acting as the primary caretaker for children in a household, concern for the community at large, a recent history of mental/emotional problems, and experience of a perievent panic attack. This research is significant because isolating the factors that increase the likelihood that women will develop PTSD may allow early identification and treatment of those at risk, reducing both the emotional and economic burden of PTSD after disasters.

COPING SKILLS FOR STRESS: PREVENTION, MANAGEMENT, AND TREATMENT

Social Support

One of the best buffers against stress is a satisfactory support system. Friends and family members who offer positive support can greatly diminish the impact of stress. In fact, research with undergraduate college women has shown that the presence of another woman who is perceived to offer nonevaluative, positive support to the research subject during an acutely stressful performance situation resulted in a significant reduction in the subject's cardiovascular responses to the stressor.[72] Women without a support person present had significantly greater cardiovascular responses (meaning a greater stress response). The perceived quality of the support modulated the impact of the stressor in that the more supportive the subject perceived the support person to be the less was the subject's stress response.

You Are What You Think

When an event occurs, you may make a judgment about that event that may impact how much stress you will or will not experience as a result of that event. If you take time to examine this process, you can understand it better and use it to your advantage; this is known as the technique of cognitive appraisal. **Cognitive appraisal** is the process of categorizing an encounter with respect to its significance for well-being.[73] The two main evaluative issues of cognitive appraisal are "Am I in trouble or being benefited, now or in the future and in what way?" and "What, if anything, can be done about it?"

Because the amount of stress experienced is so dependent upon how a stress-eliciting event is perceived, one obvious technique for managing stress is to learn to alter your destructive thought patterns. There are numerous methods for altering negative patterns of thinking.[74] One important technique is **thought stopping.** Each time a negative thought comes to mind, you immediately say to yourself "stop." The command "stop" acts as a distractor and interrupts the flow of self-defeating thinking. Thought stopping can be followed by substitutions of positively reassuring or self-accepting statements. Positive affirmations are self-statements that accentuate positive feelings or actions. Affirmations can be applied to any area of life. Example affirmations might be "I am confident and strong," "I feel good about myself," "I am calm and relaxed," "I am a beautiful and worthwhile person," and so on. You may not believe the statements at first, but with continued daily practice you will eventually begin to act as if you believe the statements. Before long, you will begin to, consciously or unconsciously, create the feeling or behavior you desire. Self-suggestion, whether it be positive or negative, has a powerful influence on the state of your mind and body. Complete *Journal Activity:* "Stop the Negative, Accentuate the Positive" to help accomplish this behavior.

Stress and Nutrition

Maintaining a well-balanced and nutritious eating pattern is vital for maintaining health and well-being and for countering the ill effects of stress. Although comprehensive coverage of nutrition is provided in Chapter 10, it is important to note here that certain food substances can contribute to stress by stimulating the sympathetic stress response. Certain substances act as **vasoconstrictors,** in that they constrict the blood vessels of the body causing an elevation in blood pressure

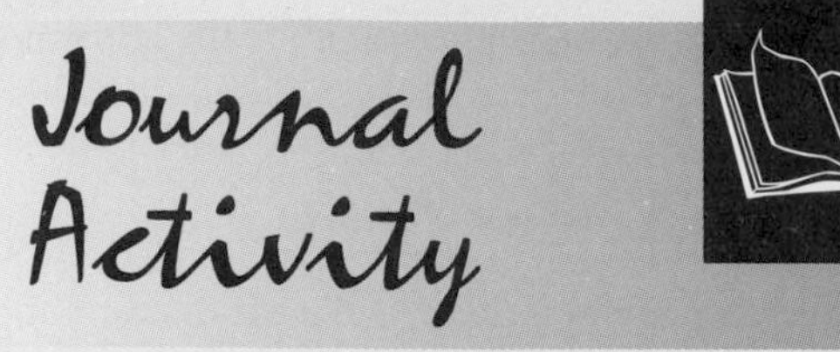

Stop the Negative, Accentuate the Positive

Make a list of the self-defeating thoughts you say to yourself. Now take index cards and on each one write a positive self-suggestion to replace each self-defeating thought. Carry the cards with you during the day. Once a day repeat the positive affirmations to yourself. At first, you may want to focus on just one affirmation at a time to get used to the process. The more you practice a positive self-suggestion, the quicker you will change in the desired direction.

and heart rate.[75] They also create a temporary elevation in mood or energy level. Some of these stimulants are commonly present in our everyday life such as caffeine, found in coffee, tea, sodas, and some diet pills; chocolate or cocoa; processed sugar; and nicotine. These substances tend to interfere with the ability to reduce stress and anxiety levels. When the effects of these stimulants wear off, the individual often experiences a crash period. The body is exhausted from the pressure placed on it during the period of physiological elevation. These substances create elevations in stress or anxiety levels, and they also lead to greater fatigue and exhaustion. There is sometimes a temptation to take more of these substances in order to re-elevate the energy or mood level. Thus, these substances not only increase the stress and anxiety level, but for many people, they can be a part of an extremely detrimental addictive cycle. Reductions in types and amounts of these substances from one's diet should be gradual. These substances can produce such a strong physiological response in the body that some withdrawal symptoms may be present. If withdrawal symptoms become too uncomfortable, then an individual should consult with a health care provider for assistance in reducing and eliminating these substances from her diet.

Women under stress may crave foods high in fat and sugar. These foods can cause a person to feel lethargic. Stress can also lead to bouts of overeating or undereating. Special attention should be paid to one's eating patterns during stressful times.

Some vitamins are thought to be helpful for cushioning the blow of stress on the body. The vitamin B category may be effective in countering stress and depression, and some women take a form of stress B complex for these purposes. Ask your health care provider about incorporating a regimen of healthy vitamins into your daily routine.

The intake of appropriate amounts of water is necessary to maintain a healthy body. When an individual is under stress, toxins seem to build up more in the body. Because water flushes the waste products from your body, an increase in water consumption during stressful periods may be advised.

Use of Herbs

Native healers from many continents have used herbs for healing since ancient times. The World Health Organization also recognizes the potential benefits to using herbal medicines.[76] Medicinal plants and herbs are important to the health of many communities; between 35,000 and 70,000 species have at one time or another been used for medical purposes, and international use of herbal medicines and natural products is steadily increasing. Today, healing herbs can be found in many local health food stores. Many herbs have healing and soothing effects on the nervous system.[77] In various combinations, the following herbs (plants and oils) can be used for relaxing baths: oatmeal, lime flowers, chamomile flowers, lavender, rosemary, thyme, and yarrow. Some herbal teas and tonics can also have a relaxing and soothing effect. It is important to consult a trained herbalist or herbal guide before utilizing these herbal baths, teas, or tonics. Also, if you have allergies, exercise caution in using these substances.

Aromatherapy is the use of the scent or aroma from essential oils produced from certain herbs that benefit the individual. The use of essential oils can enhance recovery from particular mental and physical ailments. Essential oils can be used in baths, massage, as room fragrances, or as inhalants. Essential oils affect the body through the olfactory system. The olfactory system, used in the sense of smell, has a direct link to the limbic system, the part of the brain that deals with emotions. Herbalists claim that the scent from certain oils can directly impact the brain, stimulating certain systems in the body that may facilitate healing.

Essential oils are very potent. It takes only a few drops of an essential oil in several ounces of a base oil for a massage, or a few drops of essential oil in bath water, to get the desired effect. Several essential oils can be helpful in countering stress and anxiety disorders, including jasmine, eucalyptus, rosemary, lavender, chamomile, clary sage, rose, and ylang ylang.[78] An individual who wishes to utilize aromatherapy should consult an aromatherapist or aromatherapy guide.

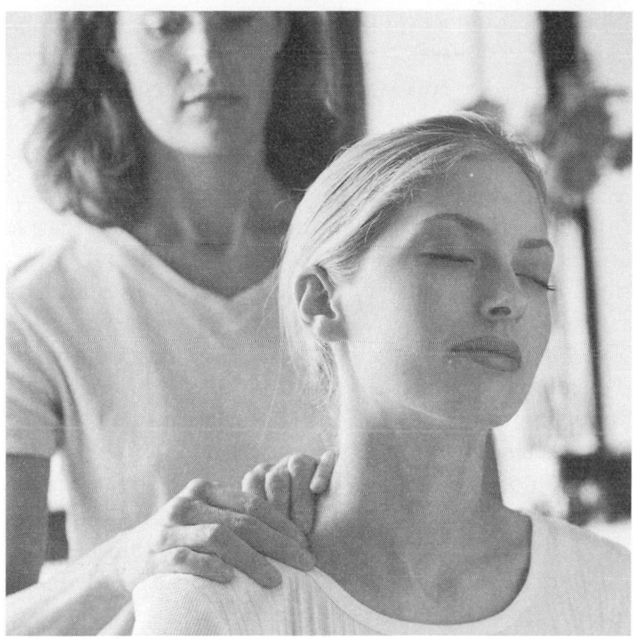

Massage therapy is good for helping the body to relax.

Massage and Reflexology

Massage involves systematically stroking, kneading, and pressing the soft tissues of the body to induce a state of total relaxation.[79] Massage works mainly on the muscles, ligaments, and tendons and affects particularly the body's balance of blood and fluids. A most effective massage can be obtained by visiting a certified massage therapist. However, individuals can learn some simple techniques to share with one another at home using a massage guide.

Reflexology is the use of compression massage on designated areas on the hands and feet. Reflexology is based on the principle that there are areas, or reflex points, on the feet and hands that correspond to each organ, gland, and structure in the body.[80] Reflexology is a means of helping the body attain balance in all its functions. It influences areas where weakened circulation has allowed waste matter to interfere with functioning. Through reflexology, the body is encouraged to renew itself so that all its processes are working in harmony. A basic understanding of human anatomy is vital for doing proper reflexology. Improper use of reflexology can be harmful, so it is recommended that you receive treatment from a trained reflexologist.

Acupressure and Acupuncture

Acupressure is a relaxing natural therapy that teaches the body to identify and release patterns of holding tension.[81] Acupressure has been used by Chinese healers for several centuries and is now in common practice in many cultures, including the United States. Acupressure treatments consist of slow, gradual finger pressure applied to designated sites on the body. These sites correspond with neural receptor sites. Acupressure is sometimes used to support conventional medical treatment. It can be used to recover from shock or trauma. Acupressure is frequently used for relaxation, improved circulation, tension release, and pain control.

Acupuncture, a therapy related to acupressure, is also an ancient art that has been practiced for centuries in Asia. It utilizes fine needles inserted into acupressure points to stimulate relaxation and healing. Consumers around the world utilize acupuncture; 90 percent of the pain clinics in the United Kingdom and 77 percent in Germany use acupuncture.[82]

Exercise

A regular exercise routine is a very effective approach to stress management. Exercise allows us to release pent-up anxiety and to stimulate and flush out the body's systems through movement. Exercise techniques are covered in Chapter 11 of this book. It is important to remember that simply taking the time to go for a walk can be an effective stress reducer.

Tai Chi is an exercise system specifically designed to calm the mind and emotions. It is a low-impact exercise appropriate for any age group and is especially popular among older adults. Tai Chi is very effective at stretching muscles and enhancing flexibility of joints. It is also a form of meditation.

Time Management

Managing one's time effectively can reduce stress. This often requires some planning, prioritizing, and structuring. High-achievement-oriented persons may not have trouble with the planning and structuring part, but they often have difficulty with prioritizing. They feel the obligation to get everything done. It takes some discipline to accept the idea that sometimes not everything will get done. Weighing the most important tasks (such as time with family versus time at work, or time for self versus time with the family), putting them in the order of most importance, and then just doing the best you can and not worrying about the rest is a healthy and realistic attitude. (See *Journal Activity:* "Time Management.")

Mind–Body Medicine: An Overview

The National Institutes of Health's National Center for Complementary and Alternative Medicine (NCCAM) advocates for the potential health benefits of mind–body medicine. As described by the NCCAM, mind–body medicine focuses on the interaction among the brain, mind,

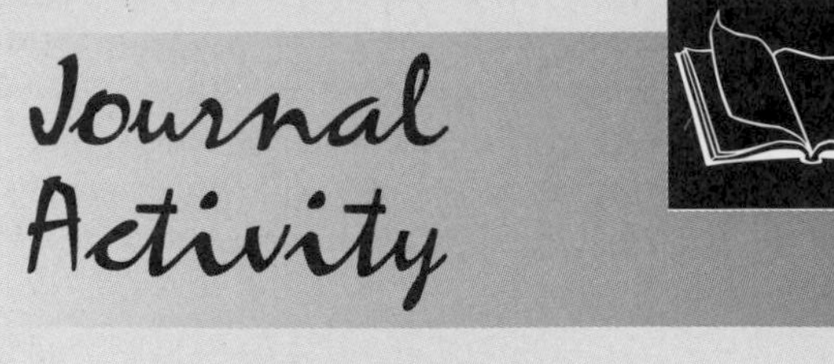

Time Management

Record how you use your time for one week. Study your record, and try to reduce those activities that take too much time or are less important than other activities. Now make a schedule by dividing your time into blocks so that similar activities can be scheduled together. (Purchasing a date book might be helpful here.) Classify activities into a few major areas of responsibility, such as chores, course work, job, recreation, and socializing. Schedule activities within each block of time. Schedule related activities in the same time block if possible. Complex activities need to be broken down into small steps or tasks so that you have a better chance of completing them. Be sure to schedule time for short breaks during long blocks of concentrated effort to minimize stress and fatigue. Reassess your time management activities occasionally and make adjustments when necessary.

body, and behavior, and the powerful ways in which emotional, mental, social, spiritual, and behavioral factors can directly affect health.[83] It regards as fundamental an approach that respects and enhances a person's capacity for self-knowledge and self-care, and it emphasizes techniques that are grounded in this approach.

Mind–body medicine typically focuses on intervention strategies that are thought to promote health, such as relaxation, hypnosis, visual imagery, meditation, yoga, biofeedback, Tai Chi, cognitive-behavioral therapies, group support, calming self-talk, and spirituality. The field views illness as an opportunity for personal growth and transformation, and health care providers as catalysts and guides in this process. Certain mind–body intervention strategies, such as group support for cancer survivors, are well integrated into conventional care (and thus are mainstream approaches) and, while still considered mind–body interventions, are not considered to be complementary and alternative medicine (CAM).

Mind–body interventions constitute a major portion of the overall use of CAM by the public. In 2002 more than 30 percent of the adult U.S. population used at least one form of mind–body intervention, including relaxation techniques and imagery, biofeedback, and hypnosis. Prayer was used by more than 50 percent of the population.[84] The following is a presentation of selected research reviewed by the NCCAM that demonstrates some of the benefits of mind–body medicine.

Mind–Body Influence on Immunity There is considerable evidence that emotional traits, both negative and positive, influence people's susceptibility to infection. Following systematic exposure to a respiratory virus in the laboratory, individuals who report higher levels of stress or negative moods have been shown to develop more severe illness than those who report less stress or more positive moods.[85] Recent studies suggest that the tendency to report positive, as opposed to negative, emotions may be associated with greater resistance to colds. These laboratory studies are supported by longitudinal studies pointing to associations between psychological or emotional traits and the incidence of respiratory infections.[86]

Mind–Body Interventions and Disease Research on mind–body medicine stretching across 20 years has provided considerable evidence that psychological factors contribute to the development and progression of coronary artery disease.[87] There is evidence that mind–body interventions can be effective in the treatment of coronary artery disease, enhancing the effect of standard recurrences of cardiac rehabilitation in reducing mortality and recurrences of cardiac events for up to 2 years.[88] Multiple studies with patients who have various types of cancer suggest that mind–body interventions can improve mood, quality of life, and coping, as well as lessen disease and treatment-related symptoms, such as chemotherapy-induced nausea, vomiting, and pain.[89] Some studies have suggested that mind–body interventions can improve the function of the immune system; but it is unclear whether the improvement is large enough to have an impact on disease progression or prognosis.[90,91] Mind–body interventions have been applied to various types of pain associated with disease. Research demonstrates that these interventions may be particularly effective as complementary treatment in the management of arthritis, with reductions in pain maintained for up to 4 years and reductions in the number of physician visits.[92] Mind–body interventions have also been shown to be effective with more general acute and chronic pain management, headache, and low-back pain.[93]

Mind–Body Interventions for Surgical Preparation Research has demonstrated that mind–body interventions can better prepare patients for the stress associated with surgery. Randomized controlled trials—in which some patients received audiotapes with mind–body techniques (guided imagery, music, and instructions for improved outcomes) and some patients received audio tapes without such techniques—found that subjects receiving the mind–body intervention recovered more quickly and spent fewer days in the hospital.[94] Mind–body interventions have been shown to reduce discomfort and adverse effects during vascular and renal procedures. Pain increased linearly with procedure time in a control group and in a group practicing structured attention, but remained flat in a group practicing a self-hypnosis technique. The self-administration of analgesic drugs was significantly higher in the control group than in the attention and hypnosis groups.[95]

The preceding body of research was reviewed by the NCCAM to demonstrate both preventive and recovery health benefits of mind–body medicine. The ultimate capacity for humans to consciously utilize the mind–body connection for healing and wellness has not yet been determined. It is clear that humans can use thoughts and emotions to affect health, yet relative to other areas, science has barely begun to explore this avenue of medicine. Much more research is required to help us understand the full potential for preventing illness and facilitating recovery with mind–body techniques.

Body Awareness

Your body talks to you. It tells you when it is getting too stressed. When you do not listen to it or choose to ignore what it is telling you, then it will start "screaming" at you with various aches, pains, and disorders. A body scream can take many forms. Many of these are listed in earlier sections of this chapter as stress symptoms and disorders. The longer it takes the body to get your attention, the more severe the manifestation of the body's scream.

You can refine your listening skills and respond to the body's needs before it gets to the screaming stage. Focus on your forehead. Stay aware of when you create lines or wrinkles due to tightening the forehead (frontalis) muscles. You do not need to "scrunch" the forehead while concentrating or focusing and certainly not while worrying. Keep the forehead as smooth and relaxed as possible at all times.

Be aware of your jaw. When you are truly relaxed, there should be a slight space between your upper and lower teeth while your mouth is closed. Tension in the jaw (masseter) muscles will prevent this. If you have carried high levels of tension in your jaw for a long time, it may take a while, sometimes several days, for it to completely relax.

Be aware of your neck and shoulders. As tension builds during the day, many people tend to start moving their shoulders gradually up toward their ears without even realizing it. Keep your shoulders down and relaxed. This will minimize the tension in those neck and shoulder (trapezius) muscles.

The few suggestions given regarding awareness refer directly to the body. However, a more relaxed body can also lead to a more relaxed mind and vice versa. The state of the body affects the mind and the state of the mind affects the body. They are interconnected. Attention to both the mind and the body will promote more holistic health.

Relaxation Exercises

Relaxation exercises are designed to calm the body, mind, and emotions.[96] Practiced daily, they can be most effective in managing stress. Most relaxation exercises take only about 15 minutes or less, so it is possible to incorporate at least one into your daily routine. **Progressive relaxation** is one of the most commonly used relaxation techniques.[97] This technique involves alternately tensing and releasing the muscles, beginning with the feet and slowly working through each section of the body. This technique enhances awareness of tension and facilitates relaxation in each part of the body. Many people are not aware that they are tense until they engage in a relaxation exercise.

Autogenic phrases is another commonly used relaxation exercise.[98] These are self-statements designed to calm the body and mind. (See *Journal Activity:* "Relaxation Exercise.")

It is possible to set aside only a minute or so and receive substantial benefits using certain brief techniques. The **relaxation response** is a technique through which one learns to quiet the body and mind by using long, easy exhalations allowing the body to relax while sitting in a comfortable position.[99] Upon perceiving a stressful event, the "quieting reflex" is a set of specific responses, such as striving for a positive mental state, an "inner smile," and a deep exhalation with the tongue relaxed and the shoulders relaxed, which should be used immediately.[100] (See the example in *Journal Activity:* "Quieting Reflex.")

Biofeedback

Biofeedback is the use of electronic equipment to monitor the physiological state of the body while the individual learns techniques to voluntarily regulate the body's systems and reduce unwanted symptoms. Biofeedback for stress reduction is used with relaxation exercises. It enhances the learning of techniques for reducing mental, emotional, and physical tension. With biofeedback equipment, an individual can immediately

Journal Activity

Relaxation Exercise

Find a partner. Try this version of an autogenic training exercise. Sit in a comfortable position and close your eyes. Now have your partner read to you the phrases listed below. Be sure and have her read very slowly, pausing 5 seconds between each phrase, and read in a relaxed and mellow tone of voice. You can also record the script onto a tape and listen to it.

> I feel quite quiet . . . I am beginning to feel quite relaxed . . . My feet feel heavy, heavy and relaxed . . . My ankles, my knees, and my hips feel relaxed and comfortable . . . The whole central part of my body feels relaxed and quiet . . . My hands, my arms, and my shoulders feel heavy, relaxed, and comfortable . . . My neck, my jaws, and my forehead feel relaxed . . . My whole body feels quiet, comfortable, and relaxed . . . My arms and hands are heavy and warm . . . I feel quite quiet. . . My arms and hands are relaxed, relaxed and warm . . . Warmth is flowing into my hands, they are warm, warm . . . I feel quite quiet . . . My mind is quiet . . . I withdraw my thoughts from my surroundings . . . I feel serene and still . . . I am awake but in an easy, quiet, inward-turned way . . . My mind is calm and quiet . . . I feel an inward quietness . . .

Maintain the inward quietness for about another minute or so and ask yourself the following questions: (1) What were your physical sensations during today's practice? (2) What were your feelings? and (3) What were your thoughts? Were they in words, images, or both? Reactivate by taking five slow, full breaths. Stretch and feel energy flowing through your body. Open your eyes. Write your experience in your journal.

Journal Activity

Quieting Reflex

Think of using four S's to help you remember to relax: smile, slack, sag, and smooth. As you take a deep breath in, put a smile on your face. Now, as you exhale slowly, let your jaw go slack and loose, sag your shoulders, and relax and smooth the muscles in your forehead. When you are confronted with a stressful event, try doing this slowly, three or four times in a row. Note any differences in the way you felt before the exercise and after. Write your experience in your journal.

see the negative effects of stressful thoughts and feelings and the positive effects of relaxation techniques on the body. Immediate and accurate feedback about the effects of stress and relaxation on the body facilitates the learning of voluntary control over the autonomic nervous system. Biofeedback is a noninvasive and painless therapy. Disorders or conditions that are effectively treated with biofeedback therapy include migraine and tension headaches, high blood pressure, neck and back pain, irritable bowel syndrome, Raynaud's disease (chronic cold fingers, toes, ears, nose, etc.), phobias, panic and anxiety, jaw pain, teeth grinding, and other stress-related disorders.

There are many types of biofeedback. The modality used depends on the nature of the presenting problem.[101] Biofeedback is used to teach a person to voluntarily warm the hands and feet, which lowers blood pressure; to relax muscle tension, which reduces and eliminates pain; to facilitate healthy breathing for relaxation; and to alter brain wave patterns thereby allowing the individual to achieve and maintain a state of alert relaxation that is ideal for learning and performance. Brain wave biofeedback, or **neurotherapy** (neurofeedback), is frequently used to treat learning disabilities, attention deficit disorder, and addiction disorders. Biofeedback therapy is available from mental or physical health therapists who have received specific education and training in biofeedback techniques.

Meditation

Meditation, one of the most common mind–body interventions, is a conscious mental process that induces a set of integrated physiological changes termed the relaxation response. It is a common technique utilized to foster health and well-being. It can facilitate feelings of personal balance and harmony, relaxation, and increased awareness of oneself and one's environment. It can assist with the development of intuition, self-insight, and greater self-trust. An expansion of consciousness often occurs from meditation that replaces feelings of isolation, provides

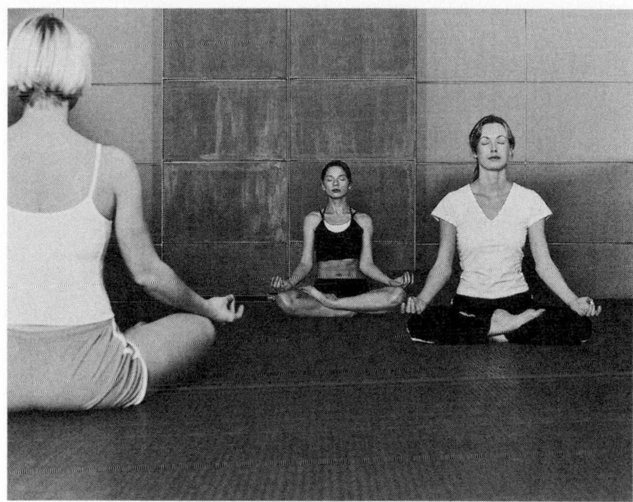

Meditation fosters health and well-being

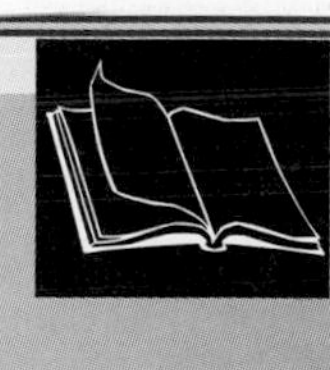

Journal Activity

Meditation Exercise

Try this beginning-level meditation exercise using the following steps: (1) lie in a comfortable position with eyes closed and breathe deeply, relaxing your mind and body; (2) imagine a very powerful presence within you and all around you that is totally loving, strong, and wise and that is nurturing, protecting, and guiding you; (3) relax and enjoy the feeling that you are being totally taken care of by the universe; (4) conclude the meditation with the following affirmation—"I feel and trust the presence of the universe in my life."[104]

This type of meditation encourages individuals to turn within for intuitive insight and creative ideas. What experiences did you have during this exercise?

greater personal security, and creates a sensation of being in communion with the universe. (See *Journal Activity:* "Meditation Exercise.")

Meditation can be a guided exercise or can take the form of completely blanking one's mind to allow for spontaneous imagery or insight. Meditations designed for healing purposes may involve a focus on the body and its healing mechanisms. A healing meditation may also be more abstract such as to visualize a swim in healing waters or to be showered by a colorful rainbow that symbolically represents the chakras, hypothetically the main energy centers in the body. Tai Chi is utilized as a meditation of movement that simultaneously aligns the body with mind and spirit. A variety of schools or types of meditation exist.[102]

Numerous benefits can be gained by the individual from the practice of meditation: (1) meditations can bring about an increase in ego strength; (2) meditations can be applied to special problem areas and can be used to help explore a specific area and help loosen defenses (resistance to insight or change); (3) meditations assist with centering, the quality of feeling at ease with oneself and with one's environment; (4) meditations facilitate growth by teaching the individual to regard his or her being as something of real value and to give serious attention to the totality of being; and (5) meditations assist with growing beyond the ability to function in everyday life while being relatively pain-free.[103]

Functional magnetic resonance imaging (fMRI) has been used to identify and characterize the brain regions that are active during meditation. This research suggests that various parts of the brain known to be involved in attention and in the control of the autonomic nervous system are activated, providing a neurochemical and anatomical basis for the effects of meditation on various physiological activities.[105] Studies involving imaging are advancing the understanding of mind–body mechanisms. For example, meditation has been shown in one study to produce significant increases in left-sided anterior brain activity, which is associated with positive emotional states. Moreover, in this same study, meditation was associated with increases in antibodies to influenza vaccine, suggesting potential linkages among meditation, positive emotional states, localized brain responses, and improved immune function.[106]

Yoga

Yoga involves the practice of body postures and poses to improve health by bringing the body into balance and reducing stress and tension. Hatha Yoga was developed in ancient India as a simple system of eight to ten poses that have evolved into the elaborate technique of today.[107] Yoga techniques range from very simple stretches to more complex twists and headstands. Yoga is an activity that can be used by persons of varying mobility and age.

Proper Breathing

Breath is life. Breathing is a variable rhythm that is linked to all metabolic functions.[108] Although breathing is automatic, it is affected by emotional and physiological

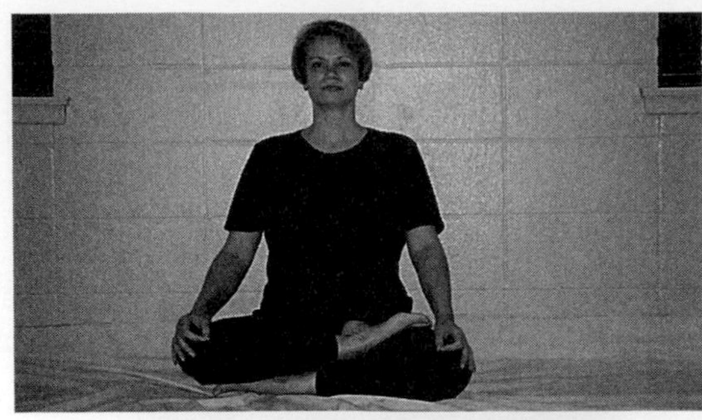

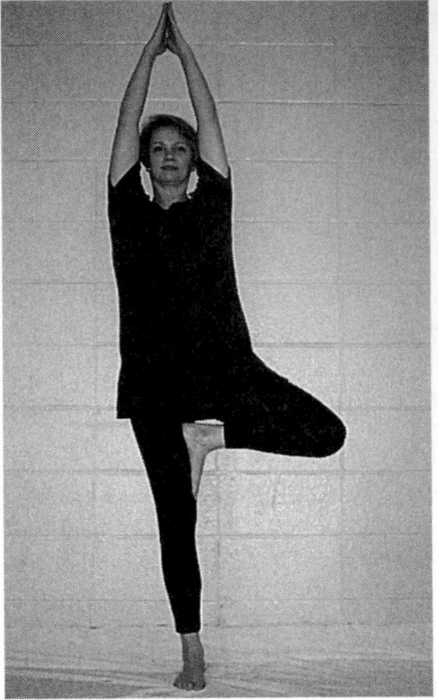

Yoga is good for relaxation, and is a great fitness activity too.

Her Story

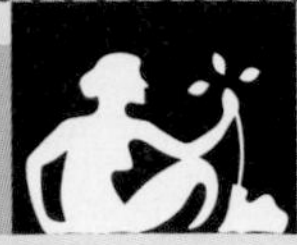

Natalie: The Benefits of Stress Management

Natalie went to a stress management workshop and then never tried any of the techniques in her daily life. She said she was too busy and eventually admitted that she had a low opinion of people who did not work hard all of the time; she thought they were lazy. So she resisted relaxing. Natalie realized that her misconceptions about herself and others were interfering with her own health and well-being. After a personal attitude adjustment, Natalie tried some of the techniques and was amazed at how much better her life became. She had fewer emotional and physical discomforts, and she could manage her busy schedule much better. She also reported having a more worry-free and relaxed attitude about life. She was enjoying life more now that she was managing her stress better.

- Do you know someone who finds excuses not to practice relaxation?
- Why do you suppose they put relaxation as such a low priority in their lives?
- Do you think that relaxation practice is important for your health?

demands on the body. Short, quick, and shallow breathing that originates mostly from the chest area is the least effective pattern for full oxygenation of red blood cells. In chest breathing, known as thoracic breathing, the rib cage spreads and the chest goes up. In spite of its appearance, this breathing mode results in very little air entering the lungs. This type of breathing is most common under stress.

Abdominal breathing, referred to as **diaphragmatic breathing,** is a healthy type of breathing. This is accomplished by alternately contracting the diaphragm and abdominal muscles that increase the space in the chest into which the lungs can expand to accept air.

Sometimes the individual is unaware of her breathing pattern. Training for proper breathing should begin with heightened awareness of current breathing patterns and then practice to create longer, deeper, and fuller breaths. For fuller benefits, breathing should be initiated from the abdomen (diaphragm), filling up the bottom of the lungs in the upper diaphragm with air and completing the task by filling up the top of the lungs in the chest. Exhaling reverses this pattern. Healthy, relaxing breaths should be easy and unlabored. When sitting quietly, a woman's breathing rate should be about 14 to 15 breaths per minute or less.

CONCLUSION

Many people claim they have no time for stress management. This simply implies that they have no understanding of what stress management is. Stress management makes life easier, not harder. It does not entail more work. Instead, it is fun and relaxing. Think of it as a form of entertainment and recreation. If you claim to have no time for stress reduction or management, then you should consider the reasons you are hesitant to relax. Now, go out and try some stress management for yourself. Remember, you are worth it. (See *Her Story:* "Natalie: The Benefits of Stress Management."

Chapter Summary

- Stress is the physical, mental, and emotional response to the presence of a perceived stressor.
- The primary anatomical areas that are involved in the stress response are the cerebral cortex, the hypothalamus, the adrenal glands, the hormone ACTH, corticoids, and adrenalin.
- Life stressors fall into five major categories: social, psychological, psychosocial, biochemical, and philosophical.
- The immediate stress response is the mobilization of the body for confrontation or avoidance of challenge; this is referred to as the fight-or-flight response.
- The general adaptation syndrome is the long-term response to stress and consists of three stages: alarm, resistance, and exhaustion.
- There is good stress and bad stress. Eustress is considered good stress because it is motivational stress, whereas distress is debilitating stress. When stress is too great, it can become distress.
- The effects of stress are cumulative; symptoms may begin as relatively minor body aches and pains and gradually progress to more severe disorders and diseases. Major life events as well as daily hassles can produce stress.
- A variety of coping techniques can be easily learned and may prove to be beneficial in reducing stress.
- A positive attitude and taking time to play may protect some people from the potentially damaging effects of stressors.

Review Questions

1. What is stress and why do people perceive stressors differently?
2. What is optimal stress and what is the impact of going beyond this?
3. How does the stress response impact the endocrine system and the autonomic nervous system?
4. What are the three stages of the general adaptation syndrome?
5. What are some of the disorders or conditions that may result from prolonged stress?
6. Which stress-related disorders are more common in women than men?
7. What types of stressors exist for women in various roles?
8. What types of stressors are more specific to multicultural issues?
9. What are some effective strategies for coping with stress?

Resources

Organization

Association for Applied Psychophysiology and Biofeedback
10200 West 44th Avenue, Suite 304
Wheat Ridge, Colorado 80033
Phone: 303-420–2902

Audiotapes and CDs

Calm Down: Relaxation and Imagery Skills for Managing Fear, Anxiety, Panic (1995)
Countdown to Relaxation (1993)
Daydreams and Get-Aways (1993)
Relax . . . Let Go . . . Relax (1982)
Stress R–E–L–E–A–S–E (1983)
Take a Deep Breath (1992)
Warm and Heavy (1994)
Worry Stoppers: Breathing and Imagery to Calm the Restless Mind (1995)
Whole Person Associates, Duluth, MN. Phone: 800-247-6789, Web site: www.wholeperson.com

Videotapes/DVDs

The Science of Stress (2001)
Stress Hurts! A Wake-Up Call for Women (2001)
Films for the Humanities & Sciences, Box 2053, Princeton, NJ 08543-2053, Phone: 800-257-5126, Web site: www.films.com

Web Sites

American Council for Headache Education
www.achenet.org
American Headache Society
www.ahsnet.org
American Institute of Stress
www.stress.org
Biofeedback Certification Institute of America
www.bcia.org
Healthcite
www.healthcite.com
International Headache Society
www.i-h-s.org
Magnum, Migraine Awareness Group: A National Understanding for Migraineurs
www.migraines.org
National Headache Foundation
www.headaches.org

National Institute of Neurological Disorders and Stroke (NINDS)
www.ninds.nih.gov
World Headache Alliance
www.w-h-a.org

Suggested Readings

Allen, J., and R. Klein. 1996. *Ready, Set, Relax: A Research Based Program of Relaxation, Learning and Self-Esteem for Children.* Watertown, WI: Inner Coaching.

Babior, S., and C. Goldman. 1995. *Overcoming Panic, Anxiety & Phobias.* Duluth, MN: Whole Person Associates.

Bassett, L. 2001. *From Panic to Power: Proven Techniques to Calm Your Anxiety, Conquer Your Fears, and Put You in Control of Your Life.* New York: HarperCollins.

Bohensky, A. 2003. *The Self-Esteem Workbook for Teens.* New York: Growth.

Bourne, E. 2005. *The Anxiety and Phobia Workbook.* Oakland, CA: New Harbinger.

Bourne, E. 2003. *Coping with Anxiety: Ten Simple Ways to Relieve Anxiety, Fear and Worry.* Oakland, CA:New Harbinger.

Davis, M., E. Eshelman, and M. McKay. 2000. *The Relaxation and Stress Reduction Workbook.* 5th ed. Oakland, CA: New Harbinger.

Greenberg, J. S. 2008. *Comprehensive Stress Management.* 10th ed. New York: McGraw-Hill.

Greenberg, J. S. 2006. *Your Personal Stress Profile and Activity Workbook.* 4th ed. New York: McGraw-Hill.

Hanson, J. 2002. *The Women's Book of Yoga and Health: A Lifelong Guide to Wellness.* Boston: Shambhala.

Lusk, J. 1992. *30 Scripts for Relaxation Imagery & Inner Healing.* Vols. I & II. Duluth, MN: Whole Person Associates.

McKay, M., and , P. Rogers 2000. *The Anger Control Workbook.* Oakland, CA: New Harbinger.

Schiraldi, G. 2002. *The Self-Esteem Workbook.* Oakland, CA: New Harbinger.

Seaward, B. 1997. *Managing Stress: Principles and Strategies for Health and Wellbeing.* 2nd ed. Boston: Jones & Bartlett.

Williams, M., and S. Poijula 2002. *The PTSD Workbook.* Oakland, CA: New Harbinger.

References

1. Curtis, J. D., and R. A. Detert. 1981. *How to relax: A holistic approach to stress management.* Mountain View, CA: Mayfield.
2. Selye, H. 1975. *Stress without distress.* New York: New American Library.
3. Cannon, W. 1932. *The wisdom of the body.* New York: Norton.
4. Selye, *Stress without distress.*
5. Torkelson, E., and T. Muhonen. 2004. The role of gender and job level in coping with occupational stress *Work & Stress* 18 (3): 267–74.
6. Taylor, S., L. Klein, B. Lewis, T. Gruenewald, R. Gurung, and J. Updegraff. 2000. Biobehavioral responses to stress in females: Tend and befriend, not fight-or-flight. *Psychological Review* 107 (3): 411–29.
7. Taylor, S. E. 2002. *The tending instinct.* New York: Henry Holt.
8. *Mosby's medical, nursing, and allied health dictionary* 4th ed. 1994. St. Louis: Mosby-Year Book.
9. Cohen, S. 1996. Psychological stress, immunity, and upper respiratory infections. *Current Directions in Psychological Science,* 5: 86–90.
10. Cohen, S., W. Doyle, D. Skoner, B. Rabin, and J. Gwaltney, 1997. Social ties and susceptibility to the common cold. *Journal of the American Medical Association* 277 (24): 1940–44.
11. Markovitz, J. H., K. A. Matthews, M. Whooley, C. E. Lewis, and K. J. Greenland, 2004. Increases in job strain are associated with incident hypertension in the CARDIA study. *Annals of Behavior Medicine* 28 (1): 4–9.
12. Gupta, M. A., and A. K. Gupta 2004. Stressful major life events are associated with a higher frequency of cutaneous sensory symptoms: An empirical study of non-clinical subjects. *Journal of the European Academy of Dermatology and Venereology* 18: 560–565.
13. Epel, E. S., E. H. Blackburn, J. Lin, F. S. Dhabhar, N. E. Adler, J. D. Morrow, et al. 2004. Accelerated telomere shortening in response to life stress. *Proceedings of the National Academy of Sciences* 101 (49): 17312–15.
14. Ibid.
15. Farabaugh, A. H., M. Mischoulon, M. Fava, C. Green, W. Guyker, and J. Alpert. 2004. The potential relationship between levels of perceived stress and subtypes of major depressive disorder (MDD). *Acta Psychiatrica Scandinavica* 110: 465–70.
16. Freeman, L. M. Y., and K. M. Gil. 2004. Daily stress, coping, and dietary restraint in binge eating. *International Journal of Eating Disorders* 36: 204–12.
17. Kudielka, B. M., R. Von Kanel, M. L. Gander, and J. E. Fischer. 2004. *Work & Stress* 18 (2): 167–78.
18. *Mosby's medical, nursing, and allied health dictionary.*
19. Doctor's guide: Global edition. 1996. DG News: New study shows migraine hits women harder. www.docguide.com (retrieved September 22, 2006).
20. Eikermann, A. 2000. Headache, menstruation and oral contraceptives. *Headache World 2000—Headache and Hormones.* World Headache Alliance. http://w-h-a.org/wha2/Newsite/print.asp?idContentNews=26 (retrieved March 23, 2006).
21. Ibid.
22. MacGregor, E. A., et al. 2003 Estrogen supplements may help prevent menstrual migraine: Study results encouraging. World Headache Alliance. http://w-h-a.org/wha2/Newsite/print.asp?idContentNews=645 (retrieved March 23, 2006).
23. Eikermann, Headache, menstruation and oral contraceptives.

24. Stewart, W. F. R. B. Lipton, E. Chee, J. Sawyer, and S. D. Silberstein. 2000. Menstrual cycle and headache in a population sample of migraineurs. *Neurology* 55: 1517–23.
25. Dzoljic, E., et al. 2002. Prevalence of menstrually related migraine and nonmigraine primary headache in female students of Belgrade University. *Headache* 42:185–93.
26. Ibid.
27. Massiou, H. 2000. Headache and pregnancy. *Headache World 2000—Headache and Hormones*. World Headache Alliance. http://w-h-a.org/wha2/Newsite/print.asp?idContentNews=26 (retrieved March 23, 2006).
28. MacGregor, A. 2000. Headache, the menopause and HRT. *Headache World 2000—Headache and Hormones*. World Headache Alliance. http://w-h-a.org/wha2/Newsite/print.asp?idContentNews=26 (retrieved March 23, 2006).
29. Ibid.
30. HealingWell.com. 2001. *Migraine medication.* www.healingwell.com/migraines (retrieved October 2001).
31. Ibid.
32. Ibid.
33. Whitman, N., D. Spendlove, and C. Clark. 1984. *Student stress: Effects and solutions.* Washington, DC: ERIC Clearinghouse on Higher Education.
34. Campbell, R., L. Svenson, and G. Jarvis. 1992. Perceived level of stress among university undergraduate students in Edmonton, Canada. *Perceptual and Motor Skills* 75 (2): 552–54.
35. Kanner, A., J. Coyne, C. Schaefer, and R. Lazarus. 1981. Comparison of two modes of stress management: Daily hassles and uplifts versus major life events. *Journal of Behavioral Medicine* 4 (1): 1–39.
36. Barko, N. 1983. Stress in professionals and nonprofessionals, men and women. *Innovation Abstracts* 5 (9).
37. Canam, C. 1986. Perceived stressors and coping responses of employed and non-employed career women with pre-school children. *Canadian Journal of Community Mental Health* 5 (2): 49–59.
38. Lennon, M. 1994. Women, work, and well-being: The importance of work conditions. *Journal of Health and Social Behavior* 35 (September): 235–47.
39. Bird, C. 1999. Gender, household labor, psychological distress: The impact of the amount and division of housework. *Journal of Health and Social Behavior* 40 (1): 32–45.
40. Ibid.
41. Bost, B. 2001. *The hurried woman syndrome: Healing for the 50 million women who suffer.* New York: Vantage.
42. Cacioppo, J. T, M. H. Burleson, K. M. Poehlmann, W. B. Malarkey, J. K. Kiecolt-Glaser, G. G. Bernstein et al. 2000. Autonomic and neuroendocrine responses to mild psychological stressors: Effects of chronic stress on older women. *Annals of Behavioral Medicine* 22 (2): 140–48.
43. Moen, P., J. Robison, and V. Fields. 1994. Women's work and caregiving roles: A life course approach. *Journal of Gerontology* 49 (4): 176–87.
44. MacEwen, K., and J. Barling. 1988. Multiple stressors, violence in the family of origin and marital aggression: A longitudinal investigation. *Journal of Family Violence* 3 (1): 73–87.
45. Wheatley, D. 1991. Stress in women. *Stress and Medicine* 7 (2): 73–74.
46. Walters, V. 1993. Stress, anxiety and depression: Women's accounts of their health problems. *Social Science and Medicine* 36 (4): 393–402.
47. Siegel, B. 1986. *Love, medicine and miracles.* New York: Harper & Row; Borysenko, J. 1988. *Minding the body, mending the mind.* New York: Bantam.
48. Castro, F., P. Furth, and H. Karlow. 1984. The health beliefs of Mexican, Mexican American and Anglo American women. *Hispanic Journal of Behavioral Sciences* 6 (4): 365–83.
49. Snapp, M. 1992. Occupational stress, social support, and depression among black and white professional managerial women. *Women and Health* 18: 41–79.
50. "Koroshi"—Overwork—Taking its toll on women in Japan. *WIN News,* 1992. Winter, p. 61.
51. Kenney, J. W. 2000. Women's 'inner-balance': A comparison of stressors, personality traits and health problems by age groups. *Journal of Advanced Nursing* 31 (3):639–50.
52. Francis, M., and C. Sacra. 1994. Stressed out? *Mademoiselle* (September): 190–93.
53. Logue, B. 1991. Women at risk: Predictors of financial stress for retired women workers. *Gerontologist* 31 (5): 657–65.
54. Minkler, M., and R. Stone. 1985. The feminization of poverty and older women. *Gerontologist* 25: 351–57.
55. Survey. 1994. *Orange County* (California) *Register,* October.
56. Blau, F. D., and M. Kahn. 2000. Gender differences in pay. *Journal of Economic Perspectives* 14 (4): 75–99.
57. U.S. Department of Labor, Women's Bureau. 2001. www.dol.gov/dol/wb/public/wb_pubs/20/fact00.htm (retrieved September 2001).
58. Bird, C., and M. Fremont. 1991. Gender, time use, and health. *Journal of Health and Social Behavior* 32 (2): 114–29.
59. Presley, B. 1993. Women pay more for success. *New York Times,* July 4.
60. Marcus, A., T. Zeeman, and C. Telesky. 1983. Sex differences in reports of illness and disability: A further test of the fixed role hypothesis. *Social Science and Medicine* 17: 993–1002; Nathanson, C. 1980. Social roles and health status among women: The significance of employment. *Social Science and Medicine* 14a: 463–71; Verbrugge, L. 1983. Multiple roles and physical health of men and women. *Journal of Health and Social Behavior* 24: 16–30; Waldron, I., and J. Jacobs. 1988. Effects of labor force participation on women's health: New evidence from a longitudinal study. *Journal of Occupational Medicine* 30: 977–83.

61. Ross, C., and C. Bird. 1994. Sex stratification and health lifestyle: Consequences for men's and women's perceived health. *Journal of Health and Social Behavior* 35 (June): 161–78.
62. Isaacson, L., and D. Brown. 1993. *Career information, career counseling, and career development.* 5th ed. Boston: Allyn & Bacon.
63. Lawler, K., and L. Schmied. 1992. A prospective study of women's health: The effects of stress, hardiness, locus of control, Type A behavior, and physiological reactivity. *Women and Health* 19 (1): 27–41.
64. Rogers, S. 1990. *Tired or toxic? A blueprint for health.* Syracuse, NY: Prestige.
65. Dow, C. 1988. Monitor tone generates stress in computer and VDT operators: A preliminary study. Presentation at the Annual Meeting of the Association for Education in Journalism and Mass Communications, Portland, OR.
66. American Psychiatric Association. 2000. *Diagnostic and statistical manual of mental disorders.* 4th ed., text revision (DSM-IV-TR). Washington, DC: APA.
67. McKee, D. B., and J. Dingee, 2003. Treatment of anxiety disorders. In M. Kopala and M. Keital (eds.), *Handbook of counseling women,* pp. 458–81. Thousand Oaks, CA: Sage.
68. Ibid.
69. Ibid.
70. Ibid.
71. Pulcino, T., S. Galea, J. Ahern, H. Resnick, M. Foley, and D. Vlahov. 2003. Posttraumatic stress in women after the September 11 terrorist attacks in New York City. *Journal of Women's Health* 12 (8): 809–20.
72. Fontana, A. M., T. Diegnan, A. Villeneuve, and S. J. Lepore, 1998. Nonevaluative social support reduces cardiovascular reactivity in young women during acutely stressful performance situations. *Journal of Behavioral Medicine* 22 (1): 75–91.
73. Lazarus, R., and S. Folkman. 1984. *Stress, appraisal, and coping.* New York: Springer.
74. Chandler, C., and C. Kolander. 1988. Stop the negative, accentuate the positive. *Journal of School Health* 58 (7): 295–97; Peale, N. 1990. *The power of positive thinking.* New York: Doubleday.
75. Block, K., and M. Schwartz. 1995. Dietary considerations: Rationale, issues, substances, evaluation, and patient education. In Mark Schwartz (ed.), *Biofeedback: A practitioner's guide.* 2nd ed. New York: Guilford.
76. Zhang, X. 1996. Traditional medicine and WHO. *World health* (March/April): 4–5.
77. Mabey, R., M. McIntyre, P. Michael, G. Duff, and J. Stevens. 1988. *The new age herbalist: How to use herbs for healing, nutrition, body care, and relaxation.* New York: Macmillan.
78. Devereaux, C. 1993. *The aroma therapy kit: Essential oils and how to use them.* Boston: Charles E. Tuttle.
79. Lidell, L., S. Thomas, C. Cook, and A. Porter. 1984. *The book of massage: The complete step-by-step guide to Eastern and Western techniques.* New York: Simon & Schuster.
80. Bayly, D. 1988. *Reflexology today.* Rochester, VT: Healing Arts Press.
81. Bauer, C. 1991. *Acupressure for everybody.* New York: Henry Holt.
82. Zhang, Traditional medicine and WHO.
83. National Center for Complementary and Alternative Medicine. 2005. Mind–body medicine: An overview. August. http://nccam.nih.gov/health/backgrounds/mindbody.htm (retrieved March 26, 2006).
84. Ibid.
85. Cohen, S., W. J. Doyle, R. B. Turner et al. 2003. Emotional style and susceptibility to the common cold. *Psychosomatic Medicine* 65 (4): 652–57.
86. Smith, A. and K. Nicholson. 2001. Psychological factors, respiratory viruses and exacerbation of asthma. *Psychoneuroendocrinology* 26 (4): 411–20.
87. National Center for Complementary and Alternative Medicine, 2005.
88. Rutledge, J. C., D. A. Hyson, D. Garduno et al. 1999. Lifestyle modification program in management of patients with coronary artery disease: The clinical experience in a tertiary care hospital. *Journal of Cardiopulmonary Rehabilitation* 19 (4): 226–34.
89. Mundy, E. A., K. N. DuHamel, and G. H. Montgomery. 2003. The efficacy of behavioral interventions for cancer treatment–related side effects. *Seminars in Clinical Neuropsychiatry* 8 (4): 253–75.
90. Irwin, M. R., J. L. Pike, J. C. Cole, et al. 2003. Effects of behavioral intervention, Tai Chi Chih, on varicella-zoster virus specific immunity and health functioning in older adults. *Psychosomatic Medicine* 65 (5): 824–30.
91. Kiecolt-Glaser, J. K., P. T. Marucha, C. Atkinson, et al. 2001. Hypnosis as a modulator of cellular immune dysregulation during acute stress. *Journal of Consulting and Clinical Psychology* 69 (4): 674–82.
92. Luskin, F. M., K. A. Newell, M. Griffith, et al. 2000. A review of mind/body therapies in the treatment of musculoskeletal disorders with implications for the elderly. *Alternative Therapies in Health and Medicine* 6 (2): 46–56.
93. Astin, J. A., S. L. Shapiro, D. M. Eisenberg, et al. 2003. Mind–body medicine: State of science, implications for practice. *Journal of the American Board of Family Practice* 16 (2): 131–47.
94. Tusek, D. L., J. M. Church, S. A. Strong, et al. 1997. Guided imagery: A significant advance in the care of patients undergoing elective colorectal surgery. *Diseases of the Colon and Rectum* 40 (2): 172–78.
95. Lang, E. V., E. G. Benotsch, L. J. Fick, et al. 2000. Adjunctive nonpharmacological analgesia for invasive medical procedures: A randomized trial. *Lancet* 355 (9214): 1486–90.
96. Davis, M., E. Eshelman, and M. McKay. 2000. *The relaxation and stress reduction workbook.* 5th ed. Oakland, CA: New Harbinger.
97. Jacobson, E. 1978. *You must relax.* New York: McGraw-Hill.

98. Luthe, W. 1969. *Autogenic training*. Vols. 1–3. New York: Grune & Stratton.
99. Benson, H. 1975. *The relaxation response*. New York: Avon.
100. Stroebel, C. 1978. *Quieting response training*. New York: BMA.
101. Schwartz, M. 2003. *Biofeedback: A practitioner's guide*. 3rd ed. New York: Guilford Press.
102. Novak, J. 1989. *How to meditate*. Nevada City, CA: Crystal Clarity.
103. LeShan, L. 1974. *How to meditate*. New York: Bantam.
104. Gawain, S. 1986. *Living in the light*. Mill Valley, CA: Whatever Publishing.
105. Lazar, S. W., G. Bush, and R. L. Gollub et al. 2000. Functional brain mapping of the relaxation response and meditation. *Neuroreport* 11 (7): 1581–85.
106. Davidson, R. J., J. Kabat-Zinn, J. Schumacher, et al. 2003. Alterations in brain and immune function produced by mindfulness meditation. *Psychosomatic medicine* 65 (4): 564–70.
107. Folan, L. 1981. *Lilias, yoga, and your life*. New York: Collier Books.
108. Fried, R. 1990. *The breath connection: How to reduce psychosomatic and stress-related disorders with easy-to-do breathing exercises*. New York: Plenum Press.

Sexual and Relational Wellness

Chapter Six
Preventing Abuse against Women

Chapter Seven
Building Healthy Relationships

Chapter Eight
Examining Gynecological Issues

Chapter Nine
Designing Your Reproductive Life Plan

Part Three

Chapter Six

Preventing Abuse against Women

CHAPTER OBJECTIVES

When you complete this chapter, you will be able to do the following:

- Identify the extent of violence and abuse against women in the United States
- Categorize the various types of abuse committed against women
- Develop protective plans to avoid the possibilities of rape
- Summarize the characteristics of women who are abused
- Explain common elements present in all types of abuse
- Categorize the types of consequences abused women experience
- Develop strategies for leaving an abusive relationship
- Utilize information and methods necessary to heal from the wounds of an abusive relationship
- Determine methods by which violence and abuse against women can be reduced and prevented
- Evaluate the various sources of assistance available to abused women and their children

THE REALITY OF VIOLENCE AGAINST WOMEN

Maria gently pressed the cold towel against her cheek and ear. Painfully she removed the numbing cold compress and looked at her inflamed swollen face in the mirror. Why? . . . she asked herself . . . why does this happen to me? She hated it. She hated him, yet, here she was, and remained, an abused wife. As she looked once again at her physical wounds, she knew that her most profound wounds were hidden within.

In the beginning, if one were to read the Bible, women were instructed to be subservient to men, ". . . the desire shall be to thy husband, and he shall rule over thee."[1] The word "woman" is derived from the Anglo-Saxon *wifman,* which literally means "wife-man," a term implying that wifehood and woman are inseparable—that woman exists to be of service to man. The concept and treatment of women as the lesser sex is documented throughout history. For example, during the Stone Age, duties essential to survival—working the land, finding shelter, preparing food—were, for a time, shared by men and women. As metals were discovered and agriculture using heavy tools increased, man used the strength and labor of other men, reducing some men to slaves and diminishing the role of women to the position of servitude. Thomas Aquinas, the thirteenth-century Christian theologian, stated that woman was created to be man's helpmate, but her unique role is in conception . . . since for other purposes men would be better assisted by other men.[2] The attitude of a woman "belonging" to and serving the needs of man too often has led to men "controlling" or "disciplining" women by punishment in whatever manner was deemed necessary or appropriate. According to an old English common law doctrine, a husband could punish his wife for any behavior he considered inappropriate. This law, called the "Rule of Thumb," permitted a husband to beat his wife with a stick no larger than the circumference of his thumb.

In the early history of the United States, violence, especially domestic violence, was met with varying degrees of concern. Scholars who have studied domestic violence believe there is a direct relationship between the degree of male dominance in a society and the extent of violence toward women.[3] Female servants in the South in the eighteenth and nineteenth centuries often fell victim to rape by their "owners"; prostitutes often are beaten by a man who "owns" them for the brief period of time for which he paid.

Historical records of U.S. court proceedings reveal that husbands tended to batter their wives less in the nineteenth century than in the late twentieth century.[4] Prior to our mobile and transient society of today, families, long-time neighbors, and friends sometimes intervened against violent husbands and offered a buffer and a place of refuge for the abused woman and her children.

Abuse of women encompasses a wide spectrum of behaviors, from sexually derogatory remarks to rape and from battering to murder. Tragically, in the United States every 2 minutes one rape or sexual assault occurs and every hour, 50 women are victimized by an intimate.[5] More than half of these women are raped by a family member, friend, or acquaintance.

Prevalence of violence against women varies little among all cultures, among unmarried and married couples, and among socioeconomic groups. The wife of a Fortune 500 company president is just as likely to be abused as is the wife or partner of a blue-collar laborer. One in four women will experience domestic violence sometime in her lifetime.[6] Abused women of all races and cultures seek refuge in safe shelters, utilize community agencies, and seek the support of the legal system.

Violence and abuse against women is a perplexing phenomenon. The perpetrator is usually someone the victim knows—and often loves—the husband, boyfriend, father, or other relative. Nearly 5.3 million incidents of intimate partner violence (IPV) occur each year against U.S. women aged 18 and older, and 3.2 million occur against men.[7] Former surgeon general Antonia Novello, at the 1991 American Medical Association National Leader-ship Conference, stated, "Domestic violence is a cancer that gnaws at the body and soul of the American family. It is the number one cause of injury to women. . . ."[8] An adult female today is more likely to be raped, beaten, and/or stalked by her current or former husband, her boyfriend, or her date than by any other person.[9] Incidents, such as the following, are recounted in state and federal government reports and illustrate the extent of violence and abuse inflicted against females. A 9-year-old girl in Texas reports that she was raped by her father; a 15-year-old Connecticut girl was stabbed by her boyfriend; an Idaho woman was raped by her boss; a 46-year-old woman in New Mexico was thrown out of a moving car by her husband; a 31-year-old Baltimore woman was beaten, choked, and raped by a former friend who was helping her move; and an Arizona woman, 8 months pregnant, fled from her home after her husband beat her with a broomstick and threatened to kill her. The wide diversity of these incidents reveals that no one is immune; violence happens to women from all walks of life, old and young, rich and poor, homemakers and homeless, and it is usually inflicted by someone they know. These incidences are called **acquaintance violence,** meaning violence and abuse committed by a parent, relative, coworker, neighbor, or friend.

Women may be victimized more by individuals they know due to the fact that society and/or the legal system has not, in the past, disapproved of acquaintance violence. Abuse committed in the home, called **domestic abuse,** is often perpetrated by an individual whose belief system is grounded in extremes—it can only be right or wrong: the dinner was prepared or it was not, performance of some duty was carried out or it was not. Family violence, according to Dobash and Dobash,[10] has existed for centuries and has been accepted as being a part of a "patriarchal terrorist" system. By virtue of observation and/or experience, children often perpetuate family traditions by engaging in and/or accepting those behaviors that they have seen or experienced in their own family environment. Children from abusive families are more likely to grow up to be abusive parents.[11] In addition to witnessing family violence, children witness more than 100,000 acts of violence on TV by the time they complete elementary school and 200,000 acts of violence on TV by the time they graduate from high school.[12]

THE EXTENT OF THE PROBLEM

Statistics about IPV vary because of differences in how different data sources define IPV and how data are collected. Most IPV incidents are not reported to the police, with only 20 percent of IPV rapes or sexual assaults, 25 percent of physical assaults, and 50 percent of stalking directed toward women being reported. Even fewer IPV incidents against men are reported.[13] Astoundingly, one out of four women will be the victim of a violent crime sometime during their lifetime. Violent crimes against women are consistent across racial and ethnic groups: Hispanic, non-Hispanic, black, and white.

Intimate partner violence is primarily a crime against women. In the United States each year, approximately 1.5 million women and more than 800,000 men are raped or physically assaulted by an intimate partner.[14] Estimates indicate that more than 1 million women and 371,000 men are stalked by intimate partners each year.[15] Of as much concern, male violence against women

FYI

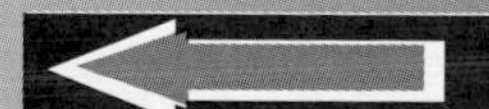

The Violence Against Women and Department of Justice Reauthorization Act 2005[16]

The Violence Against Women Act was reauthorized in the fall of 2005 and signed into law by President Bush in January 2006. This act

- enhances core programs and policies in the criminal justice and legal systems and reaffirms the commitment to reform systems that affect adult and youth victims of domestic violence, dating violence, sexual assault, and stalking;
- makes new strides to end domestic and sexual violence and stalking by addressing currently unmet needs;
- provides practical solutions to improve response of the criminal justice and legal systems for local groups, to enhance collaboration between victim service organizations and civil legal assistance providers, and to enforce protective orders;
- includes the reauthorization of critical programs and the development of new services that respond to evolving community needs; and
- works to provide transitional housing options, protect the safety and confidentiality of homeless victims, and ensure that victims can access the criminal justice system.

inflicts much more damage than female violence inflicts against men. Crandall et al.[17] found that 44 percent of women murdered by their intimate partner had visited an emergency department within 2 years of the homicide and, of these women, 93 percent had at least one injury visit. See *FYI:* "The Violence Against Women and Department of Justice Reauthorization Act 2005" to learn about the latest federal legislation to reduce and prevent violence against women and children.

Why Women Stay in Abusive Relationships

Virginia, married 23 years to an abusive executive, remained in the relationship because she was, for many years, economically dependent upon her husband. Forgoing her education to assist him through college, she maintained the house and raised the children. Over the years, Virginia developed few job skills, had no training outside the home, and had no other place to live. When Virginia talked about leaving, her husband threatened her with more abuse and the possible loss of the children. Feeling trapped and fearing physical and legal retaliation, Virginia felt she had no choice but to remain in the relationship.

Situational factors such as financial dependency, lack of education, lack of job skills, or job inexperience are all too real for women involved in abusive relationships. Statistically, a woman with children who leaves the home has a 50 percent probability that her standard of living will drop below the poverty level. Moreover, a woman is often in greater physical danger when she attempts to leave the relationship. She fears for her safety, her children's safety, and sometimes the safety of anyone who attempts to help her. Fear is the major reason that women stay in an abusive relationship.

Emotional factors such as fear of social isolation and lack of emotional and financial support from family and friends may contribute to women staying in unhealthy and abusive relationships. Abused women frequently lose touch with supportive friends and family due to the isolative nature of abuse. Cultural constraints (for example, men are the dominant sex) and religious beliefs (for example, divorce is a sin) may also keep women from leaving these relationships. Women generally accept the responsibility for success or failure of the relationship; to leave is to feel like a failure.

Love for the abuser is one reason for not reporting abuse inflicted by a partner. Laura, a woman who had been abused by her husband for a number of years, cried as she said, "I love him; I don't want him arrested; I don't want to hurt him, but I don't want him to hurt me either. I don't know what to do." The partner may be the father of her children; they love him, therefore, she is reluctant to eliminate his presence from the home.

Curiously, abused women often are concerned about their husbands' inability to survive on their own. They might ask themselves, "If I should die, would he be able to survive?" The answer is, of course, "Yes!" Concerns about survival if she remains in the abusive relationship and the fears associated with having independence and major life changes if she leaves create much ambivalence about the situation. And she can live with the false hope that he will change. Feeling trapped in the relationship, women may determine that some place to live, even if abusive, is better than no place to live, especially if children are involved. (See *Her Story:* "Pat: Choosing to Leave an Abusive Marriage.") Society's view of domestic violence is often a barrier to a woman's willingness to admit that she has been abused.

People may not understand why abused women do not leave the relationship, or think they may deserve the abuse or even enjoy it. The fact is that many barriers exist that discourage this abuse from being reported. Even the legal system may create a barrier to gaining a proper perspective concerning the actual incidences of violence and abuse. Slow to respond to the needs of violated women, the legal system in some states doesn't even consider spousal violence and abuse a felony until after the second conviction of the abuser.

Her Story

Pat: Choosing to Leave an Abusive Marriage

It wasn't easy for me to leave my spouse because, first of all, I still loved him. We had invested 24 years in our marriage, and I had never been totally on my own. Therefore, I was afraid I couldn't make it on my own financially. Until finally after several breakups, numerous arguments, and fights with some of them being near fatal on both our parts, I realized it was time for "Me" to do something different, and healthy. So I moved out for the last time. Since that time I have grown so much more spiritually and mentally. I've learned how to become an optimistic person, which means for me: things will be and are bad at times, but things won't be and aren't bad all the time. Marriage is a good example of that statement because so many years of my marriage were bad, but out of all of that, he and I have a daughter and son who we love. Through our children we were blessed with two precious and loving grandsons.

I thank God and every person who helped and encouraged me: the residential shelter, my adult children, the counseling center. Even with all of that help, it would not have worked had I not made the decision to help MYSELF, even though it took time and extreme courage. I thought I would never reach a serene point or fulfill my life goals, but I did and I have. I started college in the spring, I have a job, a car, an apartment, but most of all, I have peace of mind! Thank you God, thank you everybody.

- What type of feelings do you have as a result of reading this story?
- What do you think was the impetus for Pat leaving the relationship?
- What do you think of Pat's explanation of being an optimistic person?

Once violence becomes part of a relationship, it usually escalates in severity and frequency. An innocent remark, a push, or a criticism often initiates a response that ranges from a slap, kick, or punch to permanent damage (physically and/or psychologically) or even death. The resulting consequences negatively affect the victim/survivor, her children, and perhaps the perpetrator. (See *Journal Activity:* "Do You Know Someone in an Abusive Relationship?")

Journal Activity

Do You Know Someone in an Abusive Relationship?

Are you acquainted with someone who has experienced some form of abuse? Answer the following questions in the context of knowing a woman who has experienced abuse. Have you noticed any negative attitudes or behaviors this person exhibits? If so, what are they? Could these negative characteristics be due to her abusive environment? Has she shared this information with you? Do you have enough information to draw a connection between incidents of abuse, behaviors, and attitudes?

TYPES OF ABUSE

Abuse against women takes many forms, each with varied and far-reaching consequences. Perhaps an awareness and understanding of the major types of violence and abuse inflicted upon women and the resultant consequences may be helpful in the prevention of abuse. Perhaps a clearer understanding of the destructive effects will motivate women to take action and resolve the abuse or dissolve the relationship, either through family counseling or by leaving. Following is a brief description of the major types of violence that women may experience during various stages in their lives.

Childhood Abuse

One of the most serious problems in our society is abuse inflicted on children. It is often the root of abusive adult relationships. **Childhood abuse** consists of maltreatment of a child before age 18 through physical or mental injury, sexual abuse or exploitation, and/or negligent treatment by the individual(s) who are responsible for the child's welfare. There are four different types of childhood abuse: physical abuse, neglect, emotional abuse, and sexual abuse.

- *Childhood physical abuse* can result in cuts, burns, contusions, frequent pain without obvious injury, bites, or any other intentional pain that results in injury. Slapping, hair pulling, even tickling—especially to the point of hysteria—are also forms of childhood abuse. Physical abuse may begin as physical punishment and escalate into injurious, painful acts. Implements such as belts, switches, or paddles may be used to hit the child anywhere on the body. Frequent use of enemas or laxatives, unnecessary medical probing, and other intrusive procedures physically intrude on a child's right to privacy and respect.

- *Childhood abuse by neglect,* which is a less obvious form of physical abuse, is described as not providing a child with basic necessities (for example, shelter, food, clothing, medical needs, or a hygienic environment). Obvious malnourishment, fatigue and listlessness, lack of personal cleanliness, or habitually dressing in torn and/or dirty clothes are noticeable signs of neglect. Less obvious types of neglect are being unattended for long periods of time; needing glasses, dental care, or other medical attention; and not receiving emotional support or attention.
- *Childhood emotional abuse* is the most perplexing type of child abuse. Although there may be no physical evidence of emotional abuse, there are telltale indications that this type of abuse is occurring. Parents can inflict emotional abuse on a child by depriving her or him of an essential sense of self-worth. Emotional abuse includes continually criticizing or belittling the child, talking perpetually to the child in negative terms, threatening severe punishment or abandonment, and ignoring the child. Demanding perfection (for example, a perfect appearance or performance), excessive control by denying spontaneity and creativity, and disallowing social peer interactions are further types of emotional abuse. Learning problems, behavioral extremes such as isolation or aggressiveness, expressions of depression, and apathy are often consequences of emotional abuse.
- *Childhood sexual abuse* refers to oral, anal, or vaginal intercourse, fondling, unwanted touching, and/or using instruments on a child's genitalia. Forcing a child to view adult genitalia, to watch a pornographic scene or movie, or to undress or expose herself or himself to an adult are also forms of child sexual abuse. Eighty-five percent of childhood sexual abuse is done by an individual the child knows (for example, a parent, relative, or neighbor). Harmful and serious physical, emotional, behavioral, and social consequences often are the result of childhood sexual abuse. High-risk behaviors, depression, anxiety, alcohol or illicit drug abuse, eating disorders, which can lead to long-term physical health problems such as STIs, cancer, or heart disease, often result from childhood abuse.[18] If it is early, severe, and repeated, childhood sexual abuse may result in a permanently fragmented identity such as multiple personality disorder. This condition incorporates images of the perpetrator and possibly other individuals as well as one's self; the victim may not even be aware of the existence of the other personalities.[19] (See *Women Making a Difference:* "Teri Hatcher, Actress.")
- Children who experience sexual abuse often have a poor sense of self-worth. They withdraw, isolate themselves, and may be suicidal. One common result of childhood sexual and physical abuse is **posttraumatic stress disorder (PTSD).** PTSD develops over a period of time as a result of some traumatic event, such as war, a violent act, or abuse. Symptoms such as irritability, edginess, and insomnia among others do not arise at the time of the trauma but occur at a later time in life. These are similar to the PTSD symptoms people experience as a result of being at war as well as going through other traumatic life events. As adults, women can begin to experience these symptoms and may not understand why the symptoms are developing. Children who experienced childhood sexual abuse may, as adults, develop PTSD and have involuntary memories, flashbacks, nightmares, and physical reactions when exposed to reminders of the events.

Women Making a Difference

Teri Hatcher, Actress

Teri Hatcher, actress and new author, has had a rocky road to stardom and to personal growth. She is currently the best-known *Desperate Housewife* in America, but until recently has had a hidden part of her past. Teri is the victim of childhood sexual abuse, and she reveals in her book, *Burnt Toast,* that the victimization of her as a child profoundly damaged her throughout her entire life and produced a spirit of shame. Starting at age 5, Teri was sexually molested by her uncle—an uncle that made her feel loved and special. This continued until she was 9 years old, when her parents, suspecting something was amiss, no longer allowed the aunt and uncle around the family. The willingness to deal with the devastation of this abuse occurred when Teri learned, 35 years after her own abuse, that a 14-year-old girl committed suicide after being abused by this same uncle. Teri, through much soul-searching, decided that she must come forward and give a deposition against this man so that he would be prosecuted. She did and he was.

In *Burnt Toast,* Teri Hatcher states: "Are you the kind of person who tries to scrape off the black?" . . . Maybe you don't want to be wasteful, but if you go ahead and eat that blackened square of bread, then what you're really saying—to yourself and to the world—is that the piece of bread is worth more than your own satisfaction. Up "til now I ate the burnt toast." Teri Hatcher wrote the book to help women stop the pattern of taking less than what they deserve, to help stop the "burnt toast" syndrome for their daughters.

FYI

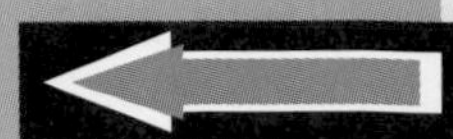

The Cycle of Abuse[20]

Phase I—Tension or Buildup
This phase is characterized by increasing arguments and minor forms of verbal or physical abuse. The perpetrator attempts to keep the woman under control, and she is aware of the consequences if she does not "obey or carry out" his demands. During this phase, the woman may be more willing to be helped by assistance from community resources or to listen to a trusted friend, relative, or member of the clergy about the reality of the relationship.

Phase II—Battering Incident
In the perception of the perpetrator, situations that cause tension or anger exceed his ability to cope and result in angry and violent responses. A former batterer will know that these violent responses serve either to reduce this stress or to change "her" behavior. Intervening factors such as police involvement or injury requiring medical attention may occur during this phase.

The perpetrator and the woman may be more amenable to intervention following the battering event. She may be hurt, angry, or frightened; he may feel shame and/or guilt. Both may want the violence to cease. Arrest of the batterer and the immediate consequences are good intervention factors that may keep the violence and abuse from recurring.

Phase III—Calm or "Honeymoon" Phase
During this phase, the couple experiences feelings of reconciliation, calmness, and reminders of earlier, more loving periods in their relationship. This phase is usually shorter than the tension phase, and it usually disappears over time as battering incidents become more frequent and severe. The man attempts to justify his behavior by blaming others: the victim or use of alcohol or drugs. Promises that it will never happen again are made. He usually means it, at least until the next time there is tension or disagreement.

The woman is often not amenable to assistance or counseling during this phase, especially if the battering cycle has not occurred often. During this phase, the woman receives the most rewards (for example, loving attention, flowers, gifts) for remaining in the relationship. The perpetrator is well-behaved and caring. The woman is most receptive to this behavior and responds to his overtures for reconciliation. Both partners may minimize, forget, or distort the incident(s), which will eventually result in the cycle being repeated.

Intervention directed toward the perpetrator may be possible in this phase due to remorsefulness and the desire to please his partner. However, as this phase passes and the batterer believes his partner will remain in the relationship, he becomes less willing to be involved in any intervention process and the cycle begins again.

More than 3 million referrals concerning the welfare of 5.5 million children were reported to U.S. Child Protective Services agencies in 2004.[21] Of the 903,000 children who were found to be victims of child maltreatment, 57 percent were victims of neglect, 2 percent suffered medical neglect, 19 percent were physically abused, 10 percent were sexually abused, and 7 percent were psychologically abused. These children were from all ethnic groups: 50 percent were white, 25 percent were African American, 15 percent were of Hispanic origin, and 2 percent and 1 percent were of American Indian/Alaska Natives and Asian/Pacific Islanders, respectively. Sadly, women (59 percent) were more likely than men (41 percent) to be the perpetrators of abuse against children. More than 1,300 children died as a result of abuse or neglect during 2001, and the younger the child, the more vulnerable she or he was to abuse. Children under 6 years of age accounted for 85 percent of child fatalities.[22] This is a sad commentary on our society, and it is a problem that has far-reaching consequences because children, both males and females, who are abused very often grow up to be child and/or spousal abusers themselves.

Abuse and Adult Women

Females who are abused during childhood often expect to be abused or feel they deserve abuse during their adult relationships. Prevention and treatment programs often address the worthiness and respect of self as a way to overcome this misconception. Abuse inflicted on adult women often takes forms similar to child abuse.

Physical Abuse Physical abuse, or battery, is the most overt type of domestic violence adult women encounter. Being kicked, hit, bitten, choked, pushed, having hair pulled, being thrown across the room or down on the floor, and/or being assaulted with some type of weapon are examples of battery. Perpetrators may target certain areas of the body for abusing, such as the breast, face, hairy areas of the body where bruises or abrasions are difficult to detect, or even the abdomen of a pregnant woman.

Abuse, especially physical abuse, tends to be cyclic in nature and typically involves three stages: increased tension building, the acute battering incident, and finally, the "honeymoon" phase, a loving, calmer, less tense period of time. The cyclic nature of this tragedy predicts that it will be repeated over time. Further explanation of these phases is found in *FYI:* "The Cycle of Abuse."

Psychological Abuse

Psychological abuse, unlike physical abuse, is clandestine and insidious. It is traumatic, often long-lasting, more difficult to assess, and less likely to lead to intervention and/or prosecution of the perpetrator.

Psychological abuse comes in many forms and can include some or all of the following conditions:

- *Financial disadvantages.* This is characterized by the perpetrator having control over household finances. The woman may not be allowed to work, and therefore she becomes entirely financially dependent on her partner. If she is working, she may have to account for all the money she earns, thus reducing her sense of freedom or independence outside the relationship.
- *Young children at home.* This includes threatening to take children from their mother, abusing the children, or using the children to degrade or belittle their mother. Statements such as "You're stupid, just like your mother," or "How can you ever amount to anything, just look at who your mother is," produce a psychological environment that hinders the development of worthiness and positive self-concept, degrading both the mother and the children.
- *Fear for herself and her children.* A woman may be frightened by her partner's looks, gestures, voice, destruction of property, or harming of children or pets. The worry that he may explode and express verbal degradation, curse, and call her or the children names can further contribute to her humiliation and fear. The home as a safe environment no longer exists.
- *Threatening harm.* The perpetrator inflicts harm on the children or threatens to take them away. He may even allude to committing suicide. The perpetrator may also threaten to kill her, the immediate family, other relatives, or close friends. His threats are designed to create anxiety and fear in his partner and the children.
- *Ultimate control of behavior.* The perpetrator may limit his partner's activities by controlling her freedom to join organizations, limiting contact with companions, and not allowing her to go on errands or to travel. He fears the loss of control and influence over her life if she is absent too often or too long from the home. His extreme possessiveness or jealousy creates the need to know with whom and where his partner is at all times.
- *Isolation.* The perpetrator controls all social contacts and movements of a woman. Severe jealousy and frequent accusations serve to isolate the woman, keep her psychologically off balance, and contribute to the abusive environment. The systematic destruction of a woman's self-esteem results from continual psychological abuse. This type of abuse is often present when physical and/or sexual violence are also present.

Sexual Assault

Sexual assault is a term used to describe numerous forms of sexual improprieties and sexual violence toward another individual. It can result from manipulation or coercion as well as through physical force. Rape, a type of sexual assault, is sexual intercourse that is forced on women and is considered an act of violence, aggression, power, and control rather than an act of sexual desire. Psychologists who work with sex offenders see numerous types of offenders, including those for whom rape is a desire to dominate or control, those for whom it is an extension of anger, and those who seem to have been motivated by sex.[23]

The prevalence of rape is astounding. Sexual violence is a serious problem that affects millions of people every year. One in six women (17 percent) and one in thirty-three men (3 percent) *reported* experiencing an attempted or completed rape at some time in their lives.[24] Three out of four who reported being raped and/or physically assaulted since age 18 stated that a current or former husband, cohabiting partner, or date was responsible.[25] Women who were raped by a stranger were more likely to report the rape to police.

Police estimate that only 34 percent of stranger rape and 13 percent of acquaintance rape are reported. The United States is the most rape-prone contemporary society in the world. These tragic numbers reflect a dark and shameful side of human nature. Each statistic is reflective of a woman whose life is forever changed as a result of a violation inflicted on her by another human being. The number of reported and unreported sexual assaults is staggering. But even *one* sexual assault is one too many.

A woman may be raped by a male who she knows or by a male who is a stranger to her. Each type of rape presents its own set of circumstances and consequences. **Acquaintance rape** is the sexual assault of a woman by a man whom she knows, such as a man who is in her class or lives in her residence hall. **Date rape,** a form of acquaintance rape, refers to the rape of a woman by a man who she has agreed to see socially. Some rapists prefer to know their victims because they are able to get closer to them or trap them in a vulnerable position without creating alarm. Acquaintances are also able to gain more information about the routine, friends, and living conditions of the intended victim, and perhaps believe that a woman will be less willing to report the rape if she knows the rapist.

Date and acquaintance rape are characterized by physical attacks on the woman's breasts or genitals, sexual sadism, and forced sexual activity. Acquaintance rape occurs more frequently among college students, especially freshman women, than among any other age group. According to research conducted on a number of campuses, approximately 20 percent of college women reported being raped while on a date.[26] One study revealed that one in two college women said they had experienced some type of sexual aggression, and one in four or five reported being the victim of rape or attempted rape. Nine out of ten victims of rape knew their attackers as dating partners or acquaintances at the time of the assault,[27] with the majority taking place in living quarters. Yet only 5 percent of completed or attempted rapes of college women were reported to law enforcement.[28]

Acquaintance rape can often be prevented by being aware of certain male behaviors. A man who demonstrates a disrespectful attitude toward other individuals, especially women, may indicate that he sees women as second-class citizens. Furthermore, the potential acquaintance rapist often lacks concern for a woman's feelings, may express extreme jealousy, or may attempt to be domineering. He often is highly competitive and may use physical violence as a means of coping with stress-filled situations. He may also speak negatively about women's rights or tell jokes that are demeaning to women. *FYI:* "Characteristics of a Rapist" summarizes characteristics to be aware of in a potential rapist.

Women should avoid individuals who exhibit these behaviors and seek out companions who display behaviors that are conducive to developing a healthy and enjoyable relationship. *Health Tips:* "Avoiding Date Rape" offers guidelines to use to avoid being placed in a position of possible danger. Four main factors increase the risk of being sexually assaulted:

- Frequently drinking enough to get drunk
- Being unmarried
- Previously being a victim of sexual assault
- Living on campus (for on-campus victimization only)

Marital rape appears to be mainly an act of violence and aggression, in which sex is the method used to humiliate, hurt, degrade, and dominate the spouse, usually the female partner. The violence and brutality in the sexual relationship of the couple seem to escalate with time. The sexual violence is frequently accompanied by life-threatening acts or warnings.

Compassion, caring, and believing a woman are important responses offered by supporters who are involved with assisting someone following an act of rape. *Health Tips:* "What to Do If You Are Raped" provides suggestions for what to do if you find yourself or a friend to be the victim of a rape.

Use of alcohol can set a woman up to be the victim in a rape. Over one-half of women who were raped and almost three-fourths of men who raped had been drinking or using drugs prior to the assault. Alcohol can cause distortion of thinking and reasoning abilities, and it lessens the ability to recognize danger signals such as changes in a man's voice, his behaviors, and suggestions for being alone together. A woman may be less able to communicate her feelings about what she does and does not want to do sexually. The chance that words such as "no" or "maybe" will be interpreted to mean "yes" is more

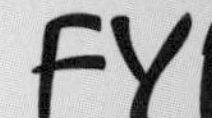

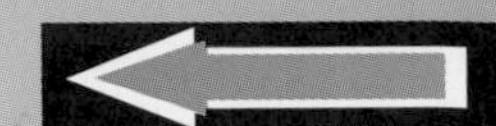

Characteristics of a Rapist

Companionship is usually welcomed, desired, and healthy. Unfortunately, not everyone is a safe companion. When deciding to associate with another person, it is important to know the traits of a person who may commit rape. Watch for the following characteristics as indicators of a potential rapist.

Rapes for power over women

- Needs to completely dominate and control (for example, *he* makes all decisions, gives all instructions, and makes the commands and demands)
- Covers feelings of inadequacy by acts of power
- Is possessive of female friends
- Often ridicules, criticizes, and insults partners
- Wants every moment of his partner's time accounted for
- Checks on partner by constantly following her, calling her friends, questioning her all the time
- Believes that women should be passive and submissive

Rapes due to anger at women

- Expresses contempt, hostility, and hatred toward women
- Has an explosive temper
- Verbally abuses companions
- Becomes angrier or more physically aggressive when using alcohol or other drugs
- Thinks of women as sex objects
- Blames others for his anger or misfortunes

Health Tips

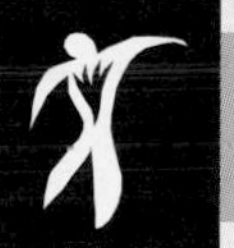

Avoiding Date Rape: Guidelines for Men and Women[29]

Men

- *Know your sexual desires and limits.* Communicate them clearly. Be aware of social pressures and realize it's okay not to score.
- *Being turned down when you ask for sex is not a rejection of you personally.* Women can express their desire not to participate in a single act of sex. You may think your desires are beyond control. However, your actions are certainly within your control.
- *Accept a woman's decision.* "No" means "no." Don't read other meanings into the answer. Don't continue after you are told "No!"
- *Don't assume that just because a woman dresses in a sexy manner and flirts that she wants to have sexual intercourse.*
- *Don't assume that previous permission for sexual contact applies to the current situation.*
- *Avoid excessive use of alcohol and other drugs.* Alcohol and other drugs interfere with clear thinking and effective communication.

Women

- *Know your sexual desires and limits.* Believe in your right to set those limits. If you are not aware, stop and talk about it with your date.
- *Communicate your limits clearly.* If someone starts to offend you, tell him so firmly and immediately. Polite approaches may be misunderstood or ignored. Say "no" when you mean "no."
- *Be assertive.* Often men interpret passivity as permission. Be direct and firm with someone who is sexually pressuring you.
- *Be aware that your nonverbal actions send a message.* If you dress in a sexy manner and flirt, some men assume you want to have sex. This does not make your dress or behavior wrong, but it is important to be aware of a possible misunderstanding.
- *Pay attention to what is happening around you.* Watch the nonverbal clues. Do not put yourself into a vulnerable situation.
- *Trust your intuition.* If you feel you are being pressured into unwanted sex, you probably are.
- *Avoid excessive use of alcohol and other drugs.* Alcohol and other drugs interfere with clear thinking and effective communication.

Health Tips

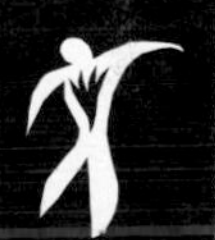

What to Do If You Are Raped

- Contact a friend or someone for support. There is always someone who will help you.
- Seek medical attention at once. All injuries are not immediately present.
- Do not bathe, douche, change your clothes, or rinse your mouth. If there is any possibility that you will report the crime, you don't want to destroy any evidence. Take a clean change of clothes with you to the hospital. Ask for tests to detect any sexually transmitted infections.
- You have the option of reporting the crime to the police. There are trained personnel who can assist you in making that decision. They will explain the legal process to you.
- Write down what happened, in your own words. This will be helpful to you if charges are filed, the case goes to trial, and you decide to testify.
- Even if you decide not to testify, provide information about the rapist to the police which could help solve other rape cases.
- Get follow-up help and support. Counseling centers, rape centers, and health centers may be of help.
- Do not blame yourself for the incident.

likely if either the man or woman has been drinking. Sometimes men urge women to drink to increase the chances that the women will be unable to resist pressure to have sex. A man may even feel that a woman who has several drinks is asking to have sex, regardless of what she says. Under the influence of alcohol, men are more likely to be more aggressive in regard to sex and women are more likely not to recognize some of the danger signs.

To compound the concerns related to alcohol and sexual assault, specific drugs, usually slipped into a woman's drink, can produce disinhibition and amnestic effects for the potential victim. Rohypnol (roofies), gamma hydroxy butyrate (GHB), and ketamine hydrochloride (Special K), described in detail in Chapter 13, are used as an accessory to date or acquaintance rape on or near college campuses.[30] Easy to place in the potential victim's drink, these drugs are tasteless and odorless and difficult to detect. Effects include increased confusion, relaxation or a dreamy state, and eventual unconsciousness; the victim usually is unable to remember what happened, which makes prosecution difficult.

Murder In this country, in 2003, 21 percent of murder victims were killed by their spouse or intimate partner. Seventy-nine percent of those victims were women.[31] More than half the defendants accused of murdering their spouses had been drinking alcohol at the time of the murder.[32] These women were the victims of the one person in their life who professed to love and honor them—their partner. Unfortunately "until death do us part" came all too soon for the female partner. Murder is frequently the ultimate end to long-term and escalating abuse—abuse that, for unknown reasons, had been tolerated over time and was neither punished nor treated. Consider the fate of Monique in *Her Story.*

Crisis centers across the United States report case after case of deadly outcomes of abusive relationships. For example, Christine in New Mexico was stabbed twenty times by her former husband; Louise was shot to death by her estranged husband as she picked up their children after a weekend with their father; Joycelyn's throat was slashed by a former boyfriend as she left a restaurant with a date. Although the manner in which each woman was killed differed, the underlying circumstances were quite similar: each woman was killed by a past or present husband or lover. Murder may be the final statement men make to their partners. A violent end to a relationship is often marked by desperate and barbarous acts on the part of the male partner.

> Men often hunt down and kill wives who have left them; women hardly ever behave similarly. Men kill wives as part of planned murder-suicides; analogous acts by women are almost unheard of. Men kill in response to revelations of wifely infidelity; women almost never respond similarly, although their mates are more often adulterous. Men often kill wives after subjecting them to lengthy periods of coercive abuse and assaults; the roles in such cases are seldom, if ever, reversed. Men perpetrate familicidal massacres, killing spouse and children together; women do not.[33]

The highest profile criminal and civil murder case of all time may well be that of O. J. Simpson. Simpson, a well-recognized professional athlete, TV personality, and actor, was accused of murdering his former wife and her male friend. In the development of the murder case against Simpson, prosecutors uncovered a history of harassment and verbal and physical abuse of his wife. Other "well-known" men have faced similar charges. Jeffrey MacDonald, a physician and Special Forces Green Beret, was convicted of killing his wife and two daughters; Claus von Bulow was tried and convicted of murdering his wealthy wife and then won a reversed decision on appeal; actor Robert Blake was eventually acquitted of murdering his wife, Bonny Lee Bakley; and Scott Peterson was convicted of murdering his wife and unborn son and is now on death row at San Quentin Prison. (The Unborn Victims of Violence Act, making it a crime to harm an unborn, viable fetus, was signed into law in April 2004.)

Her Story

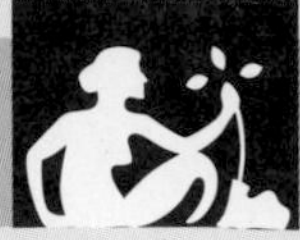

Monique: Abuse and Murder

Monique, after years of abuse often witnessed by her three children, finally left Kent, her husband of 9 years. As she began to make a life of her own for herself and her children, Kent became more and more resentful and angry. One cool October evening, Kent went to Monique's house with the idea of reuniting. Monique refused; Kent became enraged, and while their children watched, he beat his estranged wife to death with his son's baseball bat.

- Are there actions that Monique could have taken to protect her family from Kent?
- Remembering what you read earlier in this chapter about children witnessing abuse in the home, what behaviors do you think may be exhibited by these children?

Same-Sex Domestic Violence Violence against gay individuals and gay partners has increased significantly in recent years according to a study by the National Gay and Lesbian Task Force. Incidents of victimization include verbal harassment and threats, physical assaults, murder, and abuse by police. In 2003, lesbians, gays, bisexuals, and transgender people experienced 6,523 incidents of domestic violence. Six of these incidents resulted in murder.[34]

In *Hate Crimes: Confronting Violence against Lesbians and Gay Men,*[35] the authors state that the link between the victimization of gay men and lesbians is due to the underlying, societally based message that the gay lifestyle is unacceptable and that violence is a just and rewarding punishment for homosexual behavior. Domestic violence is usually discussed as a concern of heterosexual partners, but domestic violence occurs at similar rates in lesbian, gay, bisexual, and transgender (LGBT) relationships.

Numerous barriers exist for LGBT partners who are dealing with domestic violence. Already experiencing condemnation, discrimination, and denial, revealing additional "dirty laundry" may place same-sex partners in an even more precarious position. LGBT relationships are often condemned and exist in secret, and partners are often denied the rights of married couples; to reveal that domestic violence occurs in these relationships provides more ammunition to people who already condemn same-sex partnerships. Therefore, the wall of silence grows stronger.

Care and assistance for LGBT victims of domestic violence is limited, and few shelters around the country reach out to victims of same-sex violence. People who are not "out" may be reluctant to report violence at the hands of their partners, and laws may make it difficult to obtain protective orders. An excellent assistance program is the Los Angeles Gay & Lesbian Center's STOP Partner Abuse/Domestic Violence Program. This center provides intervention and prevention services that address the unique needs of youth and adults in the LGBT community. Services include survivors' groups, a court-approved batterers' intervention program, crisis intervention, individual counseling, specialized assessment, education and consultation, and a multifaceted prevention program.[36] Educating mental health service providers and medical and law enforcement personnel about the special issues related to violence in LGBT partners will ensure that services are sensitive, appropriate, and accessible.[37] More shelters, more resources, and better training for professionals who work with LGBT victims of violence are critical needs.

Sexual Harassment Although **sexual harassment** is not violent in nature, it is abusive. It represents abuse of power and position, and, furthermore, it is a criminal offense. Taking place most often in the workplace or educational setting, it can also be a type of domestic abuse, wherein the abuser dominates his partner so that she feels unable to refuse sexual requests.

Types of sexual harassment include unwanted and unwarranted comments with sexual overtones or sexual innuendos, unwanted and uninvited touching or staring, and requests for sexual favors. Jokes, comments, or personal questions with sexual overtones that are offensive to the listener are also considered sexual harassment. Sexual harassment includes working, being, or living in a hostile, offensive, or intimidating environment in which actions or talk of a sexual nature exists because of gender. Female college students may be asked to provide a sexual act in return for a favor or preferential treatment provided by a professor. Men as well as women may be victims of sexual harassment; however, more commonly women are harassed by men. (See *Viewpoint:* "Is This Sexual Harassment?")

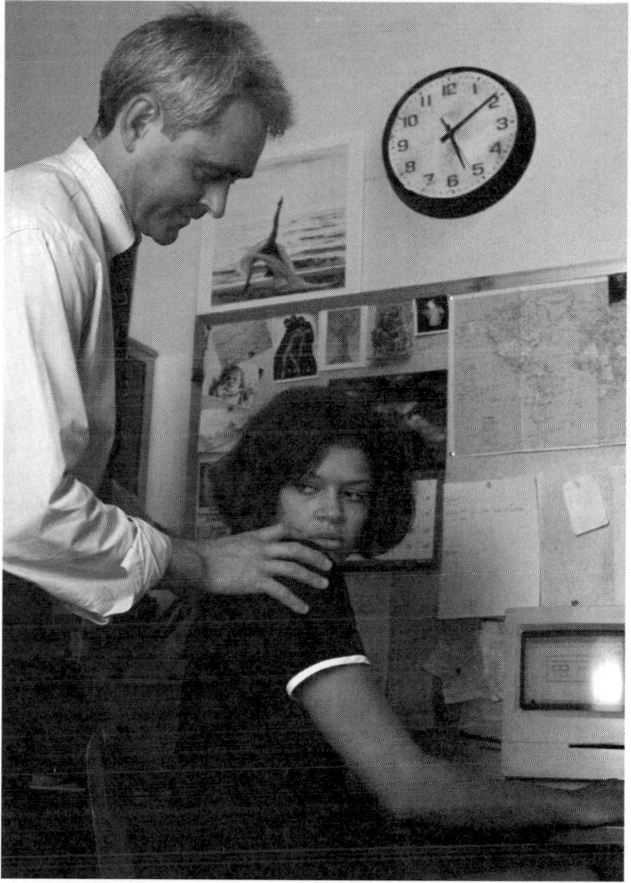

Unwanted touching is a type of sexual harassment.

Viewpoint

Is This Sexual Harassment?

Michelle worked in a department dominated by males. She brought to this job prior sales experience and qualities that made her effective in working with employees and customers. Her immediate supervisor developed a habit of telling his stories of sexual conquests to male employees when Michelle was near enough to hear. She politely asked him to wait until she was unable to hear the conversations before sharing the details of his sexual ventures. He refused, stating that he was not talking to her in the first place, and secondly, if she found the conversations so disturbing, to move far enough away so that she was unable to hear. If you were in Michelle's position, would you consider this a sexual harassment situation? If yes, what would you do about it? If you don't consider it sexual harassment, do you find it offensive?

Health Tips

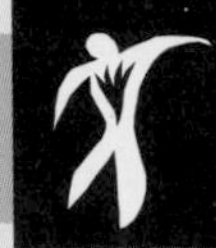

Strategies for Addressing Sexual Harassment

- Do not ignore innuendos or degrading statements; otherwise, they will not stop. Clearly and firmly state your objections immediately. (Perhaps the harasser did not understand that the words or gestures were offensive.) You may need to share the incident(s) with a trusted individual in case you file charges later.
- Write down any incident(s) or written communication made by the harasser; date and file the information. Be sure to include the time, place, date, and witnesses, if any were present. Include what occurred and your response.
- Give the written information to another trusted individual as well as verbally share the incident with her or him. This person may be needed for verification if you elect to file charges either now or in the future.
- Confront the harassment by reporting it to authorities; you may be able to keep this from happening to others. If desired, talk to a professional counselor who can help you deal with any emotional distress related to the incident.
- Be truthful and accurate about the incident. Do not place the reputation of yourself and someone else in jeopardy if you are unsure about what happened. The fallout for you and the accused can have serious and embarrassing consequences.

Health Tips: "Strategies for Addressing Sexual Harassment" contains suggestions for resolving concerns of sexual harassment. Have you ever experienced sexual harassment? If so, do you think these suggestions are beneficial?

INCIDENTS OF VIOLENCE AND ABUSE

Having just read about the many types of violence and abuse against women, it is easy to see that incidents of abuse appear in many forms and range from minimal to very severe. A woman may quite easily experience several incidents, such as obscene telephone calls or being stalked, during her lifetime. No such experience should be considered inconsequential. Complete *Journal Activity:* "Incidents of Abuse" to evaluate how you would handle this situation. Unwanted touching is a type of sexual harassment.

Journal Activity

Incidents of Abuse

Having just read about abusive and violent acts against women, write down any incidents that you have experienced. Did you respond in any way to the perpetrator? If so, what did you say or do? Did you share the incident with anyone? Was the incident serious enough that you needed to involve the legal system? Was there a way to handle the situation better than you did? If so, what would that have been?

COMMON ELEMENTS IN ALL TYPES OF ABUSE

All forms of abuse share four common elements and are linked with concerns regarding resolution of abusive situations. These elements reflect common thought that influences public opinion and often hinders effective legal and societal resolutions, delays the victims' efforts to seek help and counseling, and/or slows the process of healing. These common elements are discussed below.

Minimization

The public often thinks that violence and abuse are rare and that official statistics accurately represent prevalence. Violence against women can be likened to an iceberg: the tip of the iceberg represents the reported amount of violence; the larger portion of the iceberg, which remains unseen, is the actual occurrence and is estimated to be two to three times greater than abuse that is reported.

Directionality

Violence occurs largely in one direction; men victimize women. Incest is generally from father or stepfather to daughter or stepdaughter; generally men make obscene phone calls to women; date rape almost always involves men assaulting women.

Trivialization

Violence against women is often viewed in a joking way: "Incest is the game the whole family can play," "If you're going to be raped, just lie back and enjoy it." Remarks and jokes tend to negate the impact and seriousness of violence against women and promote a sporting aspect to men's violence.

Blaming the Victim

This occurs not only in violence but in such crimes as car theft or house burglaries as well. Worldwide, studies identify events that purportedly "trigger" violence. Examples of these includes not obeying her husband, talking back, not having food ready on time, not caring for children or home as instructed, questioning him about money or girlfriends, refusing sex, or going somewhere without permission.[38] Little girls are accused of behaving "seductively," and women are held responsible for not stopping men sooner when kissing leads to an assault. An underlying assumption is that women are careless, men are not responsible for their actions, and self-control is much more difficult for men than for women.

CHARACTERISTICS OF BATTERED WOMEN

What are the traits of women who have been abused or violated? Why do they often remain in abusive relationships, either unable or unwilling to leave or seek assistance? Do these women develop these traits prior to experiencing abuse, or as a result of the abuse?

Personal Beliefs

Battered women tend to feel degraded, worthless, isolated, and depressed and to have low self-esteem.[39] Mistaken personal beliefs, such as "Battering is part of a loving relationship," or "If only I didn't make him mad, I wouldn't get hit," may originate in childhood and develop further in subsequent abusive relationships. These beliefs interfere with development of self-worth and prevent the victim from developing life-enhancing behaviors. Abused women often watched when their mothers or sisters were abused. They equate abuse with love and believe that this is how women are supposed to be treated by husbands, fathers, and other men. They come to believe that those who love you, abuse you.

Abused females usually hold to the traditional belief that the man is the head of the household and the woman is to be subservient. Whatever her perception of marriage is before the union, his violence eventually convinces her that yielding to him, maintaining the household, and/or taking care of the relationship and the children is safer than behaviors exemplified in "liberated" marital partnerships.

Personal Feelings

Adult female victims who experience varied forms of abuse often have or will develop low self-esteem and beliefs of worthlessness. Abused women often underestimate their abilities. A woman may assess her worthiness as it relates to her success as a wife or mother. If she is involved in a stormy, abusive, and dysfunctional relationship, even if she is successful in other areas of her life, feelings of inadequacy and poor self-concept soon develop. Therefore, her perception is that her lack of abilities causes the abuse to occur. The woman often believes she is deserving of the abuse because the batterer may camouflage abusive acts under a cloak of discipline. He teaches her a lesson, just as her parents did and just as her father taught her mother during violent episodes that she may have witnessed during her childhood.

Abused women, often blaming themselves for causing the partner's violence, are socialized to believe they are responsible for maintaining the relationship. Therefore, if the relationship is unhappy, disturbed, or abusive, she feels it is her responsibility to "repair" it or soothe whatever is bothering the abuser. She believes that if only she were a better lover, wife, mother, or worker, she would not be abused. This self-blame often leads to depression if the abuse continues. However, studies indicate that as abuse increases in severity and frequency, women become less likely to blame themselves and more likely to blame their partner.

The feeling of hopelessness may be a trait of the female both before and during the abusive relationship. She may believe she cannot "do any better" than the partner she is currently with, or she may be so emotionally and financially dependent on the partner that she feels afraid and/or unable to resolve the abusive situation. A woman may feel helpless in terms of her ability to move out of the relationship. She may be unaware of any type of available assistance to help her deal with the abuse. Feeling emotionally and psychologically helpless, she becomes indecisive and unable to trust her ability to think or act outside of the relationship with her partner.

Codependency

Women often have a codependent relationship with the abuser. **Codependency** means developing a dependency with the abuser and the abuser's problem(s) to the point of self-neglect. Codependent women think and feel responsible for the needs of other people. These responsibilities may include their feelings, thoughts, actions, choices, wants, needs, well-being, lack of well-being, and ultimate destiny. Therefore, a codependent woman who is in an abusive relationship often feels responsible for the abuse and is willing to endure it so that she can be available to care for the abuser.

Perception of Partner

An abused woman's perception of her violent partner is often one of need; that is, the perpetrator needs her. She may believe that she is the only person who can help him overcome his problem; therefore, she feels compassion and pity. If her partner is a chemically dependent batterer, she may believe he will stop the abuse if he stops using alcohol and/or other drugs. She may believe that if she leaves him, he may abuse alcohol and drugs to the point of illness or death. Even in relationships having a history of long-term battering, women often love the batterer and are emotionally dependent upon the relationship.

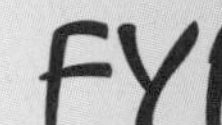

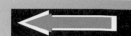

Physical Abuse Scale[40]

These acts of violence are listed in priority from less severe to most severe. The progression of physical abuse can be used in domestic abuse evaluations to determine the level of violence at which the perpetrator is operating and acts as a guide to determine the level of protection needed by the victim.

1. Throwing things; punching the wall
2. Pushing, shoving, grabbing, throwing things at the female
3. Slapping with an open hand
4. Kicking, biting
5. Hitting with a closed fist
6. Attempted strangulation
7. Beating up (pinning the victim to the wall or floor, repeatedly kicking or punching her)
8. Threatening with a weapon
9. Assault with a weapon

CONSEQUENCES OF ABUSE

Consequences of abuse are varied and depend on the duration, type, and severity of the abuse. Over time, continual abuse will result in one or more of the following consequences.

Physical Consequences

Depending on the type of abuse inflicted, a woman can experience a plethora of physical consequences. Cuts, burns, punctures, bites, bruises, bleeding, dislocations, and bone fractures are physical manifestations of abusive encounters. Over time, physical abuse usually escalates in both severity and frequency. Abused women usually have a history of many visits to emergency rooms. Medical care providers are trained to screen injuries that may indicate various types of abuse. (See *FYI:* "Physical Abuse Scale.")

Physical wounds inflicted on women may eventually result in chronic, long-term disorders and disabilities. Conditions such as chronic arthritis, hypertension, gastrointestinal disorders, or asthma, which can develop because of stress, may be consequences of long-term physical abuse.

Emotional and Psychological Consequences

Women are likely to experience negative psychological effects as a result of abusive relationships. Continual abuse will cause women to feel depressed and worthless, experience anxiety attacks, and feel they are going crazy. As a result of these feelings, women experience major emotional distress. The most devastating psychological effects appear as a result of being abused by a trusted person who was known to the victim (for example, a father, stepfather, or brothers).

As children, girls who have been sexually abused may develop feelings of anxiety, depression, anger, hostility, guilt, shame, and/or inferiority. These feelings can develop as an immediate response to the abuse, or they may develop in adulthood. As adults, these women often experience nightmares, relationship distress, and sexual dysfunction. Women who were sexually abused as children may have problems relating to their own parents as well as to both men and women; these women also experience difficulty in responding to their own children in a healthy manner. The severity of emotional and psychological consequences depends on the length of time since the abuse, the length of time the abuse lasted, the woman's age at the time of abuse, and her relationship to the perpetrator. (See *Her Story:* "Sue Anne: Surviving Incest.")

Another young woman, describing the emotional pain she experienced as a result of abuse, proclaimed her self-hatred by saying, "I had an oil slick oozing goo inside me. I knew I was filled with something evil, and that evil rubbed off on everyone I came in contact with. So I didn't let anybody really get near me."[41]

Women who have been victimized will experience an immediate postvictimization distress response that includes a pattern of fear and avoidance, disturbances of self-concept and self-esteem, and sexual dysfunction.

Spiritual Consequences

The very basic values of meaningful life and meaningful relationships are undermined as a result of early abuse, especially when the abuse is inflicted by individuals who are supposed to nurture and protect (for example, father, stepfather, grandfather, uncle). Females may find that

Her Story

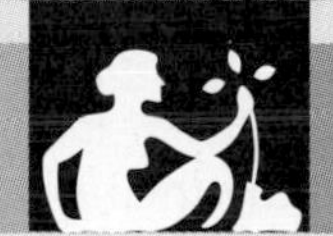

Sue Anne: Surviving Incest

Sue Anne recounted the incestuous relationship with her father that always occurred in the mornings. After her mother left early for work, her father would come into the room as she was dressing for school. As the incest continued, it became broader in its scope, until Sue Anne had all but become her father's full-time lover. She escaped as much as possible by participating in as many school functions as possible. Sue Anne did not date until well into her college years, then married someone who was emotionally distant and withdrawn. She reported that as a married adult it was impossible to have sexual relations with her husband in the morning, and they continually argue about sexual issues. Sue Anne has difficulty with other intimate relationships even to the point of feeling uncomfortable holding her own children, believing that she will "infect" her children if she is physically too close to them.

- What are some positive steps Sue Anne could take to begin healing from the abuse she experienced from her father?
- How can Sue Anne establish a support system that can assist her in this issue?
- Can Sue Anne's husband play a role in the process of her healing from her early experiences?

core values such as trust, honesty, respect, and concern are impaired or lost as a result of abusive relationships, especially abuse inflicted by supposedly caring men. Abused women report an inability to trust and respect others, especially men. Perhaps of greater concern is the fact that these women may mistrust their *own* perceptions of other people's behaviors and motives. Abuse in the family destroys the very foundation on which healthy functioning relationships are built.

Social Consequences

Violence and abuse manifest themselves with a variety of societal consequences. For example, increased use of dwindling health care resources causes the costs of medical care to rise, overloads medical personnel, and may lead to hasty diagnoses and sometimes too-aggressive treatments for many disorders. Emergency care is the most costly and most frequently used form of medical care following incidents of abuse. Communities experience overburdening of police, judicial, and human resources systems that lead to increases in taxes and increases in social problems such as drug abuse, violence, and homelessness. Society as a whole suffers from abusive relationships—not just monetarily—but with the negative consequences of violence cycling into the next generation, violence of all types is continued. In general, abuse contributes to decreases in the quality of life for everyone, not just for those in abusive relationships.

LEAVING THE ABUSIVE RELATIONSHIP

Deciding to Leave

Some women stay in abusive relationships, but others leave. Abused women typically leave an abusive environment five to seven times before they feel safe enough and have accumulated the resources needed to leave for good. Women frequently return to perpetrators following a visit to a safe shelter or a relative's home. Following her return, methods for eliminating the abuse without terminating the relationship, if both partners desire, need to be developed. However, if the abuse continues following each return, then she should seek assistance to leave the relationship permanently.

During the course of abuse, women may have involved the legal system in a number of ways. Calling the police during bouts of abuse, gaining protection for children, and obtaining restraining orders to keep the abuser at a distance are all proper and probable ways to use the legal system. As a woman prepares to leave a relationship, she may need to again use the resources of the legal system. Occasionally a safe escort out of the home is required, as well as accompaniment to secret and safe housing for her and her children. Community resources can be invaluable to a woman who has decided to remove herself and her family from an abusive environment.

Developing a Safety Plan

Once a woman makes the decision to leave the relationship, perhaps her most critical concern is developing a safety plan and determining a means of survival. The safety plan needs to include a means of leaving, a list of people to call in case of emergency, and a suitcase containing clothing, personal items, money, Social Security cards, bankbooks, children's birth certificates and school records, and other important documents. Immediate survival needs consist of locating a safe place to live once she has left the relationship, being able to feed and clothe herself and the children, and determining a way to become financially self-sufficient. Long-term survival may include finding a job, completing some type of education, or developing necessary job skills. It may also include locating dependable and quality child care.

Answering the following questions may assist women in determining the essential elements necessary for their survival and their children's survival. Are there family or friends where she can stay? If not, does she know how to access alternative means of shelter? Does she need to contact the police or obtain legal aid? Does she need counseling services? What other community agencies might assist her? Let's take a close look at some possible answers to these questions.

Locating Safe Shelter

This can be as simple as calling the police and asking for help. Currently there are several thousand safe shelters throughout the United States in which women can find safety, as well as advocacy, support, and other needed services. Check the phone book under "domestic violence," "women's shelter," "shelter for battered or abused women," and "crisis hotline" to locate the nearest safe shelter. In rural areas where safe housing may not be available, women can contact a local church or community center for assistance in locating temporary safe shelter.

Knowing what to expect is beneficial and may lessen the anxiety of leaving the abusive environment. Safe-shelter personnel will usually transport women and their children from an emergency room, the police station, or any other designated place to the shelter and away from the abusive partner.

Women and their children often arrive at the shelter with only the clothes they are wearing and return to their home to retrieve their belongings only when their partners are absent. They may need to utilize the shelter's resources for a time. Women and their children are usually allowed to remain in the safe shelter for 30 days with the option of increasing the time if the situation warrants it, unless other women are waiting to move in. During their stay, women help with the routine care and maintenance of the shelter, cook meals for themselves and their children, and wash and care for personal clothing.

Planning for the future without the abusive partner is also an important task during a woman's stay at the shelter. Depending on their individual needs, women may receive personal, group, and/or job-related counseling. Shelter personnel provide access to government assistance programs such as Women, Infant and Children (WIC), food stamps, and drug abuse counseling, if needed. Women may also receive help obtaining Medicaid and Social Security benefits. Other important tasks may include seeking employment, locating child care, filing protective orders, and starting divorce proceedings.

Locating Other Resources

Because safe shelters are temporary and serve only as a short-term bridge, other resources beyond the abusive environment, the abuser, and the former belief system are essential. Financial assistance may be temporarily obtained from Aid for Dependent Children (AFDC), the American Red Cross, the Social Security Administration, or local church charities. Phone numbers and addresses for these agencies can be found in local telephone directories. (See *Health Tips:* "Locating Local Resources.") A multitude of resources can be found on the Internet, and it is possible to "hide" Web site searches so no one can discover the search.

Housing can often be found through the local housing authority, Housing and Urban Development Office (HUD), or local property management offices, which often have apartments for rent at lower rates. Addresses and information for agencies that provide child care are usually provided to women during their stay at the safe shelter. Child care arrangements, sometimes at a reduced rate, are often made between the shelter and child care providers. Additionally, churches often have day care centers that are made available to local safe-shelter children on a temporary basis. Women who are making the effort to move forward following an abusive relationship may elect to share child care responsibilities, caring for one another's children while each works at different times.

Job training is available through a variety of sources. Communities offer adult learning centers with computer classes, Graduate Equivalence Diploma (GED) classes, and literacy volunteers. Social services departments offer job counseling, skill testing, and contact persons for job location through state or county employment commissions. Many temporary personnel agencies provide on-the-job training programs, which can lead to employment opportunities for women who already possess job

Health Tips

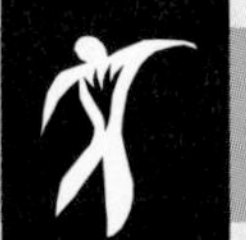

Locating Local Resources

Locate addresses and phone numbers for the following list of helpful resources in your town that can be used by women who are in need of assistance. Add any additional agencies or individuals who can be beneficial. Attach a city map and highlight helping agencies.

Agency	Phone #	Address
Emergency		
Crisis hotline		
Police		
Ambulance		
Safe house		
Legal Aid		
Child protective service		
Doctor		
Friend		
Other:		
Other:		

skills. Many towns and cities have community colleges at which job training or job-skill refresher courses are available for women who seek assistance. State, county, and local agencies provide emotional and financial counseling, often without charge.

HEALING FROM ABUSE

Healing from violence and abuse is possible. In fact, it is probable if a woman makes the choice to heal and then takes the steps, sometimes long and painful steps, to move forward and to thrive. Thriving means to flourish, bloom, to become whole, whole in one's own life and also in friendships, family relationships, and love relationships. Healing means moving beyond repair of the damage to body, mind, and soul. It also means being able to feel at peace, to feel genuine love, and to gain satisfaction with one's life and contribute to one's immediate and expanding environment.

One survivor said that healing and recovery are beautiful parts of life. Her healing "family" not only consisted of her present, nonabusive husband, her children, and grandchildren, but also included her fellow travelers—other survivors she learned to love and trust. The gift she had given herself was to allow all of her healing family to express love, warmth, and kindness.

Survivors of abuse recount the stages and feelings they experienced as they progressed toward healing and moved forward with their lives. These women have come to realize that they survived the traumatic time of abuse and became adults. From this awareness, women can move forward through the necessary stages into a life of satisfying relationships and contributions.

In their book *The Courage to Heal,*[42] Bass and Davis identify fourteen stages that women experience as they progress toward healing and recovering from abuse. It should be noted that survivors may not experience every stage and may not go through them in any particular order. *FYI:* "The Process of Healing" is a paraphrased summary of these stages.

HOW TO HELP

Helping a woman who is leaving an abusive relationship and is attempting to move forward with her life may not always be the responsibility of the legal, judicial, or social systems. Women often turn to friends and family first for support and assistance. Family, friends, and professionals who are available and knowledgeable about how to help these women can go a long way in aiding their chance to develop a healthy and contributing lifestyle.

How can friends and family help? How can you help? Consider the following suggestions developed by the U.S. Center for Mental Health Services titled *Supporting the Survivor.*[43]

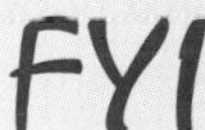

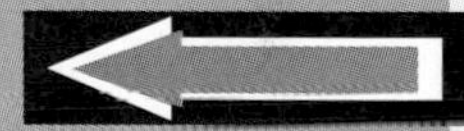

The Process of Healing

- Commit to heal, and begin to move toward self-change.
- Processing memories of the abusive incidents and the accompanying feelings is often painful and depressing; remember that it is transitional and will go away.
- Admit to yourself that the abuse did occur. Share this essential step with a trusted person who can help you with any feelings of shame associated with the incidents.
- Place the heavy blanket of guilt and shame on its rightful owner—the perpetrator. In no way was the abuse the fault of the victim.
- Develop realistic and appropriate feelings toward other people by getting in touch with the vulnerable child within—that child you may have lost in the process of coping with the agony that can accompany abuse.
- Listen to your instincts; listen to your own feelings, mind, and body. This promotes learning to trust oneself and builds a foundation from which to approach life situations.
- Recognize and feel all the losses related to an abusive relationship: loss of childhood, loss of trust, loss of idealized relationship, loss of respect, loss of joy, and so much more. This enables you to confront the pain, feel it, express it, and move forward.
- Use the freeing emotion of anger, considered the back bone of healing, and direct it to where it belongs: toward the perpetrator and the individuals who were not protective.
- Confront the perpetrator and disclose the abuse, if possible, because this can be an empowering and freeing activity for women who choose to do it.
- Forgiving the perpetrator is highly recommended, though it is not necessary for healing. But forgiving yourself is a must.
- Spiritual renewal through religion, nature's beauty, meditation, and/or contributing to society is important to the process of resolution and moving forward.

- *Listen.* Talking about the experience, when the survivor is ready, will help validate what happened to him or her and can reduce stress and feelings of isolation. Let the survivor take the lead in conversations and respond when appropriate.
- *Research.* If the victim/survivor wants more information, would like to report a crime, or has other concerns, help her find the answers and resources.
- *Reassure.* As strange as it may sound, survivors often question whether an incident was their fault or wonder what they could have done to prevent the crime against them. They may need to hear that it was not their fault and be assured that they are not alone.
- *Empower.* Following trauma, victims can feel as though much of their lives is beyond their control. Aiding them in maintaining routines can be helpful, as well as offering options or possible solutions.
- *Be patient.* Every journey through the healing process is unique. Try to understand that it will take time, and do what you can to be supportive. The healing process has no predetermined timeline.
- *Ask.* The survivor may need help with any number of things or have questions on many different topics. Even a favor as mundane as running a few errands or keeping the children temporarily can be helpful.
- *Encourage.* Suggest that the survivor seek professional support in addition to your support.

Time and space will be required for a woman to proceed through the stages of healing. As a friend or family member, express compassion for and validation of her feelings, such as feelings of fear, anger, guilt, and pain. Also, helping her through the stages of healing will produce changes in your relationship with her. Be prepared to make some changes in your attitude and behaviors toward her.

Equally important, children must be taught that the use of violence to resolve problems and exert control over others is unacceptable behavior. Children may need as much emotional support as their mother after leaving an abusive environment. Many of the same support systems that have been discussed for women also offer opportunities for healing and growth for children. Children need both healthy role models and structure and discipline without abuse.

MOVING FORWARD

I kept working on change . . . slowly, slowly I moved ahead. My body cells replace themselves. . . . I can replace and remove the damage, the pain. Yes, I have more work, but I have come a long way, baby! I now have the skills and the desire to move ahead; I will use them and I will find peace.

A SURVIVOR

Women can develop skills that enable them to heal from abusive relationships. Moreover, they can engage in activities that foster resolution of the abuse and promote progression toward a joyful and fulfilling life.

Building Resiliency

Resiliency is the ability to recover, to overcome adversity, to bend and bounce back like a willow tree in a windstorm. Resiliency can be developed as a skill and utilized to recover from the adverse effects of an abusive relationship. Finding and developing support systems outside the abusive environment can assist women in recognizing characteristics of healthy relationships. Having contact with "healthy" individuals who believe in the woman will promote belief in herself. These supportive relationships also provide conditions that enable women to feel worthwhile and valued. Susan, leaving home as a young teen following years of incest, found support and acceptance in a church group. She told of how the church group assisted her in developing a sense of purpose and value. Spirituality, too, can promote the development of resiliency because it fosters a sense of worthiness and a purpose for living. As a result, women should seek to discover and fulfill that purpose. Abused women report recognizing potential personal power as a way to take control of their lives and develop resiliency. Becoming self-directed, making personal decisions, taking responsibility for oneself, and being self-sufficient are methods by which personal power can be discovered.

Even though the history of the abuse cannot be erased, moving through and acting on these stages allows a woman to discover stability, develop a positive perspective, experience peace, and move forward to a satisfying and contributing life.

Self-Caring

"Why would I care for myself when no one else cared for me? Besides, I was too busy taking care of everyone else. Caring for myself made me think I was 'selfish,'" stated one survivor of domestic abuse. **Self-caring** or self-nurturing means taking care of one's own physical, emotional, and spiritual needs. Having concern for others should not be neglected, but concern for others should not be at the expense of oneself. Self-caring is often a major change in behavior for women who have been in abusive relationships. Self-care enables women to recognize the value of self and to act accordingly by making healthy, nurturing choices. Engaging in fun and enjoyable activities is indicative of moving ahead with life and practicing the art of self-care.

What would you do if you were asked to demonstrate self-care activities? Answers to this question often reflect the stage of healing and growth that survivors are in at any given point. "Having a quiet meal or a complete

Assess Yourself

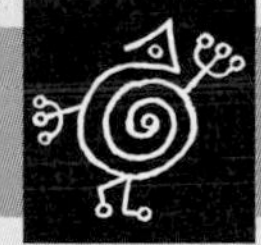

Recognizing and Meeting Personal Needs

Identify and briefly explain some of the things a woman can do to meet the various needs that are important to moving forward with her life.

Needs	Who	How	Where
Survival			
Security			
Love/acceptance			
Self-worth			
Self-actualization			

night's sleep" may be indicative of initial stages of moving ahead with life. Women who, perhaps, have moved further through the healing and growth process may provide such answers as enjoying a hot tub, working in the garden, watching movies, reading books, exercising, cooking a favorite meal, buying flowers, or sharing loving embraces. Whatever the method, engaging in self-care activities is an important move away from former negative beliefs and toward a healthier life.

Meeting Needs

Except for the most basic survival needs, such as food, shelter, and clothing, a woman's higher level needs often go unmet in an abusive relationship. Moving forward certainly means moving beyond survival needs and toward needs that promote progression and growth. Abraham Maslow, whose hierarchy of needs model was introduced in Chapter 3, provides an excellent guide to determining human needs. The need for security, love and acceptance, self-worth, and self-actualization (the fulfillment of a woman's potential) are discussed by Maslow as necessary for basic well-being and continual growth. Adhering to the suggestions found in the section titled "Leaving the Abusive Relationship" and utilizing the resource information presented here can provide the means by which these needs can be recognized and met. Now complete *Assess Yourself:* "Recognizing and Meeting Personal Needs."

PREVENTING ABUSE

Preventing abuse against women must be addressed at all levels: personal, community, state, and federal. Support and advocacy can be addressed at each level as can strategies that enable women to stop abusive episodes or, even better, prevent abusive patterns from ever occurring.

Personal Level

At the personal level, consider the following suggestions that provide empowerment for women, enabling them to recognize and partner in a nonabusive and whole relationship.

- Teaching women to be intolerant of any form of abuse inflicted upon them or their children is an essential component of prevention.
- Educating girls and boys from an early age about the characteristics of healthy and long-lasting relationships will set the foundation for preventing abuse in adulthood. These characteristics include respect, love, shared values, trust, honesty, commitment, mutual caring, and communication.
- Improving the self-worth of women may assist them to think well enough of themselves and to accept that they do not deserve and should not tolerate any abusive behaviors. Personal self-worth leads to the desire to live in a healthy and whole family environment.
- Creating awareness of the negative consequences for women and children, both short-term and long-term, that result from involvement with an abusive partner can assist in preventing relationship abuse.

Healthy relationship awareness not only is a means of empowerment for females but also is a way of changing patterns of socialization for the two sexes. From an early age, boys must be taught that relationships are a partnership in which both participants share in all areas of decision making, responsibilities, and promotion of the relationship's success.

In thinking back on boys and young men in your life, can you remember characteristics that created an uneasy or skeptical feeling in you about them? Do you remember any of the following traits or behaviors that have been identified as characteristics of potential abusers: very little tolerance for others who have different ideas, opinions, or beliefs; low self-esteem; feelings of inadequacy as a man; being quick to anger; rigid and controlling behaviors or demands; overuse of alcohol and use of other drugs; blaming others for anything that doesn't work out; criticizing others; or being from a family in which there was abusive treatment of the mother and/or children.

Autobiography in Five Short Chapters

I.

I walk down the street.
There is a deep hole in the sidewalk.
I fall in
I am lost . . . I am helpless
It isn't my fault
It takes forever to find a way out.

II.

I walk down the same street.
There is a deep hole in the sidewalk.
I pretend I don't see it.
I fall in again.
I can't believe I am in the same place
but, it isn't my fault.
It still takes a long time to get out.

III.

I walk down the same street.
There is a deep hole in the sidewalk.
I see it is there.
I still fall in . . . it's a habit
my eyes are open.
I know where I am.
It is my fault. I get out immediately.

IV.

I walk down the same street.
There is a deep hole in the sidewalk.
I walk around it.

V.

I walk down another street.

by Portia Nelson[44]

Community Level

A community effort to prevent violence and abuse against women is essential because abuse is a social problem, not a private or secret problem. These community actions have been initiated in some areas to address violence and abuse against women as a major social concern:

- Coordination of agencies and programs that can serve to reach families in the community has been accomplished in some areas of the country. The legal, medical, social, and educational agencies have developed formal and, in some instances, informal linkages to educate and provide services to families.
- Parenting classes, relationship-building skills, and stress management seminars are a few of the components that communities offer that can promote healthy family relationships, family preservation, and support for families in need of these services. When the health and well-being of individuals and families are destroyed by family violence, the quality of community life deteriorates.
- Programs for men, especially abusive men, are being developed in which they learn to take responsibility for their actions, develop better partnering skills, and find support for change and growth among other participants.
- Extended-day programs for children and youth have been developed, either at school sites or at community centers. Providing recreational and educational activities and sometimes personal and social guidance, these centers offer a safe, fun, and caring environment for youth from all types of families.
- Increasing community awareness, speaking out about individual and victims' rights, and holding men accountable for their abusive actions is critical, not only in preventing violence and abuse against women but in stopping it as well.

State and Federal Levels

State and federal legislation, legislators, agencies, and other governing entities are making inroads into accepting the fact that women *are* abused and that not only the perpetrators but also the systems that allow this to go unchallenged must be stopped. State and federal governments are continuing to enact legislation to prevent violence and abuse against women as well as prosecuting individuals who dare to commit this crime against another human being, especially human beings whom they profess to love.

- Laws to protect the rights of women against violence and abuse are being passed at the state and federal government levels.

- Reporting any injury that medical personnel, during the time of treatment, perceive to be the result of violence or abuse is required by many states. A physician who fails to report suspected abusive wounds of any type (for example, cuts, burns, bruises, or bullet wounds) is subject to fines or even a possible jail sentence.
- Passage of the most comprehensive and expensive crime bill in U.S. history occurred in 1994, providing $13.5 billion for law enforcement, $9.9 billion for prisons, and $6.9 billion for crime prevention.[45] As a part of this crime bill, the Violence Against Women Act is a landmark mandate that continues to strengthen law enforcement strategies and promote safeguards for victims of domestic and sexual assault. This law has provisions related to safe streets, safe homes for women, civil rights and equal justice for women in the court system, rights against stalking, and protection for battered immigrant women and children. The Department of Justice coordinates efforts with other federal agencies as well as state, local, and tribal law enforcement agencies.
- The Trauma Act, passed in 2003, expands research on the psychological aftereffects of violence against women and enhances research on socioeconomic and sociocultural correlates of violence, research related to special populations, and violence screenings.[46]

It is clear that violence and abuse against women are raging crimes in this country. Varied and complex negative consequences result—not only for women, but for our children, who are possibly future victims or perpetrators. To rectify and to prevent this, actions at all levels—from the individual to the federal government—must continue. Until violence and abuse are absolutely condemned by everyone, abuse will continue and women will remain trapped in a potentially lethal cycle of violence.

Chapter Summary

- Abuse against women has been documented throughout history.
- Domestic abuse, sexual assault, child abuse, and other forms of abuse against women are an epidemic in this country and produce serious physical, mental, emotional, and social consequences for men, women, and their children.
- Financial concerns, self-blame, emotional issues, codependency, and perception of her partner are reasons women often remain in abusive relationships.
- Fear for their children's lives and safety as well as their own is sometimes the impetus for leaving an abusive relationship.
- Having a plan that includes safe facilities, a support system, and accessibility to a variety of resources are important assets when leaving an abusive relationship.
- As women heal from abusive relationships, they generally experience the healing process in a number of stages.
- Family and friends can aid women who have left abusive relationships in moving forward with their lives. Survivors can develop skills that assist their efforts to improve the quality of life for themselves as well as their children.
- Developing a widespread and comprehensive approach to prevention of abuse and violence against women must be a personal priority as well as a priority at the local, state, and federal government levels.

Review Questions

1. Historically, why have women been considered the lesser or weaker sex?
2. Why is it that women often believe they deserve the abuse they receive in a relationship?
3. How and why is the perpetrator socialized into a belief system?
4. Why are women reluctant to report domestic abuse?
5. What barriers in society reduce the likelihood that domestic abuse will be reported to law enforcement authorities?
6. What is meant by psychological abuse, and what are a number of the resulting consequences?
7. What are the behaviors of a potential rapist, and how can women avoid being in a situation where a rape could occur?
8. What are some methods that can help resolve issues related to sexual harassment?
9. What characteristics are associated with women who are abused? How do they develop?
10. What are some of the physical, psychological, spiritual, and social consequences when experiencing abuse?
11. What are the types of resources available to enable a woman to leave an abusive relationship?
12. What are the indicators of healing that show that women are moving ahead with their lives after abuse?

Maslow divided love into two primary categories: D love and B love. D love is based on deficiency, a desire to have another person meet one's unmet needs. As long as her needs are met, she is in love. D love has elements of possessiveness, jealousy, and dependence. B love is based on being. B love includes autonomy, interdependence, and mutual satisfaction. The relationship is secure and partners experience freedom to be themselves. Two other recognized theories of love are Sternberg's triangular model and Lee's six lovestyles.

Sternberg's Triangular Theory

Sternberg's triangular theory of love focuses on three components: commitment, intimacy, and passion. These components explain nine different combinations of love, but not why love occurs. One side of the triangle focuses on the emotional aspect of love (intimacy); the second side focuses on the motivational aspect of love (passion); and, the third side focuses on the cognitive side of love (commitment). The combinations of these three aspects explain different types of love, and changes in the components are illustrated by changes to the size and shape of the triangles. (See Figure 7.1.)

Liking occurs when only the emotional side of love (intimacy) is present. Two friends who trust each other, share similar values and beliefs, and communicate well form an intimate bond. They know the vulnerabilities and strengths of each other and form a close friendship. *Empty love* occurs when commitment alone is present. For example, when Julie states emphatically, "You know, I really don't like Ted anymore but I took a marriage vow. I said 'in sickness and in health, for better or for worse, until death do us part' and that's what I intend to honor. When I want to talk about intimate matters, I talk to my best friend. Besides, the children need a father and I can't find a job now." Julie's religious beliefs, the values instilled during childhood, and limited financial earning potential keep her from leaving to seek a more fulfilling relationship. She may not like Ted as a person, but she married him and intends to stay with him. *Infatuation* occurs when passion is the sole dimension in the relationship. This concept can be summarized as "a crush." Kenitra isn't worried about Andre's values, beliefs, background, job, or anything else; she doesn't care. Andre is awesome, she's never seen anyone more attractive, and she thinks about him all the time. *Romantic love* involves the dimensions of intimacy and passion. Two people who like and are physically attracted to each other but do not have a commitment to form a romantic liaison. In one study, when men and women were asked, "What constitutes a romantic act?" both sexes cited "taking walks together" most often. The women's list included taking walks together, sending or receiving flowers, kissing, candle-lit dinners, cuddling, declaring "I love you," love letters, slow dancing, hugging, and giving surprise gifts. The list for men looked similar and included taking walks together, kissing, candle-lit dinners, cuddling, hugging, flowers, holding hands, making love, love letters, and sitting by the fireplace.[9]

FIGURE 7.1 Sternberg's Triangular Theory of Love

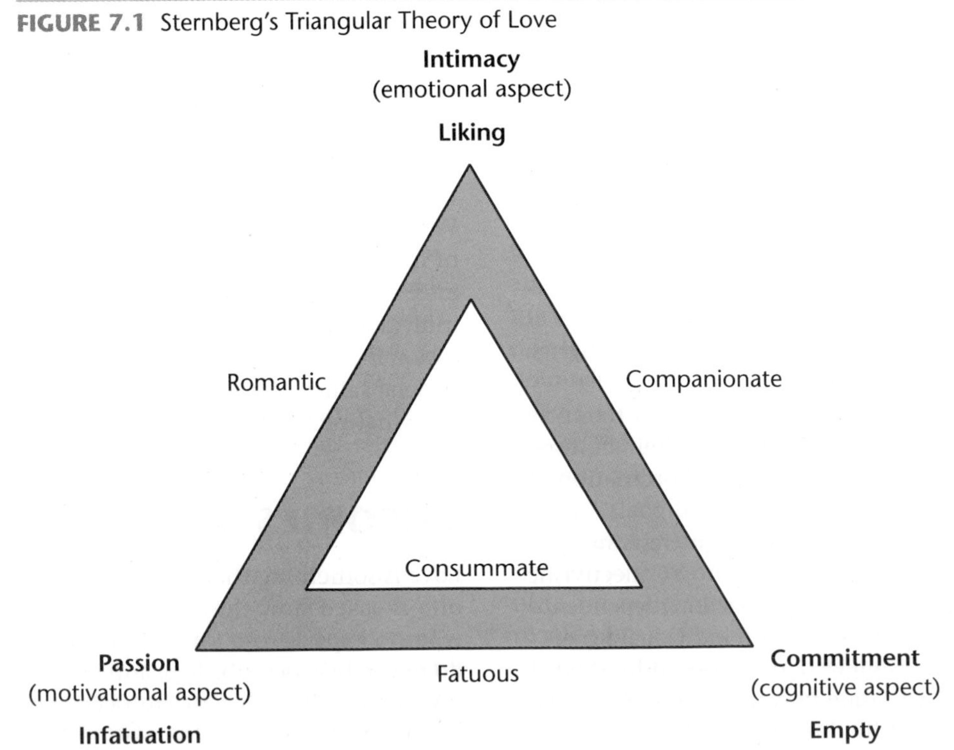

When passion and commitment result in a committed relationship without taking time to get to know each other, *fatuous love* results. Jill met Jackie at a softball game. It was the first game between their teams and the two players were immediately attracted to each other. After the game, they hugged and agreed to meet later at the bar. They ended the night at Jill's place and the sex was great. The next week, Jill asked Jackie to move into her apartment. They were "in love" and ready to commit to a lifetime together. Six months later they shook their heads, wondering how they could have possibly been attracted to each other. They ran out of things to talk about and had very little in common. *Companionate love* involves intimacy and commitment without passion. In some long-term relationships, the physical attraction may die but the intimacy and commitment provide the ingredients for a long-term friendship. The partners are best friends. When all three components are present in the relationship, *consummate love* or complete love occurs. This love is what partners strive to create and to maintain. It requires nurturing, physical attraction, vulnerability, and a commitment to growing together. When all three components are absent in the relationship, Sternberg calls this *nonlove*. These are just casual interactions that occur without any form of relationship evolving.

Lee's Six Lovestyles

I love him, but I'm not in love with him. I like him, but I'm not sure I love him. What do we mean by such words? Psychologist John Alan Lee, in *The Colors of Love,* identifies six different lovestyles.[10] He identifies three primary lovestyles (*eros, storge,* and *ludus*) and three secondary lovestyles (*mania, pragma,* and *agape*). **Erotic love** occurs when lovers get involved quickly and base their attraction on physical attributes and sexual passion. This love is based on "chemistry" and "love at first sight." Eros is a major ingredient in relationship success.

Ludic love is an uncommitted alliance with more than one partner. The partners may be very different from one another because love is based on game playing rather than romance. A partner is "kept guessing" and distancing occurs when dependency develops. Ludus tends to be negatively related to satisfaction with relationships.

Pragmatic love draws two people together for practical reasons such as financial security or parental potential. It is "pragmatic" and fills certain specifications for a partner such as similar background, good job, or good parent. It is often present in long-term relationships.

Manic love is often portrayed in the "heart throb" of Hollywood, the perfect match. The emotional highs and lows remind one of a roller-coaster ride, and possessiveness, dependency, and jealousy abound. Mania leads to total focus on and fear of losing one's partner.

Altruistic love places the needs of the partner above one's own needs. It is selfless and nondemanding, and one chooses self-sacrifice rather than hurting a partner. This love is sometimes referred to as **agape,** a more spiritual relationship.

Storgic love is more like friendship, without the passion. It provides a secure, trusting relationship that evolves from a deep, abiding friendship and leads to long-term relationships.

BIOCHEMISTRY OF LOVE

Helen Fisher is a leading researcher in the biochemistry of love. Recent functional magnetic resonance imaging (MRI) brain scans performed by her research team confirmed her hypothesis that the neurotransmitter dopamine is a major player in romantic love. The brain scans were taken while each subject stared at a picture of his or her beloved. The researchers discovered that while many brain parts became active in each subject who was experiencing love, two regions appeared to be central to the experience: the caudate nucleus and the ventral tegmental area (VTA).[11] The caudate nucleus is a large C-shaped region that lies deep near the center of the brain and is considered part of the limbic system, known as the primitive emotional brain. The brain scans showed that parts of the body and the tail of the caudate nucleus became very active as a lover gazed at the photo of a sweetheart. The caudate nucleus, according to Fisher, "is part of the brain's 'reward system,' the mind's network for general arousal, sensations of pleasure, and the motivation to acquire rewards. The caudate helps us to detect and perceive a reward, discriminate between rewards, *prefer* a particular reward, anticipate a reward, and expect a reward. It produces motivation to acquire a reward and plans specific movements to obtain a reward. The caudate is also associated with the acts of paying attention and learning." Not only did the subjects exhibit activity in the caudate, but the more passionate they were, the more active their caudate was: those who scored higher on a self-report measure taken as part of the study, the Passionate Love Scale, also showed more activity in a specific region of the caudate when they looked at the picture of their sweetheart. The researchers "also found activity in other regions of the reward system, including the septum and a brain region that becomes active when people eat chocolate. Chocolate can be addictive." Fisher maintains that romantic love is addictive, too. The other area where activity was discovered on the fMRI brain scans by Fisher's research team was the VTA, a central part of the reward circuitry of the brain.

> The VTA is a mother lode for dopamine-making cells. With their tentacle-like axons, these nerve cells distribute

TABLE 7.1 Number of Interracial Marriages in the Year 2000 (in thousands)

	RACE OF WIFE					
	WHITE*	AFRICAN AMERICAN*	AMERICAN INDIAN*	ASIAN*	BIRACIAL OR MULTIRACIAL*	HISPANIC, WHITE**
Race of Husband						
White*	—	78.77	137.16	380.47	219.77	503.15
African American*	208.79	—	7.39	27.52	33.33	16.65
American Indian*	131.25	3.75	—	2.59	5.80	4.27
Asian*	123.64	4.47	1.31	—	17.81	9.07
Biracial or Multiracial*	210.15	20.02	6.19	31.99	251.45	11.45
Hispanic, White**	410.28	6.39	4.70	12.28	9.43	—

* Persons not of Hispanic origin.

** Represents white persons of Hispanic origin. Hispanic is not considered a race classification by the U.S. Census Bureau.

SOURCE: U.S. Census Bureau 2000 data.

African American husband. In addition, a number of other configurations also exist (see Table 7.1). From these data we see that interracial marriage takes on a variety of configurations in the United States.

Most interracial dating occurs among college students, but most interracial marriages involve women who are older, previously divorced, and working in a diverse environment.[34] Current trends suggest that changes are occurring in the demographics of interracial marriages. More white women who marry African American men are now in their first marriages and are young, and most intend to have children.[35] The degree of discrimination, prejudice, and animosity these couples (and their children) will face depends, to some extent, on their socioeconomic status, the diversity within their community, and their educational status. Their relationship, particularly if they are an African American and white couple, faces demands not experienced by other couples, including other intermarriage groups. These demands create opportunities for extraordinary growth and maturity within the couple, as well as potential downfalls that can contribute to a higher than normal divorce rate. Couples who find themselves in interracial relationships need support and encouragement, not only from each other, but from friends and family. (See *Her Story:* "Michelle: An Interracial Relationship Encounters Family Bigotry.")

Children's identities are also changing, and with these changes the blurring of color lines is accelerating. Under pressure from mixed-race Americans, the Census Bureau changed its rules in 2000 to allow for selection of five race/ethnicity categories. In a 2000 survey, nearly one in three children whose fathers were non-Hispanic white and whose mothers were African American identified themselves as white, a change from 1980 when only one in four self-identified as white. Similarly, nearly half of children of non-Hispanic white fathers and Native American, Chinese, or Japanese mothers were identified as white. This emerging racial and ethnic melding will create an increasingly fluid society.

Lesbian Couples

Lesbian couples have a unique opportunity to experience the best and also the most challenging aspects of what it means to be "female" in a relationship. Previously, we discussed the psychological and sociological factors that impact individual roles in relationships. As women, lesbians have grown up with the same societal influences as their heterosexual counterparts. A major difference between the two groups is that lesbians must be more consciously aware of the influences they will accept or reject. For instance, lesbians usually accept the values of a collectivistic society, thus both partners are relationship-focused. This focus on community encourages equality and equity, regardless of whether they are in a committed, long-term relationship or an intimate friendship. By the same token, lesbians often reject the influence of income on power as exemplified in a patriarchal society. "Lesbians do not use income to establish dominance in their relationship. They use it to avoid having one woman dependent on the other."[36]

Lesbians, by virtue of being same-sex couples, encounter additional challenges in their relationships. One potential difficulty is maintaining personal boundaries, which easily can become blurred when both partners focus on emotional intimacy and exclude personal autonomy. Maintaining balance between autonomy and intimacy is an important consideration. Another potential difficulty for lesbian couples is the lack of adequate role models for "peer relationships." Within the lesbian community, long-term relationships are often "closeted," particularly among older lesbians who grew up during more discriminatory times. Many lesbian couples form committed relationships but do not receive the

Her Story

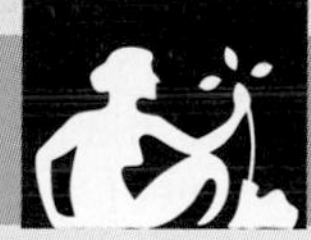

Michelle: An Interracial Relationship Encounters Family Bigotry

Michelle, a 24-year-old senior, met Tony at a nightclub. She found him physically attractive, but more important, she enjoyed talking with him. When she discussed her work, he showed genuine interest. When he asked her out on a date, she wondered what her parents would think. They never told Michelle that she could not date a black man. But she could recall a time when she was 9 or 10 years old and her father commented negatively about an interracial couple at a restaurant. However, she decided to go ahead with the date.

Michelle told her mother about Tony immediately but waited nearly 6 months before telling her dad. Her mother was pretty open-minded about it, but her father could not accept it. She had always been "Daddy's little girl," had followed the path that made him happy, and now, she just couldn't understand his feelings. Maybe with some time, he would accept it. Why didn't he trust her to make the right decisions for herself?

They had been dating for 2½ years when Michelle became pregnant. It wasn't planned, but they were excited about having a baby. Michelle would be graduating soon, and Tony had an excellent job as a business consultant. Her mother handled the news pretty well; she didn't like the idea that they weren't married. Her dad, however, went through the roof . . . he said he hadn't accepted the relationship so he most certainly wasn't going to accept this! He didn't even want her in the house anymore; he didn't want to see her. Michelle was devastated; how could he treat his own daughter this way? Would her baby ever know her grandfather? What should she tell her little girl as she grew up and wanted to know about her grandparents?

- How would your parents respond to an interracial grandchild?
- What would you do if you were in Michelle's situation?

same benefits as married couples, for example, health insurance, help in finding a job for one partner when the other is relocated, tax benefits, and family support.

In the past, lesbian couples didn't have the option of raising children unless one or both partners had children from a previous heterosexual relationship. Today, the number of lesbian couples choosing to have children is rising steadily, and their options include adoption, artificial insemination, or other arrangements. Children provide the same parental bond for lesbian couples as it does for heterosexual couples but may create some additional parenting issues. Difficulty can arise when others, particularly those opposed to lesbian lifestyles, question the ability or right of lesbians to raise children. They suggest that children raised in a same-sex household may differ from other children emotionally or that the children may be raised to be lesbians or gay. A study comparing men and women raised by heterosexual single mothers and lesbian mothers found that these young adults exhibited similar behavioral patterns regardless of the sexual orientation of the parent. Almost all (including twenty-three of twenty-five lesbian-raised adults) described themselves as heterosexual and indicated a desire for marriage and children.[37]

Single Lifestyles and Parenthood

An increasing number of women are choosing to remain single. As the number of single-female households increases, the number of households with children continues to decrease, and the age of first marriage continues to rise. Women are feeling less pressure to get married as more career opportunities, better education, and better birth control methods, have become available. Many American women are enjoying the advantages of a single lifestyle and plan to keep it that way. Those who plan to get married are waiting longer. The median age for first marriage was 25.1 years in 2000. The postponement of marriage has led to a substantial increase in the percentage of never-married women, 73 percent of 20- to 24-year-olds and 22 percent of 30- to 34-year-olds.

Another trend is the growing number of one-parent households, both male and female. Two factors seem to contribute significantly to this trend: the increase in births to unwed mothers and the growth in divorce. In the United States 13 percent of all households were single-parent in 1970 compared to 26 percent single-mother families and 5 percent single-father families in 2000. The number of single-mother families increased from 3 million in 1970 to 10 million in 2000, while the number of single-father families grew from 393,000 to 2 million. In female-maintained families, 35 percent were never married, and about 34 percent were divorced. A higher percentage of women were out of the labor force or unemployed compared to married-couple family groups (35 percent to 29 percent), and a lower percentage had attended college (40 percent to 55 percent).

Female-maintained families compared to male-maintained families tended to have more than one child, were more likely to have family incomes below the poverty level (34 percent compared to 16 percent), and were less likely to have ever married (34 percent compared to 43 percent). Children living with divorced single mothers typically had an economic advantage over those living with never-married single mothers.[38]

Among young adults (ages 18–24), the pattern of living arrangements continues to shift. In 2000, 56 percent of males and 43 percent of females lived at home with one or both parents. Only 4 percent were likely to live alone, and the majority of young adults were more likely to cohabit, live with roommates or persons other than spouses, or with their parents than to live alone or with a spouse. Thirty percent of males and 35 percent of females lived with others who were neither spouses nor parents.

Among men and women ages 65–74, men were more likely to live with a spouse (77 percent compared to 53 percent). Among older adults (ages 75+), 67 percent of men were living with spouses compared with only 29 percent of women the same age. Older women who were not currently married were more likely than men to live alone (49 percent compared to 21 percent). Another 22 percent of older women were living with someone other than a spouse. These differences reflect a higher male mortality rate.[39]

TROUBLED RELATIONSHIPS

When a relationship gets into trouble, a variety of patterns can ensue that exacerbate existing problems and prevent resolution. As conflict and distress increase, the familiar pattern occurs more quickly, and partners become more entrenched in their role of perpetuating the pattern. Couples continue to cycle through these patterns until the relationship ends or they seek help.

Love Addiction

The idea that love might be connected to "addiction" seems contradictory; however, loving relationships built on emotional and physical intimacy differ significantly from "addictive," incomplete relationships built on faulty thinking and feeling. This pattern has been described as love/avoidance addiction.[40] It occurs when one partner, the **love addict,** feels the need to be rescued and the other partner, the **avoidance addict,** attempts to avoid involvement with the partner. The primary fear of the love addict is abandonment; the primary fear of the avoidance addict is intimacy. The secondary fear of each is reversed, thus both have the same two fears: abandonment and intimacy. Unless both partners make a concerted effort to break these cycles (usually through making conscious decisions to understand and change behaviors that contribute to these patterns), the relationship will deteriorate further until one partner leaves.[41]

Terminating a Relationship

According to the U.S. Census Bureau, 52 percent of all first marriages end in **divorce,** and more than 60 percent of second marriages fail.[42] The National Center for Health Statistics reported that for 2004 the national divorce rate was 3.7 divorces per 1,000 population. The states with the lowest divorce rates were Massachusetts (2.2), Illinois (2.6), Iowa (2.8), Minnesota (2.8), and Washington, D.C. (not really a state; 1.9). The states with the highest divorce rates were Nevada (6.4), Arkansas (6.1), Wyoming (5.2), Idaho (5.0), and West Virginia (5.0). One suggested reason for such differences is that laws vary from state to state regarding dissolution of marriage. For example, Massachusetts law has traditionally required a very long waiting period between the filing for divorce and the entry of a divorce decree. In contrast, Nevada has historically been a state recognized for quick and easy divorce, requiring very short waiting periods and limited length of residency.

According to the National Center for Health Statistics, the divorce rate dropped from the years 1990 to 2004 in all but two states that reported this statistic (not reporting a divorce rate for 2004: California, Georgia, Hawaii, Indiana, and Louisiana). The divorce rates stayed the same from 1990 to 2004 for New Jersey (3.0) and Maine (4.3). States with the largest decline in divorce rate from 1990 to 2004 were Nevada (from 11.4 to 6.4), Arizona (from 6.9 to 4.2), and Oklahoma (from 7.7 to 4.9). The decline in the divorce rates from 1990 to 2004 reflects the pattern of a decreasing marriage rate over these same years.

It is well known that the emotional and financial effects of divorce are generally greater for women than for men. The group who suffers and fares most poorly is older women, especially when they are ending a long-term relationship, have limited work experience, or have relied on the husband as the wage earner. Information about the financial and emotional effects of breakups on cohabitating women supports a similar trend. Cohabitating women have the added burden of limited or no legal remedies. These women may experience more difficulty in gaining emotional support than divorcing women because their relationships are less acceptable or recognized by the general population. A breakup of a relationship (lesbian, cohabitating, or divorcing) can cause a number of disruptive consequences in women's lives, including depression, lower self-esteem, anxiety, feelings of betrayal or abandonment, as well as changes in child rearing, career decisions, finances, and housing.

Many women, with time, will choose to remarry or become involved in another relationship. Remarriages have been found to be more fragile and break up at a greater rate than first marriages. U.S. Census Bureau data show that more than 62 percent of remarriages of women under age 40 end in divorce, and when children are involved, the rate is even higher.

A major problem for a blended family is that expectations of the adults and the children are often unrealistic. When these expectations are broken (regardless of the reason), partners may experience conflict. The partner with children may find herself caught between the needs of her current partner and the needs of her children from the previous marriage or relationship. The parent–child relationship was established before this relationship, and she may feel compelled to reassure her children that they will not be abandoned again. Meanwhile, her new partner may feel slighted. He may feel like he has to compete with the children for her attention. Realistically, it takes time and patience to blend a family, and unless all parties set reasonable expectations, trouble will ensue. Conflict can also ensue if unresolved differences or unfinished business exists with an ex-partner. This tension can definitely impact and affect the new relationship.

Potential Sources of Conflict

Individual problems may also come between partners in the relationship. Some of these problems include self-absorption, excessive ambition, feelings of inferiority or superiority, criticism, contempt, or defensiveness. Self-absorbed partners always put their own needs ahead of their partner's needs. They are unable or unwilling to meet their partner's needs if those needs interfere with their own. A partner with excessive ambition will make getting ahead in the material world a higher priority than the relationship. Most women prefer intimacy and relationship, not goals connected to ambition. Whether a partner has feelings of inferiority or superiority, she is masking the underlying malady, low self-esteem. The behaviors and interaction with a partner will manifest differently, but the root cause is the same. A partner with feelings of inferiority will defer to her partner because she believes he has more rights, is more knowledgeable, or is more deserving. A partner with feelings of superiority will believe she has more rights, knows more, and "is more" than her partner. A critical partner attacks his partner for who she is rather than her behaviors. This type of attack can certainly be construed as emotional abuse of a partner and creates few opportunities for changing the pattern. A partner who feels contempt for his partner can intentionally hurt her with words or actions. A partner exhibiting defensiveness may deny responsibility or make excuses for his actions. If she complains, his complaint will be louder, stronger, worse, one better. He may "dig in" on his position and not see any alternatives. The distancer will put up a wall and shut the other person out with silence. This position inhibits emotional intimacy and keeps the other person "guessing."

A number of warning signs may signal a troubled relationship, including an increase in physical symptoms by a partner, an increase in alcohol or drug consumption, silence or emotional withdrawal by a partner, more frequent arguments, more fantasies of separation, or more divergent lives. These signs may manifest in actual behaviors such as a partner's affair, lying or other deceit, inattentiveness, lack of sexual interest, outside influences, and illegal activity. Several of these behaviors and issues are described in the following sections.

External Affair Sexual infidelity may occur for different reasons. Some affairs result because expectations were not met; others are viewed as a payback or punishment; whereas others involve emotional intimacy and closeness. The four words, "I'm having an affair" can be a wake-up call or a death knell to relationships. These words and the act itself certainly signal problems in a relationship. Affairs exacerbate the problems that currently exist, and the person isn't necessarily running to something as much as running away from something. The reason most cited as to why a woman has an affair is "I wanted more warmth and intimacy."

Women often view a partner's affair as the ultimate betrayal. It is construed as deceptive and violates the commitment between primary partners. Yet some women are known to seek an extramarital affair. In one study of dating, cohabitating, and married women, the researchers found that the length of a relationship and number of previous partners were positively related to the potential for a secondary sex partner. Women who had four or more sex partners before the current relationship were nearly ten times more likely to have another sex partner. Married women with multiple previous partners were twenty times more likely than their counterparts with no previous partners to have a secondary sex partner. And, as the length of the relationship increased, the potential for a secondary sex partner also increased. The researchers found that cohabitating women were less committed than married women to monogamy.[43] Four percent of married women compared to 20 percent of cohabiting women had a secondary sex partner.

Nonmonogamy within the relationship, whether heterosexual or lesbian, increases the likelihood of a breakup.[44] Although an affair has the potential to destroy a relationship, it doesn't have to end the relationship. The end of an affair can be the new beginning to an existing relationship. The outcome depends on the willingness of both individuals to work through broken expectations.

Money Few people openly discuss their finances or even think about their attitudes toward money before getting seriously involved in a relationship, yet numerous studies show that money is the most discussed issue in heterosexual relationships. Money issues are often a major consideration because the amount of money earned determines power within the relationship. And power equates with freedom to make important decisions. Blumstein and Schwartz found that the amount of money a person earned, in comparison to her partner, was the major factor in determining relative power in heterosexual, but not lesbian, relationships. They suggested, "Since women in this society are not accustomed to judging their own worth by how much money they make, we feel that lesbians do not fall into judging their partners by such a standard."[45] Lesbians had grown to reject the male-provider philosophy and preferred to equally share financial responsibility. For heterosexuals, power and money differed according to the male-provider philosophy. Married women who accepted the male-provider philosophy had less power in the relationship, regardless of income level between the spouses. In cohabitating couples, money equated with power but these women were more likely to believe that equal contributions were important.[46] (See *Viewpoint:* "Spending Differences Can Impact Relationships.")

The key to resolving money issues in a relationship is understanding one's own habits and communicating with a partner regarding the management of money and power within the relationship. A couple must set joint priorities and appreciate the differences that exist in philosophy and patterns of handling money.

Sexuality Sexual feelings, desires, and activities are present throughout the life cycle and profoundly shaped by culture. Differences between male and female attitudes toward sex begin early and can be seen from the first sexual encounter. When females are asked about their first sexual encounter, they usually choose to be sexual with someone they like. When males are asked about their first sexual encounter, curiosity is usually the driving force.

Physical intimacy tends to be viewed differently by men and women. Most men view sex as a way to be emotionally intimate, whereas most women want emotional intimacy before they can be sexual. Blumstein and Schwartz found considerable differences among men and women in their sexual patterns. The majority of married couples were having sex at least once a week. Lesbians, on the other hand, were far less sexual than married, cohabitating, or gay male couples, even when compared at each stage of relationship development. But lesbians were much more active in the amount of

Viewpoint

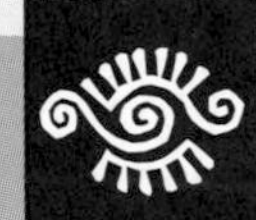

Spending Differences Can Impact Relationships

Money conflicts within relationships are common, particularly if expectations differ when it comes to the management and control of money. Money harmony is difficult to maintain and requires flexibility and communication. Olivia Mellan, author of *Money Harmony: Resolving Money Conflicts in Your Life and Relationships,* calls money harmony "a balanced state in which both partners feel free to spend, save, or invest money in ways that support their deeper desires, values, and sense of themselves."[47] Money harmony can occur only if partners are willing to discuss and explore their beliefs and behaviors related to money. Mellan identified seven common money personality types: spenders, hoarders, avoiders, amassers, money monks, worriers, and bingers. Spenders use the slogans "shop till you drop" or "power shopping." This person enjoys spending and has a hard time saving money. Hoarders are the misers, the stingy money savers who put money away for a rainy day. The miser has a strict budget and will not part with her money unless absolutely necessary. Managing money is a difficult, overwhelming task for avoiders. This person waits until the last minute to pay her bills and often is late with her payments. She is overwhelmed by the concept of budgeting and saving, thus seldom budgets or saves. Amassers base their self-worth on net worth. An amasser will accumulate money to feel good about herself, and workaholism is common. Money monks view the love of money as the "root of all evil," therefore they tend to give money to socially worthwhile projects or religious endeavors. They seldom accumulate money so as to avoid the temptation of valuing it too highly. Worriers, on the other hand, see money as a scarcity and are extremely cautious. They review the budget and expenditures over and over, looking for corners to cut or making sure to account for every dime. Bingers use money to fill an emotional need, and the "rush" that comes from spending money dissipates with the empty feelings that follow the binge.

Which pattern of money management most describes your behavior? If you are in a relationship, which pattern does your partner practice?

physical contact (cuddling, touching, hugging) between partners when compared to other couples. Genital sex was less important to lesbians even though physical intimacy, without sex, was usually an end unto itself.[48]

Keeping physical intimacy alive can be difficult for partners, particularly when schedules get busy, distractions increase, and familiarity and friendship cause the physical and sexual intimacy to wane.

The definition of **sexual function** is "the ability to experience *desire* (positive anticipation and feel deserving of sexual pleasure), *arousal* (receptivity and responsivity to erotic touch resulting in lubrication for the woman and erection for the man), *orgasm* (a voluntary response that is a natural culmination of high arousal), and *satisfaction* (feeling emotionally and sexually fulfilled and bonded)."[49] Sexual dysfunction is more common among women than men, with the most common female dysfunctions being (1) inhibited sexual desire, (2) nonorgasmic response during partner sex, (3) painful intercourse (dyspareunia), (4) female arousal dysfunction, (5) primary nonorgasmic response, and (6) vaginismus (a painful spasmodic constriction of the vagina often rendering copulation impossible).[50] The most common male sexual dysfunctions are (1) early ejaculation, (2) erectile dysfunction, (3) inhibited sexual desire, and (4) ejaculatory inhibition.[51]

The rates of sexual dysfunction and dissatisfaction continue to be high.[52] According to sex researcher McCarthy, "The number of couples with sexual dysfunction or dissatisfaction has not decreased; if anything it has increased. Of special concern is the nonsexual relationship. When the criterion of being sexual fewer than 10 times a year is used, approximately 20% of married couples and 30% of non-married couples who have been together at least 2 years have nonsexual relationships."[53] Although some sexual dysfunction has a physical pathology, much of the cause for sexual dysfunction is emotional or psychological in nature. There is a classification of sexual dysfunctions and disorders included in the DSM-IV (*Diagnostic and Statistical Manual of Mental Disorders,* Fourth Edition).[54] A tri-phasic model proposed by Kaplan in 1974 is still used to classify sexual dysfunctions as disorders of desire, arousal, and orgasm.[55] "Traditional causes of sexual dysfunction were lack of information, repressive attitudes, high anxiety, lack of sexual skill, and rigid sex roles."[56] Lack of information is no longer a common cause for sexual dysfunction today because of the availability of self-help books and sexuality courses. However, with sexual themes prevalent in today's advertising and entertainment industry, there are now unrealistic expectations and performance demands that contribute to high anxiety.

The originators of couple sex therapy were Masters and Johnson in 1970.[57] According to McCarthy, "Their model of 2-week intensive therapy by a male–female co-therapy team is almost extinct, but two of their concepts form the essence of contemporary sex therapy. First, sexual dysfunction is best conceptualized, assessed, and treated as a couple issue. Second, sexual comfort, skill, and functioning can be learned."[58] Sexual exercises are the preferred modality for helping couples develop a comfortable, functional sexual style.[59]

When a couple has good sexual relations, this contributes to the overall relationship satisfaction, but it is not a major factor.

> A clinical adage is that sexuality contributes 15–20% to a marriage, serving as shared pleasure, a means to reinforce intimacy, and a tension reducer to deal with the stresses of life and marriage. Sexuality energizes the marital bond and facilitates special couple feelings. When sexuality is dysfunctional or nonexistent, it plays an inordinately powerful role, perhaps 50–75%, draining the marriage of vitality and intimacy. . . . Paradoxically, bad sex plays a more powerful negative role than good sex plays a positive role in marriage. The most commonly cited reasons couples separate in the first 2 years of marriage are a sexual conflict/fertility problem (e.g., unwanted pregnancy or infertility), an extramarital affair, or a sexual dysfunction (especially inhibited sexual desire).[60]

There have been significant cultural shifts in recent years that are related to sexuality. There has been an increase in the frequency of premarital sex, increases in sexually transmitted diseases, continual increases in the HIV/AIDS epidemic, and heightened sensitivity to sexual trauma, especially child sexual abuse; "[t]hose kinds of changes have led to a counterreaction from religious and conservative groups, especially the 'family values' movement."[61] A paradigm shift occurred in 1998 in the conceptualization of male sexuality when Viagra, a male performance–enhancing drug, was introduced. This shift was the medicalization of male sexuality. Though some researchers have warned against this trend, it seems to be "gaining momentum not only in the treatment of erectile dysfunction, but of early ejaculation. The movement to medicalize female sexuality is now growing."[62] One has to wonder what this might mean, both positively and negatively, for couple sexuality.

Sexuality is more than simple mechanics involving genitals, intercourse, and orgasm.[63] In fact, experts recommend that sexual partners avoid rigid roles and mechanical sex and that the prescription for satisfying sex is integrating emotional intimacy, nondemand pleasuring, and erotic stimulation.

> Sexuality is an affirmation of your attractiveness, desirability, sense of masculinity or femininity. Affectionate clothes-on touching (kissing, hugging, holding hands) is integral to your marital [or relationship] bond. Sensual experiences (whole body massages, showering or bathing together, nondemand pleasuring, cuddling in bed at night or in the morning) nurture your relationship

> and serve as a bridge to sexual desire. Playful and erotic touching (seductive dancing, erotic play in the shower, mixing manual and oral stimulation) builds sexual desire. . . . The best sex is between two aware people who take responsibility for their sexuality and creatively share feelings, needs, and preferences and are open to erotic scenarios and techniques. The essence of creative sexuality is a trusting relationship in which feelings and requests are shared.[64]

Child Rearing and Household Labor Gender is the major criterion used by heterosexual couples for the distribution of household tasks and child rearing. Women do the majority of household tasks and child rearing, estimated at two to three times that of men. Even for couples who appear to divide household labor more equally, men do not assume more responsibility; instead, women, in effect, choose to do less. This condition of inequity exists irrespective of education, income, and presence of children. The assigning of tasks based on gender may be efficient, but it often relegates women to subordinate roles in the relationship, leading to depression and a sense of powerlessness. Women who feel relegated to this role and powerless to change it are more likely to experience psychological distress. This sense of inequality can lead to marital distress, and in a larger sense, gender inequalities within the relationship (unpaid household labor and child care) may produce gender inequalities outside the relationship.[65] Researchers have found that lesbian couples are more careful to divide household labor equally (maybe because few women enjoy doing these tasks) than married or gay couples.[66] This equal sharing of responsibility for menial tasks and sense of personal power in choosing to share the tasks acts as a protective factor in preventing emotional distress.

Children represent another challenge for couples. A large percentage of households (41 percent of unmarried and 46 percent of married) have children under 18 years of age. It is important for parents to agree on discipline and child-rearing practices, and compromise is sometimes required. Another household trend is the decrease in family size. In 1970, 17 percent of households had four or more children compared to only 6 percent of households in 2000.

Inattentiveness Once a woman enters a committed relationship, she faces a variety of challenges to keeping the relationship alive. One danger she may face in a relationship is getting too busy or too tired to exercise the skills necessary to keep the relationship healthy and functional. These skills include effective communication, such as good listening skills, conflict resolution, and the ability to work toward mutual compromise.

Couples tend to slip into inattentiveness unknowingly, being too busy with taking the kids to soccer, meeting deadlines, or juggling added responsibilities. These demands are conditional real demands on the relationship, but if they continue to build, problems can begin. At some time the couple needs to prioritize these demands or the relationship may terminate. Ideally, the relationship needs to be nurtured on a daily basis the same way the self needs nurturing. However, at minimum, specific time must be set aside at least once a week to focus on nurturing the relationship, time to have dinner and talk, enjoy a movie, or engage in mutually enjoyable activities. The key to success is to manage time, rather than letting time manage the partners.

Resolving Conflicts—Fighting Fair

Some experts suggest that how couples fight or handle fundamental disagreements is a major predictor of whether the relationship will last. Robert Levenson and John Gottman studied numerous couples and monitored physiological responses to determine the impact of the disagreements. They found that successful couples find a way to put a conflict behind them, whereas troubled couples leave the argument unresolved, thus eroding the bond that holds them together. They found that couples who had the same fighting style were most successful. The three fighting styles they saw were validators, volatile reactors, and conflict avoiders. Validators would discuss their differences, attempting to understand the other's viewpoint, and strive to reach a compromise. Volatile reactors shouted at each other and attempted to outmaneuver their partner to a position of submission. Conflict avoiders, the least successful of the three types, did everything possible to avoid conflict. When disagreements occurred, these couples just agreed to disagree, not looking for compromise or a change in stance of the other partner. Levenson and Gottman also conducted a 12-year longitudinal research study of twenty-one gay couples and twenty-one lesbian couples. Their research showed that these couples, compared to straight couples, used more affection and humor when discussing a disagreement. They were less belligerent and domineering and used fewer fear tactics than straight couples. Lesbians were more expressive—positively and negatively—quite likely a by-product of society's acceptance of expressiveness in women.

In *The Dance of Anger,* psychologist Harriet Lerner discussed some ineffective techniques women may use to handle anger.[67] These techniques (silent submission, ineffective fighting and blaming, and emotional distancing) are used by women to keep a relationship harmonious, but often at the expense of authenticity. These patterns happen during times of stress or overload and may change depending on the individual with whom the woman is arguing. The patterns of expressing anger are classified as pursuers, distancers, underfunctioners, and overfunctioners. Pursuers value talking through an

Health Tips

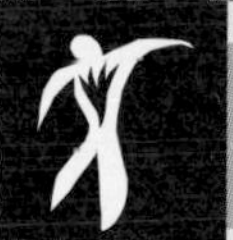

Fighting Fair

Successful negotiation requires that both partners must

- Clearly state the problem or complaint
- Agree to discuss the problem or complaint
- Commit to: +Change the pattern
  +Find an acceptable compromise
  +Disagree

issue and want a partner to do the same. They seek closeness when disagreements occur and feel hurt when the other person seeks distance. Distancers want to be left alone, emotionally and physically, when disagreements occur. They attempt to figure things out away from the pressure of the moment. They address the issue again when they are ready. Underfunctioners appear weak and submissive, fragile, or irresponsible. They fall apart under stress and become disorganized or nonfunctional. They have difficulty appearing competent to those close to them. Overfunctioners are the "fixers" who give advice and move in quickly to resolve a dispute.

Couples can learn to negotiate for their needs in a fair manner. (See *Health Tips:* "Fighting Fair.") The first step in fair fighting requires that both partners agree to engage in the discussion. The partner who is angry should ask her partner if he or she is willing to engage in a fight for change. When they are willing to engage in the discussion, the partner with the complaint should state it clearly and ask for what she needs or wants. When the other person has heard and restated the complaint, she has several options: she can agree to the request, she can ask for clarification, she can offer an alternative, or she can agree to disagree (say no). Successful negotiation occurs when both parties have heard each other and have committed to change the pattern, found an acceptable compromise, or have reached an agreement to disagree.[68] Difficulties arise in all relationships; the difference between successful and unsuccessful resolution is the willingness of both partners to openly share their concerns and negotiate for change.

POSITIVE PARENTING RELATIONSHIPS

The responsibility of every parent is to protect and nurture a child and also to prepare that child for success and happiness in family relations, school achievement, work satisfaction, and other life challenges. (See *Women Making a Difference:* "Joy A. Thomas: Working Mother of the Year.") The style of parenting used to attempt to fulfill parental responsibilities is vital to the success or failure of that goal. There are three common types of parenting, two of which are dysfunctional and one that is recommended.[70] One dysfunctional parenting style is referred to as "Giving Orders"—to be too controlling by giving orders, setting unreasonable limits, and giving children little or no freedom. Another dysfunctional parenting style is referred to as "Giving In"—to be too permissive by giving children lots of freedom but no limits. The most functional parenting style is referred to as "Giving Choices"—to help children learn a balance between freedom and limits by offering them choices and allowing them to experience the natural and logical consequences of those choices. "Giving Choices" is a **democratic parenting style** and will help parents raise a responsible child by (1) setting limits for children and (2) giving

Women Making a Difference

Joy A. Thomas: Working Mother of the Year[69]

The International Association of Working Mothers (IAWM) and the Moms in Business Network (MBN) named Joy A. Thomas as the 2006 Working Mother of the Year. Joy is the senior director of business planning and development for the renal division of Baxter Healthcare Corporation where she has worked for 12 years. She leads strategy teams to ensure the delivery of vital drugs to kidney patients in the United States and abroad, bringing much-needed health care to people in developing nations. She is a dedicated mother of three children aged 7, 6, and 3 and volunteers for a number of school and community activities to spend even more time with them. According to Gina Robison-Billups, president and founder of MBN and its sister association IAWM, there are more than 80 million mothers in the United States and approximately three-quarters of them work. Robison-Billups feels that Joy Thomas is a good example of a successful career woman who can put her family first while excelling in her career and contributing to her community. Do you think that working mothers must deny their family's basic needs to create and maintain a professional career or to get or keep a job? What factors may allow some working mothers to dedicate more time to their family? What factors keep some working mothers from dedicating more time to their family?

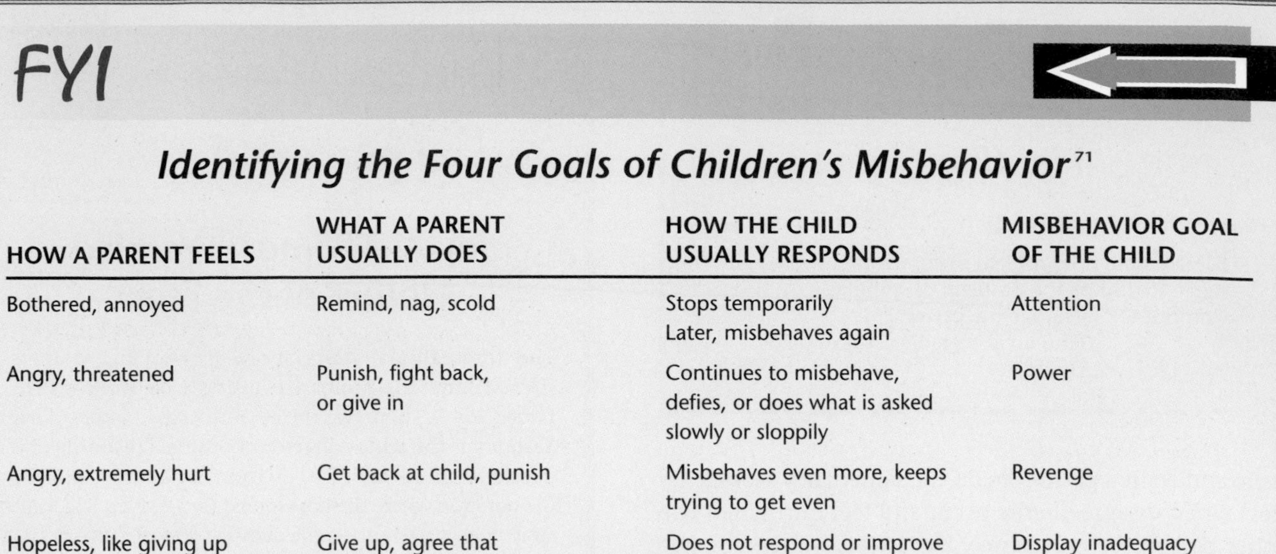

FYI

Identifying the Four Goals of Children's Misbehavior[71]

HOW A PARENT FEELS	WHAT A PARENT USUALLY DOES	HOW THE CHILD USUALLY RESPONDS	MISBEHAVIOR GOAL OF THE CHILD
Bothered, annoyed	Remind, nag, scold	Stops temporarily Later, misbehaves again	Attention
Angry, threatened	Punish, fight back, or give in	Continues to misbehave, defies, or does what is asked slowly or sloppily	Power
Angry, extremely hurt	Get back at child, punish	Misbehaves even more, keeps trying to get even	Revenge
Hopeless, like giving up	Give up, agree that the child is helpless	Does not respond or improve	Display inadequacy

children choices within those limits. For example, "You have math and science homework. Which would you like to do first?" or "You may choose to remove your muddy shoes, or you can choose to clean the muddy tracks from the floor. You decide."

All children need to feel accepted, to have a sense of belonging in a family, and to be acknowledged as a significant member of that family.[72] Children need guidance, encouragement, and support to develop and thrive and to feel as if they belong. A child who chooses negative behavior as a way of feeling she or he belongs is a **discouraged child.** A discouraged child often misbehaves to accomplish one of the following goals: (1) to gain attention, (2) to achieve power, (3) to seek revenge, or (4) to display inadequacy. (See *FYI:* "Identifying the Four Goals of Children's Misbehavior.") Understanding and recognizing which one of the four goals of misbehavior the child is seeking will help a parent to respond adequately to the child's needs thereby moving the child from a state of discouragement to one of encouragement. A key to successful parenting is to remember that if what you are doing is not working, then change your response to the child's behavior.

Therapists recommend four ingredients for forming strong relationships with children: (1) showing respect, (2) having fun, (3) giving encouragement, and (4) showing love. Giving encouragement means believing in children. "We must believe in our children if they are to believe in themselves:

- To feel capable and loved, children need lots of encouragement.
- To be ready to truly cooperate, children need to feel good about themselves."[73]

The democratic parenting style is successful because it provides opportunities for a child to succeed. Children who experience success will begin to believe in themselves again and be willing to cooperate.

Chapter Summary

- Statistics suggest that relationships are more difficult to maintain in today's society. Over one-half of all first marriages end in divorce.
- Relationships have undergone a number of changes as gender roles and attitudes have converged.
- Sternberg's triangular theory of love suggests that relationships can be envisioned as the sides of a triangle. The sides include commitment, intimacy, and passion.
- Healthy relationships are characterized by attributes such as trust, respect, honesty, and authenticity.
- Unhealthy relationships are characterized by traits such as self-absorption, jealousy, feelings of inferiority or superiority, and distancing.
- Marriage, cohabitation, same-sex unions, and remarriages are different types of relationships.
- People spend money according to different personality profiles.
- Sexuality plays an important role in relationship satisfaction.
- Resolving conflicts by fair fighting is important to the happiness of partners in a relationship.
- The four ingredients for forming strong relationships with children are show respect, have fun, give encouragement, and show love.

Review Questions

1. What gender-role attributes seem best suited to relationships?
2. What are the differences between individualistic and collectivistic societies?
3. What are the key components of each stage of dating?
4. What is the difference between physical and emotional intimacy?
5. What is consummate love based on Sternberg's theory?
6. Which two areas of the brain are most active during the early stages of romantic love, and what two additional areas of the brain are most active with longer romantic involvement?
7. Which neurotransmitter has been identified by Fisher to be actively involved in the experience of romantic love?
8. Which hormone stimulates sexual desire?
9. Name the male hormone and the female hormone that produce behaviors associated with emotional attachment.
10. What are the lovestyles described by John Alan Lee?
11. What are the differences between vitalized and devitalized marriages?
12. What is a peer marriage?
13. What characteristics do cohabitators share with married couples? with singles?
14. What are some challenges to lesbian couples?
15. What characteristics are exhibited by love addicts? by avoidance addicts?
16. What are the major issues in troubled relationships?
17. What is the definition of sexual function?
18. What are the most common female sexual dysfunctions?
19. Kaplan classifies sexual dysfunction into what three areas of disorder?
20. What is the most effective parenting style?
21. What are the four goals of misbehavior for children?
22. What are the four ingredients for forming a strong relationship with children?

Resources

Organization

American Association for Marriage and Family Therapy.
800-374-2638
www.aamft.org

Suggested Readings

Angier, N. 1999. *Woman: An Intimate Geography*. Boston: Houghton Mifflin.

Bernstein, R. 2003. *Straight Parents, Gay Children: Keeping Families Together*. New York: Thunder's Mouth Press.

Berzon, B. 2004. *Permanent Partners: Building Gay and Lesbian Relationships That Last*. Rev. ed. New York: Plume/Penguin.

Borhek, M. 1993. *Coming Out to Parents: A Two-Way Survival Guide for Lesbians and Gay Men and Their Parents*. Cleveland, OH: Pilgrim Press.

Clunis, D. M., and G. D. Green. 2003. *The Lesbian Parenting Book: A Guide to Creating Families and Raising Children*. New York: Seal Press.

Clunis, D. M., and G. D. Green. 2005. *Lesbian Couples: A Guide to Creating a Healthy Relationship*. Emeryville, CA: Seal Press.

Costello, C. B., A. J. Stone, and V. R. Wight. 2003. *The American Woman 2003–2004: Daughters of a Revolution—Young Women Today*. New York: Palgrave Macmillan.

Dinkmeyer Sr., D., G. McKay, and D. Dinkmeyer Jr. 1997. *The Parent's Handbook*. Circle Pines, MN: American Guidance Service.

Faber, A., and E. Mazlish. 2002. *How to Talk so Kids Will Listen & Listen so Kids Will Talk*. New York: Perennial/HarperCollins.

Fairchild, B., and N. Hayward. 1998. *Now That You Know: A Parent's Guide to Understanding Their Gay and Lesbian Children*. Harcourt Brace.

Fisher, H. 2004. *Why We Love: The Nature and Chemistry of Romantic Love*. New York: Henry Holt.

Gilligan, C. 2003. *The Birth of Pleasure: A New Map of Love*. New York: Alfred A. Knopf.

Griffin, C., and M. Wirth. 1996. *Beyond Acceptance: Parents of Lesbians and Gays Talk about Their Experiences*. New York: St. Martin's Press.

Hendrix, H. 2001. *Getting the Love You Want: A Guide for Couples*. New York: Henry Holt.

Hendrix, H. 2003: *Getting the Love You Want Workbook: The New Couples' Study Guide*. New York: Atria Books.

Johnson, S. 2001. *For Lesbian Parents: Your Guide to Helping Your Family Grow Up Happy, Healthy and Proud*. New York: Guilford.

MacKenzie, R. J. 2001. *Setting Limits with Your Strong-Willed Child*. New York: Three Rivers Press.

McCarthy, B., and E. McCarthy 2006. *Getting It Right This Time: How to Create a Loving and Lasting Marriage*. New York: Informa/Routledge.

Moles, K. 2001. *The Relationship Workbook: Activities for Developing Healthy Relationships and Preventing Domestic Violence*. Plainview, NY: Wellness Productions.

Nelsen, J., L. Lott, and H. S. Glenn. 1999. *Positive Discipline A–Z: 1001 Solutions to Everyday Parenting Problems*. New York: Three Rivers Press.

Schultheis, G. M., B. O'Hanlon, and S. O'Hanlon. 1999. *Brief Couples Therapy: Homework Planner*. New York: John Wiley & Sons.

White, J., and M. C. Martinez, eds. 1997. *The Lesbian Health Book: Caring for Ourselves*. Seattle: Seal Press.

References

1. Presented by Michel Ann Fultz, Louisville Center for Adult Children, Louisville, Kentucky, 1996.
2. Adams, G. R. 1982. The physical attractiveness stereotype. In A. G. Miller (ed.), *In the eye of the beholder: Contemporary issues in stereotyping*. New York: Praeger; Berscheid, E. 1985. Interpersonal attraction. In G. Lindzey and E. Aronson (eds.), *Handbook of social psychology*. New York: Random House.
3. Lerner, H. G. 1990. *The dance of intimacy: A woman's guide to courageous acts of change in key relationships*. New York: Harper & Row.
4. Sacher, J. A., and M. A. Fine. 1996. Predicting relationship status and satisfaction after six months among dating couples. *Journal of Marriage and the Family* 58:21–32.
5. Peplau, L. A., C. T. Hill, and Z. Rubin. 1993. Sex role attitudes in dating and marriage: A 15-year follow-up of the Boston couples study. *Journal of Social Issues* 49 (3): 31–52.
6. Antill, J. K. 1983. Sex role complementarity versus similarity in married couples. *Journal of Personality and Social Psychology* 45:145–55.
7. Hui, C. H., and H. C. Triandis. 1986. Individualism-collectivism: A study of cross-cultural researchers. *Journal of Cross-Cultural Psychology* 17:225–48.
8. Dion, K. K., and K. L. Dion. 1993. Individualistic and collectivistic perspectives of gender and the cultural context of love and intimacy. *Journal of Social Issues* 49 (3): 53–69.
9. Livermore, B. 1993. The lessons of love. *Psychology Today* 27:30–39.
10. Lee, J. A. 1976. *The colors of love*. New York: Prentice-Hall.
11. Fisher, H. 2004. *Why we love: The nature and chemistry of romantic love*. New York: Henry Holt, pp. 68–72.
12. Ibid., pp. 68–72.
13. Ibid., pp. 72–73.
14. Ibid., pp. 72–73.
15. Ibid., pp. 81–82.
16. Ibid., pp. 81–82.
17. Ibid., p. 82.
18. Ibid., p. 88.
19. Ibid., p. 89.
20. Ibid., p. 89
21. Wallerstein, J. S., and S. Blakeslee. 1995. *The good marriage: How and why love lasts*. Boston: Houghton Mifflin.
22. Evans, P. 1996. *The verbally abusive relationship*. Holbrook, MA: Adams Media, pp. 36–37.
23. Ibid., p. 37.
24. Ibid., p. 123.
25. Ibid., p. 122.
26. Fields, J., and L. M. Casper. 2001. America's families and living arrangements: March 2000. *Current Population Reports*. Washington, DC: U.S. Census Bureau.
27. Lavee, Y., and D. H. Olson. 1993. Seven types of marriage: Empirical typology based on ENRICH. *Journal of Marital and Family Therapy* 19:325–40; Olson, D. H., D. Fournier, and J. Druckman. 1986. *PREPARE/ENRICH Counselor Manual*. 2nd ed. Minneapolis, MN: PREPARE/ENRICH, Inc.
28. Fowers, B. J., K. H. Montel, and D. H. Olson. 1996. Predicting marital success for premarital couple types based on PREPARE. *Journal of Marital and Family Therapy* 22:103–19.
29. Schwartz, P. 1994. Modernizing marriage. *Psychology Today* 27:54–59.
30. Fields and Casper, America's families and living arrangements.
31. Brown, S. L., and A. Booth. 1996. Cohabitation versus marriage: A comparison of relationship quality. *Journal of Marriage and the Family* 58:668–78.
32. Wu, Z. 1996. Childbearing in cohabitational relationships. *Journal of Marriage and the Family* 58:281–92.
33. Besherov, D. J., and T. S. Sullivan. 1996. One flesh: America is experiencing an unprecedented increase in black–white intermarriage. *New Democrat* 8 (4): 19–21.
34. Solsberry, P. W. 1994. Interracial couples in the United States of America: Implications for mental health counseling. *Journal of Mental Health Counseling* 16 (3): 304–17.
35. Besherov and Sullivan, One flesh.
36. Blumstein, P., and P. Schwartz. 1983. *American couples: Money, work, sex*. New York: William Morrow.
37. Tacker, F., and S. Golombok. 1995. Adults raised as children in lesbian families. *American Journal of Orthopsychiatry* 65:203–15.
38. Fields and Casper, America's families and living arrangements.
39. Ibid.
40. Mellody, P., A. W. Miller, and J. K. Miller. 1992. *Facing love addiction: Giving yourself the power to change the way you love*. San Francisco: HarperCollins.
41. Ibid.
42. National Center for Health Statistics, Centers for Disease Control and Prevention. 1995. *Monthly Vital Statistics* 43 (13).
43. Forste, R., and K. Tanfer. 1996. Sexual exclusivity among dating, cohabitating, and married women. *Journal of Marriage and the Family* 58:33–47.
44. Blumstein and Schwartz, *American couples*.
45. Ibid., pp. 109–111.
46. Ibid.
47. Mellan, O. 1994. *Money harmony: Resolving money conflicts in your life and your relationships*. New York: Walker.
48. Blumstein and Schwartz, *American couples*.
49. McCarthy, B. 2002. Sexuality, sexual dysfunction, and couple therapy. In A. S. Gurman and N. S. Jacobson (eds.), *Clinical handbook of couple therapy* (3rd ed., pp. 629–652). New York: Guilford Press, p. 634.
50. Ibid., p. 634.
51. Ibid., p. 634.
52. Laumann, E., J. Gagnon, R. Michael, and S. Michaels. 1994. *The social organization of sexuality*. Chicago: University of Chicago Press.
53. McCarthy, Sexuality, sexual dysfunction, and couple therapy, p. 630.
54. American Psychiatric Association. 2000. *Diagnostic and statistical manual of mental disorders*. 4th ed., text revision *(DSM-IV-TR)*. Washington, DC: APA.

55. Kaplan, H. 1974. *The new sex therapy*. New York: Bruner/Mazel.
56. McCarthy, Sexuality, sexual dysfunction, and couple therapy, p. 629.
57. Masters, W., and V. Johnson. 1970. *Human sexual inadequacy*. Boston: Little, Brown.
58. McCarthy, Sexuality, sexual dysfunction, and couple therapy, p. 629.
59. McCarthy, B., and E. McCarthy. 2002. *Sexual awareness*. New York: Carroll & Graff.
60. McCarthy, Sexuality, sexual dysfunction, and couple therapy, p. 630.
61. Ibid., p. 630.
62. Ibid., p. 630.
63. McCarthy, B., and E. McCarthy. 2006. *Getting it right this time: How to create a loving and lasting marriage*. New York: Informa/Taylor & Francis, pp. 75–76.
64. Ibid.
65. Major, B. 1993. Gender, entitlement, and the distribution of family labor. *Journal of Social Issues* 49:141–59.
66. Blumstein and Schwartz, *American couples;* Kurdek, L. A. 1993. The allocation of household labor in gay, lesbian, and heterosexual married couples. *Journal of Social Issues* 49:127–39.
67. Lerner, H. G. 1989. *The dance of anger: A woman's guide to changing the patterns of intimate relationships*. San Francisco: HarperCollins.
68. PAIRS International, Inc. *PAIRS for love—for life: Resolving anger nondestructively*. Pembroke Pines, FL. Info@pairs.org.
69. PR Newswire Association. 2006. Baxter Executive Named Working Mother of the Year. www.prnewstoday.com (retrieved September 7, 2006).
70. Dinkmeyer Sr., D., G. McKay, and D. Dinkmeyer Jr. 1997. *The parent's handbook*. Circle Pines, MN: American Guidance Service, pp. 3, 6.
71. Dinkmeyer, McKay, and Dinkmeyer, *The parent's handbook*, pp. 14–15.
72. Ibid., p. 10–11.
73. Ibid., pp. 19.

Chapter Eight

Examining Gynecological Issues

CHAPTER OBJECTIVES

When you complete this chapter, you will be able to do the following:

- Describe the female reproductive anatomy
- Demonstrate the proper breast self-examination technique
- Describe the phases of the menstrual cycle
- Recognize the signs and symptoms of uterine fibroids
- Contrast the stages of the female sexual response cycle
- Explain the advantages and disadvantages of hormone replacement therapy

This chapter covers female reproductive anatomy and physiology, breast health, and the human sexual response cycle. It looks at the changes you can expect to experience from menarche to menopause. This information is important in raising awareness about your body and how it functions.

FEMALE REPRODUCTIVE ANATOMY AND PHYSIOLOGY

The chapter begins with a discussion of the female reproductive anatomy, particularly the external genitals, the internal genitals, and the breasts.

External Genitalia

The external genitalia, termed the pudendum or **vulva,** refers to those parts that are outwardly visible. The vulva includes the mons pubis, labia majora, labia minora, clitoris, urethral opening, vaginal opening, and perineum. Individual differences in size, coloration, and shape of the external genitalia are common. (See Color Plate 1.)

Mons Pubis The **mons pubis** is a triangular, mounding area of fatty tissue that covers the pubic bone. During adolescence, pubic hair begins to appear on the mons pubis as a result of increased sex hormones. This hair, varying in coarseness, curliness, amount, and thickness, covers the mons and may extend to the navel. The mons protects the pubic symphysis (the place where the pubic bones join) and cushions the woman's body during sexual intercourse.

Labia Majora The **labia majora** are two longitudinal folds of adipose tissue covered with skin. They are sometimes referred to as the "outer lips" and have darker pigmentation than the labia minora. The labia majora protect the vaginal and urethral openings and are covered with hair and sebaceous (oil) glands. The inner surfaces tend to be smooth, moist, and hairless. After childbirth, the labia majora may separate and no longer fully cover the vaginal area. The labia majora become more flaccid as a woman gets older.

Labia Minora The **labia minora,** sometimes referred to as the "inner lips," consist of erectile, connective tissue that darkens and swells during sexual arousal.

The labia minora, located inside the labia majora, are more sensitive and responsive to touch than the labia majora. The labia minora enclose the clitoris. The upper folds form the prepuce, while the lower folds form the frenum of the clitoris. At the bottom, the folds blend together to form the fourchette, the anterior edge of the perineum.

Clitoris The **clitoris** is a highly sensitive organ composed of nerves, blood vessels, and erectile tissue. It is covered with a thin epidermis. It can be found under the prepuce, clitoral foreskin, by separating the folds of the labia majora. The clitoris consists of a shaft and a glans that becomes engorged with blood during sexual stimulation. It is homologous to the penis in males, meaning that they develop from the same embryonic tissue. The clitoris is the key to sexual pleasure for most women, and consequently, some misogynist cultures practice female circumcision

Urethral Opening The urethral opening is located directly below the clitoris. It is the opening through which a woman urinates. The urethral opening, urethra, and bladder are unrelated to reproduction. Urinary tract and bladder infections can occur with transmission of bacteria from the vagina or rectum.

Vaginal Opening The vaginal opening, or introitus, may be covered by a thin sheath called the **hymen.** Hymens vary in size, shape, and thickness, and usually have an opening in the center through which menstrual blood flows. A common myth is that an intact hymen indicates virginity and that it breaks during a young woman's first sexual intercourse. Using the presence of an intact hymen for determining virginity is erroneous. The hymen can be perforated by many different events, such as the first menstrual blood, the use of a tampon, strenuous exercise, or some mishap. Some women are born without hymens, and some women retain intact hymens despite several experiences of sexual intercourse.

Perineum The **perineum** is the part of the muscle and tissue located between the vaginal opening and the anal canal. It holds up and surrounds the lower parts of the urinary and digestive tracts. The perineum contains an abundance of nerve endings that make it sensitive to touch. A common practice in Western medicine was to perform an **episiotomy,** an incision of the perineum, for widening the vaginal opening to facilitate childbirth. However, the American College of Obstetrics and Gynecologists now urges limiting its use and no longer considers the procedure routine. The number of episiotomy procedures in the United States has declined from more than 1.6 million in 1992 to 716,000 in 2003.[1] Women's advocates and medical researchers challenge the need for the practice as a routine procedure, suggesting that the incision greatly increases the probability of tears into and through the anus. Some women consider episiotomies a form of female genital mutilation.

Internal Genitalia

The internal genitalia consist of the vagina, cervix, uterus, fallopian (uterine) tubes, and ovaries. (See Color Plate 1.)

Vagina The **vagina** connects the cervix to the outer body and lies between the bladder and the rectum. The vaginal canal serves three important functions. First, the menstrual flow and uterine secretions pass through the vagina to the vaginal opening. Second, the vagina serves as the birth canal during labor and can expand during childbirth to several inches in width. Third, the vagina is lubricated by two Bartholin's glands and is the female organ of copulation. During puberty, the vagina begins to produce a clear or white discharge. This self-cleaning process, called leukorrhea, gives the vulva its characteristic smell. Douching or hygiene products are unnecessary and may actually disturb the normal pH balance. Unpleasant odors may be a sign of infection, and if they continue, a health care provider should be contacted.

A common myth is that the size of a penis contributes to sexual satisfaction. In reality, the vagina expands to accommodate the size of any penis. Another myth is that a penis may become trapped within the vagina. In fact, unlike animals with a bone in the penis, a male's penis becomes flaccid after ejaculation and cannot be trapped in the vagina.

Cervix The **cervix** is the portion of the uterus that protrudes into the vaginal cavity. It has a smooth, glistening mucosal surface. The cervical opening to the vagina is small, thus preventing tampons and other objects from entering the uterus. During childbirth, the cervix dilates to accommodate the passage of the fetus. The dilation of the cervix is an early sign that labor has begun. The cervical opening is small and round in a nulliparous (never having given birth) woman but becomes wider after one or more deliveries. When a woman has a Pap smear, the cells are scraped from the cervix and examined under a microscope to detect cancer or precancerous conditions. A Pap smear is both a visual inspection and a cell culture.

Uterus The **uterus** is often described as being pear shaped and about the size of a clenched fist. The powerful muscles of the uterus expand to accommodate a growing fetus and contract strongly to begin the birth process and push the fetus through the birth canal. The **endometrium,** the complex, inner lining of cells,

Women Making a Difference

Dr. Susan M. Love: A Pioneer in Women's Breast Health and Menopause Research

Susan M. Love is one of the founding mothers of the breast cancer advocacy movement and serves on the Boards of the Y-ME, the National Breast Cancer Coalition, and the Young Survivor's Coalition. She is an adjunct professor of surgery at UCLA and the founder and director of the Dr. Susan Love Research Foundation, whose mission is to eradicate breast cancer within 10 years. This effort can be achieved only if new solutions are created to overcome existing research barriers.

Dr. Love is best known for her groundbreaking books: *Dr. Susan Love's Breast Book* and *Dr. Susan Love's Menopause and Hormone Book*. Her lectures have always been visionary and challenging to existing medical practices. Her continued work in the area of breast cancer research provides hope for the many women who live with breast cancer today.[2]

consists of blood-enriched tissue that sloughs off each month during the menstrual flow if fertilization does not occur. It is the organ in which the fertilized egg becomes implanted and the fetus matures. An endometrial biopsy can be used to detect diseases or infertility problems.

Fallopian (Uterine) Tubes The fallopian tubes, or oviducts, serve as a pathway for the ovum (egg) to the uterus and as the site of fertilization, typically in the upper third of a fallopian tube. The sperm travel through the vagina, cervix, and uterus to fertilize the egg in one of the fallopian tubes. The fertilized egg takes approximately 6 to 10 days to travel through the fallopian tube to implant in the uterine lining.

Ovaries The **ovaries** are the female gonads (sex glands) that develop and expel an ovum each month. A woman is born with approximately 400,000 immature eggs called follicles. The majority of the follicles disappear before puberty. Usually none are found after menopause. Very few of these follicles reach full maturity; about 400 to 500 are developed and released for possible fertilization during a woman's reproductive years. The follicles in the ovaries produce the female sex hormones progesterone and estrogen, which are important in preparing the uterus for the implantation of a fertilized egg. The ovaries are homologous to the male's testes.

FIGURE 8.1 Structures of the breast

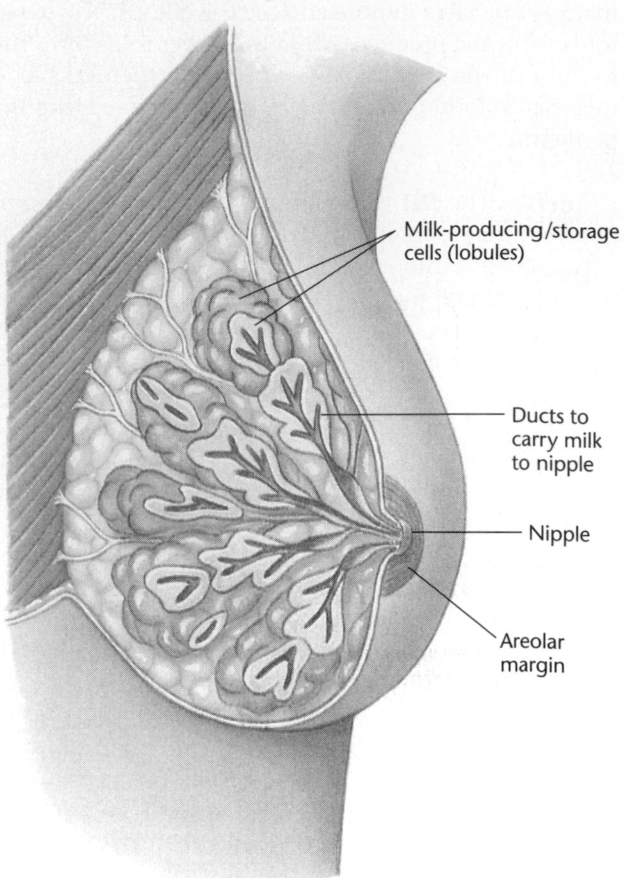

Breasts

The breasts function as organs of sexual arousal, contain the mammary glands that nourish a newborn baby, and consist of two main types of tissues, glandular and stromal (supporting). Glandular tissues house the milk-producing lobules and ducts. Each breast contains fifteen to twenty-five clusters called lobes, which have smaller sections called lobules. Lobes and lobules are connected by ducts opening into the nipple. The ducts join together to form ampulla, the collecting sacs located just behind the nipple. The nipples, composed of erectile tissue, become temporarily erect with cold temperature, sexual stimulation, or lactation. The pigmented portion around the nipple of each breast is called the areola, which usually darkens during pregnancy and in women who have had children. The core of the nipple is the opening of the fifteen to twenty-five ducts and contains sebaceous glands that keep the nipple lubricated during breast-feeding. Figure 8.1 shows the structures of the

FYI

Benign Breast Conditions

Benign breast conditions are common changes in breast tissue with no cancerous breast abnormality. Some of the more common changes are discussed.

Nipple discharge: Fluid coming from the nipple(s). Typically spontaneous milky, clear, yellow, or green discharge from both nipples. Persistent discharges should be evaluated by a health care provider, but in most cases the condition is benign.

Lobular carcinoma in situ (LCIS): Not classified as a cancer but, rather, a precancerous condition. LCIS begins in the lobules and is typically monitored closely by a health care provider.

Fibrocystic breast condition: Describes a variety of changes in glandular and stromal tissues in the breast(s). Symptoms include cysts, fibrosis (excess fibrous connective tissue), lumpiness, areas of thickening, tenderness, and breast pain.

Cysts: Accumulations of fluid in the breast. Cysts are noncancerous and present as smooth, rounded lumps that are movable. They respond to the body's hormone levels and are most common in premenopausal women.

Fibroadenomas: Common benign breast tumors that are found more often in African American women than in other women. They are usually too small to feel by self-examination. Fibroadenomas tend to be round and have borders.

Intraductal papillomas: Noncancerous wartlike growths inside the breast. These often involve the large milk ducts near the nipple.

Mastitis: Most commonly affects women while they are breast-feeding. Bacteria enter the breast duct and attract inflammatory cells.[3]

Health Tips

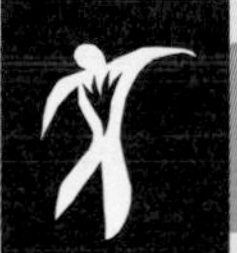

Treatment of Fibrocystic Breasts

Women with fibrocystic breasts should consult a health care provider for recommendations. Suggestions may include:

- Wear extra support bras.
- Avoid caffeine.
- Use oral contraceptives.
- Use aspirin, acetaminophen, or Motrin.
- Maintain a low-fat diet.
- Apply heat.
- Reduce salt.
- Take vitamin E, vitamin B-6, niacin, or other vitamins.
- Have breast lumps removed surgically.
- Take prescribed medications[4]

breast. The supporting structure of the breasts is connective tissue, composed mainly of collagen, a material that also makes up bone and tendons. Stromal tissues include fatty and fibrous connective tissue.

Breast size is determined primarily by heredity and depends on the existing amount of fat and glandular tissue. Breasts may exhibit cyclical changes, including increased swelling and tenderness just before menstruation.

Benign Breast Conditions Benign breast conditions are often detected by clinical breast examination, routine mammography, or breast self-examination. The most common benign breast conditions include fibrocystic breast condition, benign breast tumors, and breast inflammation. (See *FYI:* "Benign Breast Conditions.")

Fibrocystic breast condition is a catchall phrase for any signs or symptoms not related to breast cancer. It is not a disease but, rather, a variety of changes in the glandular and stromal tissues of the breast. Women may have cyclic periods of pain, tenderness, and swelling in the breast tissue, particularly during the 1 to 2 weeks before menstruation. (See *Health Tips:* "Treatment of Fibrocystic Breasts.") These symptoms may occur concurrently with lumps or masses of overgrown breast tissue. Benign (noncancerous) breast changes are most common in the upper-outer quadrant of the breasts, followed by the lower-outer quadrant of the breasts. Many women, nearly 70 percent, experience benign breast changes, that is, breast lumps, pain, tenderness, or nipple discharge during the menstrual cycle. The American Cancer Society suggests that nine out of every ten women have some type of abnormality when breast tissue is examined under a microscope. The diagnosis of whether a mass is benign (noncancerous) or malignant (cancerous) is usually confirmed by observing the lump over time, imaging tests, or biopsy. Approximately 10 percent of the women who get mammograms will require a breast biopsy to determine whether the mass is benign or malignant. Just remember, 85 to 90 percent of lumps are benign and most do not require biopsy.

Lumps, breast pain, and nipple discharge are the three most common breast complaints of women seeking medical attention. Nipple discharge, fluid from the nipple(s), is typically caused by hormonal imbalances or papillomas. Nearly 20% of women may experience spontaneous fluid nipple discharge. Bloody or watery nipple discharge, especially if it is from one side or a single duct, is considered abnormal. Only around 10 percent of abnormal discharges are cancerous. The following discharge may be of concern:

- Bloody or watery with a red, pink, or brown color
- Sticky or clear in color
- Brown to black in color (opalescent)
- Appears spontaneously without squeezing the nipple
- Persistent
- On one side
- A fluid other than breast milk[5]

Researchers at the Mayo Clinic conducted a retrospective study of over 9,000 women who had been diagnosed with benign breast conditions. They found that the risk of breast cancer increased with diagnosis of benign breast conditions. The findings were translated for women as follows: If 5 in 100 women in the general population were to get breast cancer, the study predicted that 1 more woman (6 in 100) with nonproliferative breast lesions would get cancer. For women with proliferative breast lesions or atypical changes, 10 in 100 or 14 in 100 would get cancer. The risk doubles or nearly triples depending upon the benign breast condition. Family history was an independent variable that increased a woman's risk of developing cancer, depending on the closeness of the relationship. And age at diagnosis of benign breast conditions was also a factor, with younger women having a greater risk.[6]

Breast Self-Examination Women can take a proactive approach to ensuring general breast health by examining their breasts monthly. Figure 8.2 shows the breast self examination (BSE) technique endorsed by the American

FIGURE 8.2 How to examine your breasts[7]

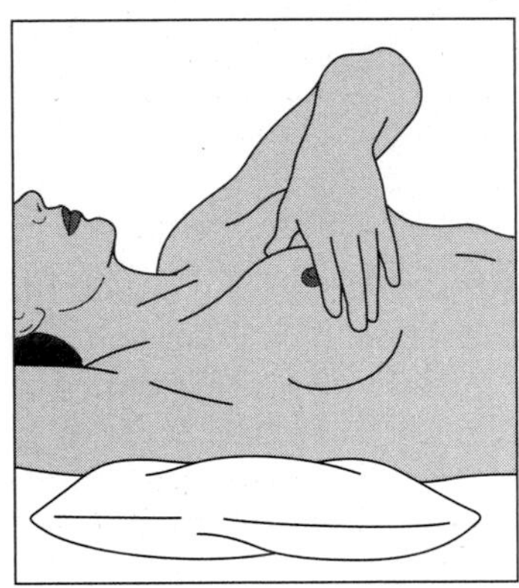
A

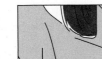

Lie down and place your right arm behind your head (A). The exam is done while lying down, not standing up. When lying down the breast tissue spreads evenly over the chest wall and it is as thin as possible, making it much easier to feel all the breast tissue.

Use the finger pads of the three middle fingers on your left hand (B) to feel for lumps in the right breast. Use overlapping, dime-sized, circular motions of the finger pads to feel the breast tissue.

Use three different levels of pressure to feel all the breast tissue. Light pressure is needed to feel the tissue closest to the skin, medium pressure to feel a little deeper, and firm pressure to feel the tissue closest to the chest and ribs. A firm ridge in the lower curve of each breast is normal. If you're not sure how hard to press, talk with your doctor or a nurse. Use each pressure level to feel the breast tissue before moving on to the next spot.

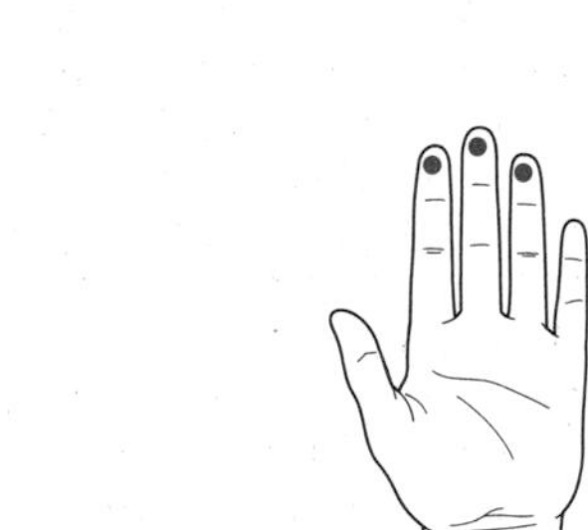
B

Move your fingers around the breast in an up and down pattern, beginning with an imaginary line drawn straight down your side from the underarm and moving across the breast to the middle of the sternum (C). Be sure to check the entire breast area going down until you feel only ribs and up to the neck or collar bone (clavicle).

There is some evidence to suggest that the up and down pattern (sometimes called the vertical pattern) is the most effective way to cover the entire breast without missing any breast tissue.

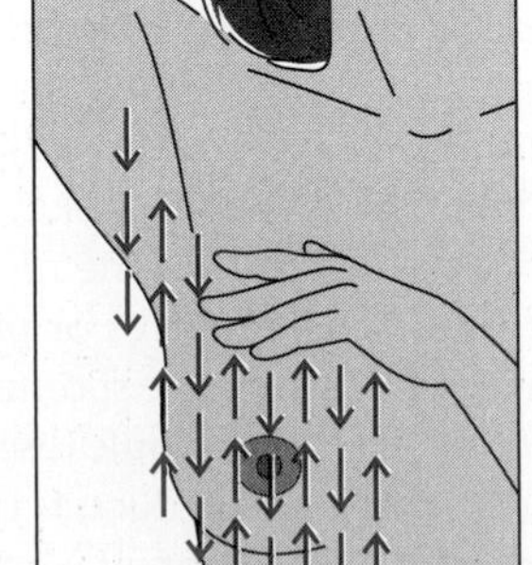
C

Repeat the exam on your left breast, using the finger pads of the right hand.

While standing in front of a mirror with your hands pressing firmly down on your hips, look at your breasts for any changes of size, shape, contour, dimpling, pulling, or redness, or scaliness of the nipple or breast skin. (The position of pressing down on the hips contracts the chest wall muscles and enhances any breast changes.) Continue to look for changes with your arms down at your sides and then with your arms raised up over your head with your palms pressed together.

Examine each underarm while sitting up or standing and with your arm only slightly raised so that you can easily feel in this area. Raising your arm straight up tightens the tissue in this area and makes it difficult to examine.

Cancer Society (ACS). Monthly breast self-examination is important for raising your level of awareness regarding changes that could be abnormal. However, the ACS guidelines now suggest that while BSE is important to general breast health, it has a limited role in early detection of cancer. Breast self-examination can be conducted on a regular basis so that you become familiar with the shape and feel of your breasts. If a change occurs (lumps, dimpling changes, skin irregularities, or nipple discharge), you should *immediately* contact your health care provider.

The best time for you to conduct BSE is about a week after menstruation because breasts are less tender at this time. Women who are postmenopausal may choose the first day of each month or a special date, such as their birth date or anniversary date of every month. Although BSE is important, it is only one component of breast health and early detection of cancer: mammography and clinical examinations are essential for early detection of changes.

Mammography Mammography remains the gold standard for early detection of breast cancer. Researchers are confident of the benefits of mammography, thus keeping previous basic screening recommendations outlined by the ACS. However, a number of technologies, such as breast ultrasound and MRI (magnetic resonance imaging), that, when used with mammography, appear to increase the effectiveness of screening and diagnosis. Women are advised to have an annual mammogram, starting at age 40. However, the ACS now emphasizes education, knowing the benefits and limitations of mammography. The guidelines are also more specific about who is at increased risk. "Now, women and their doctors are encouraged to discuss the possibility of beginning screening earlier (at age 30, or in rare cases even younger). Another option might be to consider screening with breast ultrasound or MRI in addition to their regular mammogram."[8]

Cosmetic and Reconstructive Breast Surgery

Breast augmentation surgery is the insertion of saline (saltwater) implants. Women who have augmentation are encouraged to practice monthly BSE and have yearly clinical breast exams. Mammography on women with implants involves special views to see both the breast tissue and the implant.

Breast reduction surgery is performed to reduce the size of the breasts. Women who have reduction surgery should practice BSE and have yearly mammography after the age of 40 or if they are at high risk for breast cancer. With any type of surgery, certain risks should be considered. The most common complication with breast augmentation is capsular contracture (a feeling of breast hardness). Other complications for any surgery can include bleeding, fluid collection, excessive scar tissue, infections, and problems with anesthesia.[9]

MENSTRUATION

Changes in the physiology of the body brought about as the result of hormonal influences signal the end of childhood and the beginning of puberty. Young adolescent females experience their bodies becoming much fuller in the breasts, hips, and thighs and they move from girlhood to womanhood with the initiation of monthly menstrual cycles. Biologically, all of these changes occur to prepare the female body for potential reproduction. The onset of menstruation, **menarche,** is a central focus of body politics. Menarche not only is a physiological happening, but also is viewed as "a gendered sexualized happening, a transition to womanhood as objectified other."[10]

Menarche sets the stage for how a young woman perceives her sexuality. Most young girls anticipate their period with a range of emotions from fear, disgust, and embarrassment to joy and excitement. Indeed, researchers have suggested that a young woman's attitude toward menstruation is influenced and shaped by how the media, popular culture, and others portray it.[11]

Over the past century, a decrease of about 3 to 4 months in age of onset of menstruation has occurred every decade.[12] Today, the average preadolescent's body begins to change around age 10 or 11, but for some young girls, it begins much earlier. Data suggest that 48 percent of African American and 15 percent of non-Hispanic white girls show pubic hair and develop breast buds by the age of 8. However, the average age for the onset of menarche is 12.8 years, and this beginning age seems to have stabilized. The onset of menstruation can be affected by a variety of factors, including genetics, socioeconomic conditions, nutritional status, and in some cases, exercise regimens. Overweight and obesity also are known risk factors for early puberty. The emotional, as well as physiological, changes can have a huge impact on young girls. They may feel "different" from their friends, and it can seem as if the world changed overnight. What are your personal recollections of menarche? Record them in the *Journal Activity:* "Your Recollection of Menarche" or discuss them with friends. Were your experiences the same as your friends'?

Six primary hormones are involved in regulating the female reproductive system: gonadatropin releasing hormones (follicle stimulating hormone releasing factor (FSH-RF) and luteinizing hormone releasing factor (LH-RF)) from the hypothalamus, follicle stimulating hormone (FSH) and luteinizing hormone (LH) from the pituitary gland, and estrogen, progesterone, and the male hormone testosterone from the ovaries. Puberty begins when FSH and LH are released from the pituitary gland (the master gland), which stimulates the ovaries to produce more estrogen. Estrogen is responsible for developing the secondary sex characteristics of puberty. These changes may include an increase in body hair, the beginning of breast growth, distribution of body fat, size of larynx and its

Journal Activity

Your Recollection of Menarche

The menstrual cycle is something that every young person, male or female, should understand. Sharing our stories about menarche can take away the secrecy that some of us experienced. Write a paragraph or two about your experience with menarche. If it was positive, write about the events that made it positive. If it was negative, write about how you would have liked the experience to have been.

influence on the voice, and a widening of the hips or pelvic area. A growth spurt of several inches may occur at this time. For many girls, the first few menstrual cycles may not be associated with ovulation. However, once menstruation begins, a young woman must assume that ovulation and fertility can occur.

The menstrual and ovarian cycle are generally divided into phases: follicular (or proliferative), ovulatory, luteal (or secretory), and menstrual. The **follicular phase** begins when FSH-RF is released by the hypothalamus and the pituitary gland is activated to secrete FSH and a small amount of LH, which cause the follicles to begin maturing. When the maturing follicles release estrogen, the endometrium thickens and cervical mucus changes. This phase lasts 10 to 14 days and includes the eggs' maturing in the ovaries. Every month, a blisterlike structure (graafian follicle) develops on one or the other ovary. This structure holds the ovum, which triples in size. The follicular phase is the most variable part of the cycle as the endometrium continues to build up and thicken. When the estrogen level reaches a certain point, LH-RF causes the pituitary to release a large amount of LH. The surge in LH causes the mature follicle to burst open and release an egg. (Many types of birth control pills block this surge in LH, thus inhibiting ovulation.) Just before ovulation, an abundance of clear, stretchy mucus is secreted by the cervix. This mucus facilitates the movement of the sperm toward the egg. During the **ovulatory phase,** the largest follicle bursts, and the mature egg is released into one of the fallopian tubes. The cell and tissue changes following ovulation are quite constant through the next 14 days. Once an egg is released, menstruation will occur in about 14 days unless fertilization has occurred. The corpus luteum (a temporary structure formed from an ovarian follicle following the release of a mature egg) accounts for the relatively stable time between ovulation and menstruation. The basal body temperature upon awakening in the morning is lower during the first part of the menstrual cycle, but rises with ovulation and remains about 4°F higher through the luteal phase. Progesterone, from the corpus luteum, is responsible for the rise in basal body temperature. After ovulation, the egg stays alive for about 24 hours. Sperm can stay alive inside a woman's body for 3–4 days, but possibly as long as 6–7 days. Intercourse, before or after ovulation, can result in pregnancy. The time frame is about 7–10 days in the middle of a cycle, which we know can be 20–35 days in length.[13] The only safe infertile interval is after ovulation has occurred and the ovum is no longer viable. The empty follicle becomes the corpus luteum during the **luteal phase.** The corpus luteum (yellow body) secretes estrogen and larger amounts of progesterone, which are necessary to maintain a pregnancy by preparing the endometrium for a fertilized egg. If the egg is fertilized, the thickened blanket of blood vessels becomes the placenta. If the egg is not fertilized, the corpus luteum disintegrates and becomes the corpus albicans (white). The spiral arteries of the endometrium close off, and the blood pools along with the endometrium for the menstrual flow. The final phase is **menstruation.** Estrogen and progesterone levels drop and the sloughing off of the endometrium occurs. The amount of menstrual bleeding varies from woman to woman, and the expulsion of blood clots (pooled blood in the vagina) is common. The blood can vary in color from bright red to dark brown. Normal menstrual periods can range from 4 to 8 days, and cycles can vary from 20 to 40 days. (See Color Plate 2.) Some women experience little discomfort during this time, but others have fluid retention, cramping, mood swings, weight gain, breast tenderness, diarrhea, or constipation.[14]

Irregular uterine bleeding or excessive bleeding at menstruation can be caused by a number of factors. If irregular or unusual bleeding occurs, a health care provider should be consulted.

Pelvic Examination and Pap Test

Pelvic Examination Regular screening with a pelvic examination and Pap test is important for any sexually active woman. A pelvic examination should be conducted annually for 3 consecutive years for all women who are or have been sexually active or are over age 18. If the results are negative (no abnormalities), less frequent examinations can be conducted at your discretion in consultation with your health care provider. Women with a history of abnormal Pap smears or who have been treated for cervical abnormalities should be screened every 2 to 4 months for 1 to 2 years and then annually. Women who have had hysterectomies for treatment of a malignant lesion should be screened annually to ensure that a tumor has not recurred. Women at high risk for cervical cancer due to HPV or HIV infections, cigarette smoking, or sexual activity with multiple partners should be screened annually.[15]

The pelvic examination includes a visual screening to ensure that the reproductive organs look normal in size, shape, and location, a Pap test to screen for cervical cancer, and a bimanual check of the ovaries, fallopian tubes, and uterus. The health care provider visually checks the vaginal area for signs of herpes, tumors, or genital warts. She then gently inserts a speculum into the vagina to view and check the internal organs for abnormalities. It is helpful if a woman can remain relaxed during the examination. Many women feel embarrassed or apprehensive about the pelvic examination, but relaxing the stomach and vaginal muscles makes the pelvic examination easier. A Pap test and then a bimanual examination follow the visual examination. The bimanual examination requires the health care provider to place two gloved fingers (with lubricating jelly) into the vagina to feel for abnormalities in the fallopian tubes, ovaries and uterus, sometimes followed by a rectal examination. She checks for tumors, tenderness to the area, and the location of the organs.

When a woman is making an appointment for her first pelvic examination, she should inform the nurse or health care provider that it is her first exam. The young woman should NOT use vaginal creams or douche, or have sex, for 48 hours before the examination. At the exam, she will be weighed, her height will be measured, and her blood pressure will be taken; then she will be given a gown to put on and a sheet to put over her stomach and legs. The exam table has stirrups (holders for the feet) and with the woman's knees bent, the health care provider will conduct the examination. The exam may include the external (visual) exam, the speculum exam, and the bimanual exam.

Pap Test The Pap test is a standard part of any pelvic examination. The best time to have a Pap test is 10 to 14 days after the first day of the last menstrual period. A woman should avoid using douches, using lubricants and having sex for 48 hours before the examination. The Pap test is conducted by taking a sample of cells from the cervical area, called the squamous epithelium. This area is the site where 90 percent of all cervical cancers begin. The speculum separates the vaginal walls and exposes the cervical opening. A brush or Thin-Prep is used to scrape some cells from the part of the cervix that protrudes into the vagina, and then the cells are smeared onto a slide. Another sample is taken from the endocervical canal and wiped onto another slide; then the speculum is removed.[16] Both slides with samples are sent to a lab for analysis. Sometimes a woman will spot blood after a pelvic examination; this is normal and does not require treatment unless the area remains tender. Until recently, health care providers relied on the Pap test to reveal any cellular abnormalities such as human papilloma virus (HPV) infection. Health care providers now use the ViraPap test as an adjunct to the Pap test to detect HPV. Test accuracy of the ViraPap for genital HPV is almost 95 percent. If the test results are positive, a woman has an increased risk of developing precancerous lesions. Further tests will most likely be conducted to determine if cervical cancer is present.

The primary purpose of having a Pap test is to prevent invasive cancer from occurring. Precancerous cervical lesions (or dysplasia) can be detected when small and easily treated. If left untreated, the normal history of progression is from dysplasia to cancer.[17] Cervical cancer develops slowly and is nearly 100 percent curable if detected when localized. A minute or two of discomfort (whether emotionally or physically) is well worth the benefit of early detection. A woman's failure to undergo an annual examination is more common than a failure by the physician to obtain an accurate smear or the lab technologist to misread a slide. The most important preventive measure is to comply with the American Cancer Society and National Cancer Institute guidelines for annual pelvic examinations.

Menstrual Disorders

Endometriosis **Endometriosis** occurs when the endometrium (the lining of the uterus) fragments and lodges in other parts of the body, most commonly in the pelvic cavity. It also lodges on the uterosacral ligaments, on the ovaries, fallopian tubes, and supporting broad ligaments. The fragments build up tissue each month and then break down and bleed, causing inflammation, scarring, and adhesions. The cause of endometriosis remains unclear, but scientists are continuing to explore possible causes including reverse flow of menstrual blood and tissue, immune system problems in destroying endometrial tissue, and blood and lymphatic transport of endometrial tissue outside the uterus. Treatment of endometriosis includes hormonal therapy, laparoscopic surgery, pain medication, and major surgical management, depending upon the needs of the woman.[18] Treatment may alleviate the symptoms, but removal of endometrial tissue does not mean a woman is cured. Chronic endometriosis can be frustrating and disabling for women and is a common cause of dysmenorrhea, dyspareunia (painful intercourse), chronic pelvic pain, and infertility.

Dysmenorrhea Painful menstrual cramps, dysmenorrhea, is the most cited reason for missing school or lost workdays for young women. Although most women occasionally experience menstrual cramps, 5 to 10 percent of women will experience painful, incapacitating cramps for several hours to a couple of days. Primary **dysmenorrhea,** painful menses without evidence of a physical abnormality, is believed to be a normal body response to uterine contractions that result from increased production of prostaglandins. Prostaglandins cause the forceful, frequent uterine contractions associated with the pain of menstruation. A number of other symptoms may occur as well, including nausea, vomiting, gastrointestinal disturbances, and fainting. Dysmenorrhea typically begins several hours before menstrual bleeding and can last several days. Some women alleviate painful cramps with OTC medications such as ibuprofen (Advil, Nuprin, Motrin IB), with drugs designed specifically for menstrual symptoms (Midol, Pamprin), or with prescription nonsteroidal anti-inflammatory drugs such as naproxen or Indocin. If these medications do not work, oral contraceptives that contain both estrogen and progesterone may be prescribed. Some women try to increase their physical activity, cut down on salt to reduce possible fluid retention, or rest more because of feelings of fatigue. Secondary dysmenorrhea is usually due to anatomic abnormalities such as a congenital abnormality of the uterus, presence of fibroids or endometrial polyps, an IUD, pelvic inflammatory disease, or endometriosis. Secondary dysmenorrhea is diagnosed during a pelvic exam, ultrasound, or laparoscopy, and treatment depends on the type of disease.

Amenorrhea It is not unusual for women to miss some periods during their lifetime because menstruation is tied to emotional, biological, and environmental conditions. Primary **amenorrhea** indicates a significant physical disorder characterized by delayed puberty, the failure to menstruate by age 16, or lack of menses by age 14 along with the absence of secondary characteristics such as breast development and increased body hair. The incidence of primary amenorrhea in the United States is only 2.5 percent. Multiple causes for the disorder have been identified including the normal delay of onset (up to ages 14–15), drastic weight reduction or malnutrition, chronic illness, extreme obesity, and a number of congenital defects and abnormalities such as Turner's syndrome and hermaphroditism. The treatment of amenorrhea depends on the cause but often includes hormonal supplementation, surgery, or both. Certain conditions are unlikely to be corrected by any intervention. As long as the young woman has a uterus, it may be possible to cause pseudomenstruation with medications. Secondary amenorrhea is failure to menstruate for more than 6 months after prior establishment of menstruation. Some missed periods are quite normal, such as after childbirth or after discontinuing birth control pills. The most common cause of secondary amenorrhea in premenopausal women is pregnancy or the onset of menopause.

The prevalence of amenorrhea in young female athletes, particularly dancers, gymnasts, and long-distance runners, has received considerable media attention. The Female Athlete Triad is identified as disordered eating, amenorrhea, and osteoporosis. The combination of restrictive eating, excessive training, extreme stress, and low body-fat percentage all predispose a female athlete to amenorrhea. A young, elite athlete who participates in sports for which a slender appearance or low body fat is advantageous is at greatest risk. (See *Her Story:* "Shelly:

Her Story

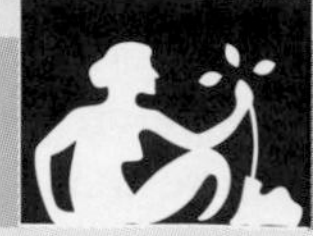

Shelly: Negative Self-Image, Overtraining, and Amenorrhea

Shelly, a 5′9″, 110-pound, Division I volleyball player, remembers the first time she dropped weight. It was the summer after her sophomore year and a new coach had been hired. She reported for the first practice and hadn't even attempted her first set to a teammate when the coach yelled, "Shelly, you're slow. What took you so long? Have you always weighed this much? I don't want a setter who can't move!"

Shelly remembers how embarrassed she felt! No one had ever said anything about her weight before, and she was faster than anyone else on the team when it came to sprints. She had even lifted weights all summer, was feeling strong, and was looking forward to the season. Doubt began to creep into her thinking. Maybe she was too fat! Maybe the coach was right!

Shelly had only known success until now. She had been a standout setter during high school, was heavily recruited by top universities, and had easily transitioned to college volleyball because she and the coach clicked. They understood each other! She couldn't believe it when her coach accepted another position. Then the university hired a high-profile coach, and she decided to stay. Shelly not only excelled in sports, she was a top-notch student as well. She had a 4.0 GPA in political science and planned to attend law school. If the new coach wanted her to drop weight, she would! If this coach thought she'd be a better setter at a lower weight, she'd do whatever it took to excel. She dropped 15 pounds in a month, going from 125 to 110 pounds. She stayed after practice and ran sprints. She dropped to 1,000 calories a day and didn't eat meat anymore. She thought the laxatives were helping too! She still felt fat and slow, and had not menstruated in 6 months.

The coach noticed that Shelly seemed fatigued during practice. Her performance seemed to be slipping; she was moving more slowly to the ball. He thought Jamie, an incoming freshman, might earn the starting position.

- What are the warning signs that indicate Shelly was suffering from the Female Athlete Triad?
- What would you say to her if you were her friend?

Negative Self-Image, Overtraining, and Amenorrhea.") The endocrine profile of this athlete may show an estrogen deficit similar to that in menopausal women. This profile has implications for infertility, premature osteoporosis, and poor psychological well-being.[19] Some studies suggest that up to 60 percent of young female athletes have episodes of amenorrhea compared to 2 to 5 percent of the general female population.[20]

Polycystic Ovarian Syndrome

Polycystic ovarian syndrome (PCOS) occurs when the ovaries produce excessive amounts of male hormones (androgens) and multiple small cysts develop. Among nonpregnant women, ovarian conditions (PCOS and ovarian failure) are the most common causes of amenorrhea. PCOS is diagnosed when women have two of the following: clinical or biochemical evidence of hyperandrogenism (excessive amounts of androgens) menstrual irregularity due to too few or no ovulatory cycles, or polycystic-appearing ovaries on ultrasound. PCOS is suspected when menstrual irregularities begin following puberty and include signs of hyperandrogenism (excess body hair following a male pattern, male pattern balding, or acne). Health care providers also screen for glucose tolerance and type 2 diabetes because of the association of PCOS with insulin resistance. Treatment for PCOS depends upon the symptoms and may include laser hair removal, electrolysis, waxing, or oral contraceptives.[21]

Assess Yourself

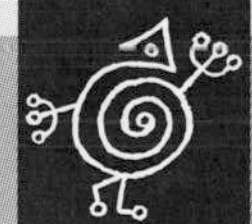

Physical and Emotional Symptoms and PMS

Over 150 symptoms have been associated with PMS, a disorder that women can experience 1 to 2 weeks before menstruation. Listed below are some common symptoms associated with PMS. Keep a daily diary of the changes in your physical and emotional state for 1 month, using a severity index of 1 to 10, with 10 being the most severe. Divide symptoms into physical and emotional and begin on day 1 of menstrual bleeding. Record any of the following symptoms you experience before menstruation: acne, anxiety, depression, dizziness, fatigue, headaches, irritability, panic, swelling, rashes, nausea, weight gain, hives, breast swelling, irregular heartbeats, joint pain, mood swings, muscle aches, paranoia, gastrointestinal symptoms, water retention, food cravings, moodiness, insomnia, withdrawal, sadness, crying, impatience, overreactivity, self-criticism, extreme sensitivity, distractibility, indecision, suicide ideation, violence.

- Did you experience any other symptoms during your menstrual cycle?
- Do you practice any nutritional or health behaviors to alleviate these symptoms?
- What other suggestions might you try?

Premenstrual Syndrome (PMS)

Premenstrual syndrome (PMS) is a politically charged and "culture-bound" issue. Some feminists believe this is another medicalization of a woman's normal cyclical pattern. The syndrome was officially recognized in the medical literature in 1931, was labeled PMS in 1953, and gained notoriety in the 1980s when several women committed violent acts attributed to the PMS syndrome. Women who suffer from PMS tend to experience groupings of symptoms. For this reason, PMS symptoms are categorized under four main headings:

- *Type A.* A stands for anxiety. This type of PMS is most notable for its emotional symptoms of anxiety, irritability, and mood swings.
- *Type C.* C stands for carbohydrate cravings (you fall into this category if you absolutely can't live without chocolate in the week before your period!). Along with the sugar cravings are exhaustion and headaches (all symptoms of low blood sugar).
- *Type D.* D stands for depression. Depression is accompanied by mental confusion, an inability to think clearly, and poor memory.
- *Type H.* H stands for hyperhydration, which is like waterlogging. You suffer from Type H PMS if you swell up like a balloon, none of your clothes fit you, and your rings cut into your fingers when your period is due. The fluid retention will also cause your breasts to swell and become tender.[22]

PMS symptoms may fall into one or a combination of these categories. Type A is the most common, accounting for 80 percent of PMS sufferers. Most symptoms of PMS taper off with the onset of menstruation although some women may continue to experience symptoms throughout the period. Changes in symptoms of PMS can be attributed to factors such as aging, childbearing, and the approach of menopause. Now complete *Assess Yourself:* "Physical and Emotional Symptoms and PMS" to determine which symptoms you experience.

Some researchers believe that the cyclical trigger for biochemical events contributing to PMS are due to normal ovarian function, not imbalances in hormones, prostaglandin, vitamins, or minerals. Suppressing the

Health Tips

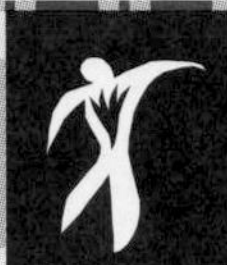

Eating Healthy to Avoid PMS[23]

Poor nutrition and low-quality foods contribute directly to the incidence of PMS. Some foods are known to worsen your problems.

Foods to Avoid

- Refined carbohydrates such as white bread, cakes, cookies, refined breakfast cereals, crackers, candy, and chocolate
- Foods that are high in fats, including dairy products and red meat
- Synthetic foods that are highly processed and full of chemical additives
- Caffeinated drinks such as coffee, tea, and soda
- Alcohol
- Salt and heavily salted foods

Foods to Add to Your Diet

- Complex carbohydrates, such as whole-grain bread, brown rice, whole-grain pasta, and whole-grain cereals
- Plenty of fresh fruits and vegetables
- Low-fat protein sources, such as fish, chicken, and vegetarian proteins
- Vegetable oils rich in essential fatty acids

ovulatory function of the ovaries, through either prescription drugs or surgery, may relieve symptoms. Other researchers point to a deficiency in serotonin as a contributing factor to psychological symptoms. Psychotropic drugs, particularly selective serotonin uptake inhibitors, have provided encouraging results.[24] Some neurotransmitter deficiencies are linked to anxiety and susceptibility to seizures, and a number of studies have linked progesterone and estrogen to worsening symptoms of PMS. Nearly half of women with PMS have symptoms unrelated to a cycle dependent pattern. Health care providers diagnose PMS by eliminating coexisting medical disorders and charting symptoms through several consecutive menstrual cycles. Symptoms that consistently occur during the second half of the menstrual cycle may be caused by PMS, and these symptoms can worsen with age before tapering off after menopause.

The best approach to dealing with PMS symptoms is to alleviate them through noninvasive strategies such as relaxation techniques, biofeedback, nutritional changes, and exercise. (See *Health Tips:* "Eating Healthy to Avoid PMS.") Suggested nutritional changes include vitamin and mineral supplements, reducing salt intake, eliminating caffeine and refined sugar, and increasing foods that are high in fiber and complex carbohydrates. Medications can help alleviate most premenstrual abdominal cramping, headaches, nausea, vomiting, and diarrhea. A health care provider can work closely with a woman experiencing PMS to alleviate discomforting symptoms. In rare instances, severe emotional symptoms may require antidepressant or antianxiety medication.

Premenstrual Dysphoric Disorder (PMDD)

Why is PMDD defined as a clinically pathological disorder while PMS is seen as normal? That's the question many feminists have asked. While women are seeking relief from feeling "bad," specialists choose to label it mental illness, which raises questions about the social construction of a disease. **Premenstrual dysphoric disorder (PMDD)** is defined as a severe form of PMS, including marked disruption of quality of life and bouts of significant premenstrual depressed mood, anxiety, sadness, or anger that occur one week before menses and impair a woman socially or occupationally.[25] The disorder, according to the *Diagnostic and Statistical Manual of Mental Disorders–IV,* must have five or more of eleven symptoms during the last week of the luteal phase in most menstrual cycles. The symptoms often resolve within a few days after menstruation begins. PMS may affect as many as 80 percent of all women, whereas PMDD affects less than 5 percent. The symptoms of PMDD include the following:

- Feelings of sadness or hopelessness, possible suicidal thoughts
- Feelings of tension or anxiety
- Mood swings marked by periods of teariness
- Persistent irritability or anger that affects other people
- Disinterest in daily activities and relationships
- Trouble concentrating
- Fatigue or low energy
- Food cravings or bingeing
- Sleep disturbances
- Feeling out of control
- Physical symptoms such as bloating, breast tenderness, headaches, and joint or muscle pain[26]

Feminists and many health care professionals have voiced concern that normal behavior in women may be labeled inappropriately or explained away as "that time of month." They believe that a condition that exists normally for most women should not be labeled "clinically pathological" or lead to stigmatizing a woman. Furthermore, the scientific research that supports the existence of premenstrual mental illness (in contrast to normal PMS) is questionable. The inclusion of the disorder in the DSM was controversial from the beginning, with more than 6 million individuals and professionals disapproving of its inclusion. Some experts were concerned that the inclusion of PMDD in the DSM-IV misrepresented the full problem and restricted research only to psychiatric areas rather than to possible physiologic causes. The symptoms for PMDD must be unique, not an exacerbation of a preexisting condition such as depression or psychosis. When PMDD is diagnosed, the recommended first line of psychiatric therapy for PMDD is selective serotonin reuptake inhibitors (SSRIs). However, a 1998 study found that 55 percent of the women in a study experienced relief within 3 months of taking calcium carbonate on a regular basis. The main point: Whether PMDD exists or not, a woman who is experiencing hormonal symptoms should be validated for her experience of those symptoms.

Uterine Fibroids

Uterine fibroids are common tumors of the uterus composed of muscle and fibrous tissue. Nearly 80 percent of all women have uterine fibroids, and 25 percent of them have severe enough symptoms to require treatment. Fibroids may cause heavy vaginal bleeding, pelvic discomfort, and pain. They may also put pressure on other organs and cause constipation or hemorrhoids. There is no known etiology or reasons for why some women have severe symptoms while others have none. Age, race, lifestyle, and genetics play a role in who gets uterine fibroids, which often begin in women between the ages of 35 and 50. African American women are two to three times more likely to be at risk than non-Hispanic white women. The first goal of treatment is to alleviate the symptoms. Bleeding can be treated with hormones or surgery. Constipation may be alleviated by increasing dietary fiber and water intake. Surgical removal of the fibroid, shrinking the tumors, or a hysterectomy is sometimes required to alleviate the symptoms.[27]

Hysterectomy

Every minute, a hysterectomy is performed in the United States, and nine of twelve of them may not meet the guidelines of the American College of Obstetricians and Gynecologists.[28] Hysterectomies are the second most common major surgery performed in the United States (the most common are cesarean sections). The most common reason for this surgery is uterine fibroids, followed by endometriosis and uterine prolapse. A **hysterectomy** is an operation to remove a woman's uterus and, sometimes, the fallopian tubes, ovaries, and cervix. A hysterectomy is performed through an incision in the abdomen (abdominal hysterectomy, or laparoscopic hysterectomy) or the vagina (vaginal hysterectomy). Hysterectomies should be performed vaginally if possible, but abdominal hysterectomies remain the more commonly performed procedure. Vaginal hysterectomies require less hospital and recovery time, and there is a quicker return to normal activities. Preferably, surgeons have equal training and success with vaginal and abdominal hysterectomies.[29]

The most common type of hysterectomy is a complete or total hysterectomy, which entails removal of the cervix as well as the body of the uterus. A subtotal hysterectomy removes the upper part of the uterus but not the cervix. When both ovaries and fallopian tubes are also removed, the surgery is known as a bilateral salpingo-oophorectomy. A radical hysterectomy removes the uterus, the cervix, the upper part of the vagina, and supporting tissues. This surgery is usually reserved for advanced cases of cancer. Whenever possible, the ovaries should be conserved. Ovarian conservation for benign conditions benefits long-term survival for women, whereas removal increases risk of death due to premature heart disease and hip fractures. However, estrogen replacement is used to counter these effects. Parker and colleagues estimate that 18,000 women a year may die prematurely because of removal of their ovaries.[30] Survey data show great variations by state and age, with Mississippi and Alabama having the highest percentages of women with hysterectomies (over 50 percent of all women 65+).[31] New York and New Jersey have the lowest percentages of women with hysterectomies (about 30 percent of all women 65+). The average percentage of women 65+ years who have had a hysterectomy is 45 percent. The average age of women undergoing hysterectomy is 42, and nearly three-quarters of all women who have hysterectomies are between 20 and 49.

Women today are recognizing that many conditions that previously called for hysterectomies may be treated with alternative therapies. For instance, type 1 von Willebrand disease is a genetic bleeding disorder that manifests itself by menstrual bleeding or bleeding during childbirth and affects 1 to 3 percent of women. Most women who have this disease are undiagnosed or treated with dilation and curettage (D+C) and hysterectomies rather than proper treatment.[32] Hysterectomy may be the best choice for certain conditions, particularly cancer, but women should seek a second opinion, ask about alternative options to try first, and ask about possible complications of surgery. A woman should make an informed decision and choose her best option.

Toxic Shock Syndrome

Toxic shock syndrome (TSS) is a rare and sometimes fatal disease caused by a toxin produced by the bacterium *Staphylococcus aureus*. It usually affects menstruating young women who use highly absorbent tampons and occurs within 5 days of the onset of a menstrual period. Skin wounds or infections elsewhere in the body may cause TSS. The best protection against TSS is using sanitary napkins. If you choose to use tampons, you can protect yourself by

Health Tips

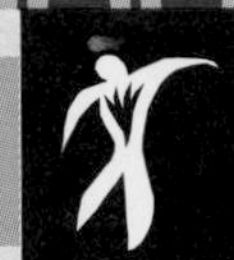

Toxic Shock Syndrome

The following are warning signs and symptoms of toxic shock syndrome. If you experience these symptoms, remove the tampon and contact your physician *immediately*.

- Sudden fever over 102 degrees Fahrenheit
- Vomiting
- Diarrhea
- Dizziness
- Fainting or near fainting
- A sunburn-like rash
- Sore throat
- Bloodshot eyes
- Rapid drop in blood pressure resulting in shock

changing tampons frequently (every 4 to 6 hours), avoiding super absorbent tampons, alternating tampons with sanitary napkins, and avoiding use of tampons between periods. Women who have had a "staph" infection should not use tampons because the recurrence rate for TSS is 30 percent. Knowing the signs and symptoms of TSS can save your life. If you experience the symptoms found in *Health Tips:* "Toxic Shock Syndrome," immediately remove the tampon and contact a health care provider.

MENOPAUSE

Natural Menopause

Menopause and hormone replacement therapy are the hottest women's health topics of the baby boomer generation. An unprecedented number of American women, about 1.25 million annually, are experiencing menopause. This generation of women has grown up believing that informed decisions are based on adequate information. They want answers to questions that previously were not asked. They want to know what to expect physiologically and psychologically as they enter this next life transition. This generation has removed the shroud of secrecy around a number of health topics, from breast cancer to menopause.

Physiologically, menopause is the time when ovulation and menstruation cease, but in the social context menopause includes the entire time period from 3 to 7 years before the last menstrual period to a year after the last period. Physically, the four stages of menopause include premenopause, perimenopause, menopause, and postmenopause. During **premenopause,** menstrual periods are beginning to be irregular but the classic symptoms of hot flashes and vaginal dryness have not occurred. A simple blood test and Pap-like smear can accurately determine the stage of menopause. Follicle stimulating hormone (FSH) levels rise dramatically as the ovaries begin to shut down, and these levels can be measured through a simple blood test. Vaginal atrophy can be determined by a Pap-like smear from the vaginal walls.

Menopause normally occurs between the ages of 40 and 58, with premature menopause occurring before 40 and delayed menopause occurring after 58. Nearly half of American women experience menopause by 50. Can a woman predict when menopause is going to occur? Not really. The premature shutting down of the ovaries may occur with autoimmune diseases such as lupus or rheumatoid arthritis, cigarette smoking, exposure to high levels of radiation in the pelvic area, or chemotherapy. There is no apparent relationship between the age of menarche and the age of menopause. Physical characteristics such as height and weight or childbearing and marital status are not related to age of menopause.

Perimenopause is the period of time (3 to 7 years) before and after the last menstrual period during which the menstrual cycle becomes erratic and hot flashes begin. During this phase, the ovaries begin to shrink and follicle stimulating hormone (FSH) is slightly elevated and the luteinizing hormone (LH) stays within the normal range. This phase covers the first 2 years prior to the final menstrual period and the 2 years following the last menstrual period. A woman may skip one or two periods, she may experience lighter or heavier menstrual flow, and the length of the menstrual period may be shorter or longer than usual. **Hot flashes,** sudden bursts of intense heat, often accompany irregular bleeding. Nearly 85 percent of all pre- and perimenopausal women experience hot flashes. Hot flashes alter skin and core temperature and precede increases in LH and FSH. Symptoms may include feelings of warmth in the face or upper body, profuse sweating, and even tremors or shaking. Some women experience anxiety, tenseness, dizziness, heart palpitations, or nausea before the hot flash. The actual cause of hot flashes is unknown, but researchers believe that mixed signals from the hypothalamus cause skin temperatures to rise while internal body temperature drops. Other symptoms include night sweats, mood disturbances, vaginal dryness, and reduced skin elasticity.

Menopause results from the normal aging of the ovaries, when estrogen levels fall and ovulation and menstruation have ceased for 12 months. A significant increase in both FSH and LH occurs due to the rapid depletion of ovarian follicles. Estrogen depletion contributes to other body changes, including varying degrees of atrophy of the internal and external genitalia. The uterus, uterine cavity, fallopian tubes, vagina, and clitoris all become smaller. The breasts may become less firm and full. Bone loss accelerates, and osteoporosis with accompanying risk of fractures becomes more

FIGURE 8.3 Disease rates for women on estrogen plus progestin or placebo.

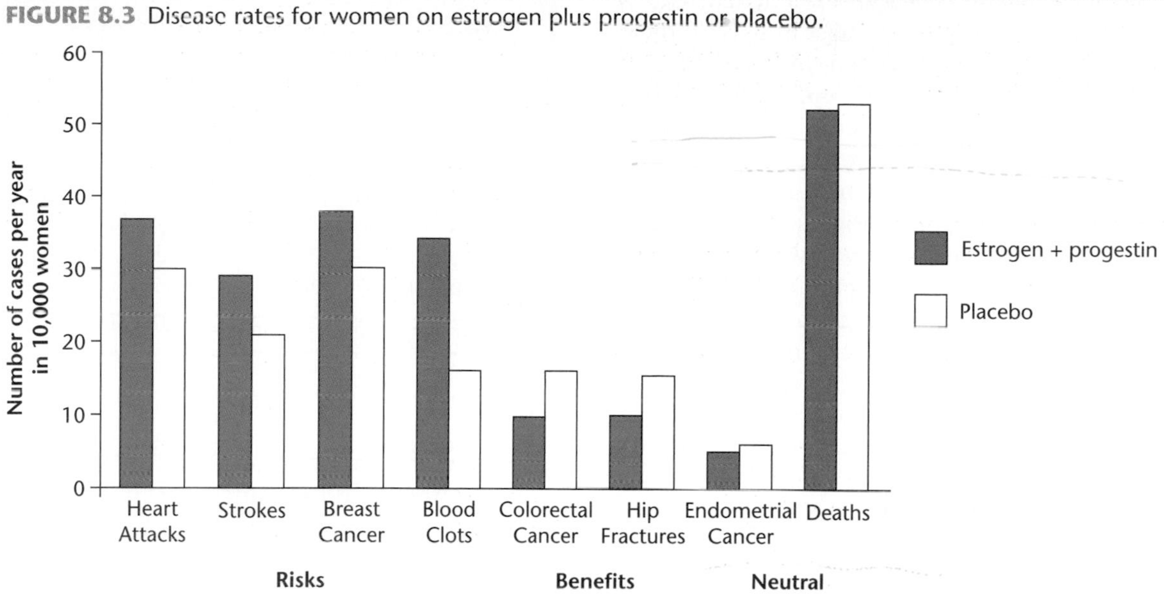

likely. Other possible changes include vaginal dryness, less vasocongestion, and decreased vaginal expansion.[33] Any vaginal bleeding after this time is considered abnormal and should be reported to a health care provider.

Postmenopause begins when menstruation has ceased for one year. Emotionally, some women view postmenopause positively as the life stage when they have more time to be creative and autonomous, to evaluate prior life choices, and to plan for future choices. Once a woman is past menopause, she will be postmenopausal for the rest of her life. Regular exercise is especially important during this phase of a woman's life. Exercise prevents or delays osteoporosis and heart disease, enhances sleep, and contributes to overall well-being.

Surgical Menopause

In contrast to natural menopause, surgical menopause, or removal of the ovaries, causes an immediate leap into menopause. Surgical menopause results from removal of both ovaries or failure of the ovaries due to surgical trauma, radiation, or chemotherapy. The body immediately stops producing estrogen and progesterone, causing an array of physical symptoms of menopause such as hot flashes, night sweats, arrhythmias and rapid heart rate, irritability and mood swings, insomnia and fatigue, and vaginal dryness. The woman, regardless of age, enters postmenopausal status with concomitant symptoms and concerns. If a woman has had a hysterectomy without removal of the ovaries, she no longer will have a period and she will go through menopause naturally.[34]

Hormone Replacement Therapy

The National Heart, Lung, and Blood Institute (NHLBI), a division of the National Institutes of Health (NIH) announced in July 2002 that it had stopped a major clinical trial of the risks and benefits of combined estrogen and progestin in the treatment of the symptoms of menopause. Data reviewed by the Data and Safety Monitoring Board had revealed that, after an average follow-up period of 5.2 years, a marked increase in invasive breast cancer, and some increase in coronary heart disease, stroke, and pulmonary embolism, occurred in women taking a combination therapy (Prempro) compared to women taking a placebo. At the time the Heart and Estrogen-Progestin Replacement Study was initiated, more than 6 million women were using Prempro daily, and no long-term clinical trials of the hormone combination had been conducted. The study involved 16,608 women aged 50 to 79 who were mostly healthy and ethnically diverse and had not undergone a hysterectomy. Study findings for the combination estrogen/progestin group compared to the placebo group (after an average of 5.2 years) included the following:

- 41 percent increase in strokes
- 29 percent increase in coronary heart disease (CHD)
- 100 percent increase in blood clots
- 26 percent increase in breast cancer
- 37 percent reduction in colorectal cancer
- No effect on endometrial cancer
- 33 percent reduction in hip and clinical vertebral fractures
- Increased risk of urinary incontinence

The long-term Women's Health Initiative (WHI) studies were initiated to answer a number of questions that had arisen over the years. (See Figure 8.3.) Does postmenopausal hormone therapy prevent heart disease and, if it does, what are the risks? What are the long-term effects of estrogen plus progestin on hip fractures? Were there potential increased risks for breast and colon cancer?

The study found that **hormone replacement therapy (HRT)** was unlikely to benefit the heart and that with long-term use the risks outweighed any potential benefits. Women currently taking the combination therapy were encouraged to discuss their status with their health care providers. The numbers of women who had hip and other fractures or colorectal cancer were lower in women taking estrogen plus progestin. The reduction in hip and other fractures was consistent with observational data of the ability of estrogen to maintain bone mineral density. However, safer medications and other strategies are available for reducing the risk of osteoporosis and subsequent hip fractures. The study found no differences in the number of women who had endometrial cancer (cancer of the lining of the uterus) or in the number of deaths from that disease. The close monitoring for bleeding and treatment of hyperplasia (increase in the number of cells) may have contributed to the absence of increased risk of endometrial cancer.[35] Another study conducted as part of the WHI has determined that older women on HRT had twice the rate of dementia, including Alzheimer's disease, when compared to women who did not take the combination therapy. These findings have reversed many of the beliefs commonly held by women regarding the benefits of HRT that were based on anecdotal evidence or less rigorous scientific studies.

In February 2004, the NIH instructed women who were participating in the oral equine estrogen–alone study to discontinue taking Premarin. The women in this study had had a hysterectomy and took estrogen alone or a placebo. The increased risk of blood clotting and stroke was similar to that found in the HRT (estrogen plus progestin) study. Women in both trials will be followed closely to monitor changes in health outcomes. An ancillary study, the WHI Memory Study (WHIMS), involved women aged 65 and older. The WHIMS study provided data that suggested a trend toward twice the risk of dementia and no protection against mild cognitive impairment in women taking the combination therapy. The women taking estrogen-alone therapy (ERT) also experienced increased risk of mild cognitive impairment plus dementia.[36] The most significant finding for both studies was that long-term use was contraindicated for cardiovascular disease.

The WHI studied women who were postmenopausal. A more recent study (2005) of women who were just beginning menopause suggests that some peri- and postmenopausal women with moderate to severe vasomotor symptoms (hot flashes) associated with estrogen deficiency may benefit from HRT. However, further study is needed.

While the WHI did not make specific recommendations about other hormone medications, most women are seeking alternatives to HRT and ERT to reduce the symptoms of menopause, including hot flashes, insomnia, and mood swings. (See Table 8.1.)

TABLE 8.1 Common Side Effects of Hormone Replacement Therapy

ESTROGENS	PROGESTINS
Breast tenderness	Symptoms similar to PMS
Breast enlargement	Headaches or migraines
Bloating	Depression
Water retention	Irritability and moodiness
Symptoms similar to PMS	Abdominal bloating
Nausea	Cramping

Given the recent findings from the WHI, women are exploring natural strategies, nutritional products, and exercise. Dietary changes such as limiting foods high in saturated fats and nitrites and avoiding red meat, coffee, tea, chocolate, soft drinks, and alcohol may help alleviate some symptoms. Nutritional soy products and herbal remedies may reduce hot flashes, irritability, and insomnia, but have not been studied for health consequences. Vitamin E, folic acid, and vitamin B-6 may help with heart health, and calcium supplements may retard bone loss. Regular exercise is encouraged for creating a sense of well-being, reducing stress, and aiding in sleep. Dressing in layers, avoiding clothing with high necks and long sleeves, and avoiding synthetic clothing (e.g., polyester) that traps perspiration also can help a woman deal with hot flashes. Vaginal dryness may be treated with topical vaginal products (gel or cream applied locally). Many postmenopausal women also report a marked increase in sleeping problems; these nearly 61 percent of women report insomnia. A health care provider may offer additional suggestions for alleviating or managing the symptoms of perimenopause, particularly those related to mood changes, sleep disorders, or a decrease in sexual libido. If HRT is used at all, it should be used at the lowest doses for the shortest duration possible. (See *Viewpoint;* "Pitting Women's Health against the Interests of Giant Pharmaceutical Companies.")

HUMAN SEXUAL RESPONSE CYCLE

The human sexual response cycle was first described by Havelock Ellis and later elaborated on by Alfred Kinsey and colleagues.[37] It is the research of William Masters and Virginia Johnson that remains the most cited when it comes to discussion of the human sexual response cycle.

Viewpoint

Pitting Women's Health against the Interests of Giant Pharmaceutical Companies[38]

In the early 1960s, Dr. Robert Wilson extolled the benefits of estrogen replacement therapy (ERT) in a book titled *Feminine Forever.* His research was supported and encouraged by Wyeth Laboratories. During the ensuing years, as research evidence called into question the potential risk of ERT, Wyeth modified its medication, Premarin, by adding progestin and/or reducing the levels of hormones. Wyeth pushed Prempro for reducing heart disease and osteoporosis without any clear evidence that it worked.

In 1990 the Nurses' Health Study reported that women taking ERT had an increased risk of breast cancer. During this same time period, the FDA refused to support Wyeth's claim that ERT (or HRT) demonstrated benefits in the prevention of cardiovascular disease. In 1997 Dr. Susan Love emphasized the link between HRT and breast cancer, and in 2002 the National Women's Health Network published *The Truth about Hormone Replacement Therapy,* focusing on hype versus science. In 2006 Wyeth launched its Web site, KnowMenopause, to extol the benefits for some women. HRT is not the first medication pushed by the pharmaceutical companies at the expense of women's health. The Dalkon Shield, thalidomide, and DES also exploited women. Thalidomide, a drug first marketed in the late 1950s as a sleep aid, was later found to cause severe birth deformities in the babies of women who had taken the drug during pregnancy. Diethylstilbestrol (DES), a drug given to pregnant women to reduce the risk of miscarriage, was found to increase cancer and reproductive problems for their daughters. What can women do to prevent future life-threatening health problems caused by supposedly safe drugs? How can pharmaceutical companies be held accountable for their science and research protocols? Are government health policies failing women?

With the exception of Kinsey's study, little, if any, empirical research has been conducted regarding the physiological response of women during orgasm. Masters and Johnson reported their controversial findings in their book, *Human Sexual Response.*[39] Several of their key findings are that, unlike men, women experience a variety of differing orgasmic responses and can experience multiple orgasms and that, physiologically, orgasms are the same regardless of whether initiated by penile penetration or masturbation.

Masters and Johnson determined that the human sexual response cycle includes four predictable phases: excitement, plateau, orgasm, and resolution. The sexual response cycle follows a pattern through the four stages with individual variability in duration and intensity. Figure 8.4 shows the human sexual response cycle experienced by women. Differing models of the human sexual response cycle have also been recognized, although not nearly as frequently as Masters and Johnson's. Helen Singer Kaplan developed a tri-phasic model of sexual response consisting of (1) desire, (2) excitement, and (3) orgasm.[40] She argues that Masters and Johnson's model neglects the importance of sexual desire. She also believes that the plateau phase is indistinguishable from the excitement phase. Here, the brain plays the key role in determining whether the sexual response occurs and/or continues. The desire phase is triggered by some thought, emotion, fantasy, or sensation that activates the cerebral cortex. The excitement phase includes vasocongestion and ends in maximum arousal. The orgasm phase follows the pattern described by Masters and Johnson and is the most distinguishable and identifiable event for women. Susan Walen and David Roth proposed a cognitive model of sexual response that emphasizes the importance of perception.[41] A sexual stimulus is only erotic if it is perceived as such. And Bernie Zilbergeld and Carol Ellison suggest a five-phase sexual response cycle.[42] The first phase is interest/desire, followed by arousal, physiologic readiness, orgasm, and satisfaction.

The subjective and cognitive components of these models differ from the purely physiologic response described in the Masters and Johnson model. Sexual desire continues throughout the life span, but women's perceptions of relationship qualities provide a strong indicator of the level of sexual desire women attain throughout the aging process.

Orgasms

Can all women experience orgasm? It is impossible to say that all women can experience orgasm, but it is true that more women would experience orgasms (including multiple orgasms) if their partners knew how to provide adequate stimulation. Inhibited female orgasm is the term used to describe the persistent delay or absence of orgasm. Researchers have proposed a variety of reasons women may not experience orgasms. The inability to have an orgasm is rarely related to a physical cause unless alcohol or medications are involved.

Most anorgasmic experiences have psychological and sociological roots or can be caused by a lack of proper technique. Some women may not feel comfortable expressing their needs and desires, and expect their partners to know what to do to satisfy them. Feeling

FIGURE 8.4 Female sexual response cycle

Excitement Vaginal lubrication begins within 10 to 15 seconds of stimulation. Labia majora and minora darken. Clitoris engorges with blood and increases in size and length. Uterus and cervix pull away from the vagina. Breasts swell and nipples become erect. Sexual tension heightens. Sex flush (darkening of the skin) may occur.

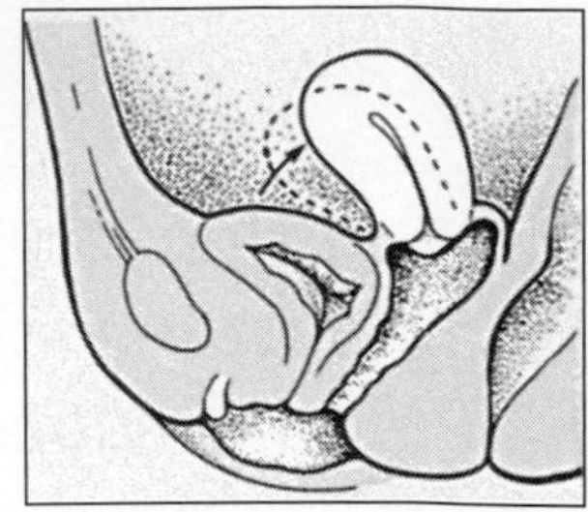

Plateau Vagina continues to expand and outer third fills with blood. Uterus elevates into abdomen. Tenting (distending of inner two-thirds of vagina) takes place. Cervix elevates. Clitoris retracts under clitoral hood. Secretion occurs from Bartholin's glands. Breasts continue to enlarge and areola engorges with blood. Sex flush may continue and spread.

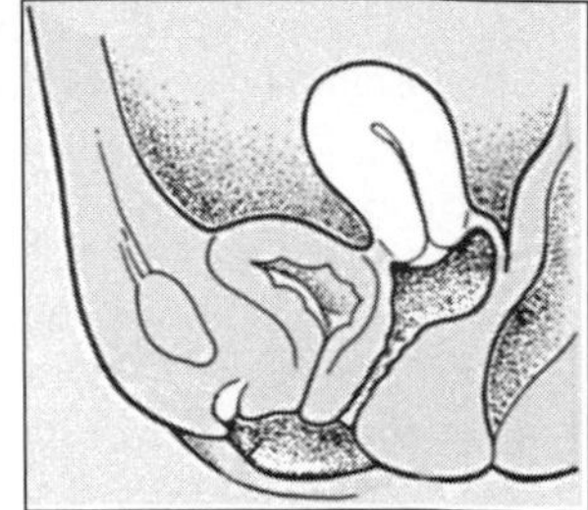

Orgasm Rhythmic contractions (3–15) of uterine walls, first 3–6 are most intense. Involuntary muscle spasms. Clitoris remains retracted under clitoral hood. Vasocongestion and myotonia (muscle tension) release. Respiration and heart rate increase frequency. Blood pressure increases.

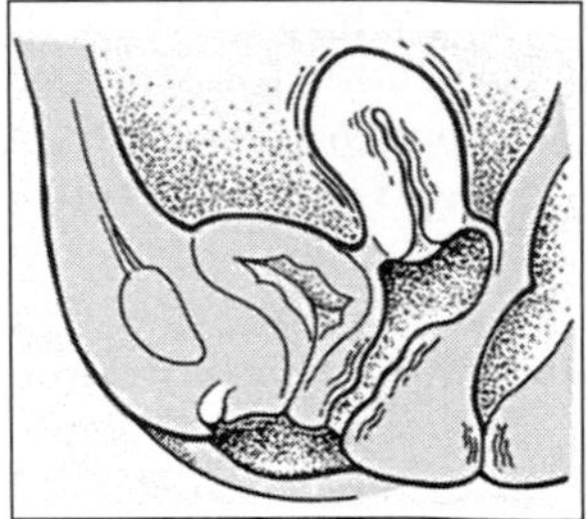

Resolution Vasocongestion and myotonia dissipate rapidly. Vaginal color returns shortly. Uterus returns to unaroused state. Labia major and minora return to normal size and shape. Swelling of breasts disappears.

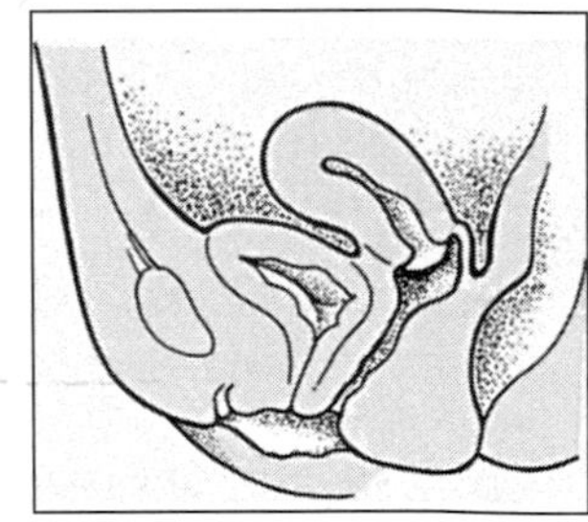

comfortable enough to communicate openly with your partner during sexual interactions is extremely important. Most women need continuous clitoral stimulation to experience an orgasm; otherwise, they stay in the plateau phase without adequate sexual tension to create an orgasm. Some women experience guilt, shame, or feelings of being "bad" as a result of strict religious upbringing. They also may have experienced socialization in stereotypical beliefs about the feminine role, such as that a woman should be submissive, pleasing, and passive. These sociological and psychological experiences can be a source of inhibited female orgasm. Most women can experience orgasm with adequate stimulation, whether through masturbation, mutual masturbation, or intercourse.

Aging and Sexual Response

Researchers are continuing to study the hormonal, relationship, and life-event factors that contribute to sexual responsiveness in older women. The aging process brings physiological changes in the human sexual response cycle. Physiologically, the excitement phase takes longer because it takes more time to lubricate the vaginal area. The orgasmic phase is shorter in duration and contractions may be less intense. And the resolution phase has also been found to be longer.[43] The work of Masters and Johnson, as well as that of other sex researchers, has been criticized for focusing primarily on the biomedical changes that come with aging and menopause. A more woman-centered approach toward female sexuality focuses on the complex psychological and sociological factors that impact sexual functioning in later years. For instance, women tend to be more relationship and intimacy focused and less genitally and orgasm focused than men. While sexual desire continues in later years, a woman's perceptions of relationship qualities provide a strong indicator of the level of sexual desire she attains throughout the aging process. Nonhormonal factors that can have a negative impact on women's sexual responsiveness include career concerns, changing family relationships, a partner's incapacity to function sexually, not having a partner, and changing priorities. As the baby boomer generation enters menopause, further research will provide better information about the effects of aging and menopause on female sexual responsiveness.

Chapter Summary

- The vulva refers to the external genitalia, those parts that are outwardly visible.
- The hymen is a thin sheath that covers the vaginal opening.
- The perineum is the muscle tissue found between the vaginal opening and the anal canal.
- An episiotomy is a surgical incision that widens the vaginal opening during childbirth.
- The vaginal opening serves as the opening for menstrual flow and the birth canal during labor, and it receives the penis during intercourse.
- The endometrium is the inner lining of cells of the uterus that is sloughed off each month during the menstrual flow if fertilization does not occur.
- The ovaries produce and expel eggs each month and also the female sex hormones, progesterone and estrogen.
- Breasts can exhibit cyclic changes including benign lumps or masses of overgrown breast tissue.
- The average age of menarche, the onset of the first menstrual cycle, is 12.8 years.
- The sex hormones involved in menstruation include follicle-stimulating hormone, luteinizing hormone, estrogen, and progesterone.
- A Pap test is the best method of detecting cervical cancer.
- Primary dysmenorrhea is painful menses without evidence of a physical abnormality.
- Secondary dysmenorrhea is usually due to anatomic abnormalities.
- Primary amenorrhea indicates a significant medical disorder.
- The causes of secondary amenorrhea remain unknown.
- The cause of endometriosis is unknown.
- Polycystic ovarian syndrome and ovarian failure are the most common causes of amenorrhea.
- PMS has physical and emotional symptoms that are associated with the luteal phase of menstruation.
- Uterine fibroids are common tumors of the uterus.
- Toxic shock syndrome occurs when a woman uses super absorbent tampons.
- Menopause is the time when ovulation and menstruation cease.
- The human sexual response cycle includes four phases: excitement, plateau, orgasm, and resolution.

Review Questions

1. What are the anatomic parts of the vulva?
2. What are the anatomic parts of the internal genitalia?
3. How are the four sex hormones involved in the menstrual cycle?
4. What are the components of the Female Athlete Triad?
5. Describe the differences between primary and secondary dysmenorrhea.
6. Describe the differences between primary and secondary amenorrhea.
7. What would you expect to occur during a pelvic examination?
8. What are some emotional and physical symptoms of PMS?
9. What are the changes that occur during the four phases of the human sexual response cycle?

Resources

Organizations and Hotlines

Endometriosis Association
8585 N. 76th Place
Milwaukee, WI 53223
414-355-2200
www.endometriosisassn.org

National Women's Health Network
514 10th St. NW, Ste. 400
Washington, DC 20004
202-347-1140
www.nwhn.org

National Women's Health Resource Center
157 Broad Street, Ste. 315
Red Bank, NJ 07001
877-986-9472
www.healthywomen.org

Web Sites

Imaginis, The Breast Cancer Resource
www.imaginis.com

National Women's Health Information Center
U.S. Department of Health and Human Services
Office on Women's Health
www.4women.gov

North American Menopause Society
www.menopause.org

Planned Parenthood Federation of America
www.ppfa.org

Dr. Susan Love Research Foundation
www.susanlovemdfoundation.org/index.asp

Suggested Readings

Barbach, L. 2000. *For Yourself: The Fulfillment of Female Sexuality.* New York: Signet.

Baron-Faust, R. 1998. *Being Female: What Every Woman Should Know about Gynecological Health.* New York: William Morrow.

Gittleman, A. C., and J. V. Wright. 1998. *Before the Change: Taking Charge of Your Perimenopause.* New York: HarperCollins.

Greer, G. 1993. *The Change: Women, Aging and the Menopause.* New York: Fawcett Columbine.

Love, S. M. 2005. *Dr. Susan Love's Breast Book: New Edition 2005* (Paperback). Cambridge: Perseus Books Group, Da Capo Press.

Love, S. M., and K. Lindsay. 2003. *Dr. Susan Love's Menopause and Hormone Book: Making Informed Choices.* Rev. ed. New York: Crown Publishing.

Northrup, C. 2002. *The Wisdom of Menopause: Creating Physical and Emotional Health and Healing during the Change.* New York: Bantam Books.

Northrup, C. 2002. *Women's Bodies, Women's Wisdom: Creating Physical and Emotional Health and Healing.* Rev. ed. New York: Bantam Books.

Seaman, B. 2003. *The Greatest Experiment Ever Performed On Women.* New York: Hyperion.

Wider, J., and P. Greenberger, eds. 2006. *The Savvy Woman Patient: How and Why Sex Differences Affect Your Health.* Society for Women's Health Research. VA: Capital Books.

References

1. American College of Obstetrics and Gynecology. 2006, March. ACOG recommends restricted use of episiotomies. www.acog.org/from_home/publications/press_releases/nr 03-31-06-2.cfm (retrieved October 2, 2006).
2. *Dr. Susan M. Love: Biography.* www.susanlovemdfoundation.org/html/bio.html (retrieved September 30, 2006).
3. Imaginis. 2005. Breast health (noncancerous breast issues). http://imaginis.com/breasthealth/benign.asp (retrieved March 27, 2006).
4. Ibid.
5. American Cancer Society. 2004. *Noncancerous breast conditions.* Cancer Reference Information. www.cancer.org/docrood/CRI/content/CRI_2_6X_Non_Cancerous_Breast_Conditions_59.asp. (retrieved March 27, 2006).
6. Hartman, L. C., T. A. Sellers, M. H. Frost, W. L. Lingle, A. C. Degnim, et al. 2005. Benign breast disease and the risk of breast cancer. *New England Journal of Medicine* 353 (3): 229–237.
7. American Cancer Society. 2006. *Updated breast cancer screening guidelines released.* www.cancer.org/docroot/NWS/content/NWS_1_1x_Updated_Breast_Cancer_Screening_Guidelines_Released.asp (retrieved September 30, 2006).
8. American Cancer Society. 2006. *Non-cancerous breast conditions.* www.cancer.org/docroot/CRI/content/CRI_2_6X_Non_Cancerous_Breast_Conditions_59.asp?sitearea= (retrieved September 27, 2006).
9. Imaginis. 2005. *Cosmetic/reconstructive breast surgery.* http://imaginis.com/breasthealth/reconstruction.asp (retrieved March 27, 2006).
10. Lee, J. 1994. Menarche and the (hetero) sexualization of the female body. *Gender & Society* 8 (3): 343–62.
11. Chrisler, J. C., I. K. Johnston, et al. 1994. Menstrual joy: The construct and its consequences. *Psychology of Women Quarterly* 18 (3): 375–87.
12. National Women's Health Information Center. 2002. *Menstruation and the menstrual cycle.* www.4women.gov (retrieved October 4, 2006).
13. Feminist Women's Health Center. 2003. *Menstrual cycles: What really happens in those 28 days.* www.fwhc.org/health/moon.htm (retrieved October 4, 2006).
14. Ibid.
15. National Cancer Institute. 2005, March. *What you need to know about cancer of the cervix.* www.cancer.gov/cancertopics/wyntk/cervix/page6 (retrieved October 2, 2006).
16. Ibid.
17. Ibid.
18. Lichten, E. M. 1989. *Medical treatment of endometriosis and pelvic pain.* www.usdoctor.com/endo.htm (March 27, 2006).
19. Boston College Eating Awareness Team. 2002, January. *The opponent: The Female Athlete Triad.* www.bc.edu/bc_org/svp/uhs/eating/eating-femaleathletes.htm (retrieved September 24, 2006).
20. Nattiv, A., and L. Lynch. 1994. The Female Athlete Triad: Managing an acute risk to long-term health. *Physician and Sportsmedicine* 22 (1): 61–68.
21. U.S. Department of Health and Human Services. 2004, December. *Polycystic ovarian syndrome.* www.4woman.gov/faq/pcos.htm (retrieved September 24, 2006).
22. Lark, S. 2006, September. *Types of PMS.* http://dev1.drlark.com/nc/pms_types.asp (retrieved September 30, 2006).
23. Wharton, L. 1997. *The natural guide to women's health: How a woman can be healthy at any age.* New York: MJF Books.
24. *Treating PMS.* 2006. www.pms.com/treating/Default.pmsx (retrieved October 2, 2006).
25. Wartik, N. 1995. Is it an illness? *American Health* (April): 67.
26. WebMD Health. 2004. *Premenstrual syndrome.* my.webmd.com/hw/womens_conditions/hw139442.asp (retrieved April 10, 2004).

27. U.S. Department of Health and Human Services. 2004, September. *Uterine fibroids.* www.4woman.gov/faq/fibroids.htm (retrieved September 30, 2006).
28. *Hysterectomy status by state and age, 1998–2000.* www.nuff.org/health_hysterectomystatistics.htm (retrieved March 27, 2006).
29. Johnson, N., D. Barlow, A. Lethaby, E. Tavender, L. Curr, and R. Garry. 2005. Methods of hysterectomy: Systematic review and meta-analysis of randomized controlled trials. *British Medical Journal* 330:1478–81.
30. Parker, W. H., M. S. Broder, Z. Lui, D. Shoupe, C. Farquhar, and J. S. Berek. 2005. Ovarian conservation at the time of hysterectomy for benign disease. *Obstetrics & Gynecology* 106:219–226.
31. *Hysterectomy status by state and age, 1998–2000.*
32. Kouides, P. A., P. Burkhard, P. D. Platak, et al. 1997. Type 1 von Willebrand disease causes significant obstetric-gynecological morbidity (abstract). *Blood* 90:32.
33. WebMD Health. 2006. *Issues surrounding natural and surgical menopause.* www.webmd.com/content/article/85/98754.htm (retrieved October 2, 2006).
34. Ibid.
35. Women's Health Initiative. 2003. *Estrogen plus progestin study stopped due to increased breast cancer risk, lack of overall benefit.* www.nhlbi.nih.gov/new/press/02-07-09.htm (retrieved October 4, 2006).
36. DHHS. National Institutes of Health. 2005. *Facts about menopausal hormone therapy.* NIH Publication No. 05-5200. Originally printed October 2002.
37. Ellis, H. 1904. *Man and woman: A study of human secondary sex characteristics.* New York: Scribner; Kinsey, A. C., W. B. Pomeroy, C. E. Martin, and P. H. Gebhard. 1953. *Sexual behavior in the human female.* Philadelphia: Saunders.
38. Woodman, S. 2002. The women's Enron. *Nation* (September 9).
39. Masters, W. H., and V. E. Johnson. 1970. *Human sexual response.* Boston: Little, Brown.
40. Kaplan, H. S. 1995. *Sexual desire disorders: Dysfunctional regulation of sexual motivation.* New York: Brunner-Routledge.
41. Walen, S., and D. Roth. 1987. A cognitive approach. In J. H. Geer and V. T. O. Donahue (eds.), *Theories of human sexuality.* New York: Plenum.
42. Zilbergeld, B., and C. R. Ellison. 1980. Desire discrepancy and arousal problems in sex therapy. In S. L. Leiblum and L. Pen (eds.), *Principles and practices of sex therapy.* New York: Guilford.
43. Masters and Johnson, *Human sexual response.*

Chapter Nine

Designing Your Reproductive Life Plan

CHAPTER OBJECTIVES

When you complete this chapter, you will be able to do the following:

- Prepare your own reproductive life plan
- Describe the benefits and risks of the available contraceptive choices
- Describe how to plan for a pregnancy
- Describe the major fetal development stages during each trimester
- Describe the reasons for female and male infertility
- Differentiate between Right to Life and Pro-Choice positions
- Explain appropriate and inappropriate parenting styles

FAMILY PLANNING

Family planning is more than a personal and family issue. It has health, social, and political implications and has been plagued by woeful governmental underfunding of birth control methods and family planning clinics for women. Indeed, women and children have been impacted by (1) governments that determine and prescribe acceptable birth control methods, (2) religious bodies that dictate reproductive choices, (3) unavailable or limited health care options, and (4) political agendas and laws that reduce women's options. While fertility rates have declined and contraceptive use has increased in the past decades, population control remains a twenty-first-century focus for world health. In too many developing countries, a family still averages four or five children. Here, the leading causes of death for women are complications associated with pregnancy, childbirth, and abortion. In recent years, several international agreements have been reached that include the right of couples to information and services to prevent too early, too closely spaced, too late, or too many pregnancies.[1] Governments throughout the world can reduce population overcrowding and improve the status of women by making a wider variety of birth control methods accessible and affordable rather than limiting women's choices. A woman needs access to a variety of reproductive options if she is going to control her own reproductive health, and the ability to pay must not prevent her from choosing the one that is right for her. In an ideal world, all pregnancies would be planned and all children would be wanted. (See *Viewpoint:* "The Benefits of Family Planning.")

In reality, nearly 45 percent of all pregnancies are unplanned and every year nearly 1 million U.S. teenagers become pregnant, twice the rate of England, three times that of Australia, six times that of France, and fifteen times that of Japan. These teenagers, especially those under age 18, are more likely to have problems with pregnancy and to have low birth weight babies, and nearly 80 percent will eventually go on welfare, most within 5 years of giving birth.[2] The children born to

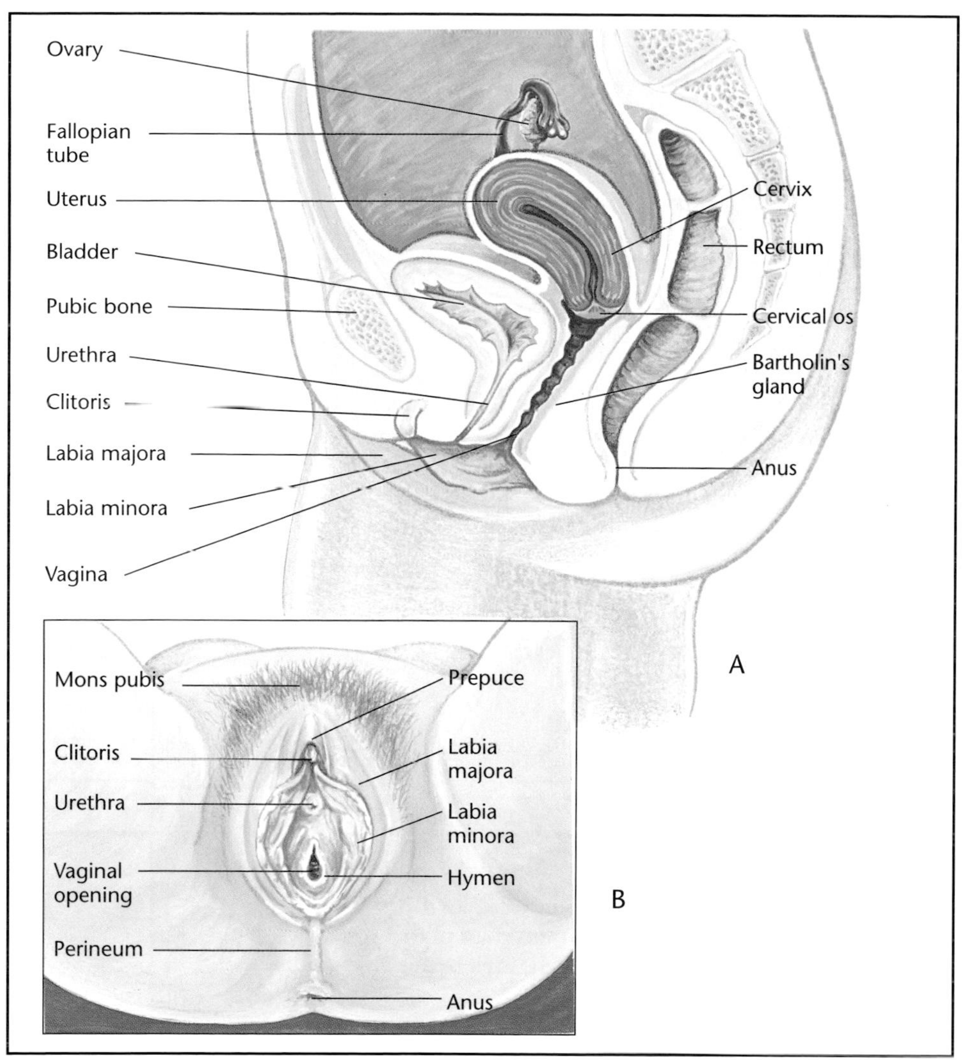

Color Plate 1
(*A*), Female reproductive structures, side view. (*B*), External view of female genitalia.

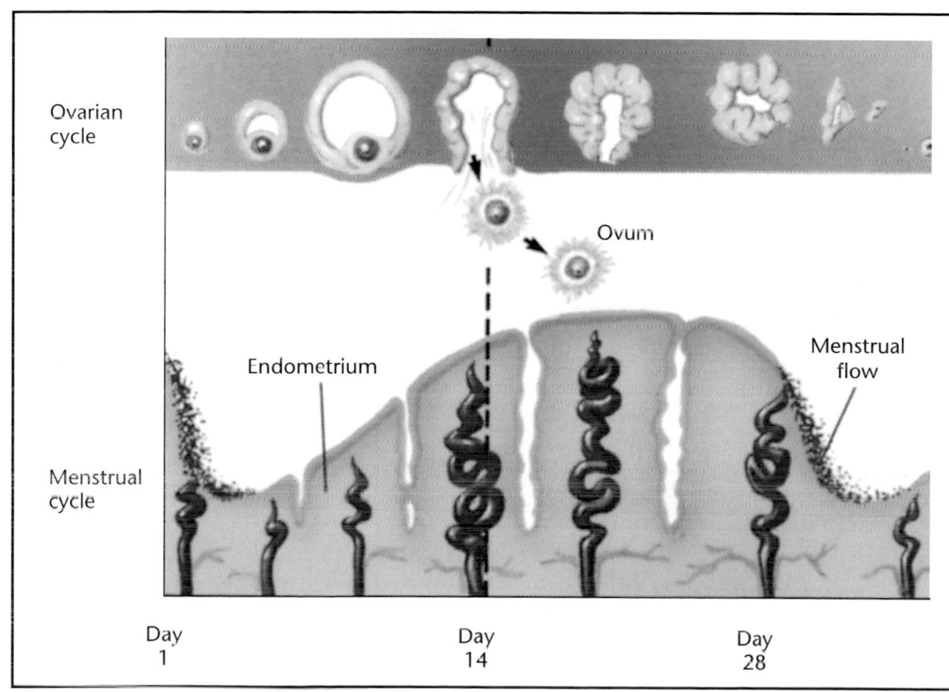

Color Plate 2
The menstrual cycle: As an egg matures in the ovary, the lining of the uterus prepares to receive a fertilized egg. The egg is released during ovulation (approximately day 14). If the egg is not fertilized, the lining is shed during the menstrual period.

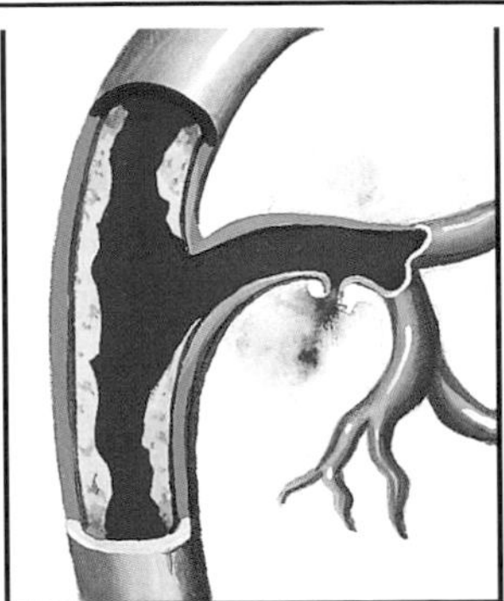

Hemorrhage
The sudden bursting of a blood vessel.

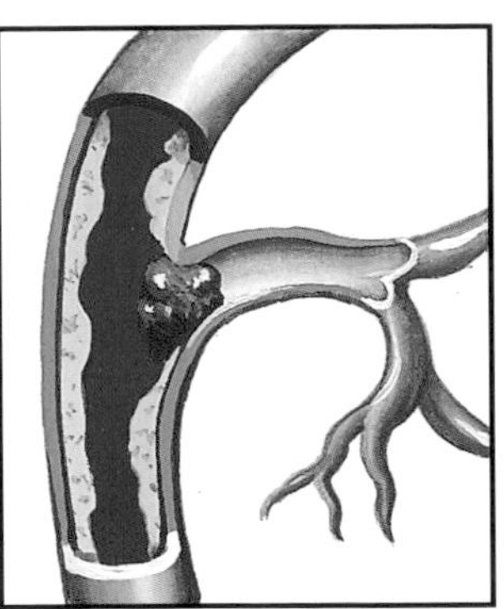

Embolus
A clot that moves through the circulatory system and becomes lodged at a narrowed point within a vessel.

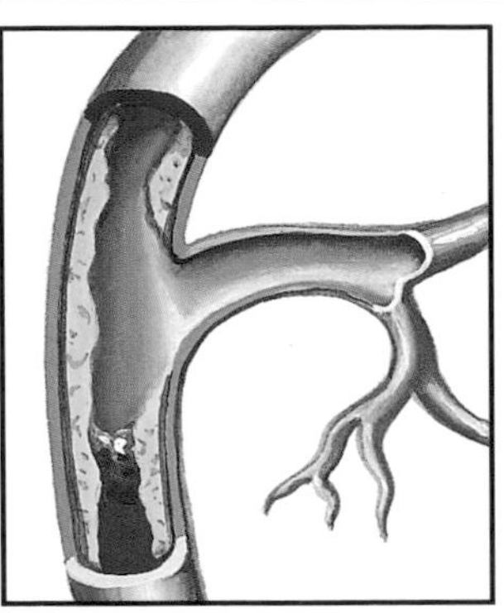

Thrombus
A clot that forms within a narrowed section of a blood vessel and remains at its place of origin.

Color Plate 7
Causes of stroke

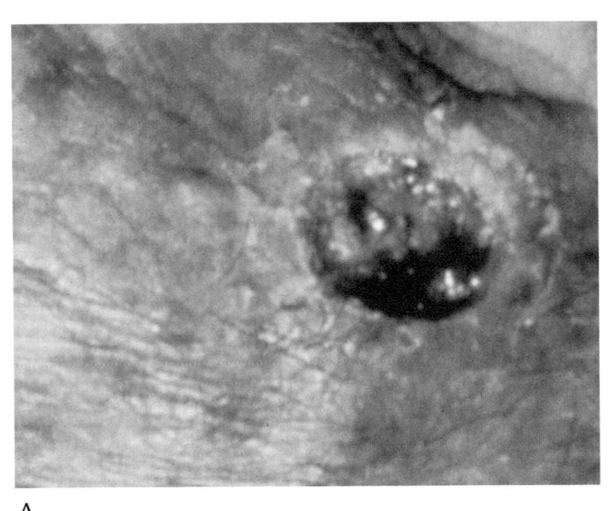

A

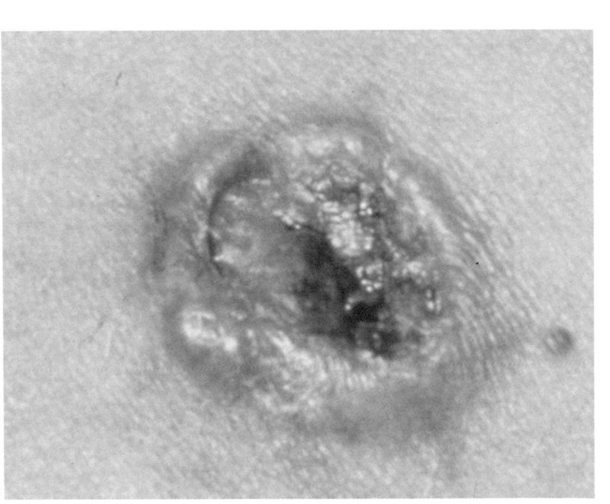

B

Color Plate 8
(*A*), Basal cell carcinoma. (*B*), Squamous cell carcinoma.

Asymmetry
One half unlike the other half

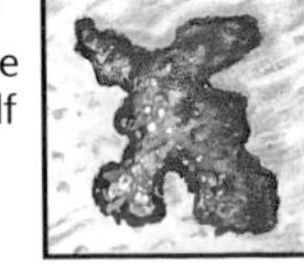

Irregularity
Border irregular or poorly circumscribed

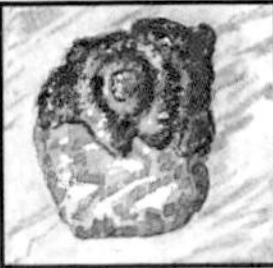

Color
Color varies from one area to another; shades of tan, brown, or black

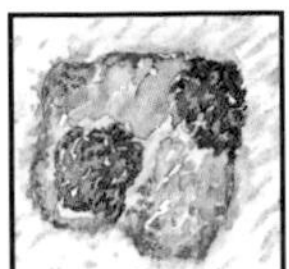

Size
Diameter larger than 6 mm as a rule (diameter of a pencil eraser)

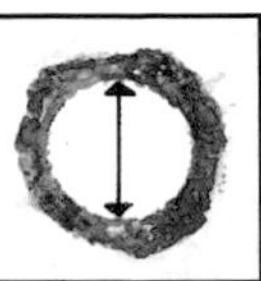

Color Plate 9
Guidelines for detecting melanoma.

Viewpoint

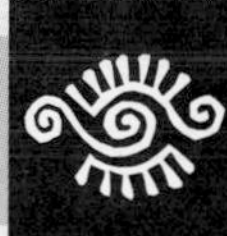

The Benefits of Family Planning

The ability to plan the number, spacing, and timing of births is essential for the empowerment of women. Family planning has a number of benefits for women, including the following:

- Family planning contributes significantly to the decrease of women who live in poverty.
- Family planning provides women with more time to spend on education and employment opportunities.
- Family planning reduces the number of maternal and infant deaths.
- Family planning reduces the global population.
- Family planning reduces the number of teenagers who give birth, thus reducing overall premature and unintended pregnancies. Teenage childbirth is associated with greater risk of dying in pregnancy and complications during delivery.
- Family planning provides adolescents with more opportunities for a better education, jobs, and income and reduces the likelihood of divorce and separation.[3]

Given these benefits and more, why does the U.S. government continue to withhold funding to the United Nations for family planning? Why does the U.S. government continue to put restrictions on the money it does provide for family planning? What should the U.S. position be regarding family planning? What funding should the U.S. government provide to teenagers for contraceptives?

these teen mothers are more likely to suffer negative outcomes such as inadequate nutrition, health care, or cognitive and social stimulation. These children are less likely to graduate from high school and, as adults, more likely to be unemployed and three times more likely to be incarcerated. On the opposite end of the spectrum, a growing number of women are postponing pregnancy until later in their life when risks for complications also increase and infertility is more common. This chapter addresses issues of reproductive health and family planning, including contraceptive choices, pregnancy, childbirth, birthing options, breast-feeding, fetal health, infertility, abortion, and adoption.

BIRTH CONTROL METHODS

A landmark decision by the U.S. Supreme Court in 1967 created the present environment of contraceptive acceptance in the United States. *Griswold v. Connecticut* held that the state law prohibiting married couples from using birth control was unconstitutional. This decision afforded married couples the right of privacy in making choices regarding the use of birth control by placing the issue beyond state intervention. Throughout this chapter, birth control and contraceptive choice are used interchangeably. While the courts have limited the definition, we define **birth control** methods as all the strategies used to keep from having a baby, including abstinence, contraceptive methods, IUDs, emergency contraception, and abortion. Contraceptive choice includes those methods that prevent fertilization of the ovum such as hormonal methods, barrier methods, and sterilization.

Choosing an appropriate birth control method requires planning and informed decision making. The first consideration is whether to *involve a partner* in the decision. A partner can assist with the choice of the appropriate contraceptive, accompany the woman to scheduled physical examinations if a prescription is required, and share the cost for the contraceptive. (See Table 9.1.)

The second consideration is *acceptability*. The method a woman selects should be congruent with her personal values and beliefs (e.g., religious) about the likelihood of pregnancy or sexually transmitted infections (STIs). If she believes that premarital sex is not acceptable, her only choice is abstinence. If she is in a monogamous relationship and her partner is STI-free, she might choose hormonal methods. If she has had a previous ectopic (outside the uterus) pregnancy, she might want to consider a method other than an IUD. Another consideration is *availability* of the method she selects. If a prescription is required, she must have access to a health care provider who can prescribe the method. If she is a minor, she may need to secure parental consent. Fourth, she needs to consider the *cost* of the method. She must weigh the cost of the method against the cost of an unintended pregnancy or unwanted STI. Can she afford this method of protection (both monetarily and in terms of method and user effectiveness)? If she chooses to use the pill, she must remember to take it at the same time every day. If she forgets, she will need to use another method during the month. Is she knowledgeable about the method, and will she use it dependably? Can she afford (financially and emotionally) to become pregnant? Another factor to consider is *health risk*. A method may be contraindicated for medical reasons. For example, women smokers over age 35 or women who are breast-feeding should choose a method other than the pill. If a woman has a family history of breast cancer, she may want to consider a nonhormonal method. If she had a previous pregnancy, the IUD may not be appropriate. If a partner has an STI, a woman may want to choose an appropriate method to reduce her risk of contracting it.

TABLE 9.1 Comparison of User Failure, Method Failure, and Cost

FERTILITY AWARENESS	USER FAILURE	METHOD FAILURE	COST
Cycle-based	20–25%	9%	Charts are free
Basal body temperature	20%	2–3%	Temperature kit $5–10
Symptothermal	20%	2–3%	Temperature kit $5–10
No method	85%	85%	
Barrier			
Spermicides	29%	15%	$8–10 kit with 20–40 applications; refills $2–5
Male condom	15%	2%	Free at clinics to $6–10/dozen
Female condom	21%	5%	$1.50–4.00
Diaphragm/cervical cap	14–16%	6%	$70–80
(with spermicide)		1–2%	
Lea's Shield	N/A	15%	
Sponge	16–32%	9–20%	
Hormonal Methods			
Oral contraceptives	6%	3%	$1.50-$30, depending on site
NuvaRing (ring)	8%	>1%	$30–35 a month
OrthoEvra (patch)	8%	>1%	$35–40 a month
Depo-Provera	3%	>1%	$30–75 every 3 months + visit
ECP (Plan B)		10–25%	$8–35
ECP (IUD)		1%	$150–500 + visit
Implanon		>1%	Unknown for insertion and removal
Other Methods			
Intrauterine device	>1%	>1%	$175–500 + visit
Tubal ligation		>1%	$1,500–6,000
Vasectomy		>1%	$350–1,000

SOURCE: Planned Parenthood Federation of America, 2006.[4]

When making a decision about the choice of birth control, a couple must have adequate information about the available **contraceptive** methods including the health benefits and drawbacks, the relative failure rates, and the cost estimate of each method. Birth control methods can be classified according to the method of protection, such as continuous abstinence, fertility awareness methods (periodic abstinence), barrier methods, hormonal methods, and emergency contraception. Now complete *Journal Activity:* "Making an Informed Decision."

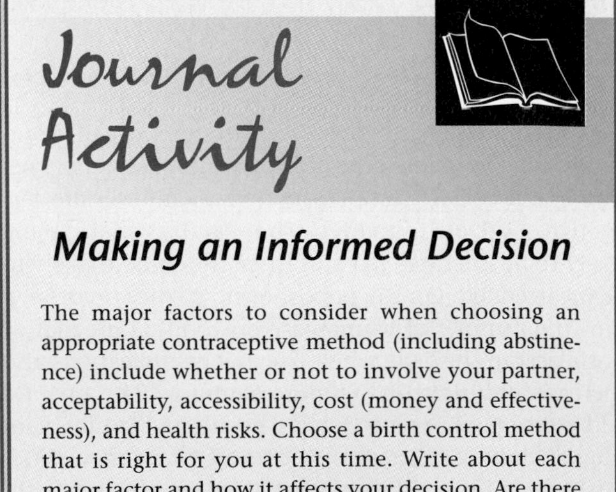

Making an Informed Decision

The major factors to consider when choosing an appropriate contraceptive method (including abstinence) include whether or not to involve your partner, acceptability, accessibility, cost (money and effectiveness), and health risks. Choose a birth control method that is right for you at this time. Write about each major factor and how it affects your decision. Are there other factors you may need to consider?

Continuous Abstinence

Continuous abstinence from sexual intercourse is the *only* sure way to prevent an unintended pregnancy. If a young woman does not want to risk pregnancy, then abstaining from intercourse is essential. Sexual activity among adolescents has gradually declined over the past decade in the United States, with the percentage of high school freshmen through seniors reporting they have ever had sexual intercourse dropping dramatically, and reported condom use among sexually active teens has increased significantly. These trends are encouraging from the standpoint of reducing STI and HIV/AIDS exposure and unplanned pregnancies. However, current federal policy, which provides millions of dollars for ineffective abstinence-only programs, has the potential

Viewpoint

Our Tax Dollars at Work?

Statistics suggest that 27 percent of females have had sexual intercourse by age 15 and that half of all females have had sexual intercourse by age 17.8. Young men and women, particularly those at greatest risk for pregnancy and contracting HIV or other STIs, need to be better informed about the risks and strategies for preventing STIs and unwanted pregnancies. They need to hear messages regarding postponement of sexual behavior and proper protection when sexually active. An assessment of sexuality education by the Sex Information and Education Council of the United States (SIECUS) found that forty-eight states either recommend or require sexuality education through state law or policy. The primary focus of this education has been abstinence-only-until-marriage programs, which are federal entitlement programs that were mandated as a provision of the welfare-reform law. Congress funneled $50 million per year for 5 years to states willing to match every $4 of federal monies with $3 of state monies. Congress has appropriated no funds for teaching sexuality education that includes discussion of contraceptive choices. Further, according to a recent press release from SIECUS, the proposed federal fiscal budget for 2007 requests an increase of 15% to $204 million for abstinence-only-until-marriage programs that have never been proven effective. If this request is fulfilled, total federal taxpayer dollars spent on these programs will top just over $1.1 billion.[5,6,7]

Abstinence-only curricula are supported by parents and community members who do not want teachers to address birth control, contraceptives, and sexual behaviors. For many of them, it is a moral issue. The debate regarding the moral versus medical/educational aspects of teaching sexuality education, particularly reproductive health, continues. What do you think about the moral and medical/educational arguments? Are schools, parents, churches, and communities doing everything they can to prevent unintended pregnancies in adolescents? How is sex defined by adolescents today (does it include oral sex)? What role should the federal government have in curricular decisions about sexuality education in the schools? What suggestions do you have for preventing or reducing STIs in adolescents?

to erode this success. (See *Viewpoint*. "Our Tax Dollars at Work.")

Abstinence-only programs have proliferated but are not supported by peer-reviewed research for prevention of STIs, HIV/AIDS, and unplanned pregnancies. Schools adopting the abstinence-only programs do not provide education about birth control, STI prevention, or sexual orientation. The outcome of this political strategy is discouraging because of the extreme detriment to many of America's impoverished adolescents who have less access to quality education regarding contraceptive protection. Comprehensive sexuality education (abstinence-plus education) differs from abstinence-only programs. Comprehensive sexuality education promotes abstinence but acknowledges that many teenagers become sexually active and need to be educated about contraceptives, condom use, emergency contraception, abortion, STIs, and HIV/AIDS. Abstinence-only education merely cites STIs and HIV/AIDS as reasons to remain abstinent and does not consistently delay sexual activity in teens. If evidence-based curricula are truly important, than comprehensive sexuality education in the schools should be supported by federal dollars.

Fertility Awareness Methods (Periodic Abstinence)

Fertility awareness methods of contraception are referred to as periodic abstinence and include the cycle-based method, the basal body temperature method, and the symptothermal method, a combination of basal body temperature tracking, cycle monitoring, and mucosal sampling. Withdrawal, referred to as coitus interruptus, is common and is mentioned, but it is not a birth control method. Natural family planning methods or fertility awareness methods help women understand their menstrual cycle better but require high motivation and cooperation by both partners. These methods have high method and user failure rates, are not suggested for couples who cannot afford a pregnancy, and offer no protection against STIs. (See Figure 9.1.)

Cycle-Based Method The **cycle-based method** (or rhythm) is a form of contraception that relies on abstinence during the period of time a woman is ovulating. It is the least user effective method of contraception and should be supplemented with another option if pregnancy cannot be tolerated. The average menstrual cycle is 21 to 35 days long, and **ovulation** can occur anytime between days 11 and 21 depending on cycle length. Ovulation occurs near the midpoint of a menstrual cycle or, put another way, approximately 14 days after ovulation, menses begins. The cycle-based method would be very effective if a woman knew the exact day of ovulation; however, pregnancy has occurred with isolated intercourse on virtually every day of the menstrual cycle. To use the cycle-based method, a woman determines the length of time between menstrual cycles,

FIGURE 9.1 Fertility awareness, also known as natural family planning, can combine each method to identify when a woman is fertile. However, it must be remembered that the cycles for most women are not consistently 28-day cycles.

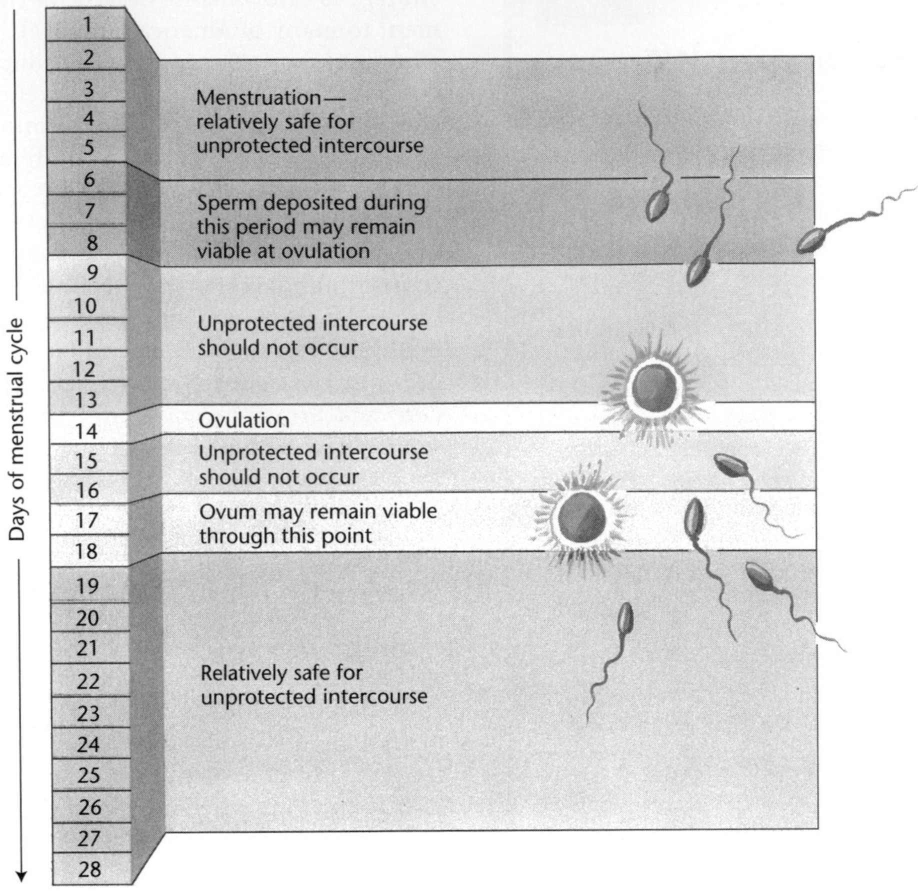

including the shortest and longest times between cycles. To be safe, a couple should refrain from intercourse during the entire time that ovulation is possible, including 5 to 7 days prior to ovulation and 3 to 5 days after ovulation. The egg can be fertilized anytime between its release by the ovary and its exit from the fallopian tube. Women with cycles shorter than 27 days should opt for another method.[8]

The cycle-based method has a 20 to 25 percent failure rate, with higher rates for single women. With perfect use, 9 in 100 women will become pregnant within a year when using this method alone. The primary advantage of this method is its acceptance by most religious organizations. The primary disadvantage is the unpredictability of a woman's menstrual cycle, particularly during stress or illness. (See *FYI:* "Factors Known to Affect the Menstrual Cycle.") Most failures of the cycle-based method have more to do with the length of viability of sperm than the day of ovulation. Sperm can be found in the cervical mucus within 20 seconds and up to 7 days after ejaculation.

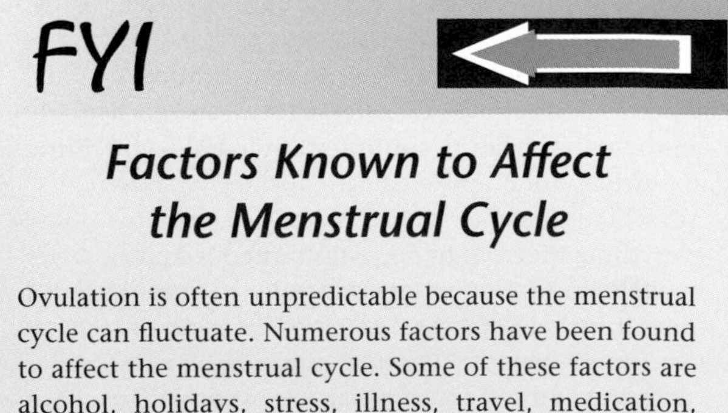

Factors Known to Affect the Menstrual Cycle

Ovulation is often unpredictable because the menstrual cycle can fluctuate. Numerous factors have been found to affect the menstrual cycle. Some of these factors are alcohol, holidays, stress, illness, travel, medication, changing work schedules, gynecological problems, excessive exercise, and perimenopausal status. What factors have impacted the length of your menstrual cycle?

Basal Body Temperature Method The **basal body temperature method** is designed to determine when a woman is ovulating. A woman's basal body temperature drops slightly 1 to 2 days before ovulation and then rises sharply by approximately one-half to 1 degree during ovulation and remains elevated until menses begins. A woman who is using this method should take her basal body temperature each morning before rising from bed for reliability. One problem with basal body temperature, as with the cycle-based method, is that sexual activity should not occur 3 to 4 days before ovulation because the sperm can remain viable in the genital tract for several days. Sexual activity also should be stopped for 3 to 4 days after the temperature elevates. Intercourse before ovulation carries a greater risk than intercourse during the postovulatory infertile phase, which is somewhat easier to determine. The sperm can remain viable for more than 72 hours, so predicting the time of ovulation is extremely important with this method. With perfect use, only 2–3 in 100 women will become pregnant within a year; however, perfect doesn't usually happen.

Symptothermal Method The **symptothermal method** is a combination of basal body temperature, cycle, monitoring, and cervical mucus monitoring. In addition to monitoring basal body temperature, a woman can detect changes in consistency of the cervical mucus at ovulation when it becomes more watery. Sexual intercourse should be avoided until the mucus thickens or dries. Monitoring basal body temperature, calendar, and mucus consistency is a better method than the cycle-based method for determining ovulation. This combination method still has a failure rate of nearly 20 percent but is preferred over any single fertility awareness method. Intercourse should be avoided or other methods considered until a woman becomes familiar with her menstrual cycle.

Withdrawal Withdrawal, **coitus interruptus,** is not a contraceptive method; it is a method that leads to many unintended pregnancies. Some young teenage women believe that pregnancy cannot occur if the penis is withdrawn from the vagina before ejaculation. In reality, the pre-ejaculate carries sperm that may be released into the vagina before withdrawal. This method has an extremely high failure rate. If a woman wants to prevent an unwanted pregnancy or protect herself from STIs, this is one method to avoid! Women who are sexually active and use no contraceptive method have an 85 to 90 percent chance of becoming pregnant during the year. If unintended intercourse occurs, women can reduce the risk of an unwanted pregnancy by using Plan B (emergency contraception, discussed later in the chapter).

Barrier Methods

Barrier methods include spermicides, condoms, sponges, diaphragms, cervical caps, and cervical shields. Spermicides and condoms are inexpensive and available over the counter. Diaphragms, cervical caps, and cervical shields require a prescription and are more difficult to use. Barrier methods have become increasingly popular because of the protection they provide against HIV and other STIs. However, their use as contraception for young women remains questionable because of high failure rates. Many health care providers recommend using a combination of the condom and oral contraceptives to protect against STIs and unplanned pregnancy.

FIGURE 9.2 Vaginal spermicides are placed deep into the vagina no longer than 30 minutes before intercourse.

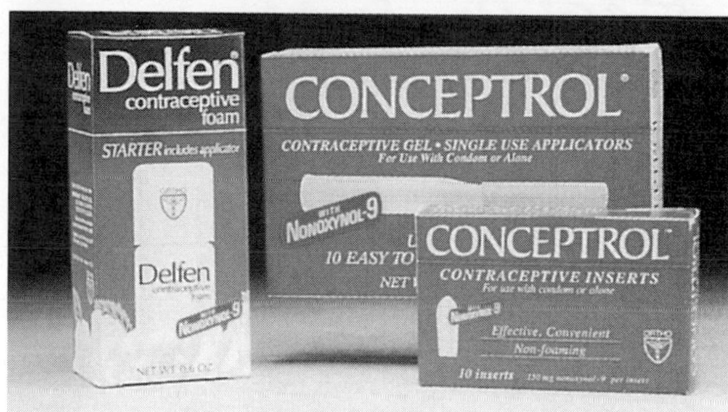

A

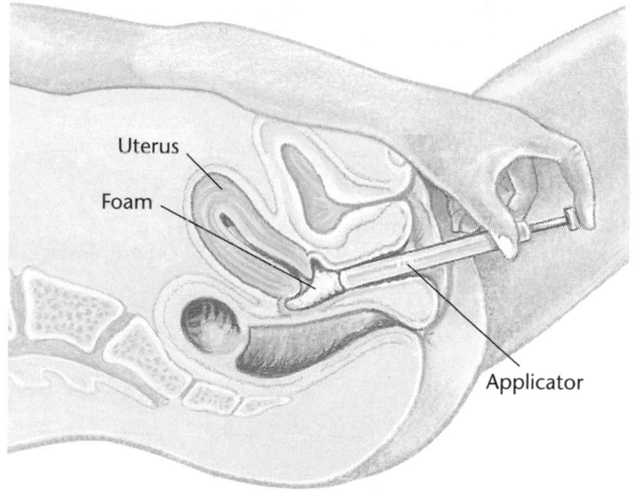

B

Spermicides Vaginal **spermicides,** a chemical method of contraceptive use, come in a variety of forms: creams, gels, films, suppositories, and foams. (See Figure 9.2.) Spermicides prevent contraception by killing or immobilizing sperm before they reach the uterus. They serve as a lubricant and can be used alone or with another barrier method, such as condoms, diaphragms, or cervical caps. Spermicides are effective within 10 minutes of application and must be reapplied before each ejaculation

Health Tips

How to Use a Condom

1. Both partners should know how to use a condom. Practice without embarrassment by using a penis-shaped object, e.g., banana, cucumber.
2. If a condom is torn, stiff, or sticky, throw it away and get another one.
3. Roll the condom down on the penis as soon as it is erect and before the penis touches the vulva. Do this as soon as possible as part of foreplay.
4. Pinch out any extra air and leave one-half inch of space at the tip of the condom. If the condom has a reservoir tip, this is easy to remember. This extra space is for the ejaculate. (See Figure 9.3.)
5. If using another lubricant, choose something like K-Y jelly, which is water based. Do not use an oil-based lubricant, which can break down the latex.
6. After ejaculation, hold the condom at the rim and withdraw the penis before it is soft. Be careful so that semen does not leak out of the condom.
7. Remove the condom, wrap it in tissue, and dispose of it safely in a waste container. Do not flush the condom in the toilet.
8. Wash the penis with soap and water before any further body contact.

FIGURE 9.3 Pinch the end of the condom to leave one-half inch of space at the tip.

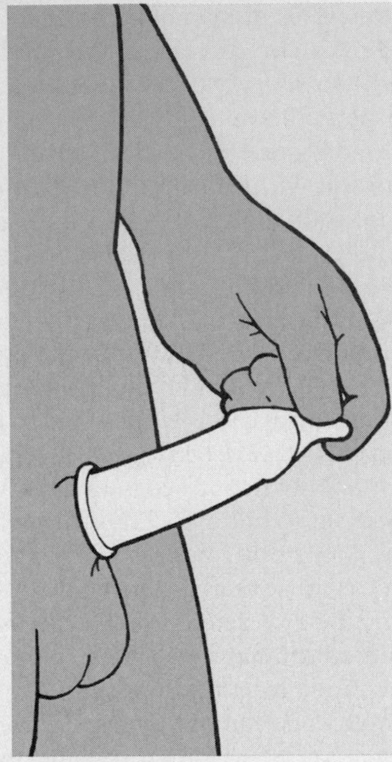

to prevent loss of effectiveness. Douching should be avoided, or if practiced, should be delayed for 8 to 10 hours after intercourse because it could force sperm into the uterine cavity. (Contrary to the messages seen in advertisements, douching does not enhance feminine hygiene or provide health benefits.) Recommendations regarding the use of the spermicide nonoxynol-9 (N-9) have changed. According to the Centers for Disease Control and Prevention, N-9 *should not* be recommended as an effective means for HIV/AIDS or pregnancy prevention in populations at high risk for HIV. In one study, women who used a condom and N-9 gel had a 50 percent higher HIV infection rate than women who used a condom and a placebo gel.[9] Method effectiveness is approximately 85 percent; user effectiveness is approximately 70 percent.

FIGURE 9.4 Condoms.

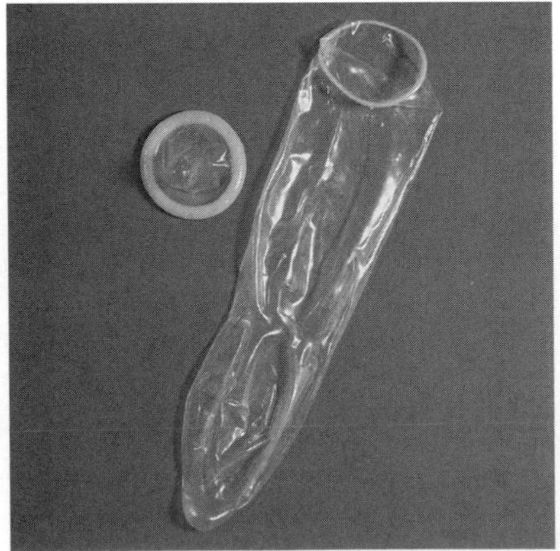

Condom, Male The latex **condom** has increased in use, primarily because it helps to protect against HIV and other STIs such as herpes simplex 2 virus, chlamydia, and cytomegalovirus. Condoms also reduce transmission of gonorrhea, hepatitis B virus, and *Trichomonas vaginalis*.[10] The condom is a thin sheath (see Figure 9.4), and it is 85 to 90 percent effective when used alone and 98 percent effective when used with a spermicide. (See *Health Tips:* "How to Use a Condom.")

Drawbacks to using a condom may include reduced spontaneity and possible allergic reactions. Using condoms as part of foreplay can help reduce a lack of spontaneity. The complaint of an allergic reaction can be addressed by a procedure called double bagging. If the male exhibits an allergy to latex condoms, he can roll a sheepskin condom onto the penis, followed by a latex condom to offer protection against HIV and other STIs. If the female exhibits an allergic reaction, the procedure can be reversed with the latex condom applied first, followed by the sheepskin condom. Sheepskin condoms, made from lamb intestines, are not recommended for preventing HIV/AIDS and other STIs because of their porousness. Polyurethane condoms could also be tried to avoid an allergic response. Regardless of what type of condom is used—latex, sheepskins, or polyurethane, it must be applied before intercourse, and a new condom should be used before each act of intercourse. Condoms should be stored in a cool place to prevent deterioration, and Vaseline and other petroleum products that contribute to breakdown of the latex should be avoided. Proper application of the condom is essential for maximizing its effectiveness. The male condom should not be used concurrently with the female condom.

FIGURE 9.5 The female condom.

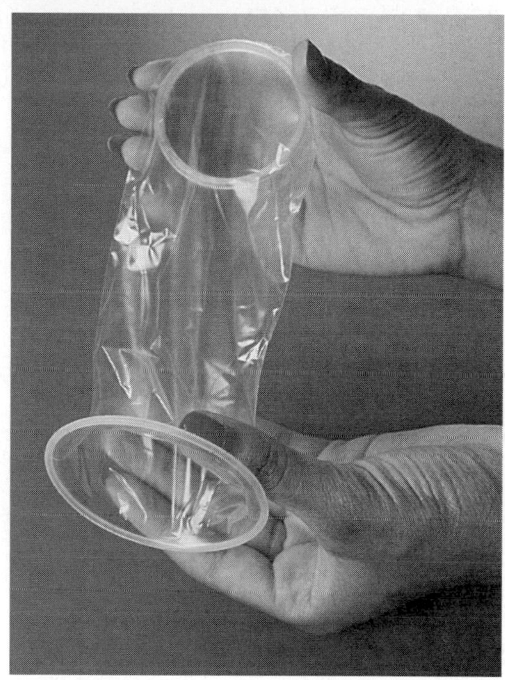

FIGURE 9.6 Diaphragm and contraceptive jelly.

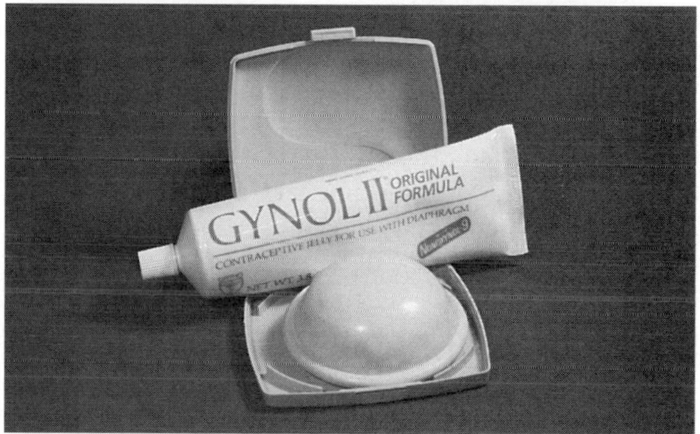

Condom, Female The **female condom** is a one-size-fits-all barrier method. It is the first barrier contraceptive for women and offers protection against HIV and other STIs. Laboratory tests demonstrate that the HIV virus and other STI viruses cannot permeate the polyurethane material. The female condom consists of a prelubricated, soft, polyurethane pouch with two flexible rings, one inserted into the vagina to cover the cervix and the other ring partially covers the labia. It is approximately $6^1/_2$ inches in length. (See Figure 9.5.) Polyurethane is strong, soft, and transfers heat, so it warms to body temperature soon after insertion. The advantage of the female condom is that it does not require fitting and its use is controlled by the woman. The major disadvantage seems to be its lack of aesthetic appeal. The female condom should be discarded in a wastebasket after one use, not flushed. The failure rate is high, 12 to 22 percent, due primarily to user error, not product failure. The restrictive labeling suggests that this method is not as effective in protecting against HIV and other STIs as the male latex condom. Some reproductive rights advocates suggest that the female condom has been subjected to much greater scrutiny and testing than the male condom.

Sponge The sponge is made from polyurethane foam and contains spermicide. It is moistened with water and then inserted deep into the vagina, and has a nylon loop attached at the bottom for easy removal. The sponge covers the cervix and blocks sperm from entering the uterus, and the spermicide immobilizes the sperm. Its method effectiveness differs for women who have not given birth and for those who have given birth: 16 compared to 32 out of 100 women will become pregnant during the first year of use. This method is easy to use once a woman learns, and the sponge can be worn for up to 30 hours without a need to be replaced and with repeated intercourse for up to 24 hours. It must be left in place for a minimum of 6 hours after last intercourse. The sponge cannot be used during any time of vaginal bleeding, including menstruation.

Diaphragm The **diaphragm** is an oval, dome-shaped device with a flexible spring at the outer edge. (See Figure 9.6.) A spermicide is applied into the dome

FIGURE 9.7 (*A*) Spermicidal cream or jelly is placed into the diaphragm. (*B*) The diaphragm is folded lengthwise and inserted into the vagina. (*C*) The diaphragm is then placed against the cervix so that the cup portion with the spermicide is facing the cervix. The outline of the cervix should be felt through the central part of the diaphragm.

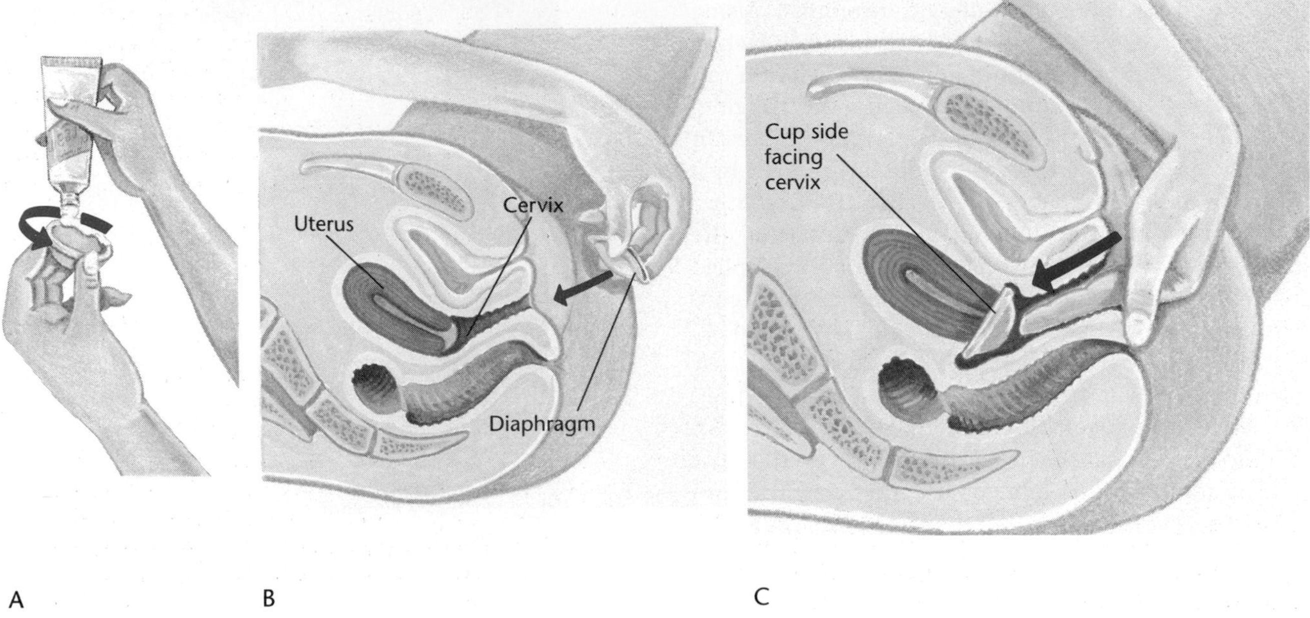

and a small amount is spread around the rim with the finger. Then the diaphragm is inserted with the back rim below and behind the cervix and held in place by the back of the pubic bone. (See Figure 9.7.) When the diaphragm is fitted properly, it is not felt by either partner. The diaphragm should be left in place for 8 hours after intercourse, and then removed. The diaphragm lowers the probability of contracting several STIs, including chlamydia and the human papilloma virus (HPV). It appears to lower the risk of cervical cancer, tubal infertility, and PID but increases the risk for urinary tract, bladder, and yeast infections. The user failure rate ranges from 6 percent to 16 percent. The diaphragm must be initially fitted by a health care provider, and refitting may be necessary after weight change, childbirth, or pelvic surgery. The diaphragm comes in many sizes and designs.

Cervical Cap The **cervical cap** is designed to fit tightly over the cervix and should be filled with spermicide before intercourse. (See Figure 9.8.) Like the diaphragm, it must be fitted by a health care provider; unlike the diaphragm, there are only three sizes: small, for nulliparous women; medium, for those who have not had an abortion or cesarean section; and large, for women who have given birth vaginally. The cervical cap can remain in place for 48 hours without spermicidal reapplication. User effectiveness ranges from 70 to 85 percent, with higher rates in younger women. The

FIGURE 9.8 After the spermicidal cream or jelly is placed in the cervical cap, the cap is inserted into the vagina and placed against the cervix.

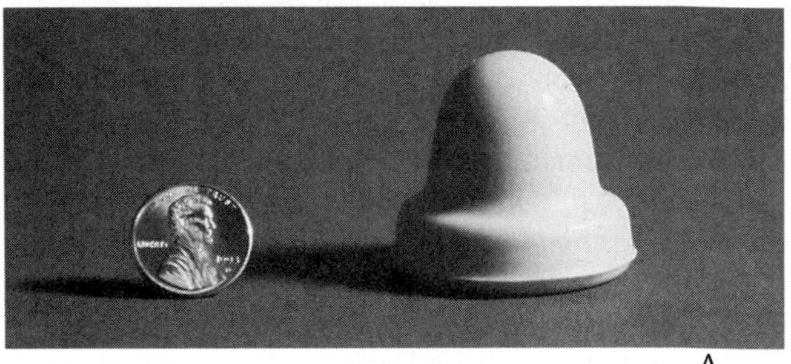

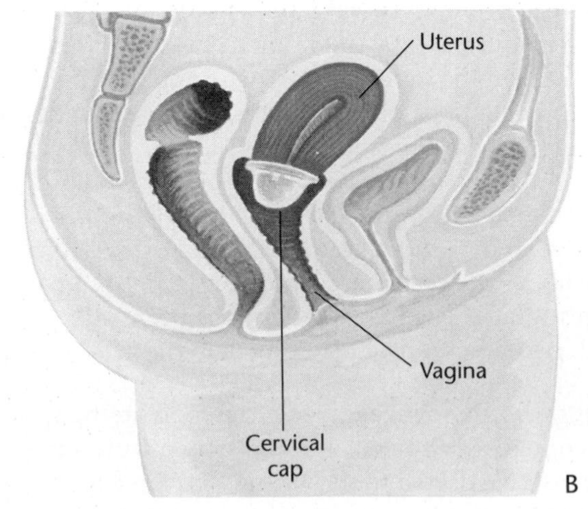

advantages of the cervical cap include its smaller size and lower cost when compared to the diaphragm, and it can be left in place up to 48 hours with no need for additional spermicide. It also provides some protection against STIs. The disadvantage for many young women is that the smaller size makes it more difficult to ensure that the cervical cap is covering the cervix properly.

Cervical Shield The **cervical shield (Lea's Shield)** is a silicone cup with an air valve that fits tightly over the cervix and comes in one size. Like the cervical cap, the shield can remain in place for 48 hours without spermicidal reapplication. It should be left in place for 8 hours after last intercourse. The user effectiveness has not been determined but appears to be slightly higher than that for the cervical cap.

Hormonal Contraceptives

Every woman who chooses to use hormonal contraceptives should know the risks and benefits of use. Hormonal methods are convenient, effective, and reversible, but they provide *no* protection against HIV and other STIs and may cause health risks and side effects in some women. They are intended solely to prevent pregnancy. The primary methods available include oral contraceptives, transdermal patches, rings, injectables, emergency contraception, and implants.

Oral Contraceptives **Oral contraceptives** (OCs) trail voluntary sterilization and IUDs in worldwide use among married women. OCs are the second most popular form of birth control in the United States with 25 percent of all women choosing this method. Among sexually active unmarried women and teens, OCs are the most widely used method of family planning because of their convenience, effectiveness, and reversibility. (See *Women Making a Difference:* "Margaret Sanger: Birth Control Activist.")

The idea of oral contraceptives dates back to the 1920s, but the pill wasn't approved by the FDA until 1960. The first OC, Enovid-10, contained 150 micrograms of ethinyl estradiol and 10 milligrams of noresthisterone (synthetic estrogen) compared to today's OCs of less than 35 micrograms of ethinyl estradiol and less than 1.5 milligrams of noresthisterone.[11,12] Oral contraceptives act primarily by inhibiting ovulation through suppressing follicle stimulating harmone (FSH) and luteinizing harmone (LH). There are basically two types: the combination pills, which contain estrogen and progestin, and the progestin-only type (mini-pills). Most oral contraceptives come in 21- or 28-day packages.

With the 21-day pack, a woman takes one pill each day at the same time for 21 days. Menstruation occurs during the 7 days that she is not taking the pill, and she begins taking the pills again after 7 days. Some women have a difficult time remembering to start taking the pills again after the seventh day, so a 28-day-cycle version is available where one pill is taken at the same time every day. The last seven pills do not contain hormones, and the woman will have her period during that time. The pill is 94 to 97 percent effective in preventing pregnancy when used properly. However, a backup method should be used in the following circumstances:

- When a woman's period begins on a day other than Sunday just before she begins taking a Sunday-start pill, she should use a backup method for the first 7 days that she takes the pill.
- When a woman is vomiting or has diarrhea, her body may not absorb the pill, and she should use a backup method for the rest of the cycle.
- When a woman forgets to take two or more pills during the cycle, she should contact her health care provider and ask for advice.
- When in doubt, use a backup.

Women Making a Difference

Margaret Sanger: Birth Control Activist

Margaret Sanger (1879–1966) was acclaimed worldwide for her founding of the American birth control movement and the Planned Parenthood Federation of America, as well as for her international efforts to encourage family planning. She was responsible for opening the nation's first birth control clinic in the Brownsville section of Brooklyn, in 1916. Sanger established these important principles: that a woman's right to control her body is the foundation of her human rights, that every woman should be able to decide when and whether to have a child, and that volunteers could organize a network of family planning centers. Today, her grandson serves as the chair of the international Planned Parenthood council and carries on the cause of ensuring that all women have the right to decide whether, when, and how many children to have. For more information on Margaret Sanger, check out this Web site: www.nyu.edu/projects/sanger.

- What are some of the ways Sanger's detractors have attempted to discredit her?
- What obstacles did she face?
- How does Margaret Sanger's story parallel some stories of women today?

When asked about the health benefits of OCs, most women cannot provide even one possible health benefit, yet research suggests that OCs provide several benefits. These health benefits include protection against epithelial ovarian and endometrial cancer, lowered risk for ectopic pregnancies and PID, lighter and less painful menstrual flow, and decreases in iron deficiency anemia.[13] Estrogen use has not been associated with increased breast cancer risk to date. A large NIH-sponsored CDC study of approximately 9,000 women between the ages of 35 and 64 who use OCs found that age at first use, higher doses of estrogen, duration of OC use, and family history of breast cancer did not increase the health risk for OC users compared to non-OC users.[14]

OCs may cause health risks and side effects for some women, however. Estrogen use is associated with a number of side effects including nausea, breast pain and soreness, and fluid retention. Progestin-only pills are associated with increased irregular menstrual cycles and vaginal bleeding, and must be taken exactly every 24 hours. If a woman becomes pregnant while on progestin-only pills, she has an increased risk of an ectopic pregnancy. Women should be advised against using hormonal methods if they are at risk for cardiovascular disease (particularly smokers over age 35) or if they have diabetes mellitus or hypertension. Other risks may include blood clots, strokes, changes in bone mineral density, and some reproductive cancers. Side effects from hormonal methods also may include headache, mood changes, dizziness, nervousness, depression, vaginal infections, and allergic skin reactions. Certain drugs may interact with hormonal methods to make them less effective. Some drugs used for epilepsy, herbal supplements such as St. John's wort, and certain antibiotics are a few examples of medications that may interfere with the effectiveness of hormonal contraceptives; however, progestin-only oral contraceptives may be used by women who smoke because they do not contain estrogen, and they may be better for women with diabetes or for those who are breast-feeding. The message is clear: Be aware and be informed! Make a wise consumer choice.

Transdermal (Skin) Patch The FDA approved Ortho Evra, the first **transdermal patch** for birth control, in 2001. Ortho Evra is a 1¾-inch square patch that releases norelgestromin (progestin) and ethinyl estradiol (estrogen) through the skin into the bloodstream. The patch is applied to the lower abdomen, buttocks, upper outer arm, or upper body (not breasts) and is worn continuously for one week. The patch is worn for 3 weeks and removed for the fourth week. A woman menstruates during the fourth week, as she would if she were using birth control pills. The patch prevents pregnancy by suppressing ovulation and also causing the cervical mucus to thicken, making sperm less viable. If the patch becomes loose for more than 24 hours, an alternative, nonhormonal method should be used during the week. Clinical trials have demonstrated 99 percent effectiveness and risks similar to those of birth control pills. Women who use the patch need to know that there is an increased risk of blood clots, heart attack, high blood pressure, stroke, liver tumors, and gallbladder disease, and the label on the package includes a warning that cigarette smoking increases the risk of serious cardiovascular side effects. Five percent of the women in clinical trials had at least one patch that did not stay attached to the skin, and 2 percent withdrew from the trials due to skin irritations. The product was found to be less effective in women weighing more than 198 pounds.[15]

The Ortho Evra patch has recently been linked to several deaths in the United States. Lawsuits are pending. Women should become familiar with the risks before considering this method of birth control. On November 10, 2005, the FDA required that a warning be added about the increased health risks due to high levels of estrogen released from the Ortho Evra patch.

The Ring NuvaRing is a clear, flexible, thin polymer **ring** that provides a continuous low dose of etonogestrel (progestin) and ethinyl estradiol (estrogen) that suppresses ovulation and causes the cervical mucus to thicken, thus preventing pregnancy. The ring is inserted into the vagina, similarly to a diaphragm, and remains in place surrounding the cervix for 3 weeks. The ring is removed at the beginning of the fourth week, and a woman menstruates 2 to 3 days after its removal, similar to the cycle for birth control pills. The used ring should be wrapped and disposed of in the a wastebasket, not flushed. A new ring is inserted on the same day of the week as the previous one was removed. NuvaRing is available by prescription and is 98 to 99 percent effective when used correctly. Side effects and contraindications similar to those of birth control pills should be expected. If the ring slips (through improper placement or some exerting force), and it has been out of the vagina for less than 3 hours, the woman is still protected from pregnancy.[16] However, using a condom as a backup for 7 days may be a wise decision.

Hormonal Injections LUNELLE monthly contraceptive injection was approved by the FDA in 2000 but is not currently available in the United States. It is a type of hormonal injection that is given in the arm, thigh, or buttock monthly to prevent pregnancy. When given monthly as prescribed, it is as effective as oral contraceptives. The failure rate of this method of birth control is less than 1 percent per year. The active ingredients are medroxyprogesterone acetate (a chemical similar to the natural hormone progesterone that is produced by the ovaries during the second half of the menstrual cycle) and estradiol cypionate (estrogen). Side effects and contraindications for users of LUNELLE are similar to those for users of oral contraceptives.

Depo-Provera (DMPA) is the most widely used progestin injection. It is injected into the gluteal or deltoid muscle of a woman once every 3 months. Depo-Provera contains depot medroxyprogesterone acetate, which prevents the egg from ripening, thus suppressing ovulation so that the egg cannot be fertilized by the sperm. It also thickens cervical mucus to keep sperm from fertilizing a viable egg. Depo-Provera lasts approximately 12 weeks and has high effectiveness (99.7 percent) and reversibility. Nearly 50 percent of women who stop using Depo-Provera because they want to get pregnant are expected to become pregnant within 10 months after their last injection, 66 percent of women are expected to become pregnant within a year, and 93 percent are expected to become pregnant within 18 months. The most common side effect is vaginal bleeding, and other side effects may include amenorrhea, weight gain, headache, nervousness, dizziness, stomach cramps, and decreased sex drive.[17] DMPA is not recommended for use of greater than 2 consecutive years, unless a woman cannot use another method, because of evidence of temporary bone thinning.

Emergency Contraception The FDA approved the first combination estrogen and progestin emergency contraceptive pill (ECP), Preven, in 1998. One year later, the FDA approved Plan B, the first progestin-only ECP. ECPs work by delaying ovulation or preventing fertilization or implantation. Postcoital contraception has been available since the early 1970s when a Canadian obstetrician/gynecologist, Dr. Albert Yuzpe, began prescribing an adaptation of the birth control pill for avoiding unintended pregnancies. ECPs contain hormones that reduce the risk of pregnancy when taken within 120 hours of unprotected intercourse. ECPs can be taken in one or two doses, 12 hours apart, and are given to delay or inhibit ovulation, alter the tubal transport of sperm or ova to inhibit fertilization, and/or alter the endometrium to inhibit implantation.[18] The sooner the regimen is begun, the better the outcome. If taken within 72 hours of unprotected intercourse, Preven has been found to reduce the risk of pregnancy by 75 percent and Plan B by 89 percent. If taken within 24 hours of unprotected intercourse, Plan B has a 95 percent effectiveness rate. In 2003 an FDA advisory panel concluded that Plan B is effective and safe for use by women and should be made available without a prescription. In 2006, Plan B was approved for over-the-counter purchase by women 18 years and older. For women younger than 18 years, Plan B must be prescribed by a health care provider. This approval makes it difficult for some of the most vulnerable young women at risk of unwanted pregnancies.

Emergency IUD (intrauterine device) insertion is also a choice within 5 days of unprotected intercourse and reduces the risk of pregnancy by 99.9 percent. It must be inserted and removed by a health care provider. The Copper T 380A IUD (ParaGard) can be left in place for up to 10 years or can be removed with the next menstrual cycle. The risks and benefits of IUDs are the same as when used for regular birth control. The cost of this method is greater than for other ECPs, around $400 for the exam, IUD, and insertion, an average of about $40 a year over the 10-year period. ECPs do not induce a medical abortion or affect the developing pre-embryo or embryo. Rather, ECPs prevent pregnancy in cases of unanticipated sexual activity, contraceptive failure, or sexual assault. Side effects of the medication include nausea and vomiting and possible breast tenderness, irregular bleeding, abdominal pain, headaches, and dizziness. Progestin-only ECP tends to have fewer side effects. The cost of the medication is minimal, and it has the potential to reduce the overall rate of abortion. Many physicians, particularly on college campuses, have been prescribing this contraceptive method for decades. ECPs are not intended to replace regular birth control, and they do not prevent pregnancy during the remaining part of the cycle.

Unfortunately, distorted information provided by-Pro-Life groups has resulted in some health care providers' refusing to write prescriptions and some pharmacists' refusing to fill prescriptions for women who request the pills. These health care providers and pharmacists believe the procedure is a form of medical abortion. However, the general medical definition of pregnancy endorsed by the American College of Obstetricians and Gynecologists in 1998 and by the U.S. Department of Health and Human Services in 1978 is that pregnancy begins when a pre-embryo completes implantation into the lining of the uterus. ECPs provide women with a viable alternative to unintended pregnancies. The best family planning methods involve pre-pregnancy planning and protected intercourse. When postcoital contraception is needed, it should be available. In the United States, a woman can call 1-800-230-PLAN to find a Planned Parenthood agency or 1-888-NOT-2-LATE for other sources of emergency contraception.

Implants In July 2006, the FDA approved a new, long-term birth control method, Implanon. Implanon is inserted subdermally on the inner side of the arm. Unlike an older implant called Norplant, which contained six matchstick-size rods, Implanon is a single-rod implantable contraceptive (etonogestrel, a progestin) that is 99 percent effective for up to 3 years. The risks associated with the implant are similar to those of other progestin-only contraceptives, including irregular bleeding, headache, acne, dysmenorrhea, and amenorrhea. Minimal local implant-site complications were noted in the clinical trials. As with all hormonal contraceptives, cigarette smoking increases the risk for serious cardiovascular and thromboembolic diseases. Implanon is currently available in 30 countries.

Norplant was developed by the Population Council and distributed in the United States by Wyeth Pharmaceuticals until 2002. Norplant (levonorgestrel) was a progestin-only implant consisting of six flexible, matchstick-like capsules filled with levonorgestrel that dissipated slowly over a 5-year time frame. The major advantage was its long-term effectiveness; the major disadvantages were the complications experienced by many women and the coercion of low-income women to use this method. By 1995 more than 200 lawsuits, including 50 class-action suits, had been filed against Wyeth Pharmaceuticals. Most of these claims were dismissed when the FDA found no basis for questioning the safety or effectiveness of Norplant when used correctly.[19] However, Norplant is no longer available in the United States, and women who wanted to have the capsules removed were able to contact Wyeth Pharmaceuticals for a referral to cover costs.

Contraindications for Hormonal Methods A woman considering any hormonal method should be asked by her health care provider whether she is pregnant and if she has active liver disease, heart problems, breast cancer, diabetes, hypertension, migraine headaches, epilepsy, or a history of blood clotting. Research regarding the effect of hormonal methods on these conditions remains mixed, and a woman may choose another method if she has any of these conditions. A woman should be asked about her sexual history, including whether she or her partner has other sexual partners. Although hormonal methods are highly effective in preventing pregnancy, they provide no protection against HIV/AIDS and other STIs.

Other Birth Control Methods

Other birth control methods also deserve consideration. These methods include intrauterine devices and sterilization. Even though intrauterine devices have lost favor in the United States, they remain one of the most common forms of birth control in other countries. And sterilization is the leading form of birth control in the United States.

Intrauterine Devices The World Health Organization and the American Medical Association call **intrauterine devices** (IUDs) one of the safest, most effective, and least expensive reversible methods of birth control available to women. Worldwide, nearly 11 percent of all married women of reproductive age use IUDs with rates in China as high as 45 percent. Contrast those statistics with the U.S. rate of less than 1 percent of all women who use contraceptive methods.[20] The IUD lost favor in the United States primarily as a result of the high risk of side effects connected to one faulty brand, the Dalkon Shield, which was withdrawn from the U.S. market in 1974 due to complaints of pelvic infections. The extensions on each side of this product were intended to prevent expulsion, but they also made insertion and removal more painful. In addition, the porous product allowed bacteria to enter the uterus, causing severe pelvic inflammatory disease (PID). The Dalkon Shield was removed from the market by the manufacturer in 1974 under pressure from reproductive rights advocates and the FDA.

Another reason for its lack of popularity was the belief that the IUD worked by preventing implantation of the fertilized egg into the uterus. Pro-Life groups viewed this as a form of abortion. Informed consensus now suggests that the IUD works by preventing fertilization. The method works by reducing the number and viability of the sperm reaching the egg or impeding the number and movement of eggs in the uterus. Current IUDs such as the Copper T380A are more effective than oral contraceptives and similar in effectiveness to implants, injectables, and voluntary sterilization in preventing pregnancies. (See Figure 9.9.)

The research now demonstrates when and why women who use IUDs might experience a higher incidence of pelvic inflammatory disease. The increased risk of PID occurs in the first month after IUD insertion and, most often, among women exposed to STIs. Risk of infection depends more on the service provided than on the IUD itself. Health care providers should be trained to use sterile practices for inserting IUDs. Overall, IUDs are no longer associated with an increased risk of ectopic pregnancies or infertility resulting from PID. The T Cu-380A (ParaGard) is now FDA-approved for effective use up to 12 years rather than the previous 4 years. ParaGard was developed by the Population Council and introduced into the U.S. market in 1988. Method effectiveness is a 1 in 100 chance of pregnancy in the first year of use and 2.1 in 100 in 10 years of use. Mirena, a hormonal IUD that remains effective for 5 years, works by releasing small amounts of the hormone progestin into the uterus. It was approved for use in the United States in 2000 and is used in more than ten other countries. Mirena may be the most effective IUD of all, and it ranks among the best family planning methods for protecting against pregnancy. Some reproductive rights advocates are hoping that it will rekindle an

FIGURE 9.9 *(A)* Progestasert IUD. *(B)* Copper T380A (ParaGard) IUD.

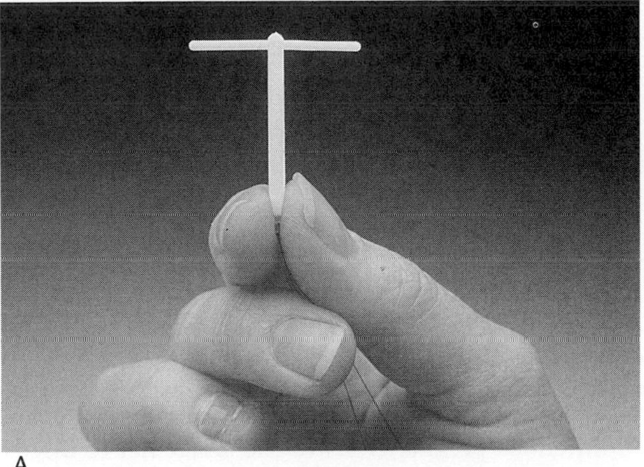

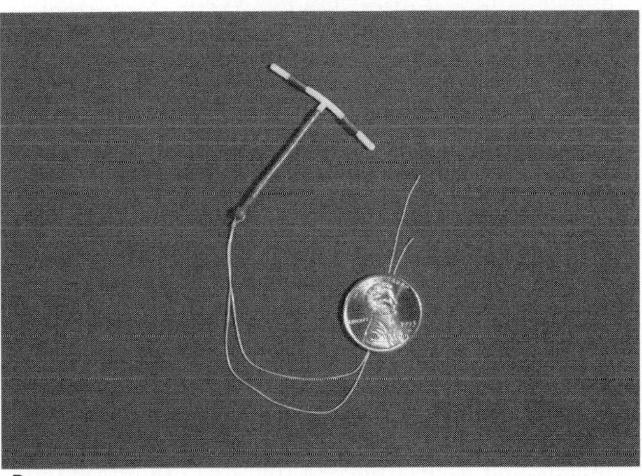

interest in IUDs in the United States. An update by the Population Council provides the following guidelines for health care providers:

- IUDs can be inserted at any time during the menstrual cycle if it is reasonably certain the woman is not pregnant.
- Current genital infection and high STI risk rule out IUD use, but past ectopic pregnancy and past PID do not.
- Only one follow-up visit is necessary—3 to 6 weeks after insertion to check for infection or expulsion. Return visits are encouraged if the woman has questions or wants the IUD removed.
- A woman of any reproductive age can use an IUD as long as she is not at risk for STIs.
- Properly trained providers can insert IUDs immediately after childbirth or early abortion.
- Nurses, midwives, and health care providers can be trained to safely insert IUDs.[21]

FIGURE 9.10 (*A*) Vasectomy. (*B*) Tubal ligation.

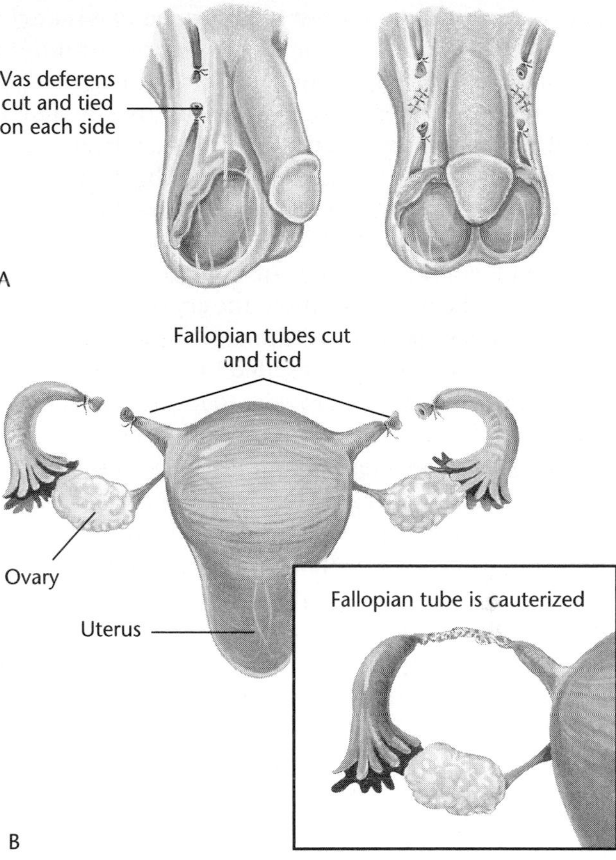

Sterilization Sterilization methods, *tubal ligation* and *vasectomy,* are the most common form of contraceptive method used by women over age 30 and by men. (See Figure 9.10.) Among ever-married women ages 15–44 years in 1995, 41 percent were surgically sterile (15.3 million women), 26 percent had a tubal ligation, 7 percent had a hysterectomy, and 12 percent were living with a partner who had a vasectomy. Since 1982 tubal ligation has become more common than vasectomy. These methods have low failure rates and low reversibility, so they should be considered only when voluntarily choosing to have no more children. Women with multiple partners or who have a partner with multiple partners still need to consider using a condom for protection against STIs and HIV/AIDS.

Tubal ligation can be performed on an outpatient basis or it can require hospitalization, depending on the type of procedure. It is the most prevalent form of birth control used in the United States. The surgery involves closing the fallopian tubes—either by inserting microinserts or by cauterizing, tying, cutting, or clamping—thus preventing the egg from becoming fertilized. A no-incision method (Essure) can be performed by a clinician who inserts two small, soft metallic coils into the fallopian tubes through the uterus. The coils cause scar tissue to grow, thus blocking the fallopian tubes. Three months after insertion, a test is performed to ensure the tubes are permanently blocked. Essure cannot be performed until 6 weeks after childbirth, miscarriage, or abortion. Advantages are numerous, but risks should be noted. Women should check with their health care provider about her or his expertise with this method. Laparoscopy, sometimes referred to as "Band-Aid" surgery, is completed through a small incision near the navel and is one of the most common methods of sterilization. Before the incision, the abdomen is inflated with a harmless gas to allow the organs to be seen more clearly.[22] A laparoscope is inserted into a small incision allowing the health care provider to locate the fallopian tube. Then, another incision is made through which the fallopian tubes are closed or an instrument is inserted through the laparoscope. This outpatient surgery takes 20 to 30 minutes to perform. Tubal ligation is most often performed immediately after childbirth. Mini-laparotomy does not require gas or a visualizing instrument. One incision is made into the abdomen through which both fallopian tubes are tied. Tubal ligation is a permanent procedure for a woman who is certain she does not want to have more children. A review of the Nurses' Health Study showed that women who underwent tubal ligation had a one-fourth lower risk of ovarian cancer.[23] Women experiencing unusual symptoms (bleeding from the vagina, fever, or discharge, bleeding or redness at the surgical site) after tubal ligation should contact their health care provider immediately.

Vasectomy is the third most popular form of contraception available, with nearly 500,000 men choosing this method each year. The traditional vasectomy is an office procedure, including one or two incisions by the surgeon to access each vas deferens. Each vas is then cauterized, tied, or sutured to prevent sperm from being ejaculated. An alternative is the no-scalpel, no incision vasectomy (NSV) procedure in which the surgeon anesthetizes the vas deferens, makes a small puncture to access each vas, and then cauterizes, lasers, sutures, or hemoclips them. NSV, when compared to conventional vasectomy, reduces the psychological barrier for many men, the surgical time from 20–30 minutes to 5–11 minutes, and the risk for infection, bleeding, and pain.[24]

After vasectomy, couples should use another form of contraceptive control until all sperm have been cleared from the ampullar storage area, which can take several weeks. A semen sample should be examined by a health care provider to determine that the sperm count has reached zero. The advantages of vasectomy, whether conventional or NSV, include its greater safety and cost effectiveness compared to tubal ligation, its low failure rate, and better rates of reversibility than tubal ligation has. The cost of a vasectomy is nearly 6 times less than the cost of tubal ligation. A common myth about vasectomy is that after the procedure males will lose their masculinity. Research shows no relationship between vasectomy and loss of masculinity or between vasectomy and prostate cancer, testicular cancer, or atherosclerosis, although studies are still being conducted.

Birth control and STI prevention are not just a woman's issue. Decisions regarding family planning and STI protection are a joint effort with both partners sharing responsibility. If a woman feels she is solely responsible for contraceptive choices, she may want to reevaluate the relationship. We strongly encourage a woman to protect her body from unwanted diseases and unintended pregnancies. We encourage her to discuss birth control considerations with her partner. Her partner should be willing to take an active and supportive role in family planning. (See *FYI:* "Male Contraception: Myths and Facts.") Remember, family planning is a joint venture.

MATERNAL AND INFANT MORTALITY

Every minute of every day, somewhere in the world, a woman dies as a result of complications arising during pregnancy or childbirth. The majority of these deaths are avoidable. **Maternal mortality** is the best indicator of the status of women, particularly their health status. Maternal mortality is defined as the death of a woman while pregnant, regardless of the site or duration of the pregnancy, from any cause related to or aggravated by the pregnancy or its management. Estimates of maternal mortality rates worldwide average 430 deaths per 100,000 pregnancies; 27 per 100,000 in developed countries compared to 480 per 100,000 in developing countries and with rates as high as 1 death per 10 pregnancies in some parts of Africa. (See *Her Story:* "Dr. Catherine Hamlin: Making a Difference for women in Africa" on page 218.)

Maternal deaths are classified as direct or indirect obstetric deaths. Direct obstetric deaths account for 80 percent of all maternal deaths and result from complications such as incorrect or inadequate treatment during pregnancy, labor, or postpartum. The most common complication is hemorrhage, usually during the postpartum phase. Infection, hypertensive disorders, prolonged or obstructive labor, and complications of unsafe abortions account for the remaining direct causes. Indirect obstetric deaths account for 20 percent of all maternal deaths and result from previous existing diseases or diseases caused by the physiological complications of pregnancy.[25] Anemia is a significant indirect

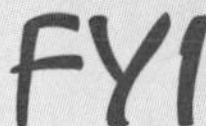

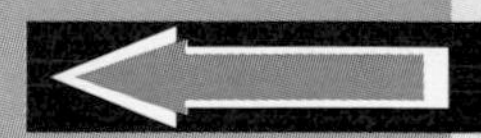

Male Contraception: Myths and Facts

When it comes to male contraception, many sayings get repeated because they *sound* good; most people haven't thought much about them. Here are some common "sound bites" and some new ways of thinking about them:

Myth	Fact
"Men aren't interested in contraception or in taking responsibility."	Men are already using their only two options, vasectomy and condoms. According to the World Health Organization (WHO), a safe new reversible, nonsurgical method could attract 41 to 75 percent of men. Several potential methods for vasectomy are being studied. These include chemical compounds (phenol mixed with alcohol) injected into each vas deferens, silicone plugs inserted into each vas deferens, and reversible vasectomy by chemicals that block the movement of the sperm.
"It's easier to stop one egg than millions of sperm."	Physically, it's easier to stop millions of sperm than one egg. The sperm travel through the vas deferens, which are easily accessed tubes where they can be incapacitated or blocked. Current tests include battery-powered capsules (implanted in each vas deferens) that emit low-level electrical currents to immobilize sperm and subdermal implants to reduce sperm counts.
"It's easier to control ovulation (one egg) than spermatogenesis (millions of sperm)."	WHO studies have shown greatly reduced sperm counts in men injected once a week with testosterone enanthate (TE), a synthetic hormone. Research also is being conducted to test a combination of TE with depot medroxyprogesterone acetate (DMPA), the progestin used in Depo-Provera. This injection may be needed only once a month. A 3-month injection (using testosterone buciclate) is being developed. A new group of drugs (gonadotropin-releasing hormone antagonists) can be used to prevent the release of FSH and LH from the pituitary glands in men and women. FSH and LH trigger ovulation and spermatogenesis. Blocking the release of these hormones may suppress fertility for men and women.
"Why develop these methods when they don't prevent the spread of HIV/AIDS?	Why develop Implanon, Depo-Provera, or transdermal patches?
"Women won't trust men to use these methods."	Unlike the "pill" concept, most nonhormonal methods are easy for a female partner to verify. She can go to the doctor with the man when he gets a shot, for example, or help him with the method herself. Also, see below.
"Men would never use this method because . . ." • It's too permanent • It's not permanent enough • It requires dedication • It requires a shot • It's not perfect for younger men • It's not perfect for older men • Etc. (Fill in the blank)	No one method is right for everybody. A "contraceptive supermarket" (a variety of choices) best suits everybody's needs.
"Why develop these methods when we're not sure they'll be completely safe and effective?"	If we never try, we'll never know.

Her Story

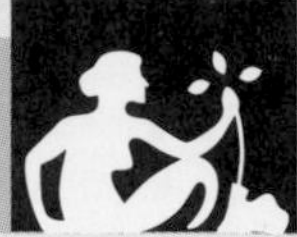

Dr. Catherine Hamlin: Making a Difference for Women in Africa

Dr. Catherine Hamlin, a native Australian who lives in Ethiopia, provides a unique and necessary medical service for Africa's poor women. In 1974 she and her husband, Dr. Reginald Hamlin, opened the only hospital then on the continent dedicated to providing surgery for *obstetrical fistulas*. Fistulas are serious childbirth injuries caused by long or obstructed labor in which blood supply is cut off to the tissues of the vagina, bladder, or rectum, causing these tissues to weaken and die. Eventually, a hole forms in the pelvis through which urine or feces passes uncontrollably, leaving a woman incontinent and malodorous as well as vulnerable to secondary infections. Fistulas are almost nonexistent in developed countries where obstetrical care and cesarean deliveries are routine. In poor and developing countries, however, this condition complicates labor and delivery for as many as 1 to 2 million girls and women per year. Girls forced to marry at young ages are more susceptible to fistulas due to physical immaturity at the time of their labor. Fistulas are rarely fatal and certainly not contagious. Nevertheless, afflicted girls and women are often rejected by their husbands and shunned by family, fellow villagers, and others who do not understand the medical facts behind the condition. Disgraced and humiliated, and often isolated from village life, these women have no chance of leading a normal life unless the fistula is repaired.

At the Addis Ababa Fistula Hospital, Dr. Hamlin and a rotating team of medical specialists provide surgery to the women who are fortunate enough to make their way to her center. The surgery repairs the fistula, enabling women to regain enough health and dignity to return to their homes and rebuild their lives. Women here receive not only reparative surgery but recovery time and counseling as well. All services are provided by the Fistula Hospital for free.

Occasionally, a woman has a fistula injury so severe or entrenched that she cannot completely recover. For such a woman, the hospital provides a 60-acre plot of land called the "Desta Mender," or "Village of Joy." Here, women unable to return to their own villages are allowed to live permanently in homes where they work land, grow food, and maintain themselves with respect. Dr. Hamlin has also trained many of her former patients in nursing, surgical, and counseling skills so that women who once suffered are now helping others.

Since its inception, The Fistula Hospital has treated over 25,000 women. While this figure is significant, sadly, it represents only a fraction of the enormous numbers of women in developing nations who need this help.

Catherine Hamlin has been named one of Australia's "National Treasures" and was nominated for the Nobel Peace Price in 1999.[26]

Questions and Discussion Points

- In what ways is Dr. Hamlin making a difference in women's lives?
- Obstetrical fistulas are largely preventable. What do you think are some of the reasons why this problem exists in poor and developing nations?
- To what other serious medical conditions do you think a woman suffering from an untreated fistula is vulnerable?
- Why do you think hospitals such as this are rare in countries where they are most needed?
- The Fistula Hospital is funded solely by private donations and operates on a meager yearly budget. If it were treating a similar condition in boys and men, do you think governmental and other groups would be more willing to provide financial aid? Why or why not?

cause of death (and may be an underlying cause of hemorrhage and infection). Other causes include malaria, hepatitis, heart disease, and HIV/AIDS. In the United States, the maternal mortality rate is higher among African American women than among white women.

The World Health Organization has determined that three interventions are essential to promote safe motherhood:

- Reducing the number of high-risk and unwanted pregnancies
- Reducing the number of obstetric complications
- Reducing deaths among women who develop complications [27]

The best mechanism for preventing maternal deaths is continuing to improve the status of women, including access to education, health care, and proper nutrition. The WHO acknowledges that maternal death is not only a health issue but also a matter of social justice. The long-term goal of bettering the status of women can be supplemented by the short-term goals of providing universal access to family planning and skilled health care.

Infant mortality, like maternal mortality, is an important indicator of a country's health status. Infant mortality is defined as the deaths of infants under 1 year old; neonatal mortality is deaths of infants under 28 days; and postneonatal mortality is deaths of infants aged 28 days to 11 months. The overall U.S. infant mortality rate is 6.9 deaths per 1,000 live births with rates of 5.8 for non-Hispanic white mothers and 14.6 for non-Hispanic black mothers. Education is another important indicator. The mortality rate is significantly higher for infants whose mothers have less than 12 years of education. The primary causes for neonatal and infant mortality are congenital anomalies, preterm/low birth weight, sudden infant death syndrome (SIDS), problems from complications of pregnancy, and respiratory distress syndrome.[28]

PROMOTING HEALTHY PREGNANCY OUTCOMES

Pre-pregnancy Planning

When a woman decides to become pregnant, pre-pregnancy planning is the first step to promote the healthiest outcome. Pre-pregnancy planning encompasses not taking any drugs without the consent of a health care provider, nutritional planning, exercise, a time lapse of one menstrual cycle between contraceptive use and conception, immunizations, and folic acid supplements. These lifestyle changes should begin as soon as a childbearing woman is contemplating pregnancy—that is, before conception and before stopping birth control. If a woman smokes cigarettes, she should quit before getting pregnant because smoking during pregnancy increases the risks of low birth weight, a premature birth, or having a newborn with increased respiratory problems. If a woman drinks alcoholic beverages, she should stop drinking before getting pregnant because alcoholic beverages can cause infertility and birth defects, and no amount is safe for a pregnant woman and her baby. Any drugs, including over-the-counter drugs, should not be taken without the consent of a health care provider. Proper nutrition and exercise includes eating appropriately from the food pyramid, avoiding megadoses of vitamins and minerals, and working out in moderation. Folic acid is a nutritional supplement that provides protection against neural tube defects (defects of the brain and/or spinal cord) to the fetus. The U.S. Public Health Service recommends 0.4 milligram of folic acid (the amount found in vitamin supplements) beginning 1 month before conception and through the first trimester. If a childbearing woman and her partner are contemplating pregnancy, it is important to discuss pre-pregnancy planning with a health care provider.

Conception

Pregnancy begins with the union of the female egg, or ovum, and the male spermatozoan. These two gametes become fused into one cell, or **zygote,** that contains the characteristics of both the female and the male. The female ovum contains 23 chromosomes, and the sex chromosome of the mature ovum is always of the X type. The mature spermatozoan contains 23 chromosomes and may have an X type or Y type, thus determining the sex of the baby. The fertilized ovum again contains 46 chromosomes, 23 from the ovum and 23 from the spermatozoan. The fallopian tubes provide the environment in which fertilization occurs and cell division begins. (See Color Plate 3.) After 3 days, the fertilized ovum is transported into the uterus. Premature expulsion from the fallopian tube could result in failure to implant, and prolonged retention in the tube could result in an ectopic pregnancy. The fertilized ovum spends another 4 days before implanting; thus, the process from fertilization to implantation is approximately 7 days. Once the chorionic villi cover the ovum, the villi begin producing hCG (the hormone tested for pregnancy). This hormone maintains the progesterone production by the corpus luteum, which supports endometrial growth. The villi decrease over time. Without hCG, the corpus luteum would degenerate, as it does in menstruation, and the **embryo** would be aborted and the woman might not even know she had been pregnant.

Twins and Multiple Births The inner cell mass, a small cluster of cells that projects into the cavity of a **blastocyst** (early embryonic cells before a cell layer has formed), may occasionally subdivide to form two separate groups of cells. Because the groups of cells have identical genes, they develop into identical twins. Fraternal twins develop when a woman ovulates two ova that are then fertilized by separate sperm. Because the sperm and ova have separate genetic codes, the fraternal twins are not identical and may be of the opposite sex. Fraternal twins are no more genetically similar than siblings from different births. Triplets and other multiple-birth babies may be either identical or fraternal depending on whether they develop from a single ovum and sperm or multiple ova and sperm.

Amnion The **amnion** (membranous sac) begins to develop even before the embryo evolves and eventually surrounds it. The amnion cavity, a fluid-filled space many of them deemed unnecessary. As a result of these reports and better monitoring, the rate of cesarean births declined and the rate of vaginal births after previous cesarean (VBAC) delivery increased from 1991 to 1996 (8 percent and 33 percent, respectively). However, since 1997, the cesarean rate has been increasing and the VBAC rate decreasing, 6 percent and 17 percent by 1999. In 1999 there were 862,068 cesarean births for a rate of 22 per 100 births, or nearly 1 in 4 or 5. Cesarean rates are lowest for teen mothers and increase steadily with maternal age. In 1999 there were 97,680 births delivered by VBAC with rates highest in teenagers and lowest in older mothers. Throughout the 1990s, women having their first child and women with diabetes, genital herpes, hypertension, eclampsia, incompetent cervix, and uterine bleeding were more likely to have cesarean deliveries.[37,38]

Data related to CNM-assisted births provide interesting comparisons to physician-assisted births. A study of differences among obstetricians, family physicians, and CNMs caring for low-risk women found that the cesarean rate for patients of CNMs was 8.8 percent compared with 13.6 percent for obstetricians and 15.1 percent for family physicians. Several other studies had similar findings of fewer cesarean deliveries by patients of CNMs.

Another interesting aspect of hospital deliveries was the dramatic decline in the average number of postpartum hospital stays for mothers and newborns. The average stay was 4 days in 1970, 2 days in 1993, and 1 day or less by 1995. A public outcry about "drive-through deliveries" prompted several states, and then the federal government, in 1996, to mandate that insurers cover minimum 48-hour hospital stays following vaginal deliveries and 96-hour stays following cesareans. One study confirmed the potential adverse impact of early postpartum discharge. Newborns discharged within 30 hours of birth were four times more likely to die within 28 days of birth, and two times more likely to die during the first year than newborns discharged more than 30 hours after birth. The potential for delayed diagnosis of curable, life-threatening conditions such as congenital heart disease and sepsis could be fatal.[39]

Birth Centers Birth centers are designed for the delivery of low-risk pregnancies. They provide a relaxed atmosphere, similar to all-in-one hospital rooms. In fact, as hospitals witnessed the growing popularity of birth centers, they began to market similar services to their patients. Birth centers emphasize collaboration between OB-GYNs, nurses, and CNMs. Some centers are freestanding and others are connected to a hospital. There are some differences between birth center and hospital deliveries. Birth centers typically do not follow hospital routines such as preps, enemas, IVs, continuous fetal monitoring, or routine episiotomies. The fetal heartbeat is monitored, but usually by a handheld Doppler instrument, which allows the pregnant woman more freedom to move. Episiotomy rates in birth centers are approximately 12 percent, compared to 90 percent in hospitals.

The philosophy of the birth center is to keep the mother and newborn together, so treatments and exams of the newborn are conducted in front of the parents. The environment is relaxed and as low tech as possible. The attending health care providers (CNM, DO or MD, and nurse) work together as a team. Most women have no complications with the deliveries, with only about 2 percent transferred to the hospital as emergency transports and 10 percent for precautionary reasons. All birth centers are linked to the acute care level of a hospital, ensuring safety for mother and baby.[40]

Birthing Positions

The traditional recumbent position, while still the norm, is being replaced by a variety of other strategies. The disadvantages of the recumbent position are compression of major blood vessels and lack of help from gravity, and the mother is more likely to need an episiotomy or to experience tearing. Better positions and supports are available that have advantages and disadvantages. Positions may include walking, sitting, getting on hands and knees, squatting, kneeling (leaning forward with support), leaning, semi-sitting, and side-lying. Supports may include birth chairs, birth balls, and sitting on a toilet. Walking has the advantages of using gravity, reducing backache, encouraging descent, aligning the baby with the pelvis, and encouraging uterine contractility. This position isn't recommended for mothers with high blood pressure and can't be used with continuous electronic fetal monitoring. Semi-sitting also uses gravity, is good for resting, can be used with continuous electronic fetal monitoring, works well in a hospital bed, and provides good viewing for others present for the birth. It presents some stress to the perineum and impairs the mobility of the coccyx (tailbone). Sitting on a toilet relaxes the perineum (reducing the risk of laceration), uses gravity, and is a familiar open-leg position for the mother. The major disadvantage is possible pain caused from the pressure of the toilet seat. Side-lying provides good fetal oxygenation, a good resting position for the mother, makes contractions more effective, and moves the labor forward. It is the best position for avoiding laceration and the need for an episiotomy and taking pressure off hemorrhoids. It is a good delivery position for a large baby and is useful if the mother has epidural anesthesia or elevated blood pressure. The disadvantages include poor eye contact with the mother and her inability to view the birth. Also, attendants may not be as familiar with this position and may have some difficulty as the baby passes through the mother's legs. Squatting is a familiar position used in many countries. It encourages rapid descent and uses gravity, allows freedom to shift weight for comfort, is excellent for fetal circulation, can increase the pelvic diameter, and provides good alignment for the baby on the descent. However, this position can be tiring for the mother and makes it difficult for the mother to assist in the delivery. It can also make listening for fetal heartbeat difficult. Other birthing positions may be used, and reviewing the advantages and disadvantages is helpful.[41]

BREAST-FEEDING

Breast-feeding has prevented nearly 6 million infant deaths each year worldwide and has the potential to prevent an additional 1 to 2 million child deaths each year. The percentage of women in the United States who are breast-feeding has been increasing, particularly among racial and ethnic minorities. The advantages of breast milk over formula are well known and include its inexpensiveness, its better nutritional quality, its ability to act as a birth control measure to limit fertility, and its role in reducing ovarian and premenopausal breast cancer.[42]

Breast milk is unique and, because of its qualities, more women should be encouraged to breast-feed their infants. Breast milk has been described as "dynamic," ever changing in content to meet the needs of a growing infant. It provides the perfect mix of nutrients, hormones, and proteins and cannot be duplicated. Lactose, the predominant sugar in milk, cannot be found in any other natural state. **Colostrum,** the initial milk produced by the mother, has numerous infection-fighting agents and is tailored to the needs of the infant. Breast-feeding plays a role in reducing obesity, helps prevent insulin-dependent diabetes and high cholesterol, and significantly decreases the risk of several acute and chronic diseases. It has been associated with better psychomotor and mental development and reduced risk of celiac disease (a malabsorption syndrome of the gastrointestinal tract), some childhood cancers, Crohn's disease (a chronic inflammatory bowel disease affecting the digestive tract), urinary tract infections, and atopic disease (a genetic disorder related to allergies and asthma). In addition, "The colostrum present in mothers delivering premature infants contains a much higher concentration of protein, anti-infection fighting components, and infection fighting cells than colostrum of full-term infants. Also, the more premature the infant, the higher the concentrations of these components."[43]

Breast-feeding has beneficial health results for the mother as well as the infant. Maternal benefits when breast-feeding begins immediately include reducing the risk of hemorrhage by helping the uterus contract; reducing the risk of breast and ovarian cancer, osteoporosis, and endometriosis; and assisting in family planning. The longer a woman breast-feeds her children, the lower her risk of breast cancer. The Lactational Amenorrhea Method (LAM), a family planning method, uses three measures to determine a woman's fertility: the return of a menstrual period, the pattern of breast-feeding, and the length of time since birth. The chance of getting pregnant is less than 2 percent if menstruation has not resumed, breast-feeding is regular and on demand, and the infant is less than 6 months old.[44]

Breast-feeding is awkward for some mothers and babies to learn. It is a specific learned skill and, given adequate assistance, both mother and infant will be successful unless unusual circumstances exist. Almost every mother can breast-feed. The Baby-Friendly Hospital Initiative is a joint project of the World Health Organization and UNICEF. Nearly 170 countries with 4,282 hospitals have participated in the program since its inception in 1991. *FYI:* "Ten Steps to Successful Breast-Feeding" presents the criteria for successful breast-feeding, which a facility must satisfy to qualify as a baby-friendly hospital.

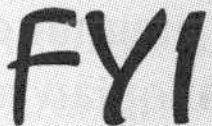

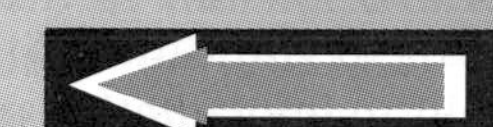

Ten Steps to Successful Breast-Feeding

Every facility providing maternity services and care for newborn infants should

1. Have a written breast-feeding policy that is routinely communicated to all health care staff.
2. Train all health care staff in skills necessary to implement this policy.
3. Inform all pregnant women about the benefits and management of breast-feeding.
4. Help mothers initiate breast-feeding within a half hour of birth.
5. Show mothers how to breast-feed and how to maintain lactation even if they have to be separated from their infants such as if they return to work.
6. Give newborn infants no food or drink other than breast-milk, unless medically indicated.
7. Practice rooming-in: allow mothers and infants to remain together 24 hours a day.
8. Encourage breast-feeding on demand.
9. Give no artificial teats or pacifiers (also called dummies or soothers) to breast-feeding infants.
10. Foster the establishment of breast-feeding support groups and refer mothers to them on discharge from the hospital or clinic.

Her Story

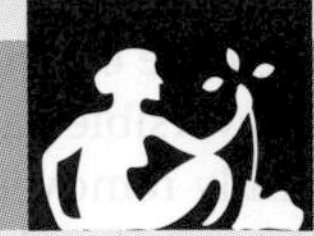

Toni and Kelly: Lesbian Parents

Toni and Kelly, a lesbian couple, chose artificial insemination as their route to having children. They have been together in a committed relationship for 8 years. When Toni decided she wanted to have a baby, she was 35 years old. Kelly thought it was a great idea and they immediately started asking friends about their options. Soon they found a health care provider who was willing to work with them and who informed them about a fertility clinic in California that would mail-order sperm to them. They contacted the clinic and received an information packet with the description and background information on a variety of sperm donors who were identified only by a code number. After careful consideration, they chose donor number 872. After working with their health care provider to determine the best time to inseminate, Toni placed a call to the clinic, and the sperm, frozen in liquid nitrogen, was delivered to their front door by UPS when the time was most optimal for fertization. Kelly and Toni carefully followed the directions, thawed the sperm, and Kelly inseminated Toni using a small plastic syringe. Toni got pregnant on the second try and gave birth to a beautiful girl, Jana.

When Jana was 2 years old, Toni and Kelly decided to have a second child. They were disappointed to learn that 872 was no longer an active donor because they wanted Jana to have a full biological sibling and they were pleased with Jana's disposition. They decided to try another donor, but Toni didn't get pregnant. When they contacted the clinic a second time, they discovered that 872 had begun donating sperm again. They were thrilled! Toni got pregnant on the first try and 9 months later, Kindra was born. Jana and Kindra are surrounded by loving parents, grandparents, and friends. The donor, 872, has provided a waiver to the clinic, giving permission to the girls to learn the identity of their father when they are 18 years old.

Although the birth of these children occurred in a loving family, Toni and Kelly know that their children may face many challenges as they grow up. Not all people are going to share Toni and Kelly's joy and happiness. Not all people are going to understand their desire to be a family.

- What do you think about this couple's desire to create a family through artificial insemination?
- What are the difficulties that Jana and Kindra may face as they grow up?
- What is the strength of this family unit?

Surrogacy

Surrogacy has been practiced throughout history and can be controversial and emotionally charged. How does this differ from selling babies? How will the non–egg donor woman feel about her partner providing sperm to impregnate another woman? In surrogacy, a woman, other than the partner, agrees to become pregnant and carry the fetus to full term. Usually the surrogate woman's own egg is fertilized by the sperm of the male from the couple seeking a baby. If IVF is attempted, the woman's fertilized egg may be placed in the surrogate woman's uterus. This child is the biological offspring of the couple.

Since 1977, nearly 4,500 children have been born to surrogate women in the United States. Few of these cases have resulted in legal battles; however, some situations have led to national attention. By 1992, many states had banned or restricted the practice of commercial surrogacy and five states had criminalized surrogacy. Most states have restricted the amount of payment the surrogate mother can receive for medical expenses and have eliminated the expenses of a broker, the person who introduced the couple and the surrogate mother. The cost of surrogacy can range from $15,000 to $40,000 and cover lawyer fees, medical costs, a possible surrogate fee, and miscellaneous expenses. Legal issues can arise if the surrogate woman tries to gain custody of the baby. Should the child be denied access to his or her biological mother? Who has the parental rights to raise this child? If a surrogate woman changes her mind and wants to keep the baby, do you think she should be allowed to do so? (See *Viewpoint:* "Surrogate Grandmothers.")

Stem Cell Issues

In recent years, the use of human stem cells in medical therapy has caused much controversy among medical scientists, bioethicists, clergy, and politicians. *Stem cells* are of two types: *adult* stem cells and *embryonic* stem cells. Adult stem cells are undifferentiated cells found among human tissues and organs. These cells are renewable and can differentiate into the specialized cell types needed in a body's tissues and organs. A stem cell's

Viewpoint

Surrogate Grandmothers

A grandmother in England gave birth to her own grandchild. Her daughter was born without a uterus, and she wanted her daughter and son-in-law to have their own child. A grandmother in South Dakota gave birth to her own grandchild. Her daughter, a librarian, was unable to have children, so the grandmother carried the fertilized embryos for her daughter and gave birth to twins. Should surrogacy remain legal? When should the children be told about this event?

primary role in a host organism is to repair and maintain the tissue in which they are found. Some scientists prefer the use of the term *somatic stem cells* in describing these cells.[52]

Somatic stem cells differ from embryonic stem cells as the term "embryonic" describes their origin. Embryonic stem cells are derived from embryos created through in vitro fertilization, which are then donated, with informed consent, for such research and are *not* drawn from an embryo already present in a woman's body. The embryos from which these cells derive are typically between 4 and 5 days old and are in the microscopic, hollow-ball stage called a *blastocyst.* The stem cells used in research are drawn from a blastocyst's inner cell mass.[53]

Scientists and medical experts working in the field of stem cell therapy believe it has the potential to alleviate many kinds of human illness and debilitating conditions, including Parkinson's disease, spinal cord injuries, blindness, deafness, birth defects, heart and cardiopulmonary diseases, and cancers. A therapy currently used is that of replacing bone marrow stem cells into individuals undergoing chemotherapy for cancer. As chemotherapy often destroys bone marrow, these cells are harvested from the individual prior to treatment, then later re-injected where they are able to replenish and rebuild fresh bone marrow.

Both types of stem cells, human adult and embryonic, have advantages and disadvantages for use in the field of medical research. Embryonic stem cells are considered *pluripotent,* able to differentiate into many types of cells needed by the body. It is thought somatic stem cells are limited into differentiating into the type of cell from which they were recovered; for example, a muscle cell can only become another muscle cell. However, some evidence suggests that adult stem cell plasticity exists, increasing the differentiation potential of a somatic cell. At present, the exact number of somatic stem cells as well as all their origins throughout the human body has not been fully discovered.[54]

For stem cells of any type to be used as medicinal therapy, they must be cultured, or grown, in a specific medium under highly controlled conditions. Large numbers of stem cells are needed for therapeutic use, and embryonic stem cells are more easily grown in laboratory culture than are mature, adult stem cells. However, if it were possible to grow large numbers of stem cells from a host, they could, like bone marrow cells, be reintroduced into a patient without fear of the body's rejecting the cells or treatments derived from them. A risk exists in using cells culled from embryos as a patient's body might reject any treatment created from such cells. Whether this would happen has not been determined in human experiments.[55]

At present, U.S. governmental funding cannot be used to initiate new embryonic stem cell lines. However, experimentation may take place on embryonic lines already in existence, and no barriers exist for private funding of research on embryonic stem cells. Some scientists believe that restricting embryonic stem cell research does a disservice to both scientific freedom and legitimate medical inquiry, as it is presently believed by many that embryonic stem cells contain much greater potential for use in medicine than other types of stem cells. However, some medical therapies using adult stem cells have been tried in other countries to varying degrees of success, but these are highly experimental and possibly dangerous and most have not been replicated in randomized, clinical trials.

The international scientific, medical, and religious communities are only beginning the debate on stem cell use in medical therapy. Some persons see the destruction of human embryos as the destruction of potential human life, and argue no matter how noble the cause, embryonic stem cells should never be used for such purposes. Others argue the rights and medical needs of human beings suffering from chronic or debilitating conditions must come before those of a microscopic cell colony. What are your thoughts on the issues regarding stem cell research? Do you believe only adult stem cells should be used for such purposes, or might there be times when using embryonic stem cells is appropriate? Or do you believe creating and using human embryos for medical research is never ethical or appropriate?

ABORTION

Not all pregnancies are planned and not all children are wanted. Worldwide, of the nearly 210 million women who become pregnant every year, not all will have live births. In fact, nearly 15 percent of pregnant women will spontaneously miscarry (usually in the second or third month) or experience a stillbirth. Another 22 percent will terminate the pregnancy by **abortion,** of which 20 million are obtained illegally.[56] These illegal abortions place a woman's health in jeopardy. The vast majority of abortions are sought for personal, not medical, reasons and include social influences (value placed on premarital chastity or marital fidelity, disapproval of having children late in life, rape, genocide), financial concerns (insufficient funds to take care of existing children, career interruption, lack of educational opportunities), or religious beliefs (from tolerance to condemnation). Figure 9.14 reports the legal abortion rate for every 1,000 women of childbearing age.

From 1986 to 2002, teen pregnancies ending in abortion declined from 46 percent to 34 percent of pregnancies among 15- to 19-year-old girls. Contributing factors include a steep decline in the pregnancy rate among sexually experienced teenagers, fewer pregnant teens choosing to have an abortion, and increased difficulty in finding clinics willing to conduct abortions. The lack of access to abortion is certainly a problem for low-income women and teenagers. Some recent barriers include

- A decline of abortion providers.
- A lack of abortion providers in the majority of all U.S. counties.
- A weakening of legal protections for women and physicians by giving states the right to enact restrictions that do not create an "undue burden" for women (*Planned Parenthood v. Casey*, 1992).
- Restrictions including parental involvement requirements, mandatory counseling and waiting periods, and limitations on public funding.
- Only 17 U.S. states pay for abortions for poor women, and about 3 percent of all abortions are paid for with public funds.[57]
- With very limited exceptions, the federal "Hyde Amendment" of 1976 has prohibited the use of federal funds for abortions for poor women. Approximately 20 percent of the women who are denied publicly funded abortions go on to bear unwanted children at considerable emotional and physical cost.

Low-income women and teenagers often face fewer options for dealing with an unwanted pregnancy than other women. (See *FYI:* "The Status of Abortion in the United States.")

The U.S. Congress has barred the use of federal Medicaid funds to pay for abortion except when the woman's life would be endangered by having a full-term pregnancy or in cases of rape or incest. In 2006 the South Dakota legislature passed a bill to ban abortion in most cases, except when a woman's life would be endangered. The legal status of this law will most likely be decided by the U.S. Supreme Court and serves as a trial balloon for the Right to Life advocates. The appointments of two conservative Supreme Court justices has led many feminists to fear that *Roe v. Wade*, which legalized abortion in 1973, is in danger of being overturned.[58] Figure 9.15 reports worldwide statistics for live births, induced abortions, and miscarriages/stillbirths.

FIGURE 9.14 Number of abortions per 1,000 women aged 15–44, by year.

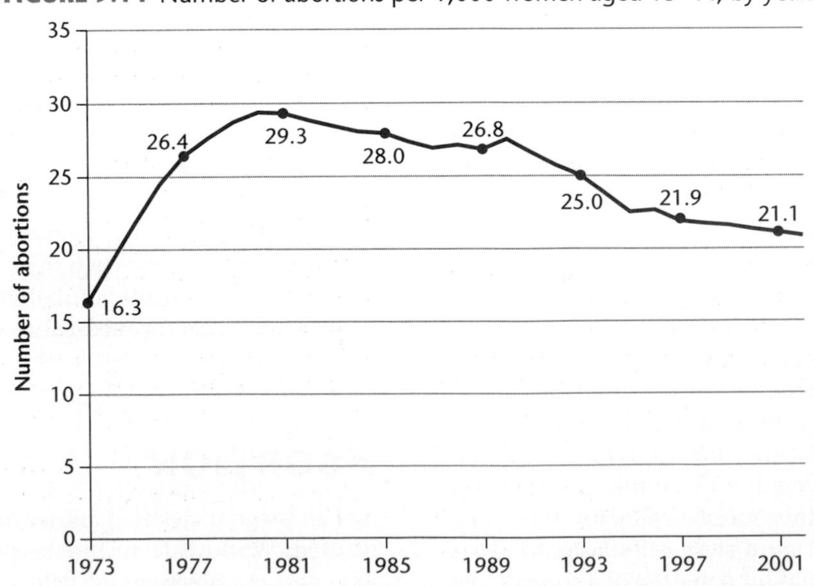

SOURCES: Alan Guttmacher Institute. 2006. *Induced abortion in the United States.* New York: Guttmacher Institute 2006. www.guttmacher.org/pubs/fb_induced_abortion.html (retrieved October 4, 2006).

FYI

The Status of Abortion in the United States

The Alan Guttmacher Institute and the Centers for Disease Control offer the most recent U.S. data related to abortion. The following findings from the Guttmacher Institute[59] are provided for your consideration:

- Two-thirds of all abortions are among never-married women.
- Nearly 48 percent of women having an abortion used a contraceptive method during the month they became pregnant.
- Black women are more than three times as likely as white women to have an abortion, and Hispanic women are two and a half times as likely.
- Black women account for 14 percent of women at risk for unintended pregnancy and they account for 26 percent of all unintended pregnancies.
- Hispanic women account for another 14 percent of women at risk for unintended pregnancy and they account for 22 percent of all unintended pregnancies.
- Thirty-four states currently have mandatory parental involvement laws in effect for a minor seeking an abortion.
- Women give at least four reasons for choosing abortion. Three-fourths say a baby would interfere with work, school, or other responsibilities; three-fourths cite responsibilities for others; two-thirds say they cannot afford a baby; and one-half say they do not want to be a single parent or are having problems with their partner/husband.
- Forty-three percent of all abortion facilities provide services only through the 12th week of pregnancy.
- The risk of death associated with childbirth is about ten times as high as that associated with abortion.
- Almost half of the women having abortions beyond 15 weeks of gestation say they were delayed because of problems with affording, finding, or getting to abortion services. Teens are more likely to delay than older women.

FIGURE 9.15 Worldwide, more than a third of pregnancies do not end in the birth of a baby.

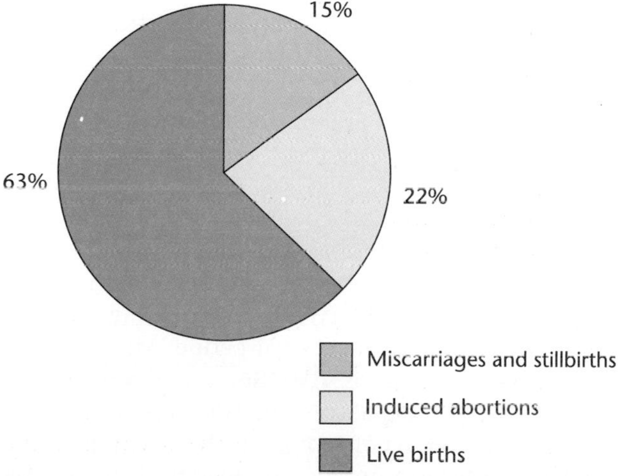

SOURCE: Alan Guttmacher Institute. 2006. *Get "in the know": Questions about pregnancy, contraception and abortion.* www.guttmacher.org/in-the-know/preqnancy.html (retrieved October 4, 2006).

Defining Abortion

Abortion is defined as the spontaneous or deliberate termination of a pregnancy. There are a number of different types of abortion including therapeutic, spontaneous, and voluntary. Spontaneous abortions (miscarriages) occur for a variety of reasons. These abortions can result from a chronic infection (i.e., PID or endometriosis), hormonal imbalances, fetal abnormalities, or problems with the uterus. Some women experience habitual abortions, which are defined as the abrupt end of three pregnancies in a row before the 20th week.

Therapeutic abortions are procedures conducted to terminate a pregnancy that threatens the life of the mother or fetus. An infected abortion is associated with an immature pregnancy that shows signs of infection of the genital tract. Fever is present and the uterus must be emptied. A septic abortion occurs when the womb is infected and the life of the mother is threatened. This abortion may be spontaneous or induced by the health care provider. A threatened abortion is a condition with symptoms of bleeding of the uterus and cramping before the 20th week. A woman with this condition requires rest and observation. Abortion may or may not occur, depending on the degree of vaginal bleeding and an undilated cervix. (See *FYI:* "Abortion Statistics.")

A voluntary (elective) abortion is the ending of a pregnancy by choice. As of 2006, forty-four states have adopted mandatory parental involvement laws for a minor seeking an abortion. Twenty-three states enforce parental consent, twelve states enforce parental notification, four states enjoin parental consent but do not enforce it, five states enjoined parental notification but do not enforce it, and six states (Connecticut, Hawaii, New York, Oregon, Vermont, Washington) and Washington, D.C., have no laws.[60] The procedures most often used in the United States for voluntary abortion include surgical techniques, vacuum aspiration or D&C, and more recently, a drug combination therapy.

Abortion Statistics

The Alan Guttmacher Institute[61] addressed the issue of abortion and teenagers. The following findings were reported:

- Abortion rates among sexually experienced teenagers have declined steadily because fewer teens are becoming pregnant, and in recent years, fewer pregnant teens have chosen to have an abortion.
- Between 2001 and 2002, almost one in five women (19 percent) who had abortions were adolescents. Most of those were among teens aged 18–19 (12 percent), with only 1 percent occurring among women under age 15.
- The reasons most often given by teens for choosing an abortion are concern about how having a baby would change their lives in a negative way, feeling that they are not mature enough to raise a child, and not having the financial resources to raise a child.
- Six in 10 teenagers who have abortions do so with at least one parent's knowledge. The great majority of parents support their daughter's decision to have an abortion.

Surgical Abortion **Vacuum aspiration,** also called suction curettage, is the most common surgical method of first-trimester abortion. Early procedures—preemptive abortion and early uterine evacuation—can be performed in a clinic or a physician's office with a local anesthetic. These procedures are typically performed in the first 4 to 8 weeks, and the most common complications may be infection or heavy bleeding for a few days. Vacuum aspiration is the procedure used for abortions in the 6th to 14th week. The cervix is dilated and a small plastic tube (or cannula) is inserted into the uterus. The cannula is attached to a pump that suctions the contents of the uterus. The procedure is completed within minutes; however, the clinical stay may be several hours to make sure there isn't any unusual bleeding or any other complications. In some situations, the uterus may be scraped with a curette to loosen and remove tissue. When a **dilation and curettage (D&C)** is performed, the cervix is dilated and the uterine lining is scraped with a curette to remove the contents. This procedure often requires general anesthesia and must be performed in a clinic or hospital. Possible complications include reaction to the anesthesia or cervical injuries. The use of D&C has declined sharply since the introduction of the vacuum aspiration procedure.

After the 14th to 15th week, abortion becomes more complicated because the fetus is larger and a greater blood supply goes to the uterus. Only 6 percent of abortions are performed between 13 and 15 weeks, and only 5 percent are performed at 16 weeks or later. A **dilation and evacuation (D&E)** procedure is an expansion of the vacuum aspiration, but a larger cervical opening is required. The method used by the health care provider determines the length of time required for dilation, from a few minutes to 2 days. The health care provider will use suction and forceps to remove the fetal parts. A curette is used to remove any remaining tissue. The D&E is usually used in the first weeks of the second trimester but can be used through the 24th week of pregnancy. The procedure takes only 10–30 minutes, with either a local anesthetic or general anesthesia.

Less than 2 percent of abortions require the induction method, and they are almost always performed in a hospital under general anesthesia. A small amount of amniotic fluid is removed and replaced with a medication (prostaglandins or pitocin) that is injected into the uterus through the abdomen. This procedure induces labor, and several hours later the fetus is expelled. Heavy bleeding, infection, or injury to the cervix can occur. A hospital stay of one or more days may be required.

Two late-term procedures, hysterotomy and intact dilation and extraction, can be performed during the end of the second trimester or during the third trimester. These procedures are major surgery and are reserved for life-threatening circumstances to the woman. All surgical abortions require an observation and recovery period. The length of time depends on the procedure and the time frame since the last menstrual period (LMP). The woman is given instructions for postoperative care, including a 24-hour number to call in case of an emergency, and an appointment for follow-up in 2 to 4 weeks.

Medical Abortion In September 2000, the Food and Drug Administration approved mifepristone (trade name Mifeprex) for the termination of an early pregnancy, defined as 49 days or less, counting from the beginning of the last menstrual period. Mifepristone, also known to some as **RU-486,** was developed by a French pharmaceutical company and approved for use in France in 1988. As of September 2002, mifepristone had been approved for use in twenty-six countries including Great Britain and Sweden. Since its approval, it has been used by more than 1 million women worldwide. A chronology of its development and introduction in the United States can be found at www.feminist.org/welcome/ru486two.html. More information on RU-486 and contraceptive research can be found at www.feminist.org/rrights/medical.html. Access to a medical abortion during the early stages of pregnancy has afforded women another option: the use of two medicines to end an early pregnancy. The regimen is effective in nearly 95 percent of women when used within 49 days from the beginning of their last menstrual period.

FYI

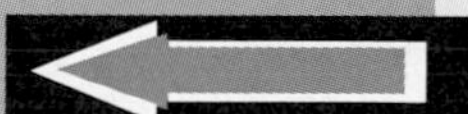

Comparison of Medical and Surgical Abortion

Medical Abortion

High success rate (about 95 percent)
Can be used in the earliest weeks following fertilization (up to 7 weeks LMP)
Requires no invasive procedure or surgery
Requires no anesthesia
Side effects other than bleeding tend to be short-lived
Does not carry risk of uterine perforation or injury to the cervix
Has the potential for greater privacy
Gives a woman greater control over her body

Surgical Abortion

High success rate (about 99 percent)
Requires only one office visit
Performed quickly (5–10 minutes)
Slightly more effective than medical abortion
Less blood loss
No awareness of the passing of the by-products of conception
Can be performed later than medical abortion (usually during the first trimester)

Medical abortion requires three visits to the health care provider for the termination of a pregnancy. The first visit includes thorough counseling, a physical examination, and determination of the length of the pregnancy. It is extremely important that the health care provider be skilled in determining the length of pregnancy and ruling out an ectopic pregnancy. The administration of 600 mg (three 200-milligram tablets) of Mifeprex in a single oral dose weakens the embryo's attachment to the uterus by blocking the action of the natural hormone progesterone. Progesterone prepares the lining of the uterus for the fertilized egg and maintains the pregnancy. In the second visit, 2 days later, misoprostol (two 200-microgram tablets) is administered if the pregnancy has not been aborted. Misoprostol has been approved by the FDA as an ulcer medicine and belongs to the class of drugs known as prostaglandins. Prostagladins work by causing contractions of the uterus, helping to expel the fertilized egg. A third visit, 2 weeks later, is required to confirm that the abortion is complete. Nearly 75 percent of women abort within 24 hours after taking misoprostol. The side effects experienced by women are typically related to misoprostol and include headaches, nausea, diarrhea, vomiting, heavy bleeding, and cramping. The bleeding may include large blood clots, unrelated to the expulsion of the conception by-products, which are approximately one-fifth of an inch.

Women who used medical abortion were highly satisfied with the procedure. Nearly 96 percent of the women in the initial study conducted by the Population Council would recommend it to others, and 91 percent would choose the method again if necessary.[62] Even in women for whom the method failed, 70 percent would try it again, and 85 percent would recommend it to others. In the initial trials, nearly two-thirds of the women felt the experience was better than expected, and three-quarters of women who had had a surgical abortion said the medical abortion was more satisfactory. The major factors contributing to satisfaction included no surgery and/or injections, noninvasive; natural, feminine, like menses or miscarriage; less painful; easier emotionally, less frightening; and easier, simpler, and faster than surgical abortion. (See *FYI:* "Comparison of Medical and Surgical Abortion.")

The drug label for Mifeprex warns that it should not be used by women with the following conditions: confirmed or suspected ectopic pregnancies; intrauterine device in place; chronic failure of the adrenal glands; current long-term therapy with corticosteroids; history of allergy to mifepristone, misoprostol, or other prostaglandins; or bleeding disorders or current anticoagulant (blood-thinning) therapy.

Postabortion Issues

Studies of women who choose abortion have found that the majority experience relief after the abortion, and the immediate feelings of guilt, loss, and/or depression usually pass quickly.[63] The circumstances leading to the decision to abort a pregnancy may include fear or threat of losing one's partner, financial hardship, missed educational opportunities or career advancement, loss of a job, detectable fetal defects, responsibility to other children, lack of social support, rape or incest, maternal age, and others.[64] A woman's feelings and emotions often are shaped by the political, religious, and social climate she experiences. Thus, support for the woman's right to choose can facilitate better recovery. (See *Her Story:* "LaShonda: An Unplanned Pregnancy and Choice.")

Like most major life events, a woman needs to handle her feelings after an abortion in her own way. She should reach a stage of accepting the loss (regardless of

Her Story

LaShonda: An Unplanned Pregnancy and Choice

LaShonda had her first child at age 15. She stayed in school during the pregnancy, but once Shamika was born she needed a job and a place of her own. So she dropped out of high school and began working at the local textile company. After 3 years of living paycheck to paycheck, she decided to finish her GED. She wanted to go to college and better her life. She met Justin in the class. He also wanted to go to college. They began dating, and 2 years later she completed her GED and was ready to apply for college—but she got pregnant. Neither Justin nor she was ready for a child.

- What should LaShonda do?
- What options did she have?

Go to the Web site www.prochoice.org and read the self-assessment guide *Unsure about Your Pregnancy? A Guide to Making the Right Decision for You.*

the reasons), rather than live in secrecy and guilt. If grief exists, the resolution of the process may be facilitated by sharing one's feelings with accepting friends and family members, health care providers, mental health professionals, or clergy. Guilt, depression, or other emotional trauma can linger if grief remains unresolved. Anti-abortion groups have attempted to document "postabortion syndrome" (PAS) with traits similar to those for posttraumatic stress disorder (PTSD). However, mainstream medical positions have never supported this assertion. Research has found that the time of greatest distress is *before* the abortion. Also, the greatest predictor of emotional well-being after an abortion was the state of well-being before the abortion. Other research by the Alan Guttmacher Institute suggests some women may develop postabortion anxiety or depression if they encounter aggressive protests during a visit to an abortion provider.[65] For the vast majority of women who have had an abortion, a mixture of feelings occurs, with a predominance of positive feelings.[66]

Political Debate

The question isn't whether abortion is a political issue; rather, the question is, Just how did it become such a major issue? Look at politicians, political appointees, and Supreme Court justices who can be elected, appointed, or denied based solely on their view of this issue. Their personal beliefs about abortion cause more political consternation than their public stance on fiscal responsibility, health care, environmental control, and other national and international issues. Look at the political platforms adopted by the political parties over the past several elections. Why is abortion such a "hot" issue? Is the issue the rights of the fetus versus the rights of the mother? Is the underlying issue "controlling" women? Is the underlying issue lack of access to contraceptives? What do you think? A variety of political maneuvers have occurred since the *Roe v. Wade* decision in 1973. In 1981 the Hyde Amendment eliminated federal funding (Medicaid) for all abortions except those in which the life of the mother would be endangered if the pregnancy should be carried to term. This measure made it more difficult for low-income women to seek assistance for an abortion, even in cases of rape and incest. As a result of public outcry, Congress did amend the law in 1993 to include federal funding for women in cases of rape and incest.[67]

In 1996 President Clinton vetoed an amendment, passed by Congress, to prevent late-term abortions. Then again, in 1997, Congress reintroduced and debated a similar amendment to prevent late-term abortions in an attempt to further restrict a woman's right to choose. The amendment was passed by the Congress, and congress*men* suggested that the debate would now shift to the issue of when life begins and protection of the unborn. The discussion about the events leading to a late-term abortion and the medical consequences for women in this situation are far different from the discussion of induced abortions for ending an unintended pregnancy. In 2005 President Bush appointed two new Supreme Court justices who may tip the balance in the Supreme Court in favor of overturning *Roe v. Wade*. What has happened since their appointments to reduce women's rights? Shouldn't the discussion focus on how to prevent unintended pregnancies rather than how to prevent abortions?

Right to Life and Pro-Choice

Is it Right to Life, Pro-Life, or Anti-Choice? Is it Pro-Choice or Pro-Abortion? Even the titles we use to describe the stances toward abortion give some indication of a person's views. What do we know about the individuals who describe themselves as Right to Life or Pro-Choice advocates? Researchers have found that Right to Life advocates tend to have a more unified attitude structure than Pro-Choice advocates. Because attitude structures are more unified, Right to Life advocates tend to be more single-minded in their beliefs. This position can best be summarized as people advocating for the rights of the fetus and as people who believe that life begins at conception. Right to

Life advocates are more dogmatic than Pro-Choice advocates and conservative religiously, politically, and socially. They view abortion as a moral issue and often will vote for political candidates on the basis of this single issue.[68]

Pro-Choice advocates tend to have less unified attitude structures, thus they are more open-minded to interpreting and organizing reality. The Pro-Choice position maintains that women should have control over their own bodies, including reproductive rights. The reasons Pro-Choice advocates give for choosing this stance are varied. They advocate for individual rights. Some may take a stance that the fetus is not a viable life, others may have strong feelings about a woman's right to choose, and still others may consider the circumstances of the pregnancy.[69] Right to Life advocates sometimes appear to be more effective politically than Pro-Choice advocates, but this is due to their single-issue politics. This appearance should not suggest that Pro-Choice advocates are less committed to their values and beliefs. Rather, Pro-Choice advocates have a variety of issues on which to focus.

Another question we might ask is, How are children being influenced by this "moralistic" (right versus wrong) debate? Look at Right to Life and Pro-Choice rallies at which children often stand next to sign-carrying parents. At Right to Life rallies, young children carry signs with graphic pictures of aborted, discarded fetuses. These children are led to believe that the women who have abortions are murderers and baby killers. At Pro-Choice rallies, children tote signs saying KEEP CHOICE LEGAL. They are led to believe that individual rights and freedoms will be sacrificed if abortion isn't legal and that all Right to Life advocates are violent. At what age did you form your opinion about abortion? How did you reach this decision? Do you think it might change? Now complete *Assess Yourself:* "Attitudes toward Induced Abortion" to determine your attitudes toward abortion.

Assess Yourself

Attitudes toward Induced Abortion[70]

For each statement about induced abortion, indicate your feelings based on the values in the following scale:

6—Strongly agree
5—Moderately agree
4—Slightly agree
3—Slightly disagree
2—Moderately disagree
1—Strongly disagree

_____ 1. Abortion is a moral issue.
_____ 2. The rights of a fetus should be protected because the unborn child can't protect herself.
_____ 3. A woman who has an abortion is selfish and self-centered.
_____ 4. Societies with high moral standards should prohibit abortions.
_____ 5. Life begins at conception.
_____ 6. If two people have unprotected sex, they should be willing to live with the consequences of their action.
_____ 7. Abortions are not an alternative when contraception has failed.
_____ 8. All abortions should be banned.
_____ 9. Parental consent should be required for all young girls under age 18 who seek an abortion.
_____10. Every young woman seeking an abortion should be required to watch a video about the procedure before making a final decision.

Total your score. Higher scores indicate a more Right to Life attitude and lower scores indicate a more Pro-Choice attitude.

Human Dimension

Reproductive rights can be debated from moral, political, health, and social dimensions. The political arena tends to make Right to Life versus Pro-Choice views seem dichotomous and bipolar opposites (much like liberal and conservative). Sometimes we forget that many men and women find themselves somewhere other than on either extreme end of a continuum. We also forget that abortions are about women (younger and older) making difficult choices. This is the human dimension of pregnant girls and women making difficult decisions. How long will this issue continue to polarize persons, communities, and countries? What will it take to focus the debate on other dimensions of reproductive rights and to forge a middle ground? Reaction to past bombings of family planning clinics in Tulsa and Atlanta indicate that Right to Life supporters have distanced themselves from the violence associated with extreme polarization. Dialog is the only strategy we can use to tolerate differences and decrease the number of unintended pregnancies and sexually transmitted infections.

ADOPTION

Adoption is an alternative to assisted reproduction or abortion. Adoption issues have changed because the rights of adoptees are now viewed as being equal to the

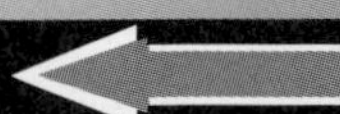

FYI

Facts on Adoption[71,72]

1. There were 21,320 foreign-born children adopted by Americans in 2003. This is more than a threefold increase from 6,536 in 1992. Adoptions by Americans while living outside the United States are not included in these numbers.
2. Since 1987, the number of yearly adoptions in the United States has remained relatively constant and ranges from approximately 118,000 to 127,000.
3. Adopted children enjoy more socioeconomic benefits than do children who remain with their biological unmarried birth mothers. They have better-educated, older mothers.
4. One to 2 million infertile and fertile couples and individuals would like to adopt.
5. Black children constitute about 14 percent of all children but account for more than 46 percent in foster care and more than 38 percent waiting to be adopted.
6. Babies, regardless of medical problems, generally do not wait long to be adopted.
7. The Web site Adoptuskids.org provides information on children waiting to be adopted.

FYI

National Adoption Registry, Inc.

The National Adoption Registry is a private registry that accepts registrations from adoptees, birth parents, and other interested individuals. Vital statistics of the adoptee are entered in the database and matched with existing information in the file. A fee is assessed for registration. (See the Resources at the end of this chapter.)

rights of birth parents and adoptive parents. Couples who are making a decision on whether to adopt a child have a variety of issues to consider. First, they need to decide on the age, race, and health status of the child they want to adopt. Do they expect to raise a normal, healthy child from infancy? Does the child's background matter? Should they consider intercountry adoption or adopting a special needs child, a minority child, or an older child? Once they decide on the kind of child they desire, they need to find an appropriate agency to meet their needs. Agencies can vary from public agencies such as county social services to private adoption arranged a lawyer, physician, or church. Services can vary from matching children and adoptive parents to educational and support services throughout the parenting years. (See *FYI:* "Facts on Adoption.")

Adoptions can be closed or open. **Closed** (confidential) **adoption** means that there is no contact between birth parents and adoptive parents. **Open adoption** means that contact occurs between birth parents and adoptive parents. This contact can vary from occasional letters to regular contact with the child. Open adoption eliminates the need for children to fantasize about their birth parents; they get actual knowledge of their ancestry. However, open adoption also brings the inherent risk of birth parents' interfering or intruding on the life of the adopted family. Bonding can become difficult if competition arises for the child's attention. Such attachment and identity issues in adopted children may not develop during the early years, especially if the child is adopted as an infant. Rather, these issues may develop during the adolescent years, when many young adults feel that they have a need to know their birth parents. This process can be difficult; the anticipation and expectation of being accepted by their birth parents are usually mixed with the fear of experiencing further rejection. The Internet has become a ready source for exchange of information between adopted children seeking birth parents and birth parents seeking information about the child they gave up for adoption years ago. (See *FYI:* "National Adoption Registry, Inc.")

Foster Care

Many children, over 100,000 in all, were once thought unadoptable. These children, labeled "special needs," live in foster care and await adoption. Special needs children include school-age or older children, children who have suffered emotional or physical abuse or neglect, children with physical or mental handicaps, siblings who desire to be kept together, children with racial or ethnic differences, or children born with HIV or other medical problems. The criteria for parents seeking to adopt special needs children are often more relaxed compared to those for adoption of infants. Foster parents, parents with large families, single parents, and others will find reduced fees and sometimes reimbursement for adopting these children.[73] To evaluate your competence to be a parent, under any or most circumstances, check *Assess Yourself:* "How Do You Rate Your Competence to Be a Parent?"

Assess Yourself

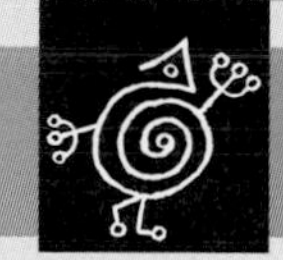

How Do You Rate Your Competence to Be a Parent?

Rate each of the items below by indicating how competent you feel about your abilities according to the following scale:

a—Very competent
b—Fairly competent
c—Somewhat competent
d—Not very competent
e—Not at all competent

How do you feel about your competence and ability to

______ 1. Care for a child when he or she is sick or upset?
______ 2. Help a child solve problems?
______ 3. Provide adequate time for a child?
______ 4. Be a good parent?
______ 5. Provide emotional support for a child?
______ 6. Maintain a close relationship with a child?
______ 7. Provide a good role model for a child?
______ 8. Discipline a child?
______ 9. Give advice to a child?
______10. Meet the needs of a child (even special needs)?
______11. Establish and enforce rules for a child's behavior?
______ 12. Obtain needed resources for a child?

Using a rating of a = 5, b = 4, c = 3, d = 2, e = 1, total your score. Which competencies are you most comfortable doing? What skills would you need to improve some of the other competencies?

Chapter Summary

- Family planning should be viewed as a health, social, and political issue.
- Fertility awareness methods include the cycle-based method, basal body temperature method, and symptothermal method.
- Withdrawal, coitus interruptus, is not a birth control method.
- Barrier methods include spermicides, condoms, diaphragms, cervical caps, and cervical shields.
- Hormonal methods include oral contraceptives, transdermal patches, injectables, and Implanon, NuvaRing.
- Emergency contraception is most effective if given within 72 hours after unprotected intercourse or method failure.
- Intrauterine devices are the most popular worldwide forms of reversible birth control.
- Sterilization methods include tubal ligation and vasectomy and are the most common form of contraception used by women over age 30.
- Choosing a birth control method should be a joint decision between a woman and her partner, but women must take precautions to protect against unintended pregnancies and sexually transmitted infections.
- Nearly 45 percent of all pregnancies are unplanned.
- Lifestyle changes should begin before pregnancy. These changes include exercise, nutritional planning and necessary supplements, nondrug use without first consulting a health care provider, a time lapse if using oral contraceptives, and appropriate immunizations.
- Early signs of pregnancy include a missed period, a light period or spotting, tender or swollen breasts, fatigue, nausea and vomiting, and frequent urination.
- One in 60 pregnancies results in an ectopic pregnancy.
- Home pregnancy tests are reliable when used properly. You must follow directions carefully when attempting to determine if you are pregnant. These tests are sensitive to the presence of hCG in the urine.
- A sequence of changes occurs to the fetus and the mother during the 40-week gestational period.
- The maternal mortality rate is higher among African American women than white women.
- Prenatal checkups are recommended monthly through the first 28 weeks, biweekly during weeks 28 to 36, and weekly thereafter.
- Certified nurse-midwives, lay midwives, and doulas provide primary care to women expecting low-risk pregnancies.
- Breast-feeding is beneficial to both mother and infant.
- Breast-feeding prevents nearly 6 million infant deaths each year worldwide.
- Primary infertility is recognized as the inability of a woman to conceive within 1 year of having unprotected sexual intercourse.
- Women and men account equally for cases of primary infertility.
- Artificial insemination involves the use of sperm from a donor or partner to fertilize an egg.
- In vitro fertilization involves the implantation of a fertilized egg into a woman's uterus.

- Multiple births are more likely to occur with assisted reproduction.
- Categories of abortion include spontaneous, therapeutic, and voluntary.
- Closed adoption is confidential and eliminates contact between birth and adoptive parents.
- Open adoption means the possibility of contact between birth and adoptive parents.
- Foster care occurs most often with special needs children.

Review Questions

1. Describe the techniques, benefits, and drawbacks for the fertility awareness methods.
2. What is the difference between method failure and user failure?
3. Discuss the procedures for applying a condom.
4. What is emergency contraception?
5. Discuss fetal development.
6. Discuss the stages of labor and delivery.
7. What are the advantages of breast-feeding?
8. What is the importance of maternal and infant mortality rates?
9. What are the arguments offered by Pro-Choice and Right to Life regarding abortion?
10. What components do couples need to consider with pre-pregnancy planning?
11. Discuss some advances in assisted reproductive technology.
12. Discuss the advantages and disadvantages of open and closed adoption.

Resources

Organizations, Hotlines, and Websites

The Alan Guttmacher Institute
120 Wall Street, 21st Floor
New York, NY 10005
212-248-1111 or toll-free 800-355-0244
www.guttmacher.org

American Association of Birthing Centers
(to locate a birthing center)
(Formerly National Association of Childbearing Centers)
3123 Gottschall Road
Perkiomenville, PA 18074
215-234-8068
www.birthcenters.org

American College of Nurse-Midwives
(directory of certified nurse-midwives)
8403 Colesville Road, Suite. 1550
Silver Spring, MD 20910
240-485-1800
www.midwife.org

American Society for Reproductive Medicine (ASRM)
(up-to-date report of fertility clinics in your region)
www.asrm.com

Dave Thomas Foundation for Adoption
4150 Tuller Road, Suite 204
Dublin, OH 43017
1-800-ASK-DTFA (1-800-275-3832)
www.davethomasfoundationforadoption.org

Doulas of North America (DONA)
P.O. Box 626
Jasper, IN 47547
888-188-3662
www.dona.org

InterNational Council on Infertility Information Dissemination (INCIID)
P.O. Box 6836
Arlington, VA 22206
www.inciid.org

NARAL Pro-Choice America
(Formerly National Abortion and Reproductive Rights Action League)
1156 15th Street N.W., Suite 700
Washington, DC 20005
202-973-3096
www.naral.org

NARAL Pro-Choice California
111 Pine Street, Suite 1500
San Francisco, CA 94111
415-890-1020
www.choice.org

National Abortion Federation
1755 Massachusetts Avenue N.W., Suite 600
Washington, DC 20036
202-667-5881
www.prochoice.org

Child Welfare Information Gateway (adoption resources)
Children's Bureau ACYE
1250 Maryland Avenue S.W., Eighth Floor
Washington, DC 20024
703-385-7565 or toll-free 800-394-3366
www.childwelfare.gov/adoption/index.cfm

National Adoption Registry, Inc.
404 a Pennsylvania Avenue, Suite 303
Kansas City, MO 64111
800-875-4347
www.nationaladoptionregistry.com

National Right to Life Committee
512 10th Street NW
Washington, DC 20004
202-626-8800
www.nrlc.org

Planned Parenthood Federation of America, Inc.
434 West 33rd Street
New York, NY 10001
212-541-7800
www.plannedparenthood.org

Population Council
One Dag Hammarskjold Plaza
New York, NY 10017
212-339-0500
www.popcouncil.org

RESOLVE, Inc.
(services for fertility problems and adoption information)
7910 Woodmont Avenue, Suite 1350
Bethesda, MD 20814
Helpline: 301-652-8585
www.resolve.org

Resources for Adoptive Parents
Internet Adoption Photolisting
(a listing of agencies, facilitators, attorneys, and exchanges for adoption services and information)
www.adoption.com

Stars of David International, Inc.
(services for Jewish and part-Jewish adoptive families)
3175 Commercial Avenue, Suite 100
Northbrook, IL 60062-1915
800-STAR-349 (800-782-7349)
www.starsofdavid.org

Wikipedia, the free encyclopedia (Stem Cell)
http://en.wikipedia.org/wiki/Stem_cell

The Stem Cell Database
http://stemcell.princeton.edu

Suggested Readings

Boonstra, H., R. Gold, C. Richards, and L. Finer. 2006. *Abortion in Women's Lives*. New York and Washington, DC: Alan Guttmacher Institute.

Brodie, J. F. 1997. *Contraception and Abortion in Nineteenth Century America*. Ithaca, NY: Cornell University Press.

Connell, E. B. 2001. *The Contraception Sourcebook*. New York: McGraw-Hill.

Curtis, G. B., and J. Schuler. 2000. *Your Pregnancy Week by Week*. Boulder, CO: Perseus.

Guillebaud, J. 2004. *Contraception*. St. Louis: Elsevier Science.

Marks, L. V. 2001. *Sexual Chemistry: A History of the Contraceptive Pill*. New Haven, CT: Yale University Press.

Murkoff, H. E., S. Hathaway, et al. 2003. *What to Expect When You're Expecting*. 3rd ed. New York: Workman.

Oudshoorn, N. 2003. *The Male Pill: The Biography of a Technology in the Making*. Durham, NC: Duke University Press.

Pipher, M. 1995. *Reviving Ophelia: Saving the Selves of Adolescent Girls*. New York: Ballantine.

Shandler, S. 1999. *Ophelia Speaks: Adolescent Girls Write about Their Search for Self*. New York: HarperCollins.

SIECUS Public Policy Office. 2006. *It Gets Worse: A Revamped Federal Abstinence-Only Program Goes Extreme*. SIECUS Special Report. Available www.siecus.org/policy/Revamped_Abstinence-Only_Goes_Extreme.pdf

Tone, A. 2002. *Devices and Desires: A History of Contraception in America*. New York: Hill & Wang.

Ulrich, L. T. 1991. *A Midwife's Tale: The Life of Martha Ballard, Based on Her Diary, 1785–1812*. New York: Random House.

References

1. World Summit for Children, 1990; Fourth World Conference on Women, 1995.
2. Lancashire, J. 1995. National Center for Health Statistics data line. *Public Health Reports* 110 (January/February): 105–6.
3. UNICEF. *Fertility and contraceptive use*. www.childinfo.org/eddb/fertility/index.htm (retrieved April 6, 2004).
4. Planned Parenthood. 2006. *Birth control*. http://www.plannedparenthood.org/birth-control-pregnancy/birth-control/effectiveness.htm (retrieved September 28, 2006).
5. Collins, C., P. Alagiri, T. Summers, and S. F. Morin. 2002. Abstinence only vs. comprehensive sex education: What are the arguments? What is the evidence? AIDS Policy Research Center and Center for AIDS Prevention Studies. *Policy Monograph Series* (March).
6. Republican National Coalition for Life. 2002. *President Bush promotes abstinence until marriage in new budget*. www.rnclife.org/faxnotes/2002/feb02/02-02-07.shtml (retrieved October 15, 2002).
7. SIECUS. 2005. *Brief history of abstinence-only-until-marriage education*. www.nonewmoney.org/history.htm (retrieved May 25, 2006).
8. Planned Parenthood. 2005. *Ways to chart your fertility pattern*. www.ppfa.org/pp2/portal/files/portal/medicalinfo/birthcontrol/pub-fertility-chart.xml (retrieved May 25, 2006).
9. Centers for Disease Control and Prevention. 2000. Notice to readers: CDC statement on study results of product containing nonoxynol-9. *MMWR Weekly* 49 (30): 717–18.
10. DaVanzo, J., A. M. Parnell, and W. H. Foege. 1991. Health consequences of contraceptive use and reproductive patterns: Summary of a report from the U.S. National Research Council. *Journal of the American Medical Association* 265: 2692–96.
11. Oral contraceptives. 2000. *Population Reports* 28 (1): Series A, number 9.
12. Planned Parenthood Federation of America. 2006. *A history of contraceptive methods*. http://www.plannedparenthood.org/uhpp/history.htm (retrieved September 28, 2006).
13. DaVanzo, Parnell, and Foege, Health consequences of contraceptive use and reproductive patterns.
14. Marchbanks, P. A., J. A. McDonald, H. G. Wilson, et al. 2002. Oral contraceptives and the risk of breast cancer. *New England Journal of Medicine* 346: 2025–32.
15. Planned Parenthood. 2004. *Smoking or—The pill, the patch, the ring*. www.ppfa.org/pp2/can/files/portal/medicalinfo/birthcontrol/pub-smoking-pill.xml (retrieved May 25, 2006).

Contemporary Lifestyle and Social Issues

Chapter Ten
Eating Well

Chapter Eleven
Keeping Fit

Chapter Twelve
Using Alcohol Responsibly

Chapter Thirteen
Making Wise Decisions about Tobacco, Caffeine, and Drugs

Part Four

Chapter Ten

Eating Well

CHAPTER OBJECTIVES

When you complete this chapter, you will be able to do the following:

- Describe the factors to consider when making food choices
- Summarize the Dietary Guidelines for Americans
- Explain the principles applied to meal planning
- Summarize the nutritional requirements needed at different life stages: adolescence, pregnancy, the older years
- Discuss the Dietary Reference Intakes necessary for proper nutrition

EATING WELL AND EATING WISELY

In the United States today, nutrition generates more attention than all other health issues. There isn't a day that goes by that we don't hear about what we should or should not eat. We often hear the mantra "You are what you eat." We read the media messages about the "fattening of America." Indeed, researchers have found a strong relationship between the foods we eat and the quality of our lives. While many questions about food and nutrition are still being researched, scientists have determined that what we eat has a strong influence on our health status. Throughout this text, we will talk about how women can protect their health by what they *don't* do, such as not smoking cigarettes, avoiding excessive use of drugs and alcohol, and being physically inactive. We also want to strongly emphasize the positive behaviors women *can* do to protect their health.

Eating well is one of those positive behaviors we can do to protect our health. Perhaps no other health practice has a greater impact on our well-being than eating wisely. As an adult woman, you are faced with many nutritional choices every day. You either plan your meals or select from a menu of some sort every time you eat, day in and day out. In our culture, eating is often a ritual—something that brings us pleasure. Unlike so many women and children worldwide, we do not eat to prevent starvation or to ensure that we survive. Our choices are often not related to nutrition but, instead, related to the emotional pleasure and other factors associated with the meal. Do the *Assess Yourself:* "Determining Your Food Choices" exercise to decide the manner in which you make your food choices. Also, see *FYI:* "Feast or Famine" for a reality check on global nutrition issues.

GUIDELINES TO GOOD EATING

What should an adult woman eat to stay healthy? Years of laboratory research and data collection from many segments of our population have revealed information that can help answer this question. These studies led to recommendations used by many meal plans, including

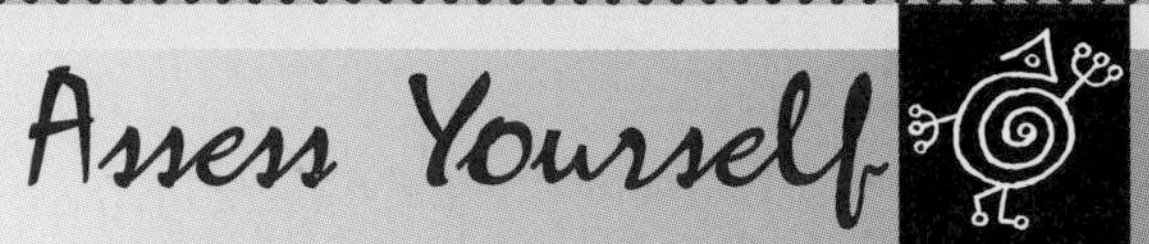

Determining Your Food Choices[1]

Look at each of the associated factors below. Consider how much each one of them influences your food choices. As you consider each one, think of it in the role it plays *most* of the time. Circle the number that best reflects your perception of the factor.

Factor	Not significant			Very significant		
Family influences	0	1	2	3	4	5
Weight control	0	1	2	3	4	5
Health	0	1	2	3	4	5
Nutrition knowledge	0	1	2	3	4	5
Convenience/time	0	1	2	3	4	5
Advertisements	0	1	2	3	4	5
Emotions/stress	0	1	2	3	4	5
Peers (friends, coworkers)	0	1	2	3	4	5
Customs/ethnic background	0	1	2	3	4	5
Physical activity level	0	1	2	3	4	5
Food costs	0	1	2	3	4	5

Interpretation: The factors that you scored as 4 or 5 influence your food choices the most. Think about each one of those, and place a "+" or a "−" sign next to it, depending on whether you think the factor is a positive or negative influence on your eating habits and your health. The first step in a mature dietary program is to evaluate the things you eat and why you eat them. Is achieving good health a reason for your food choices? Should you make it a greater priority? Through thoughtful choices, your eating experiences can be rewarding for you.

the American Heart Association's "Eating Plan for Healthy Americans":

- Total fat to meet caloric needs
  - 7–10 percent saturated fat
  - Up to 10 percent polyunsaturated fat
  - Up to 15 percent monounsaturated fat
- 55 percent or more of carbohydrates
- 15 percent protein
- Less than 300 mg per day of cholesterol[2]

How does the typical American woman's diet compare? Studies suggest that the average American eats foods from these categories:

- 15 percent of the energy value comes from protein sources.
- 46 percent of our food energy comes from carbohydrates.
- 38 percent of our energy value comes from fats.

Women with coronary heart disease (CHD), or diabetes or high LDL (low-density lipoprotein, or "bad") cholesterol, and those with fewer than two risk factors for CHD who have not met the LDL cholesterol treatment goal of less than 160 mg/dl (milligrams per deciliter) should follow the "Total Lifestyle Change" recommendation of the National Cholesterol Education Program (NCEP):

- Less than 200 mg per day of cholesterol[3]

Dietary Guidelines for Americans 2005

The Dietary Guidelines for Americans were first published in 1980 and, by law, are reviewed, updated, and published every 5 years. The *Dietary Guidelines for Americans 2005* replace the 2000 Guidelines and will be in effect until 2010. The guidelines are science-based and designed to promote health, prevent chronic disease, and serve as the gold standard of nutritional information. The guidelines empower Americans with the latest and best information on food and nutrition.[4] The 2005 report makes it clear that the major causes of morbidity and mortality are related to lifestyle issues, particularly poor diet and sedentary lifestyle. Specific diseases and conditions linked to poor diet include cardiovascular disease, hypertension, dyslipidemia (elevation of lipids, or fats, in the blood), type 2 diabetes, overweight and obesity, osteoporosis, constipation, diverticular disease, iron deficiency anemia, oral disease, malnutrition, and some cancers.[5] The prevalence of obesity has doubled in the past 2 decades. Today, 65 percent of American adults are overweight and 30 percent are considered obese, an increase from 56 and 23 percent, respectively, in 1994. Even more disturbing is the dramatic increase in overweight and obesity among children and adolescents. In order to reverse this trend, we need to consume fewer calories, become more active, and make wiser food choices. Remember: Even modest weight loss (e.g., 10 pounds) can have health benefits, and maintaining weight is better than progressive increases. The basic guidelines for Dietary Guidelines for Americans 2000 were the ABCs of Good Health: **A**im for Fitness, **B**uild a Healthy Base, and **C**hoose Sensibly. The ABCs are an easy way to remember what's important for healthy living. The 2005 Guidelines can still easily align with the ABCs: be more active, eat fewer calories, and make wiser food choices. As you can see, the key recommendations remain similar. In the following section, we have integrated the significant information and best strategies for communicating the Dietary Guidelines since 2000.[6]

FYI

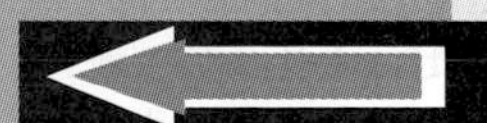

Feast or Famine

Over the past 50 years, the world's ecosystem has been impacted more by human interaction than at any other comparable time in history. The harmful effects of deforestation, degradation of ecosystems, and global climate changes disproportionately impact the poor, particularly women and children. These changes impact agriculture, freshwater resources, clean air, and animal habitats. Globally, inadequate fresh water, sanitation, and hygiene contribute to diseases that lead to 1.7 million deaths each year and the loss of more than 54 million quality life years. Malnutrition is responsible, directly or indirectly, for 60 percent of the 10.9 million deaths annually among children under the age of 5. Two-thirds of these deaths occur in the first year of life and are attributable to inappropriate feeding practices. The health and nutrition of mothers and infants are inextricably linked, and healthy child growth and development are essential for economic development. Undernutrition remains most prevalent among the poorest of the poor, whether we are talking about the poorest nations or mothers and infants within those nations. In 2003 the WHO and UNICEF called for an integrated comprehensive approach to ensure appropriate feeding for the world's children.[7]

Undernutrition seems unfathomable for many living in developed countries, with more overeating than ever before. Whether we're discussing overweight and obesity in Europe or the United States, the overabundance of high-calorie, low-nutrient-dense foods and larger portion sizes are clearly evidenced in the growing rates of overweight and obesity. The WHO findings suggest that societal advancements "have been achieved at increasing cost: degradation of 60% of ecosystem services; exacerbation of poverty for some; and growing inequities and disparities across groups of people."[8] What can you do to impact global climate change? How would you balance economic progress with increasing disparities?

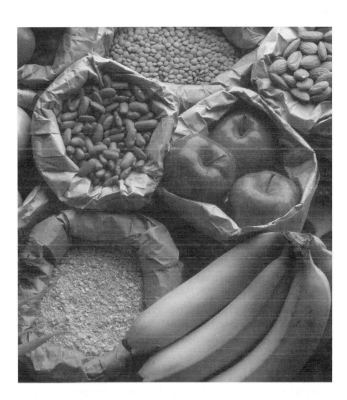

Aim for Fitness (Be more active) Aim for a healthy weight, and be physically active each day.

Aim for a Healthy Weight. Measured in terms of body fat, human beings in industrialized settings rank among the five fattest animals on earth.[9] The 1999–2002 National Health and Nutrition Examination Survey (NHANES) reported that approximately 57 percent of white women and 77.5 percent of African American women were overweight or obese.[10] Presently, the ideal "healthy weight" is not known, but women who are overweight or underweight tend to be less healthy than women who keep their weight within the current recommended ranges.

Be Physically Active Every Day. Two key factors contribute to the continual weight increase of Americans: increased daily consumption of calories and lack of consistent daily physical activity. The report *Healthy People 2010 Health Objectives for the Nation* contains numerous objectives related to maintaining healthy weight and increasing physical activity.[11] Certainly a beneficial health habit is to maintain a personal healthy weight based on sound principles of weight management by engaging in regular physical activity and monitoring calorie intake within a balanced diet. Are there saturated fats, primarily trans fats, in the food you eat? Fats are high in calories, so reduce those types of foods and increase foods lower in calories and higher in nutrients. Engage in a comprehensive and regular physical fitness program to aid in weight management. Chapter 11 provides information about developing a fitness program.

TABLE 10.1 The Fat-Soluble Vitamins, Their Functions, Deficiency Conditions, Food Sources, and Dietary Reference Intakes (DRIs)

VITAMIN	MAJOR FUNCTIONS	DEFICIENCY SYMPTOMS	PEOPLE MOST AT RISK	DIETARY SOURCES	DRI	TOXICITY SYMPTOMS
Vitamin A (retinoids) and provitamin A (carotenoids)	Promote vision: light and color Promote, healthy skin, bone growth, and tooth development Prevent drying of skin and eyes Promote immune system health Promote cell division	Night blindness Xerophthalmia (dry eye) Poor growth Diarrhea Blindness in children Dry skin (ketatinization)	People in poverty, especially preschool children (still very rare in the United States)	Vitamin A Liver Fortified milk Cheese Cream Butter Eggs Provitamin A Sweet potatoes Spinach greens Carrots Cantaloupe Apricots Broccoli Winter squash Pumpkin	Females 600–700 micrograms Pregnant women 750–770 micrograms	Nausea, irritability, hair loss, skin changes, pain in bones, fetal maiformations
D (chole-and ergocalciferol)	Facilitates absorption of calcium and phosphorus Maintains optimal calcification of bone	Rickets in children Osteomalacia in adults	Breast-fed infants, elderly shut-ins	Vitamin D–fortified milk Fish oils Sardines Salmon Egg yolks Liver Skin can make vitamin D when exposed to sunlight	Females 5–15 micrograms Pregnant women 5 micrograms*	Growth and mental retardation, kidney damage, calcium deposits in soft tissue, weight loss
E (tocopherols, tocotrienols)	Acts as an antioxidant: prevents breakdown of vitamin A and unsaturated fatty acids; protects cell walls	Hemolysis of red blood cells Nerve destruction	People with poor fat absorption (still very rare or impossible without starvation)	Vegetable oils Some greens Some fruits Wheat germ Nuts and Seeds	Females 11–15 milligrams alpha-tocopherol equivalents Pregnant women 15 milligrams alpha-tocopherol equivalents	Muscle weakness, headaches, fatigue, nausea, inhibition of vitamin K metabolism
K (phyllo- and menaquinone)	Helps form prothrombin and other factors for blood clotting	Hemorrhage, excessive bleeding	People taking antibiotics for months at a time (still quite rare)	Green, leafy vegetables Liver Milk	Females 60–90 micrograms Pregnant women 15–90 micrograms	Anemia and jaundice

TABLE 10.2 The Water-Soluble Vitamins, Their Functions, Deficiency Conditions, and Food Sources Vitamin Toxicity

VITAMIN	MAJOR FUNCTIONS	DEFICIENCY SYMPTOMS	PEOPLE MOST AT RISK	DIETARY SOURCES	RDA OR ESADDI	TOXICITY
Thiamin (Vitamin B-1)	Coenzyme involved with enzymes in carbohydrate metabolism nerve function	Beriberi, nervous tingling poor coordination, edema, heart changes, weakness	People with alcoholism, people in poverty	Sunflower seed, pork, whole and enriched grains, dried beans, brewer's yeast	1.1–1.4 milligrams	None possible from food
Riboflavin (B-2)	Coenzymes involved in energy metabolism; normal vision and skin health	Inflammation of mouth and tongue, cracks at corners of the mouth, eye disorders	Possibly people on certain medications if no dairy products consumed	Milk, mushrooms, spinach, liver, enriched grains and cereals	1.1–1.6 milligrams	None reported
Niacin (B-3)	Coenzymes involved in energy metabolism, fat synthesis, fat breakdown, skin health	Pellagra, diarrhea, dermatitis, dementia	People in severe poverty for which corn is dominant food, people with alcoholism	Mushrooms, bran, tuna, salmon, chicken, meat, peanuts, enriched grains, peanut butter	14–17 milligrams	Flushing of skin at >100 milligrams
Pantothenic acid (B-5)	Coenzyme involved in energy metabolism, fat synthesis, fat breakdown	Using an antagonist causes tingling in hands, fatigue, headache, nausea	People with alcoholism	Mushrooms, liver, broccoli, eggs; most foods have some	5–7 milligrams	None
Biotin	Coenzyme involved in glucose production, fat synthesis	Dermatitis, sore tongue, anemia, depression	People with alcoholism	Cheese, egg yolks, cauliflower, peanut butter, liver; many foods have some	25–30 micrograms	Unknown
Vitamin B-6, pyridoxine and other forms	Coenzyme involved in protein metabolism, neurotransmitter synthesis, hemoglobin synthesis, many other functions	Headache, anemia, convulsions, nausea, vomiting, flaky skin, sore tongue	Adolescent and adult women, people on certain medications, people with alcoholism	Animal protein foods, spinach, broccoli, bananas, salmon, sunflower seeds	1.3–2 milligrams	Nerve destruction at doses >100 milligrams
Folate	Coenzyme involved in DNA synthesis and making new cells	Megatoblastic anemia, inflammation of tongue, diarrhea, poor growth, mental disorders	People with alcoholism, pregnant women, people taking certain medications	Green leafy vegetables, orange juice, organ meats, sprouts, sunflower seeds; added to most refined grains	400–600 micrograms	None, nonprescription vitamin dosage is controlled by FDA
Vitamin B-12 (cobalamins)	Coenzyme involved in folate metabolism, nerve function	Macrocytic anemia, poor nerve function	Elderly, because of poor absorption, vegans	Animal foods, especially organ meats, oysters, clams (B-12 not naturally in plant foods)	2.4 micrograms	None
Vitamin C (ascorbic acid)	Immune system protection, iron absorption, protein metabolism	Scurvy: poor wound healing, pinpoint hemorrhages, bleeding gums, edema	People with alcoholism, elderly men living alone	Citrus fruits, strawberries, broccoli, greens, peppers, tomatoes	75 milligrams	Doses >1–2 grams cause diarrhea and can alter some diagnostic tests

it appears that consuming the appropriate foods and taking supplements are not harmful and are likely to be protective of our health.

Minerals

Like vitamins, minerals are needed in relatively small amounts. There are seven minerals included in the RDAs. Calcium, magnesium, and phosphorus are **macrominerals,** or major minerals. Four other minerals, iron, zinc, iodine, and selenium, are trace minerals. We obtain minerals from both plant and animal sources. Minerals obtained from animal sources possess a greater level of *bioavailability;* that is, they become more readily available to a woman's body once they are consumed. Plant sources tend to have compounds that bind the minerals, thus reducing mineral bioavailability. Minerals serve a variety of purposes within the body. (See *FYI:* "Sodium and Potassium.")

Minerals serve a variety of purposes within the body. No doubt you are familiar with the role of calcium in developing bone, and you know that iron helps to build good red blood cells. But other minerals serve many other very important functions. A healthy water balance requires appropriate levels of sodium, potassium, calcium, and phosphorus. Sodium, potassium, and calcium influence the movement of nerve impulses, and iodine is a key ingredient in the hormone thyroxin. Refer to Table 10.3 for more information about the major minerals. Two minerals of specific interest to women are calcium and iron, and these are discussed in the following sections.

Sodium and Potassium

Dietary Guidelines for Americans 2005[39]

Key recommendations

- Consume less than 2,300 mg of sodium (approximately 1 teaspoon of edible salt) per day.
- Choose and prepare foods with little salt. At the same time, consume potassium-rich foods, such as fruits and vegetables.

Key recommendations for specific population groups

- *Individuals with hypertension, blacks, and middle-aged and older adults.* Aim to consume no more than 1,500 mg of sodium per day, and meet the potassium recommendation (4,700 mg/day) with food.

Calcium About 99 percent of the calcium in the body is found in bone. The remaining 1 percent is used to stimulate muscle contractions and nerve impulses, and to regulate blood clotting.[40] For the past decade, women have become increasingly more aware of their calcium needs. Medical research has uncovered a considerable amount of information about *osteoporosis,* an age-related condition characterized by demineralization of bone. In the United States, osteoporosis is a serious threat to the health of approximately 44 million Americans. Almost 34 million Americans are estimated to have low bone mass, and more than 10 million presently have osteoporosis. Of the 10 million who have the disease, 80 percent are women.[41] Menopause and aging increase the risk of developing osteoporosis, but it is not an inevitable disease of old age. In fact, it is now known that health behaviors can greatly reduce the risk of developing osteoporosis.

Osteoporosis is perceived as a disease that afflicts old people. Research indicates, however, that the quality of a woman's bones in old age, in the absence of risk factors, is related to what a woman is able to do for herself. The development of bone mineral density (BMD) is related to calcium intake over the woman's lifetime. Specifically, it appears that the greatest influence comes during childhood and the elderly years. The intake of calcium is very important in preventing osteoporosis, but other factors also affect the development of this disease:[42]

- *Family history*—genetics is a major factor in the development of osteoporosis
- *Excess alcohol consumption*—regular consumption of 2 to 3 ounces of alcohol per day contributes to bone loss.
- *Body size*—being thin or small framed
- *Ethnicity*—Caucasian and Asian women are at highest risk; African American and Latino have lower, but still significant risk
- *Eating disorders and diet*—lifetime diet low in calcium and vitamin D
- *Medications*—use of glucocorticoids or some anticonvulsant drugs
- *Cigarette smoking*—has a deleterious effect on BMD
- *Sex hormones*—abnormal absence of menstrual periods (amenorrhea) or low estrogen level (menopause)
- *Physical activity*—sedentary lifestyle, overexercising, or extended bed rest

A woman who has a family history of osteoporosis, drinks alcohol, smokes cigarettes, and/or has an eating disorder is at a greater risk for osteoporosis. If she has a diet that is low in calcium, she is at even greater risk. Although dairy products are good sources of calcium, there are other ways of getting calcium if the woman is lactose intolerant or if she does not like dairy products.

TABLE 10.3 Water and Major Minerals

NAME	MAJOR FUNCTIONS	DEFICIENCY SYMPTOMS	PEOPLE MOST AT RISK	RDA OR MINIMUM REQUIREMENT	NUTRIENT-DENSE DIETARY SOURCES	RESULTS OF TOXICITY
Water	Medium for chemical reactions, removal of waste products, perspiration to cool the body	Thirst, muscle weakness, poor endurance, increased core temperature, decreased plasma volume	Infants with a fever, elderly persons in nursing homes	1.0–1.5 milliliter/kcal of energy expended*	As such and in foods	Seldom occurs and usually in those with mental disorders
Sodium	A major ion of the extracellular fluid; nerve impulse transmission	Muscle cramps	People who severely restrict sodium to lower blood pressure (250–500 milligrams/day)	500 mg/day	Table salt, processed foods	High blood pressure in susceptible individuals
Potassium	A major ion of intracellular fluid; nerve impulse transmission; fluid and electrolyte balance; muscle contraction	Unlikely to occur, irregular heartbeat, loss of appetite, muscle cramps	People who use potassium-wasting diuretics or have poor diets, as seen in poverty and alcoholism	750 mg/day	Spinach, squash, bananas, orange juice, other vegetables and fruits, milk and yogurt	Slowing of the heartbeat; raised blood pressure, paralysis
Calcium	Bone and tooth strength; blood clotting; nerve impulse transmission; muscle contractions; cell regulation	Poor intake increases the risk for osteoporosis	Women in general, especially those who constantly restrict their energy intake, consume few dairy products, or smoke	1000–1200 mg/day	Dairy products, canned fish, leafy vegetables, tofu, fortified orange juice	Very high intakes may cause kidney stones in susceptible people, poor mineral absorption in general, muscle rigor
Phosphorus	Bone and tooth strength; part of various metabolic compounds; major ion of intracellular fluid	Probably none; poor bone maintenance is a possibility	Elderly persons consuming very nutrient-poor diets; possibly total vegetarians and people with alcoholism	750–1200 mg/day	Dairy products, processed foods, fish, soft drinks	Hampers bone health in people with kidney failure; poor bone mineralization if calcium intakes are low
Magnesium	Bone strength; any enzyme function using ATP; nerve and heart function	Weakness, muscle pain, poor heart function	Women in general, people on thiazide diuretics	Women: 280–300 mg/day	Wheat bran, green vegetables, nuts, beans, milk	Causes weakness in people with kidney failure

*Just an approximation; best to keep urine volume at level greater than 1 liter (4 cups).

Calcium Sources

Women are often aware of their need for calcium, yet they think they must drink a lot of milk to obtain adequate amounts of calcium for their diets. Milk is not the sole source of dietary calcium, nor is it the best source. Consider some alternatives to make your diet rich in calcium.

Food (serving size)	Calcium mg
sardines with edible bones (3 oz.)	370
sesame seeds (1/4 cup)	335
skim milk (1 cup)	300
dried figs (1 cup)	287
black-eyed peas (1 cup)	211
green beans (1 cup)	165
almonds (1/2 cup)	150

(See *FYI:* "Calcium Sources" for additional calcium sources.) Additional coverage of osteoporosis can be found in Chapter 15.

Iron Humans need 10–12 mg of iron daily to manufacture **hemoglobin.** Hemoglobin is found in our red blood cells and is responsible for transporting oxygen to, and carbon dioxide away from, the body cells. Iron also helps build certain enzymes and proteins in the body. Because of the blood loss associated with menstruation, women have a greater need for iron during their reproductive years. A woman may need as much as 18 mg per day, and even more if her menstrual flow is heavy.[43] A typical adult diet contains 5–7 mg of iron per 1,000 calories.[44] Women consume about 2,000 calories per day. Therefore, it is necessary for a woman to carefully evaluate the foods she eats to ensure sufficient iron consumption. There are two forms of iron found in our diet. **Heme iron** is found in animal tissue (e.g., in red meat) and is more rapidly absorbed than **nonheme iron,** which is found in plant sources such as spinach and grains. The amount of dietary iron will vary depending on the types and amounts of the various iron-containing foods. Not all of the dietary iron will be absorbed by the body, however. Many diet-related factors tend to interfere with absorption. Zinc competes with iron for absorption. Caffeine has a negative effect on iron absorption, whereas vitamin C has a positive effect on absorption. Substances called tannins found in tea interfere with iron absorption. If a woman wants to have good iron levels, red meat should *not* be completely avoided. Foods rich in vitamin C should be consumed to take advantage of nonheme iron sources. During pregnancy, iron supplements are a must because a woman will almost double her blood volume to accommodate the growing fetus.

Water Often overlooked as a nutrient, water is, without a doubt, our most important nutrient. Depending on our fat stores, we can live for extended periods of time without foods that supply vitamins, minerals, proteins, fats, and energy, but we can expect to live only a few days without water. Most of your body is composed of water—more than 60 percent of the body's weight. Water serves a number of very important functions in the body.

- Water helps to regulate the temperature of the body. Water in the blood collects heat generated by the body and transports it to the surface of the skin. Heat energy is taken from the body as perspiration evaporates.
- Water is necessary for many of the chemical reactions that take place in the body.
- Water serves as a vehicle for removing waste products from the body. Cellular by-products are picked up by the blood and transported to the kidneys for processing and excreting the by-products with the urine.

Thirst is regulated by the concentration of sodium in the blood. When water levels drop and the percent of sodium increases, the thirst sensation is triggered.[45] A woman needs to drink at least 6 cups of water each day. She will obtain an additional 4 cups from the foods she eats. It is advisable not to rely entirely on your thirst response, however. It is not unusual, especially in cool weather, to overlook the need for water. (See *FYI:* "Water: The Overpriced Nutrient.")

Phytochemicals **Phytochemicals** are substances in plant foods that act on the body's physiology in some positive way. More and more evidence is emerging that these components tend to have health-protective qualities.[46] Table 10.4 gives some of the phytochemicals and their functions. In the future, phytochemicals may become classified as essential nutrients.

PREGNANCY AND BREAST-FEEDING

The 55th World Health Assembly and the UNICEF Executive Board have implored governments around the world to adopt a global strategy for ensuring that the feeding needs of infants and young children are met. The organizations reaffirmed that "mothers and babies form an inseparable biological and social unit,

TABLE 10.4 Food Sources and Functions of Phytochemicals

PHYTOCHEMICAL	FOOD SOURCE	ACTION
Carotenoids	Yellow and orange fruits and vegetables, dark-green leafy vegetables	Provide protection against cancer and heart disease
Allylic sulfides	Garlic, onions, chives	Help reduce the production of some enzymes associated with cancer; cardiovascular protection
Phytosterols	Green and yellow vegetables	Block the uptake of cholesterol
Phytoestrogens	Cereals, grains	Prevent diseases and conditions related to aging and menopause

Water: The Overpriced Nutrient

Although the quality of our tap water is regulated by local law and the Environmental Protection Agency, many people are dissatisfied with water that comes from the faucet. In the quest to find drinking water that is believed to be safer, more palatable, and fresher, some consumers have turned to purchasing bottled water. Worldwide, individuals consumed a total of 41 billion gallons of bottled water in 2004 while spending over $100 billion on this important nutrient.[47] This has been an exploding market, with the price increasing at a rate of 8 to 10 percent per year—twice as fast as that of other beverages. Compared to tap water, it costs from 240 to 10,000 times more per gallon to purchase bottled water, making it a very overpriced nutrient.[48]

and that the health and nutrition of one cannot be divorced from the health and nutrition of the other."[49] A woman's nutritional condition is always an important part of her life, but it takes on even greater importance when she becomes pregnant. The changes that occur within her reproductive system are profound. These changes require complex and challenging adaptations to the way she eats. In addition to her own well-being, she is faced with the nutritional demands of the fetus. Many factors influence a successful pregnancy, but a healthy and balanced diet is a major factor that influences the health of the pregnant woman and the fetus.

Energy Needs during Pregnancy

On average, a pregnant woman will need to consume approximately 300 more calories per day than she did before becoming pregnant. Some women get the impression that they are "eating for two" during their pregnancy. Such thinking leads to a greater weight gain than is necessary or healthy for the woman. The amount of weight that should be gained during pregnancy varies from woman to woman. No predetermined amount of weight gain is perfect for every pregnant woman. The average weight gain of a pregnant woman of normal weight is 20–28 pounds. Sixty percent of this weight pertains to the baby: approximately 6–8 pounds for the baby and 7.5 pounds for the placenta, amniotic fluid, breasts, and uterus. The remaining 40 percent relates to the mother's body fluids and accumulated fat.[50]

Nutrient Requirements during Pregnancy

Pregnant women need only 15 percent more calories, but up to 100 percent more nutrients, than women who are not pregnant. Ideally, a pregnant woman will make intelligent food choices that allow her to increase the intake of important nutrients without increasing her calorie intake to the point that she gains more weight than is necessary.

Protein A woman will produce about 2 additional pounds of protein during her pregnancy. About one-fourth of this increase will go to developing her blood supply, and one-half will be used to manufacture fetal tissue. The average woman, on a 2,100 cal/day diet, normally needs about 46 grams of protein. During her pregnancy, she will need to increase daily protein consumption to 71 grams. The challenge will be in her ability to increase protein without increasing fat calories, typically found in many meat sources.

Iron The most common nutrient deficiency among pregnant women is iron.[51] A woman in her childbearing years tends to have low iron stores to begin with, but during pregnancy her iron needs increase dramatically. In addition to the iron needed to build her increasing number of red blood cells, the fetus will demand iron as well. It is extremely unlikely that a woman will be able to consume enough iron in the foods she eats. It is therefore recommended that pregnant women take daily iron supplements. The current recommendation for iron intake during pregnancy is 27 mg.[52]

Folacin Folacin (also folate or folic acid) is very important during pregnancy and in women of childbearing years who may become pregnant. Folacin is necessary for the formation of tissue. One can see how important this nutrient is, given the amount of tissue being generated by the mother and the fetus. Folate deficiency has been associated with neural tube birth defects, spina bifida, and anencephaly. Neural-tube malformations, which are defects of the brain and spinal cord in the embryo, are the number one birth defect in the country today, affecting one to two infants out of every 1,000.[53] In the first few weeks of pregnancy, neural-tube defects begin to manifest themselves in the absence of sufficient levels of folacin. A daily intake of 400 μg/day of synthetic folic acid is recommended for women of childbearing years who may become pregnant. Pregnant women should consume 600 μg/day in addition to food forms of folate in a varied diet.[54] Determine your knowledge of sources of folacin by completing *Assess Yourself:* "Foods for Folacin."

Assess Yourself

Foods for Folacin

Test your knowledge of the food choices. What are the best sources of folacin? Rank-order them with "1" being the highest source and "3" being the lowest source in the group. Answers appear below.

A. 10 Triscuit crackers ____
Cap'n Crunch cereal, 1 cup ____
oatmeal, 1 cup ____

B. 1 poached egg ____
1 baked chicken breast ____
chicken rice soup, 1 cup ____

C. broccoli, 1 cup ____
yellow beans, 1 cup ____
asparagus, 1 cup ____

D. 1 hamburger ____
1 steak ____
ham, 1 cup ____

Answers: A. 3,1,2 B. 1,3,2 C. 3,1,2 D. All three low

Calcium and Vitamin D Calcium is needed to support the mineralization of bone in the fetus. Much of the calcium required for this purpose is needed during the third trimester. It is important for a woman to increase the amount of calcium in her diet early in her pregnancy. If her diet is low in calcium at the start of her pregnancy, and she makes no adjustments to improve calcium intake, calcium will be automatically removed from her own bones so that blood levels of calcium can be maintained for the fetus.[55] Along with dairy products and calcium-fortified orange juice, other sources of calcium are included in *FYI:* "Calcium Sources," presented earlier. A woman who doesn't like these kinds of foods is advised to take calcium supplements. Vitamin D is also important to the development of bone in the fetus. Studies suggest that vitamin D levels in the mother impact early bone strength and density in the newborn. The primary sources have typically been increased exposure to sunlight and use of supplements.

Vitamin and Mineral Supplements Many pregnant women, in an effort to help the growing fetus, will routinely take a complete vitamin/mineral supplement during pregnancy. The only nutrients that require supplementation are iron, folacin, vitamin D, and calcium (especially if the woman does not drink milk). All other nutrients can be obtained from the slight increase in food consumption, if a woman eats a variety of foods. High doses of certain vitamins, especially vitamins B-6, B-12, and C, are not recommended during pregnancy. Excessive amounts of these vitamins will create **rebound deficiencies.** The high amounts of vitamins place the fetus's excretion mechanisms into high gear during pregnancy. This high rate of excretion continues after delivery thus excreting the small amounts of vitamins that the infant receives.[56]

Breast-Feeding

After a woman delivers her baby, it is recommended that she make every effort to breast-feed her infant. Breast milk contains the appropriate proportion of vitamins, proteins, minerals, calories, fats, and additional amino acids. It is easier for newborns to digest and contains antibodies that help to protect them from disease and infection. In addition to providing ideal food for the healthy growth and development of infants breast-feeding is integral to the reproductive process, with important implications for the health of mothers.[57] The global public health recommendation is that infants should be exclusively breast-fed for the first 6 months of life to achieve optimal growth, development, and health.[58] Cow's milk is not recommended until the infant reaches 1 year of age. The protein and minerals in cow's milk are much too difficult for a newborn to digest, and the newborn's kidneys are not developed enough to process the high mineral content of cow's milk.[59]

A woman's nutrient needs during breast-feeding are similar to those during pregnancy. Proportionally, she will continue to require more nutrients than calories. She should continue with a nutrient-dense diet and supplement with vitamins as needed. Her calcium intake deserves special attention. If she fails to consume enough calcium in her diet, she can experience calcium loss from her bones in order to meet the needs of the infant.[60] It is also important for a woman to drink fluids after she nurses so that milk production does not diminish. A breast-feeding woman should be aware that what she takes into her body may find its way into her milk supply. Alcohol, caffeine, and other drugs can be delivered to the infant via breast-feeding. Saturated fats can also be delivered to the infant. A woman is advised to be careful about the quality of her diet if she expects to have a healthy baby.

PHYSICAL ACTIVITY

Fitness activity levels will have an effect on a woman's nutritional needs. (See *FYI:* "Physical Activity.") If a woman is a competitive athlete or happens to engage in vigorous activity for an hour or more at least 5 days per week, she could classify herself as *highly active*. As you might expect, high and low activity levels require differing food plans. Chapter 11 provides specifics regarding a comprehensive physical activity program.

Caloric Intake

Energy requirements vary according to activity level. Energy consumption is a function of the intensity of the activity and the length of time you engage in that activity. Table 10.5 provides an estimate of calorie requirements based on age group and levels of physical activity. These levels are based on estimated energy requirements for reference-sized individuals. "Reference size," as determined by the Institute of Medicine, is based on median height and weight for ages up to 18 years and median height and weight for the height to give a body mass index of 21.5 for adult females. *Sedentary* means a lifestyle that includes only the light physical activity associated with typical day-to-day life. *Moderately active* means a lifestyle that includes physical activity equivalent to walking about 1.5–3 miles per day at 3–4 miles per hour, in addition to the light physical activity associated with typical day-to-day life. *Active* means a lifestyle

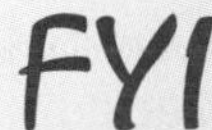

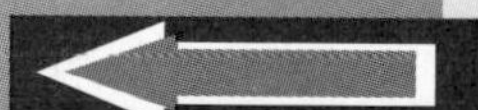

Physical Activity

Dietary Guidelines for Americans 2005[61]

Key recommendations

- Engage in regular physical activity and reduce sedentary activities to promote health, psychological well-being, and a healthy body weight.

  To reduce the risk of chronic disease in adulthood: Engage in at least 30 minutes of moderate-intensity physical activity, above-usual activity, at work or home on most days of the week.

  For most people, greater health benefits can be obtained by engaging in physical activity of more vigorous intensity or longer duration.

  To help manage body weight and prevent gradual, unhealthy body weight gain in adulthood: Engage in approximately 60 minutes of moderate- to vigorous-intensity activity on most days of the week while not exceeding calorie intake requirements.

  To sustain weight loss in adulthood: Participate in at least 60 to 90 minutes of daily moderate-intensity physical activity while not exceeding calorie intake requirements. Some people may need to consult with a health care provider before participating in this level of activity.

- Achieve physical fitness by including cardiovascular conditioning, stretching exercises for flexibility, and resistance exercises or calisthenics for muscle strength and endurance.

Key recommendations for specific population groups

- *Children and adolescents.* Engage in at least 60 minutes of physical activity on most, preferably all, days of the week.
- *Pregnant women.* In the absence of medical or obstetric complications, incorporate 30 minutes or more of moderate-intensity physical activity on most, if not all, days of the week. Avoid activities with a high risk of falling or abdominal trauma.
- *Breast-feeding women.* Be aware that neither acute nor regular exercise adversely affects the mother's ability to successfully breast-feed.
- *Older adults.* Participate in regular physical activity to reduce functional declines associated with aging and to achieve the other benefits of physical activity identified for all adults.

TABLE 10.5 Estimated Calorie Requirements (In kilocalories) for Each Gender and Age Group at Three Levels of Physical Activity[a]

		ACTIVITY LEVEL[b,c,d]		
Gender	Age (years)	Sedentary[b]	Moderately Active[c]	Active[d]
Child	2–3	1,000	1,000–1,400[e]	1,000–1,400[e]
Female	4–8	1,200	1,400–1,600	1,400–1,800
	9–13	1,600	1,600–2,000	1,800–2,200
	14–18	1,800	2,000	2,400
	19–30	2,000	2,000–2,200	2,400
	31–50	1,800	2,000	2,200
	51+	1,600	1,800	2,000–2,200
Male	4–8	1,400	1,400–1,600	1,600–2,000
	9–13	1,800	1,800–2,200	2,000–2,600
	14–18	2,200	2,400–2,800	2,800–3,200
	19–30	2,400	2,600–2,800	3,000
	31–50	2,200	2,400–2,600	2,800–3,000
	51+	2,000	2,200–2,400	2,400–2,800

[a] These levels are based on Estimated Energy Requirements (EER) from the Institute of Medicine Dietary Reference Intakes macronutrients report, 2002, calculated by gender, age, and activity level for reference-sized individuals. "Reference size," as determined by IOM, is based on median height and weight for ages up to age 18 years of age and median height and weight for that height to give a BMI of 21.5 for adult females and 22.5 for adult males.

[b] Sedentary means a lifestyle that includes only the light physical activity associated with typical day-to-day life.

[c] Moderately active means a lifestyle that includes physical activity equivalent to walking about 1.5 to 3 miles per day at 3 to 4 miles per hour, in addition to the light physical activity associated with typical day-to-day life

[d] Active means a lifestyle that includes physical activity equivalent to walking more than 3 miles per day at 3 to 4 miles per hour, in addition to the light physical activity associated with typical day-to-day life.

[e] The calorie ranges shown are to accommodate needs of different ages within the group. For children and adolescents, more calories are needed at older ages. For adults, fewer calories are needed at older ages.

SOURCE: HHS/USDA *Dietary Guidelines for Americans 2005*.

that includes physical activity equivalent to walking more than 3 miles per day at 3–4 miles per hour, in addition to the light physical activity associated with typical day-to-day life. If you are involved in some form of activity, your energy intake should match your energy expenditure unless you are attempting to lose weight.

Nutrients

It is generally believed that there is no need to increase the amount of nutrients beyond the DRIs as a person becomes physically active.[62] Exercise increases the athlete's need for more energy and water, not for more protein, vitamins, or minerals. There are, however, some aspects of nutrition and athletic performance for women that deserve special mention.

Iron deficiency has been an area of interest for some time. Investigations have revealed that iron levels are not significantly different among female athletes versus nonathletes. Those studies that report differences attribute them to poor diet rather than to physical activity.[63] Also, one of the confounding factors in measuring iron levels is the menstrual cycle, which can influence the level of iron in the blood. Vegetarian athletes or those athletes who do not eat red meat are more vulnerable to low iron levels.[64] It is strongly recommended that women who are active or highly active get at least 18 mg of iron daily, either from their diet or through supplementation.

Calcium intake is another area that has been studied among female athletes. It appears that female athletes may not be getting all the calcium they need. Many female athletes, particularly those who are concerned with being thin, have been observed with calcium intake levels that are below DRI levels.[65] If calcium levels are low, and the woman develops amenorrhea, she is likely to experience demineralization of her bones, which in turn will increase her potential for leg injuries or stress fractures. If you are physically active and follow a vegetarian diet, you should be aware of potential problems. Vegetarians, because of high fiber intake, tend to lose estrogen. A vegetarian diet may also increase the likelihood of altering a woman's menstrual cycle, particularly if the diet is low in fat, low in protein, and high in fiber.[66]

VEGETARIANISM

Women may choose to limit their diets to plant-based foods and eliminate or partially eliminate animal foods for a number of reasons: following religious beliefs, feeling that killing animals is unethical, using food resources that are low on the food chain, or eating less expensive foods. Vegetarian diet styles may vary. Vegetarians are grouped according to the animal-derived foods they eat. *Vegans* eat only plant foods; *lacto-vegetarians* eat plant foods and dairy products; *lacto-ovo-vegetarians* eat no

Her Story

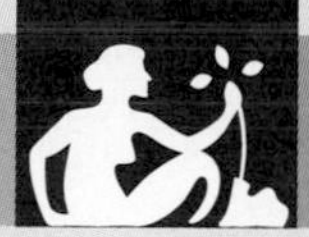

Deanne, Choosing Vegetarianism

Deanne has always been interested in environmental responsibility, including compassion to animals. When she read about the animal suffering that happens with factory farming, like greater numbers of birds being put in smaller cages, reduced square feet for hog pens, fumes from manure causing eye and respiratory infections, and slaughtering of milk cows after 5–6 years of production, she decided to read about alternatives. She thought eating free-range meat might be okay, until she read that "free range" was a meaningless term. So, Deanne decided to become a vegetarian. First, she made a list of all the meals she already ate that were meatless. Next, she made a list of the meals that could become meatless. She had a great start.

- What does Deanne need to know about eating healthy as a vegetarian?
- When Deanne takes meat out of her diet, what nutrients might she lose? What substitutes might she consider?
- What other reasons may people give for being vegetarian?

meat, poultry, or fish, but do eat eggs and milk products; and *semivegetarians* include eggs, dairy products, and small amounts of poultry and seafood in the diet. First and foremost, nutritional health is dependent on balance, variety, and moderation in the diet. Whether the diet is **omnivorous** (consuming both plant and animal food sources) or vegetarian, attention must be paid to achieving the recommended DRIs. Women considering vegetarian diets should learn about the benefits and risks before starting a vegetarian diet. (See *Her Story:* "Deanne: Choosing Vegetarianism.")

Benefits of Vegetarianism

Numerous studies have been conducted on the benefits of a vegetarian meal plan. Most studies confirm that vegetarian diets are lower in total fat, saturated fat, and cholesterol. Other beneficial outcomes of a vegetarian diet include:[67]

- *Leanness.* Vegetarians are more health conscious and more physically active.
- *Lower levels of serum cholesterol.* Vegans have lower levels than even lacto-vegetarians or nonvegetarians.
- *Lower blood pressure.* Leaner body mass contributes significantly to decreased BP.
- *Less colon cancer.* Diets high in animal tissue and animal fat tend to increase the risk of colon cancer.

Concerns of Vegetarianism

If a vegetarian encounters nutritional problems, it may be in the form of

- *Iron deficiency.* Iron levels are reportedly lower among lacto-ovo-vegetarians, and more so for women than men.
- *Insufficient levels of calcium.* Because dairy products are a good source of calcium, this nutrient can be erroneously omitted from the diet.
- *Vitamin D deficiency.* Vegans may have insufficient levels of this vitamin due to the absence of milk products and lack of sunlight. Vegans should try to get sunlight when possible and choose vitamin D–fortified products, such as orange juice and some cereals.
- *Vitamin B-12 deficiency.* Pernicious anemia develops in the absence of vitamin B-12. In fact, women can pass this deficiency on to their infants through breast-feeding.[68] Cereals and breads fortified, not enriched, with B-12 should be considered, as well as fortified soy and rice drinks.

If you have an interest in following a vegetarian dietary regimen, there are certain principles you should follow for optimal health.

- No single plant food contains all essential amino acids, but combining a variety of grains and vegetables will help vegetarians get the essential amino acids. Vegans combine foods to form meals throughout the day that become complete with the essential amino acids. Suggested substitutes for dairy products and eggs include fortified soy milk, rice milk, and almond milk; using oils as substitutes for butter; and using egg substitutes.
- Plant proteins can provide all essential and nonessential amino acids, but varied sources and a high calorie intake are recommended for adequate energy needs.
- Animal foods contain zinc, calcium, and iron.[69] Attention should be paid to consuming plant foods that contain these nutrients. For example, whole grains, soy products, nuts, wheat germ, spinach, broccoli, dark-green vegetables, and dried fruit will serve as substitutes.
- Be aware that the iron in plant foods is not as well absorbed as the iron from meat sources. Be careful, too, about consuming too much grain, bran, and soy products. These foods contain phytates (a form of phosphorus that is not readily bioavailable), which inhibit the absorption of iron, calcium, and zinc.[70] The bottom line is that vegetarianism requires intelligent planning of meals, a working knowledge of how foods interact with one another, and knowledge of the factors that influence nutrient uptake.

NUTRITION AND THE CONSUMER

We are constantly confronted with food products that claim to do amazing things. There are claims that special foods can maintain our youth, cure or prevent cancer, and supply us with an endless amount of energy. Labels on special food products and dietary supplements are usually the means by which such products deliver their claims. Understanding terminology such as "health foods," "organic," and "natural," knowing which sources of information are reliable and trustworthy, and interpreting food labels can improve a woman's ability to become a healthier consumer.

What are *health foods?* Obviously, by the term, they are foods that are meant to be beneficial to one's health! Where do we find health foods? In reality, we find them at every store that sells food, not just stores named "Health Food Stores," which is a misleading designation. When eaten in variety and moderation, and according to guidelines described in MyPyramid, all foods can be healthy. Stare, Aronson, and Barrett state:

> The term is merely a gimmick used to boost sales. . . . Some foods . . . popular as health foods are rich in nutrients, but no food has unique health-promoting properties. All foods can contribute to health when eaten as part of a varied and balanced diet. The problem with so called health foods is that they are promoted with false claims and usually are overpriced.[71] Table 10.6 lists products commonly promoted as health foods.

Additives

Many women are concerned about the amount of additives found in their foods. We tend to think of food additives as chemicals that are unnatural and added to our foods unnecessarily. The truth is that food additives play very important roles in the food we consume. Food additives are used in foods for five principal reasons:

1. *To maintain product consistency.* Anti-caking agents help products like salt flow freely. Emulsifiers prevent products from separating.
2. *To improve or maintain nutritional value.* For instance, vitamin D is added to milk to help reduce the incidence of malnutrition. Vitamin D is necessary for the appropriate absorption of calcium in order to maintain bone density.
3. *To reduce spoilage.* Preservatives will prevent spoilage caused by mold, bacteria, and fungi.
4. *To provide leavening or control acidity/alkalinity.* Leavening agents are added to help baked goods rise during cooking. Some additives modify acidity and alkalinity to improve flavor, taste, and color.
5. *To enhance flavor or provide a desired color.*

TABLE 10.6 Are the "Health" Food Claims True?

PRODUCT	CLAIMS	TRUTH
Alfalfa	Contains nutrients not found in other foods	Less than in common vegetables
	Contains all essential amino acids	Untrue
Aloe vera	Cures or alleviates asthma, glaucoma, arthritis, hemorrhoids, or anemia	Unsubstantiated
	Promotes skin softening and moisturizing	Probably true
Carob	Used in products as a chocolate substitute; lower in fat and caffeine-free	Yes; however, has similar calorie content
Coenzyme Q10	Prevents aging and increases enzyme levels in body tissue	No evidence; however, may help reduce formation of atherosclerotic formation
Fish-oil capsules	Lower blood-cholesterol and reduce heart disease	Amounts to eat are unknown; need to eat fish twice each week
Garlic	Purifies the blood, reduces high blood pressure, prevents cancer, etc.	Has lowered blood-cholesterol, but other beneficial claims are preliminary; causes bad breath and heartburn; may inhibit blood clotting
Goat's milk	Provides a highly nutritious cow's milk substitute	No more nutritious than cow's milk
	Effective against arthritis and cancer	Untrue
		Unpasteurized goat's milk can contain pathogens that cause disease
Granola	"Natural" and contains high amounts of nutrients	High in price, sugar, fats, and calories
RNA/DNA supplements	Rejuvenate old cells, improve memory, and prevent aging skin	Inactivated by the digestive process, so has none of these effects

Knowing that additives are placed in foods to maintain quality is one thing. However, concern that "unnatural chemicals" are added to our food is something else. The fear is that chemicals will harm us. Consider the ingredients in the following foods:

> *Product A:* acetone, methyl acetate, furan, butanol, methyfuran, isoprene, methyl butanol, caffeine, essential oils, methanol, acetaldehyde, methyl formate, ethanol, dimethyl sulfide, and propionaldehyde.
>
> *Product B:* actomycin, myogen, nucleoproteins, peptides, amino acids, myoglobin, lipids, linoleic acid, oleic acid, lecithin, cholesterol, sucrose, ATP, glucose, collagen, elastin, creatine, pytoligneous acid, sodium chloride, sodium nitrate, sodium nitrite, and sodium phosphate.

What do you think about these two products? Do you feel you could safely consume either of them over extended periods of time? Would you feel better knowing that product A is coffee and that product B is cured ham? The media and special interest groups have attempted to color our food supply as harmful, but the truth is that all foods we consume are made of chemicals. Calcium propionate is a common food additive. Although it may sound unnatural, it is actually a compound found naturally in swiss cheese. It is added to food to prevent bacterial growth.

Food additives are carefully regulated by the FDA and are permitted only after extensive testing. If an additive is shown to produce cancer, for example, it cannot be used—even if the additive causes cancer only when consumed in very high doses. Using it would violate the Delaney Clause in the 1958 Food Additives Amendment.[72] It is safe to say that food additives are far more protective than harmful. It would be impossible to feed everyone in this country without food additives. Additives can keep food whole some and appealing, improve the nutritional value of some foods, and improve taste, color, and texture. Diets high in fat and alcohol actually pose greater risks to health than any of the additives found in our food supply.

Organic Foods

Organic foods are one of the fastest growing sectors of the U.S. food industry. Organic foods claim to be produced, grown, and processed without use of commercial chemicals such as fertilizers, pesticides, or synthetics such as color or flavor. Organic production leads to a more sustainable environment than non-organic production. The U.S. Department of Agriculture (USDA) makes no claims that organically produced foods are safer or more nutritious than conventionally grown foods; they differ only in methods of farming, handling, and processing.[73] However, it is also true that the USDA spends less than 0.1 percent of federal agricultural research dollars on organic farming. If dollars spent are any indicator, the USDA does not necessarily value the current organic farming trend. Which organic foods might be promoted? Meat, eggs, and dairy products labeled as organic come from animals that are given no growth hormones or antibiotics. Some organic food products may be worth the extra cost; however, purchasing organic hair or cosmetic products and farm-raised fish or shellfish may be less beneficial. Take the short *Assess Yourself*: "What Do You Know about the Foods You Eat?" to determine what you know about some of the foods you eat.

Studies reveal that organic foods may cost twice as much as other foods. The USDA requires that foods labeled

Assess Yourself

What Do You Know about the Foods You Eat?

Circle the answers that you think are correct, and then check your answers below.

1. The skins of fruits and vegetables are a significant source of nutrients and fiber, but pesticides may make them less healthy. From which of the following should you always trim the peel?
   a. carrots
   b. cucumbers
   c. pears
   d. apples
2. Which of the following foods should be avoided if mold appears?
   a. yogurt
   b. peanut butter
   c. individual cheese slices
   d. all of the above
3. How soon after a meal should leftovers be refrigerated?
   a. within 1/2 hour
   b. within 1 hour
   c. within 2 hours
   d. within 3 hours

Answers:

1. A—Peel apples and cucumbers only if they have been waxed.
2. D—If you can safely remove at least 1 inch of the food along with the mold, it may be safe to eat the food. It may not be possible to completely remove all mold from products like those above.
3. C—Prepared foods can safely sit at room temperature for up to 2 hours before needing refrigeration.

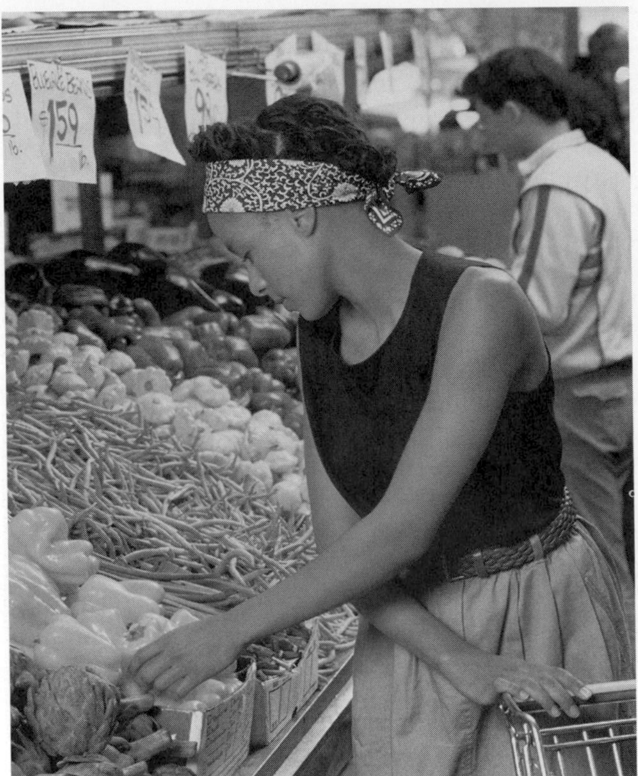

Journal Activity

Organic versus Standard-Grown Foods

Visit markets that sell organic foods and compare their claims, prices, and appearance with foods that have been grown and processed via standard agricultural methods. What are your findings? Do you receive more nutrient benefits from organic foods? How do you know? Make a chart of five foods and compare costs between the two groups. Are organic foods easy to find? How do you know foods labeled as organic are indeed organic? Do you have to travel to a special store to purchase organic foods? What were the claims of the store clerk about these foods? What is your decision about these two types of foods?

"organic" must follow the national standards of organic food production guidelines.[74] If you choose to purchase organic foods, be aware that you may be spending an unnecessary amount of money on some foods that cannot match their claims. Complete *Journal Activity:* "Organic versus Standard-Grown Foods" to help you determine whether organic foods are a wise choice for you.

Knowledge and application of this information helps us become more confident, wiser, and healthier consumers. We also need reliable assistance when we have consumer-related nutritional questions or concerns. The agencies and organizations listed at the end of this chapter provide a number of sources to obtain nutritional information. Registered dietitians in hospitals, public health departments, or clinical settings are very knowledgeable in answering consumer-related nutrition questions. Health educators, nurses, and physicians can provide reliable sources. Articles reviewed and submitted by experts in their specific professions and found in professional journals and magazines are also valuable and reliable sources of information.

Food Labeling

When you purchase or use prepared foods, do you take the time to read the labels? If so, what do you look for? Brand names, ingredients, fat content, calories? Like all consumers, you are probably interested in specific things about the product. Reading food labels has become easier because there must now be consistency in information and terminology that describe the contents of food products. As a result of the 1990 Nutritional Labeling and Education Act and regulatory actions by the FDA and the U.S. Department of Agriculture, consumers can better determine the food products that meet their individual nutritional needs.

Food manufacturers are required to place labels on their products that offer complete, accurate, and useful nutritional information. Anyone who shops can make comparisons among all foods found in grocery stores everywhere.

Food labels provide information that help women make nutritious food choices to help meet recommended DRIs. The FDA mandates that the following must be included on food labels and packages: total calories, calories from fat, total fat, saturated fat, cholesterol, sodium, total carbohydrates, dietary fiber, sugars, vitamin A, protein, vitamin C, calcium, and iron.[75] Other dietary components can be voluntarily placed on the label. The daily value (DV), which is the daily nutrient intake level recommended by nutrition authorities, is stated in percentages and reveals how much of a day's ideal total of a particular nutrient a consumer is receiving based on a 2,000-calorie-per-day diet. This reference quickly allows a woman to see how a packaged food product meets her nutritional needs.

Current food labels reveal a wealth of information by providing an easy-to-read format. The standardized serving sizes allow comparison of nutrients on similar products. Labels provide uniform definitions for terms

FYI

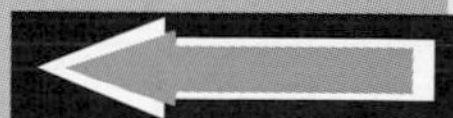

What Does a Food Label Mean?[76]

Food labels with so-called natural or organic names may not always be either "natural" or "organic." The following meaningful labels have U.S. government standards behind them while the meaningless labels do not.

Meaningful Labels

100% Organic. This designation means that, by law, no synthetic ingredients are allowed. Production processes must meet federal guidelines and have independent verification by accredited inspectors.

Organic. This means that at least 95 percent of the ingredients must meet federal standards for the term "organic." The remaining 5 percent may be inorganic or synthetic ingredients. The only exception is seafood as no current government standards for "organic" exist when referring to seafood products.

Made with Organic Ingredients. At least 70 percent of the ingredients must meet the federal standards for the term "organic." The remaining 30 percent must be from the USDA's approved list of ingredients.

Meaningless Labels

"Free-range" or "free-roaming." Often stamped on eggs, chicken, and meat, these designations may mislead consumers into thinking a farm animal has spent much of its life outdoors. However, the U.S. government standards for these labels are weak. Such labeling may mean nothing more than that a farm animal had some limited access to the outdoors, not that it spent any significant time in a healthy, outdoor environment.

"Natural" or "all natural." These designations do not mean organic. Unless these terms are used on meat or poultry products, no standard definitions for either exist, and a food manufacturer or producer may use these terms at its own discretion. The exception is meat and poultry products, for which "natural" is defined by the USDA as containing no artificial coloring, flavoring, chemical preservatives, or other synthetic ingredients.

that describe a food's nutrient content ("low-fat" or "high-fiber"), and information about the relationship between a nutrient or a food and a health-related condition, such as low-saturated fat and heart disease.[77] (See *FYI:* "What Does a Food Label Mean?")

Portion Distortion Portion size is extremely important to monitor when choosing any meal plan. Our society continues to place more value on receiving larger portions when dining out. The current trend in America is to "supersize it," "biggie size it," or "make it a grande." This, together with "all you can eat buffets" and "buy one, get one free" deals, encourages the food consumer to eat beyond meeting energy needs. Many food vendors, especially fast-food vendors, use larger portion sizes as a selling point by pricing the larger item at a better value. The perception of getting "more for less money" often keeps consumers eating or drinking more calories per meal than necessary. (See Assess Yourself: "What Do You Know about a Serving Size?")

Another way to test your knowledge about portion size is to try the interactive quiz prepared by the National Heart, Lung, and Blood Institute. Go to hp2010.nhlbihin.net/portion to test your knowledge about portion distortion.

Fast-food restaurants, whether due to time, money or convenience, are often the restaurants of choice. A woman who wants to be healthy and keep her weight at a desired level can, however, still eat fast-food by making wiser choices from the offered menus. See Table 10.7 for some healthier options at fast-food vendors. These choices may save money as well as calories.

Assess Yourself

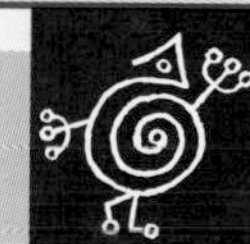

What Do You Know about a Serving Size?

One way to determine what constitutes an appropriate serving size per meal is to create a visual size comparison between a portion of food and an ordinary object.[78] Some common comparisons are

- 1 ounce of cheese = size of four dice
- 3 ounces of meat = a deck of cards or a bar of soap
- ½ cup of mashed potatoes = the amount found in an ice cream scoop
- 1 medium potato = a computer mouse
- 1 fruit serving = a baseball

Label Terminology Terms and their meanings are continually being revised. To better comprehend what you are buying, you must understand nutritional terms.

TABLE 10.7 Healthier Options at Fast-Food Vendors

FOOD CHOICE	CALORIES	POSSIBLE SUBSTITUTE	CALORIES	CALORIES SAVED
Double cheeseburger	600	Cheeseburger	320	280
Cheeseburger	320	Hamburger	270	50
Breaded chicken sandwich	515	Grilled chicken sandwich	310	205
Baked potato with cheese	570	Plain baked potato	310	260
Super fries	450	Small fries	210	240
32-oz (large) soda	310	16-oz (small) soda	150	160
32-oz (large) soda	310	32-oz (large) diet soda	0	310

SOURCE: American Cancer Society. *Restaurant eating tips*. www.cancer.org/docroot/PED/content/PED_3_2X_Restaurant_Eating_Tips_Mar_03.asp?Sitearea=PED (retrieved February 6, 2006).

TABLE 10.8 Common Food Label Terminology

The following are terms with brief explanations found on food product packaging.

Fat

- *Fat-free:* less than 0.5 gram (g)
- *Low-fat:* 3 g or less fat than found in the full-calorie product

Saturated Fat

- *Saturated fat-free:* less than 0.5 g and less than 0.5 g trans-fatty acid per serving (Trans-fatty acid is found in solid vegetable fat products, like margarine. The FDA suggests that levels of trans-fatty acid be limited in products that claim to be "saturated fat-free.")
- *Low saturated fat:* 1 g or less per serving and not more than 15 percent of calories coming from saturated fatty acids
- *Reduced or less saturated fat:* at least 25 percent less each serving than the reference food (the same product that had the original level of fat)

Calories

- *Calorie-free:* fewer than 5 calories per serving
- *Low-calorie:* 40 or fewer calories per serving
- *Reduced or fewer calories:* at least 25 percent fewer calories per serving than the full-calorie food

Calories and Fat

Light (two meanings):

- One-third fewer calories or half the fat of the full-calorie food. (If food is composed of 59 percent or more of calories from fat, the reduction has to be 50 percent of fat.)
- A "low-calorie" or "low-fat" food, in which the fat amount has been reduced by 50 percent of the full-calorie food. "Light in sodium" means that the food product has 50 percent or less sodium than the full-sodium food.

Sugar

- *Sugar-free:* less than 0.5 g per serving
- *No added sugar, without added sugar, no sugar added:* Has no sugar or ingredients containing sugars, such as fruit or fruit juice added during processing or packing. Has no ingredients made with added sugars, such as jellies or fruit juice. (If a label states "sugar-free" or "no sugar added," this applies only to a reduction in calories related to sugar, not to calories from fat, protein, or other carbohydrates.)
- *Reduced sugar:* at least 25 percent less sugar than the full-calorie food

Fiber

Note: Any food claiming increased fiber content must also meet the definition for "low-fat," or the amount of total fat per serving must appear next to the claim.

- *High-fiber:* 5 g or more per serving
- *Good source of fiber:* 2.5 g to 4.9 g per serving
- *More or added fiber:* at least 2.5 g more per serving than the full-calorie food

Food label regulations require food manufacturers to use standardized terms when describing nutrient content of foods. Descriptors such as "less," "high-fiber," "low-fat," "free," "light," "lite," or "reduced calories" must meet FDA requirements. For meat, poultry, and fish, the terms "lean" and "extra lean" apply to the fat content of these products and must meet the established percentages for fat and lean content. Table 10.8

FIGURE 10.2 How to read the food label.

Serving size

Is your serving the same size as the one on the label? If you eat double the serving size listed, you need to double the nutrient and calorie values. If you eat one-half the serving size shown here, cut the nutrient and calorie in half. Pay attention to the serving size, including the number of servings in the food package.

Calories

Do you want to lose weight? Cut back a little on calories. Look here to see how one serving of the food adds to your daily total. The number of servings you consume determines the number of calories you have eaten.

Total carbohydrate

When you cut down on fat, you can eat more carbohydrates. Carbohydrates are in foods like whole-grain bread, fruits, and vegetables. Choose nutrient-dense carbs often. They give you nutrients and energy. Reduce sugars whenever possible.

Dietary fiber

Most Americans, including women, do not get enough fiber. That goes for both soluble and insoluble kinds of dietary fiber. Fruits, vegetables, whole-grain foods, beans, and peas are all good sources and can help reduce the risk of heart disease and cancer.

Protein

Most Americans get more protein than they need. Where there is animal protein there are also fat and cholesterol. Eat small servings of lean meat, fish, and poultry. Use skim or low-fat milk, yogurt, and cheese. Try vegetable proteins like beans, grains, and cereals.

Vitamins and minerals

Your goal here is 100 percent of each for the day. Don't count on one food to do it all. Most Americans don't get enough vitamin A, vitamin C, calcum, and iron in their diets.

Nutrition Facts

Serving Size 1 cup (228g)
Servings per Container 2

Amount per Serving	
Calories 250 Calories from Fat 110	
	% Daily Value*
Total Fat 12g	18%
Saturated Fat 3g	15%
Trans Fat 3g	
Cholesterol 30mg	10%
Sodium 470mg	20%
Total Carbohydrate 31g	10%
Dietary Fiber 0g	0%
Sugars 5g	
Protein 5g	
Vitamin A	4%
Vitamin C	2%
Calcium	20%
Iron	4%

*Percent Daily Values are based on a 2,000 calorie diet. Your Daily Values may be higher or lower depending on your calorie needs:

	Calories	2,000	2,500
Total Fat	Less than	65g	80
Sat Fat	Less than	20g	25g
Cholesterol	Less than	300mg	300mg
Sodium	Less than	2,400mg	2,400mg
Total Carbohydrate		300g	375g
Dietary Fiber		25g	30g

Total fat

Aim low: Most people need to cut back on fat. Too much fat may contribute to heart disease and cancer. Try to limit your calories from fat, particularly saturated and trans fat. For a healthy heart, choose foods with a big difference between the total number of calories and the number of calories from fat.

Saturated fat

Saturated fat is part of the total fat in food. It is listed separately because it's the key player in raising blood cholesterol and your risk of heart disease. Choose foods low in saturated fat to stay healthy.

Trans fat

Trans fat is formed when liquid oils are made into solid fats like shortening and hard margarine. Trans fat raises LDL cholesterol, which increases your risk of coronary heart disease. Choose foods low in trans fat to stay healthy.

Cholesterol

Too much cholesterol—a second cousin to fat—can lead to heart disease. Cholesterol occurs naturally in the tissues of the body, and there is no evidence that dietary cholesterol is needed. Challenge yourself to eat less than 300 mg each day.

Sodium

You call it "salt," the label calls it "sodium." Either way, it may add up to high blood pressure in some people. So, keep your sodium intake low—2,400 to 3,000 mg or less each day.

The DASH (Dietary Approaches to Stop Hypertension) recommends 1,500 mg per day.

Daily Values

Feel like you're drowning in numbers? Let the Daily Value (DV) be your guide. Daily Values are listed for people who eat 2,000 or 2,500 calories each day. DVs are recommended levels of intake. If you eat more, your personal daily value may be higher than what's listed on the label. If you eat less, your personal daily value may be lower.

For fat, saturated fat, cholesterol, and sodium, choose foods with a low % Daily Value. For total carbohydrate, dietary fiber, vitamins, and minerals, your daily value goal is to reach 100% of each.

g = grams (About 28 g = 1 ounce)
mg = milligrams (1,000 mg = 1 g)

provides a review of the meanings for these terms that will increase your understanding of nutritional content of food products.[79]

Food labels have two distinct sections: a principal display panel (PDP) and an information panel. The PDP is usually on the front of the product and must contain the name of the product (not the name of the company), for example, "tuna packed in vegetable oil," and the net quantity of the product. The PDP may be where the manufacturer states certain claims, such as "low-fat," "fortified," and so forth. The information panel is the part of the label that is of greatest interest to consumers. Figure 10.2 is an example of a typical food label.

Labeling about Food Allergies Increasingly, the potential life-threatening outcomes from food allergies are being reported by the media. What exactly are they discussing, and why are food allergies more prevalent? Normally the body does not evoke an immune response. However, a food allergy is an abnormal response to a perceived toxin that evokes an immune system response. If a food is perceived as harmful, an antibody called immunoglobulin E (IgE) is created and the next time it is eaten, high levels of histamine or other chemicals (called mediation) are released to protect the body. These symptoms can affect the respiratory system, gastrointestinal tract, skin, or cardiovascular system. Symptoms can range from tingling sensations to loss of consciousness, and death. The only way to avoid the reaction is to avoid the food. While some food allergies can be outgrown, foods like peanuts, nuts, fish, and shellfish are often lifelong allergies.

Some persons equate food allergies with food intolerance. Food intolerance is an adverse food-induced reaction that does not involve the immune system. Lactose intolerance is an example. Since January 1, 2006, the FDA has required food labels to state if food products contain ingredients derived from the eight major foods or food groups that account for 90 percent of all allergic reactions: milk, eggs, fish, crustacean shellfish, tree nuts (pecans, almonds, walnuts), peanuts, wheat, soybeans. The food label must list these ingredients or say "contains" followed by the name of the source of the food allergen.[80] Check the labels on some common food products that you eat to see if any of these ingredients are present.

A skin prick test or a blood test is commonly used to determine the presence of food allergies. The type of test used by the health care provider is determined by the patient's age or health symptoms. The test results along with a history of symptoms are used to determine whether a food allergy exists. Food allergies are skyrocketing, particularly in developed and developing countries. Nearly 2 percent of adults and 5 percent of infants and children in the United States have food allergies. Some studies suggest that growing up in large families or being exposed to others in daycare may actually *reduce* the potential for developing food allergies because increased exposure strengthens the immune system. An important consideration for persons with food allergies is the potential for cross contamination when eating at a restaurant or consuming a meal prepared by someone else.

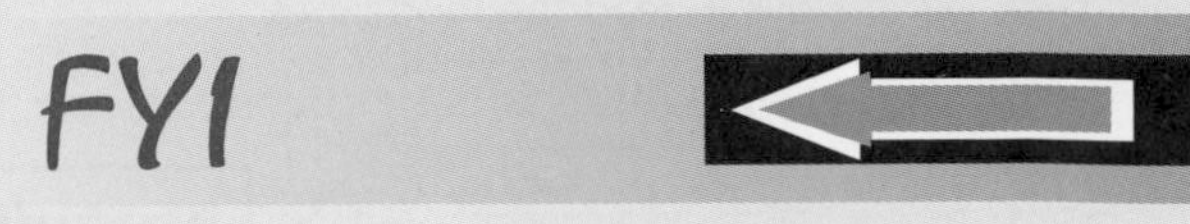

Weight Management

Dietary Guidelines for Americans 2005[83]

Key recommendations

- To maintain body weight in a healthy range, balance calories from foods and beverages with calories expended.
- To prevent gradual weight gain over time, make small decreases in food and beverage calories and increase physical activity.

Key recommendations for specific population groups

- *Those who need to lose weight.* Aim for a slow, steady weight loss by decreasing calorie intake while maintaining an adequate nutrient intake and increasing physical activity.
- *Overweight children.* Reduce the rate of body weight gain while allowing growth and development. Consult a health care provider before placing a child on a weight-reduction diet.
- *Pregnant women.* Ensure appropriate weight gain as specified by a health care provider.
- *Breast-feeding women.* Moderate weight reduction is safe and does not compromise weight gain of the nursing infant.
- *Overweight adults and overweight children with chronic diseases and/or on medication.* Consult a health care provider about weight-loss strategies prior to starting a weight-reduction program to ensure appropriate management of other health conditions.

MANAGING WEIGHT THROUGH NUTRITION

Few personal health topics have attracted the interests of the medical community as much as weight management. (See *FYI:* "Weight Management.") According to epidemiological data, women as a group are fatter now than they have ever been in our nation's history, and the percentage of overweight African American and Hispanic women is greater than that of white women.[81] At any given time, 50 percent of American women are spending billions of dollars to lose weight. Statistics like these are interesting, but what does all this mean to you? How much should you weigh? What is the best way to keep weight off?

Assessing one's risk involves using three key measures:

- Body mass index (BMI)
- Waist circumference
- Risk factors for diseases and conditions associated with obesity.[82]

A combination of BMI and waist circumference is a better descriptor than a single measure of overweight, obesity, or extreme obesity. Other, related risk factors should also be considered when assessing risk for diabetes, cardiovascular disease, hypertension, stroke, and some cancers. These risk factors include high blood pressure, high LDL cholesterol, low HDL cholesterol, high triglycerides, high blood glucose, family history of premature heart disease, physical inactivity, and cigarette smoking. Weight loss is recommended for anyone with a BMI above 25.0, a waist measurement greater than 35 inches, and any two of the risk factors mentioned above. Even a small weight loss (merely 10 percent of a person's current weight) can provide significant benefits.

Underweight, Overweight, and Obesity

More than 64 percent of adult men and women in the United States are classified as overweight (BMI between 25.0 and 29.9) or obese (BMI > 30).[84] We know more about the consequences of obesity than we do about the causes. There seem to be conflicting explanations between nature (genetic and biological causes) and nurture (those factors in the environment) as the causes of obesity. The answer lies somewhere between the two theories. As with any other human condition, it is difficult to determine the exact and singular cause. Research has linked obesity to genetic, biochemical, metabolic, psychological, and physiological factors.

Researchers continue to study the genetic causes of obesity. At least one study has uncovered a "fat gene" in mice, and it is suspected that this gene has a human counterpart.[85] Studies of identical twins separated at birth were found to have height and weight profiles similar to those of their natural parents.[86] Scientists have also isolated a specific gene that, if it undergoes mutation, interferes with the body's ability to burn fat.[87] The dietary factors related to obesity are easier to understand than the genetic factors. For example, children learn to eat to satisfy hunger, but they may also become conditioned to eat for the relief of boredom, to please their parents, or as a means to relieve stress.[88] The result is that the child does not respond well to hunger cues but, instead, responds more to the psychological and emotional signals associated with eating. Fast foods are also suspected of contributing to obesity. Fast-food outlets tend to offer high-fat, high-calorie, low-cost foods, and Americans are consuming more of these products than ever before. Obesity itself is not a life-threatening condition. However, it is a known risk factor for diabetes, heart disease, high blood pressure, gallbladder disease, arthritis, and some forms of cancer.[89] In addition, obese people have a more difficult time recovering from surgery. The health care costs associated with obesity were estimated to be $117 billion in 2000.[90]

Weight Loss

The causes of obesity are many, and so are the ways of controlling it. Millions of Americans are dieting at any given point in time and spending billions of dollars a year trying to lose weight. All of that money goes toward programs that are advertised as easy and successful, but the winners in the long run are the companies advertising their diet plans, not the women purchasing such plans. The Dietary Guidelines for Americans 2005 recommends balancing calories from foods and beverages with calories expended to maintain body weight and making small decreases in food and beverage calories and increasing physical activity to prevent gradual weight gain over time. Health care providers should be consulted before overweight children are placed on a weight-reduction diet.

Dieting versus Balanced Food Intake The major problem a woman faces when she goes on a diet is that she will eventually go *off* the diet. Herein lies the problem associated with weight loss. After realizing that she may weigh more than she feels she should, or failing to fit into clothes that she once wore very comfortably, a woman looks for ways to lose weight. The pattern becomes one in which she follows some weight-loss regimen until her weight gets to be where she would like it to be. She goes off her weight-loss regimen and returns to her previous eating habits until she gains the weight back. Then the cycle starts all over again. Dieting in this fashion leads to a weight loss–weight gain cycle known as "yo-yo" dieting. For years, data have revealed that two things happen when a woman engages in yo-yo dieting. Once weight is lost and regained, subsequent weight-loss attempts will take longer to remove the weight. Moreover, after the weight is lost and the woman goes off her diet, the lost weight comes back more rapidly than it did on previous occasions.[91] Some studies have disclosed some contradictions with these findings. It appears that women with a history of yo-yo dieting generally burn calories as fast as people who lose weight by other methods.[92] This form of weight management has been associated with poor health, especially increasing the risk of mortality.[93] Concerns surrounding the efficacy of yo-yo dieting still remain. The practice is not recommended because dieting in this fashion does not produce a weight management lifestyle for a woman.

The key to any "diet" is not to have to go on one to begin with. Regulating your weight must start when you are young. It involves a lifelong commitment to a lifestyle that balances the intake of calories with your calorie expenditure. Did you know that after your early twenties, you will require fewer calories as you age? Your **basal metabolic rate,** the amount of energy you need to maintain your body functions, will decline about 2 percent each decade after age 30.[94] If you consume a 2,000-calorie diet now, and 10 years from now you are consuming the same number of calories, you can expect to gain weight. Expect that you will need about 40 fewer calories per day per decade as you age. This will be especially important if your activity level drops off. So you can also see the value of maintaining a physically active lifestyle in addition to monitoring your calorie intake.

The goal of any weight-loss program is to burn more calories than you consume. Once you reach a comfortable and healthy weight, the goal then becomes burning the calories you consume so that your weight is maintained. Keep the following points in mind to be successful with your weight management goals.

- *One pound of fat equals 3,500 calories.* To burn 1 pound of fat, a woman must either consume 3,500 fewer calories or perform some kind of physical activity that would use 3,500 calories more than she has consumed. Conversely, if a woman eats 3,500 calories more than she burns through activity, she will gain a pound of fat.
- *Exercise is crucial to a weight management program.* In fact, research has shown that, over the long term, exercise alone will contribute more to weight management than a regimen of calorie restriction and dieting.[95] This information is very important to women, because they are more likely than men to

use food restriction to lose weight. Men are more likely to increase their exercise levels. Women say, "I need to quit eating so much." Men say, "I need to get to the gym."

- *Proper weight management is a lifetime lifestyle commitment.* It is not something undertaken because you want to fit into a particular bathing suit this summer or because you finally realize that you are 30 pounds over your ideal weight.
- *There is no fast way to weight loss.* Rapid weight loss is unhealthy, not to mention that there is often a rebound effect causing a woman to gain the lost weight back about as fast as she lost it, and then some. Weight-loss programs that advertise quick and effortless weight loss are no good.
- *Fad diets and weight-loss programs are not the answer to weight management.* Fad diets generally expect the woman to consume some special nutrient. One diet program claimed success if you ate an abundance of protein, whereas another claimed you should not eat any carbohydrates. You may remember the "Beverly Hills Diet." The dieter was to consume large amounts of fruits, especially pineapple. Weight-loss programs generally expect you to buy certain products to help you lose weight. The bottom line is that none of these programs really work. They may be good in the very short term, but their lack of behavioral change and support causes participants to eventually fail because they cannot continue the expected regimen. The dieter can then be left with considerable damage to both her self-esteem and her bank account.
- *Weight management through medications does not work.* The medical community has attempted to use certain drug regimens to combat obesity. These regimens do not work for the long term. Tolerance develops over time, and the drugs will be effective only for 4 to 6 months.[96] In addition, a number of adverse side effects may come with drug therapy, ranging from depression to hypertension. Perhaps the most significant reason for avoiding drug therapy is that it results in the avoidance of responsibility. The dieter expects a "magic bullet" to take care of the "weakness" within the person who eats too much and exercises too little.

FIGURE 10.3 Food Guide Pyramid for Older Adults

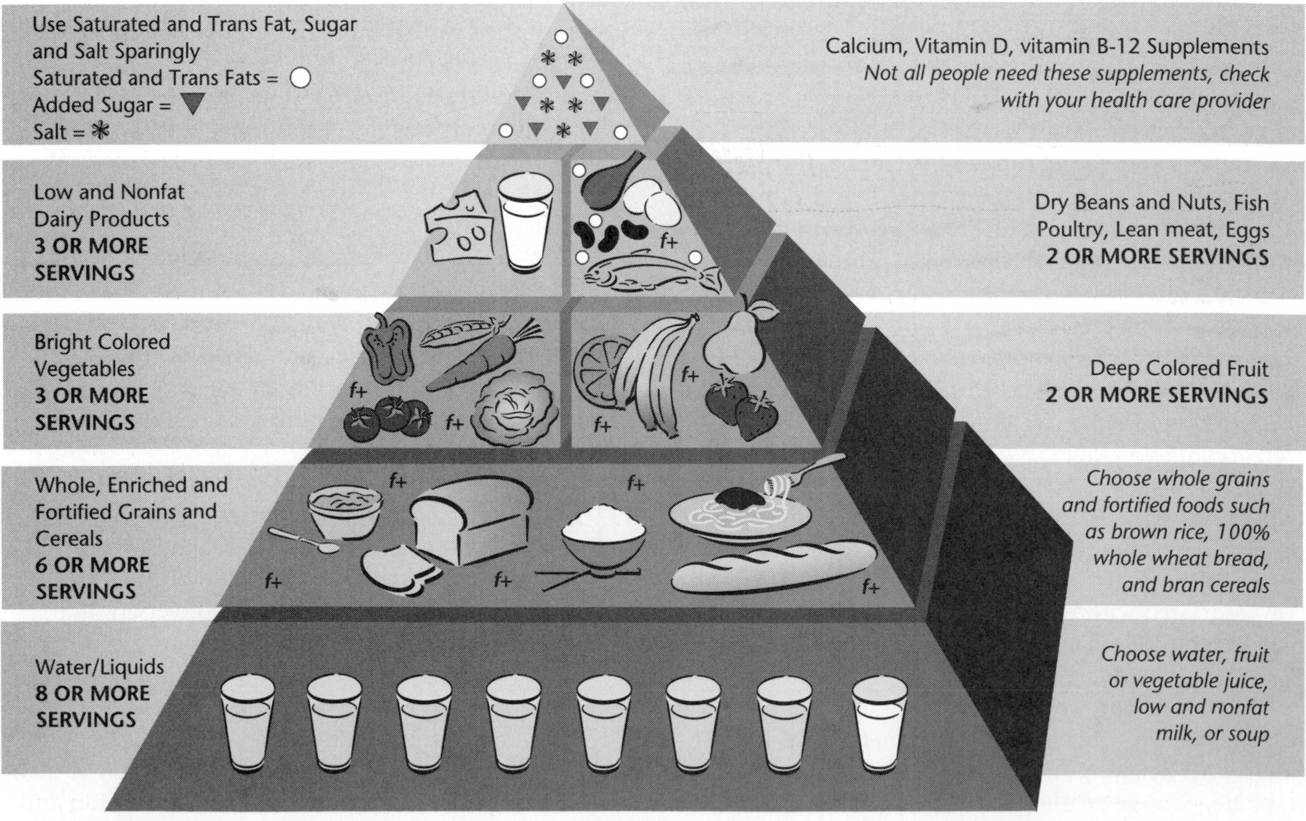

SOURCE: Copyright 2002 Tufts University.

Nutrition and the Aging Population

Proper dietary intake is essential throughout the life span, and knowledge about nutritional needs after age 65 is the first step in healthy aging. Currently, people older than 65 account for 13 percent of the U.S. population, with life expectancy for men 74 years and 80 years for women. However, the over-65 age group accounts for 50 percent of the federal health budget; 85 percent of this group have nutrition-related problems such as hypertension, osteoporosis, heart disease, and type 2 diabetes.[97] Do dietary needs change for women as they age?

Older women usually have a diet containing about 1,300 to 1,600 calories per day. Most of the Dietary Reference Intakes (DRIs) can be met through this amount of calories, but women may need supplements to obtain additional amounts of essential nutrients including vitamin D, vitamin B-12, folate, and calcium.[98] There are differences in the DRIs for women over the age of 50. For example, women under the age of 50 need 1,000 mg/day of calcium, but women over age 50 need 1,200 mg/day; vitamin B-6 needs for women under the age of 50 are 1.3 mg/day per day, but 1.5 mg/day are required for women over 50; vitamin D is needed in the amount of 5 μg/dl (micrograms per deciliter) per day for women under the age of 50, but 10 μg/dl are needed between the ages of 50 and 70, with women over 70 needing 15 μg/dl.[99] Maintaining proper nutrition during a woman's later years can be achieved by adhering to the following suggestions.

- Use the USDA MyPyramid to guide food and serving selections. (See Figure 10.3 for the Food Guide Pyramid for Older Adults (those over the age of 70).
- Drink eight or more servings of water each day to prevent constipation and dehydration.
- Decrease fat consumption and increase consumption of nutrient-dense foods such as fruits and vegetables; use food intake to obtain the most nutrients possible (consume more bright-colored vegetables and deep-colored fruits).
- Take supplements to provide needed nutrients not consumed in food intake; reduced calorie intake can reduce the potential of obtaining critical nutrients.
- Obtain higher levels of specific nutrients such as vitamin D and calcium for stronger bones and folic acid to retain mental acuity and reduce potential of stroke and heart disease.
- Maintain a physician-approved exercise regimen to strengthen bones and muscles, promote sleep, and improve appetite.

Chapter Summary

- A multitude of factors, such as family, knowledge, and emotions, influence the daily food choices we make.
- A typical American's energy values are derived from a number of sources.
- Dietary guidelines that assist American women in developing positive eating habits include the following: eat a variety of foods; balance food you consume with physical activity; select a diet with plenty of grain products, vegetables, and fruits; choose a diet low in fat, saturated fat, and cholesterol; select a diet that is moderate in sugar, salt, and sodium; and if you drink, do so in moderation.
- The Web site MyPyramid.gov provides a visual account of the variety and amount of foods that should be consumed to ensure a balanced, healthy diet.
- The six major nutrients—carbohydrates, protein, fats, vitamins, minerals, and water—provide the chemicals our bodies need for energy, building and repairing tissue, and functioning effectively.
- Most food additives pose no threat to our well-being.
- Special conditions such as pregnancy, intense levels of exercise, or chronic disease often result in the need for special foods or increased amounts of certain nutrients.
- Being overweight may not mean that a woman is overfat; however, there are serious health consequences as a result of being overfat.
- The most effective way to lose weight is to monitor calorie consumption and maintain a physically active lifestyle.
- Good nutrition consumer skills can be an important asset when selecting food products that are both beneficial and assist with weight management.
- Nutritional needs in elderly women are more specific than in younger women.

Review Questions

1. Provide four key recommendations of the foods that Americans are encouraged to eat according to the Dietary Guidelines for Americans 2005.
2. What are the Dietary Reference Intakes and the current changes that are taking place with respect to their values?
3. What is the role of carbohydrates in the body, and what are the most healthful sources to choose from?
4. What is meant by the term *nutrient density?*
5. What are the sources of the water-soluble vitamins?
6. Other than milk, what are significant sources of calcium in the diet?

7. What are the specific nutritional needs that a woman has during pregnancy?
8. What are the specific cautions a woman must recognize if she chooses to follow a vegetarian diet?
9. What changes take place in a woman's nutrient needs during exercise?
10. What are the main components required by law to appear on the information panel of a food label?
11. List and explain the various ways of measuring the amount of fat a woman has in her body.

Resources

Organizations

American Dietetic Association
120 South Riverside Plaza, Suite 2000
Chicago, IL 60606-6995
800-877-1600
www.eatright.org

American Society for Nutrition
9650 Rockville Pike
Bethesda, MD 20814-3990
301-634-7892
www.asnutrition.org

Food and Nutrition Information Center
United States Department of Agriculture (USDA)
Washington, DC 20250
202-720-2791
www.nal.usda.gov/fnic

Jean Mayer USDA Human Nutrition Research Center on Aging (HNRCA) Tufts University
711 Washington Street
Boston, MA 02111-1524
617-556-3334
www.hnrc.tufts.edu

Linus Pauling Institute
Oregon State University
571 Weniger Hall
Corvallis, OR 97331-6512
541-737-5075
http://lpi.oregonstate.edu

National Dairy Council
10255 W. Higgins Road, Suite 900
Rosemont, IL 60018-6233
312-240-2880
www.nationaldairycouncil.org/NationalDairyCouncil

Nutrition Information and Resource Center
Department of Food Science
Penn State University
8L Borland Lab
University Park, PA 16802
814-865-9714
http://nirc.cas.psu.edu/index.cfm

Oldways Preservation Trust
266 Beacon Street
Boston, MA 02116
617-421-5500
www.oldwayspt.org

Overeaters Anonymous
P. O. Box 44020
Rio Rancho, NM 87174-4020
505-891-2664
www.oa.org/index.htm

Society for Nutrition Education
7150 Winton Drive, Suite 300
Indianapolis, IN 46268
317-328-4627 or 800-235-6690
www.sne.org

U.S. Food and Drug Administration (FDA)
5600 Fishers Lane
Rockville, MD 20857-0001
888-INFO-FDA (1-888-463-6332)
www.fda.gov

U.S. Food and Drug Administration (FDA)
Center for Food Safety and Applied Nutrition
5100 Paint Branch Parkway
College Park, MD 20740-3835
www.cfsan.fda.gov

The Vegetarian Resource Group (VRG)
P. O. Box 1463, Dept. IN
Baltimore, MD 21203
410-366-VEGE (8343)
www.vrg.org/nutshell/about.htm

Videotapes

Eating for Optimal Health
The ABCs of Vitamins
Managing Your Weight
Films for the Humanities & Sciences, Box 2053, Princeton, NJ 08543-2053, Phone: 800-257-5126,
Web site www.films.com

Web Sites

Blonz Guide to Nutrition, Food and Health Sources
www.blonz.com

Body Mass Index Calculator
www.nhlbisupport.com/bmi/bmicalc.htm

Center for Science in the Public Interest
www.cspinet.org

Consumer Reports
www.consumerreports.org/cro/home.htm

Dietary Guidelines for Americans
www.health.gov/dietaryguidelines

Environmental Working Group
www.ewg.org

FDA Food Labeling
www.cfsan.fda.gov/~dms/foodlab.html

Food & Nutrition Information Center
www.nal.usda.gov/fnic

Food Safety Information Center
www.foodsafety.gov

The Food Timeline
www.foodtimeline.org

Harvard School of Public Health
Department of Nutrition
www.hsph.harvard.edu/nutritionsource
Healthy People 2010: Health Objectives for the Nation
www.health.gov/healthypeople
International Bottled Water Association
www.bottledwater.org
The U.S. Department of Agriculture, Center for Nutrition Policy and Promotion
www.usda.gov/cnpp
The USDA Food Pyramid
www.mypyramid.gov
The U.S. Food and Drug Administration (FDA)
Center for Food Safety and Applied Nutrition
CSFSN/Office of Nutritional Products, Labeling and Dietary Supplements
www.cfsan.fda.gov/~dms/transfat/html

Suggested Readings

Benardott, D. 2000. *Nutrition for Serious Athletics*. Champaign, IL: Human Kinetics.

Bren, L. 2002. Losing Weight: More Than Just Counting Calories. *FDA Consumer* (January/February): 16.

Kleiner, S. M. 1999. Water: An Essential but Overlooked Nutrient. *Journal of the American Dietetic Association* 99:20.

Nelson, M. D., and J. Knipe. 2002. *Strong Women Eat Well: Nutritional Strategies for a Healthy Body and Mind*. New York: Putnam.

Schlosser, E., 2001. *Fast Food Nation*. Boston: Houghton Mifflin.

Willett, W. C. 2001. *Eat, Drink and Be Healthy*. New York: Simon & Schuster.

Willett, W. C., and M. J. Stampfer, 2001. What Vitamin Should I Be Taking, Doctor? *New England Journal of Medicine* 345:1819.

References

1. Wardlaw, G. M., P. M. Insel, and M. F. Seyler. 1997. *Contemporary Nutrition: Issues and insights*. St. Louis: Mosby.
2. American Heart Association. 2006. *Lyon Diet Heart Study*. www.americanheart.org/presenter.jhtml?identifier=4655 (retrieved October 3, 2006).
3. American Heart Association. 2006. *Third report of the National Cholesterol Education Program*. www.americanheart.org/presenter.jhtml?identifier=11206 (retrieved October 3, 2006).
4. U.S. Department of Agriculture and U.S. Department of Health and Human Services. 2005. *Dietary guidelines for Americans 2005*. www.health.gov/dietaryguidelines/dga2005/document/html/executivesummary.htm (retrieved October 1, 2006).
5. Ibid.
6. Ibid. *Dietary Guidelines: Build a healthy base*. 2000. http://health.gov/dietaryguidelines/dga2000/document/build.htm (retrieved September 22, 2006).
7. World Health Organization. 2003. *Global strategy for infant and young child feeding*. Fifty-fifth World Health Assembly. www.who.int/entity/nutrition/topics/global_strategy/en (retrieved April 6, 2007).
8. World Health Organization. 2005. *Ecosystems and human well-being: Health synthesis: A report of the Millennium Ecosystem Assessment*. Core writing team: Carlos Corvalan, Siman Hales, and Anthony McMichael.
9. Weck, I. 1996. The dangerous burden of obesity. *FDA Consumer* (November): 16–19.
10. *Prevalence of overweight and obesity among adults: United States, 1999–2002*. National Center for Health Statistics, Centers for Disease Control. www.cdc.gov/nchs/products/pubs/pubd/hestats/obese/obse99.htm (retrieved September 22, 2006).
11. *Healthy People 2010 Health Objectives for the Nation*. U.S. Department of Health and Human Services. www.healthypeople.gov (retrieved September 25, 2006).
12. Weck, The dangerous burden of obesity.
13. National Institutes of Health. 2006, April. *Your guide to lowering your blood pressure with DASH*. NIH Publication No. 06-4082. www.nhlbi.nih.gov/health/public/heart/hbp/dash/new_dash.pdf (retrieved April 3, 2007).
14. U.S. Department of Agriculture and U.S. Department of Health and Human Services, *Dietary guidelines for Americans 2005*.
15. U.S. Department of Agriculture and U.S. Department of Health and Human Services, *Dietary guidelines for Americans 2005*.
16. Ibid.
17. Wardlaw, G. M., and A. M. Smith. 2007. *Contemporary nutrition: UPDATE*. 6th ed. New York: McGraw-Hill.
18. Consumers Union. 1991. The sugar bugaboo. *Consumer Report on Health*, 42–44.
19. Wardlaw and Smith, *Contemporary nutrition*.
20. U.S. Department of Agriculture and U.S. Department of Health and Human Services, *Dietary Guidelines for Americans 2005*.
21. Wardlaw and Smith, *Contemporary nutrition*.
22. U.S. Department of Agriculture and U.S. Department of Health and Human Services, *Dietary guidelines for Americans 2005*.
23. Wardlaw and Smith, *Contemporary nutrition*.
24. Ibid.
25. Institute of Medicine, Food and Nutrition Board. 2002. *Dietary Reference Intakes for energy, carbohydrates, fiber, fat, fatty acids, cholesterol, protein, and amino acids*. Washington, DC: National Academies Press.
26. Wardlaw and Smith, *Contemporary nutrition*.
27. Ford, E. S., and S. Liu. 2001. Glycemic index and serum high-density lipoprotein cholesterol concentration among U.S. adults. *Archives of Internal Medicine* 161:572–76; Frost, G., A. A. Leeds, C.J. Dore, S. Madeiros, S. Brading, and A. Dornhorst. 1999. Glycaemic index as a determinant of serum HDL-cholesterol concentration. *Lancet* 353:1045–48.

28. Carpenter, K. J. 1992. Protein requirements of adults from an evolutionary perspective. *Journal of Clinical Nutrition* 55:913.
29. Cristeta Comerford Named White House Executive Chef. Press release, August 2005. www.whitehouse.gov/news/releases/2005/08/20050814-1.html (retrieved October 2, 2006).
30. Whitney, E. N., and S. R. Rolfes. 2002. *Understanding nutrition.* 9th ed. Stamford, CT: Wadsworth/Thomson.
31. Consumers Union. 1994. Do we eat too much protein? *Consumer Reports on Health* (January): 1–3.
32. Wardlaw and Smith, *Contemporary nutrition.*
33. U.S. Department of Agriculture and U.S. Department of Health and Human Services, *Dietary Guidelines for Americans 2005.*
34. Mayfield, E. 1994. *Reprint from FDA Consumer* (November): 1–5.
35. U.S. Department of Agriculture and U.S. Department of Health and Human Services, *Dietary guidelines for Americans 2005.*
36. Gershoff, S. 1996. *The Tufts University guide to total nutrition.* New York: HarperPerennial.
37. Harvard Medical School. 1996. Antioxidants disappointment and hope. *Harvard Health Letter* 21 (October): 1.
38. Jha, P., M. Flaather, E. Lonn, M. Farkouh, and S. Yussuf. 1995. The antioxidant vitamins and cardiovascular disease: A critical review of epidemiologic and clinical trial data. *Annals of Internal Medicine* 123:860–72.
39. U.S. Department of Agriculture and U.S. Department of Health and Human Services, *Dietary guidelines for Americans 2005.*
40. Brown, J. E. 1991. *Every woman's guide to nutrition.* Minneapolis: University of Minnesota Press.
41. Osteoporosis and related bone diseases. 2003, February. *Fast facts on osteoporosis.* Washington, DC: National Resource Center, NIH.
42. Osteoporosis and related bone diseases 2003, January. *Osteoporosis overview.* Washington, DC: National Resource Center, NIH.
43. Institute of Medicine, Food and Nutrition Board. 2001. *Dietary Reference Intakes for vitamin A, arsenic, boron, chromium, copper, iodine, iron, manganese, molybdenum, nickel, silicon, vanadium, and zinc.* Washington, DC: National Academies Press.
44. Harvard Medical School. 1996. Vegetarian diets. *Harvard Women's Health Watch* 21 (January): 2–3.
45. Gershoff, *The Tufts University guide to total nutrition.*
46. Block, A., and C. A. Thomson. 1995. Position of the American Dietetic Association: Phytochemicals and functional foods. *Journal of the American Dietetic Association* 95 (April): 493–96.
47. Arnold, E., and J. Larson. 2006. *Bottled water: Pouring resources down the drain.* Earth Policy Institute. www.earth-policy.org/Updates/2006/Updates51.htm (retrieved September 25, 2006).
48. Beverage Marketing Association. 1998. Advertising and marketing: Waterlogged. *Los Angeles Times*, April 23.
49. World Health Organization, *Global strategy for infant and young child feeding.*
50. Insel, P. M., and W. T. Roth. 2008. *Core concepts in health.* Update. 10th ed. New York: McGraw-Hill.
51. Brown, *Every woman's guide to nutrition.*
52. Institute of Medicine, Food and Nutrition Board. *Dietary Reference Intakes for vitamin A, arsenic, boron, chromium, copper, iodine, iron, manganese, molybdenum, nickel, silicon, vanadium, and zinc.*
53. Williams, R. D. 1994. FDA proposes folic acid fortification. *FDA Consumer* (May): 11–14.
54. U.S. Department of Agriculture and U.S. Department of Health and Human Services, *Dietary guidelines for Americans 2005.*
55. Brown, *Every woman's guide to nutrition.*
56. Ibid.
57. World Health Organization, *Global strategy for infant and young child feeding.*
58. Ibid.
59. Wardlaw and Smith, *Contemporary nutrition.*
60. Brown, *Every woman's guide to nutrition.*
61. U.S. Department of Agriculture and U.S. Department of Health and Human Services, *Dietary guidelines for Americans 2005.*
62. Fahey, T, P. M. Insel, and W. T. Roth, 2007. Fit & Well Brief. 7th ed. New York: McGraw-Hill.
63. Ruud, J. S., and A. C. Grandjean. 1994. Nutritional concerns of female athletes. In I. Wolinsky and J. Hickson (eds.), *Nutrition in exercise and sport.* Boca Raton, FL: CRC Press.
64. Murray, R. G., and J. J. B. Anderson. 1994. Introduction to exercise and sport. In I. Wolinsky and J. Hickson (eds.), *Nutrition in exercise and sport.* Boca Raton, FL: CRC Press.
65. Ruud and Grandjean, Nutritional concerns of female athletes; Murray and Anderson, Introduction to exercise and sport.
66. Rudd and Grandjean, Nutritional concerns of female athletes.
67. Dingott, S., and J. Dwyer. 2003. *Vegetarianism: Healthful but unnecessary.* www.quackwatch.org/03HealthPromotion/vegetarian.html (retrieved September 22, 2006).
68. Dingott and Dwyer, *Vegetarianism: Healthful but unnecessary.*
69. Ibid.
70. Ibid.
71. Stare, F. J., V. Aronson, and S. Barrett. 1991. *Your guide to good nutrition.* Buffalo, NY: Prometheus Books.
72. Wardlaw and Smith, *Contemporary nutrition.*
73. U.S. Department of Agriculture. 2003. *Organic food standards and labels: The facts.* www.ams.usda.gov/nop/consumers/brochure.html (retrieved September 23, 2006).
74. U.S. Department of Agriculture, *Organic food standards and labels: The facts.*
75. U.S. Food and Drug Administration. 1999. *The food label.* www.cfsan.fda.gov/~dms/fdnewlab.html (retrieved September 23, 2006).
76. Consumer Reports. *Food labels can be misleading.* www.consumerreports.org/cro/food/organic-products-206/chemical-health-risks.html (retrieved January 18, 2006).
77. U.S. Food and Drug Administration, *The food label.*

78. Wart, P. J. 2005. Size matters: When you put food portions on your plate. *Health Plus*. Vanderbilt Faculty and Staff Wellness Program. http://vanderbiltowc.wellsource.com/dh/content.asp?ID=865 (retrieved February 6, 2006).
79. U.S. Food and Drug Administration. 2005. *The food label.* www.cfsan.fda.gov/~dms/fdnewlab.html (retrieved October 2, 2006).
80. U.S. Food and Drug Administration. 2005. *FDA to require food manufacturers to list food allergens: Consumers with allergies will benefit from improved food labels.* www.fda.gov/bbs/topics/NEWS/2005/NEW01281.html (retrieved September 23, 2006).
81. National Institute of Diabetes and Digestive and Kidney Disorders. 1996. *NIDDK Homepage*. NIH Pub 96–4158. www.niddk.nih.gov/ObStats/Obstats.htm. (retrieved June 16, 2003).
82. National Heart, Lung, and Blood Institute. 2005. *Aim for a healthy weight: Information for patients and the public.* www.nhlbi.nih.gov/health/public/heart/obesity/lose_wt (retrieved September 23, 2006).
83. U.S. Department of Agriculture and U.S. Department of Health and Human Services, *Dietary Guidelines for Americans 2005.*
84. *Prevalence of overweight and obesity among adults: United States, 1999–2000.* National Center for Health Statistics, Centers for Disease Control. www.cdc.gov/nchs/products/pubs/pubd/hestats/obese/obse99.htm (retrieved June 2, 2003).
85. Pellymounter, M. A., M. J. Cullen, M. B. Baker, R. Hecht, D. Winters, T. Boone, and F. Collins. 1995. Effects of the obese gene product on body weight regulation on ob/ob mice. *Science* 260:540–43.
86. Gershoff, *The Tufts University guide to total nutrition.*
87. Walston, J., K. Siler, C. Bogardus, W. Knowler, et al. 1995. Time of onset of non-insulin-dependent diabetes mellitus and genetic variation of the beta3-andrenergic-receptor gene. *New England Journal of Medicine* 333: 343–47.
88. Murray and Anderson, Introduction to exercise and sport.
89. *Do you know the risks of being overweight?* NIDDK weight control information network. www.niddk.nih.gov/publications/health_risks.htm (retrieved September 23, 2006).
90. U.S. Department of Health and Human Services, Office of the Surgeon General. 2001. *The surgeon general's call to action to prevent and decrease overweight and obesity.* Washington, DC: U.S. Government Printing Office, p. 10.
91. Brownell, K. 1988. Yo-yo dieting. *Psychology Today* 20:22–23.
92. Consumers Union. 1997. Hope for yo-yo dieters. *Consumer Reports on Health* 9 (August): 89.
93. University of Texas Health Notes. 1991. *University of Texas Health Sciences Center Lifetime Health Letter* 3:1.
94. Wardlaw and Smith, *Contemporary nutrition.*
95. Eller, D. 1997. The best way to lose weight. *Health* (May/June): 34–36.
96. National Task Force on the Prevention and Treatment of Obesity. 1996. Long-term pharmacotherapy in the management of obesity. *Journal of the American Medical Association* 276 (December): 1907–15.
97. Wardlaw and Smith, *Contemporary nutrition.*
98. Ibid.
99. Institute of Medicine, Food and Nutrition Board, *Dietary Reference Intakes for vitamin A, arsenic, boron, chromium, copper, iodine, iron, manganese, molybdenum, nickel, silicon, vanadium, and zinc.*

Chapter Eleven

Keeping Fit

CHAPTER OBJECTIVES

When you complete this chapter, you will be able to do the following:

- Describe the physical, psychological, and social benefits of fitness activities
- Distinguish between the four health-related components of fitness and explain the specifics of each component
- Analyze the relationships between chronic diseases and physical fitness programs
- Explain the importance of warm-up and cool-down activities
- Describe the methods to assess physical fitness levels
- Identify ways to make fitness programs successful
- Develop a comprehensive fitness program using the four health-related components of fitness
- Identify special considerations for exercise during pregnancy and menstruation
- Explain the dangers involved in compulsive exercising
- Describe the advantages of weight maintenance through fitness workouts
- Summarize the advantages of fitness programs for women throughout the life span

BENEFITS OF FITNESS

One doesn't have to venture far to observe people of every age, size, and culture walking, biking, or swimming their way toward improved physical condition. Today we are more aware of the increased role that fitness plays in enhancing each dimension of our health than in past decades. It could be considered both a miracle drug and a fountain of youth that is *free* for the taking! Fitness not only plays a part in reducing the risks of developing heart disease and stroke, diabetes, osteoporosis, and obesity, but also promotes the development of positive attitudes, increased energy, and well-being in general.

Is there some recreational activity you enjoy, such as tennis, racquetball, or swimming? If your fitness level were better, could you enjoy the activity more? Do you have enough energy to take care of daily responsibilities? Is stress a major part of your lifestyle, with no end in sight? Women who experience fatigue, minor aches, or lack of stamina on a regular basis need to know that improvement in each of these areas is possible by engaging in a regular and well-developed fitness program.

Physiological benefits are well documented in hundreds of research studies conducted over many years. Often the physical benefits, such as weight loss or disease prevention, are the initial reason for engaging in fitness activities, but the multitude of additional benefits a woman gains is usually the reason for continuing the program. A fitness program can produce many positive outcomes that result in prevention of the diseases that cause illness and death in women. (See Table 11.1.)

Psychological benefits gained from participating in a regular fitness program can be somewhat subjective and may vary from research study to study. These benefits

TABLE 11.1 Fitness and Disease

Cardiovascular diseases	Aerobic exercise (walking, jumping rope, cross-country/downhill skiing, swimming) strengthens and tones the heart muscle, improves blood circulation, helps control hypertension, lowers cholesterol, increases levels of high-density lipoproteins (HDLs), increases the number of red blood cells, and reduces weight, which lessens the risk of heart disease caused by obesity.
Stroke	Involvement in greater leisure-time activity is associated with reduced risk of stroke in women. Varying levels of physical activity provide varying levels of reduction in total and ischemic stroke. Walking has been shown to significantly reduce incidence of stroke.[1]
Osteoporosis	Aerobic as well as weight-bearing exercise helps to strengthen bones and prevents bone-density loss in women, helps to strengthen and tone muscle, increases muscle mass needed to support the skeletal system, and reduces risks of fracture. In older women, exercise improves strength, flexibility, and balance, which can reduce the chance of falls and fractures.
Arthritis	Exercises for range of motion (stretching), as well as water aerobics, walking, biking, and swimming, can help joints maintain strength and flexibility, and may relieve some pain.
Diabetes	After physician approval, light aerobic exercises and moderate use of weights can lower blood sugar and help the body use insulin more efficiently; it helps with weight management and reduces the risks of developing type 2 diabetes in women.[2]
Breast cancer	Engaging in physical activity lowers the risk of developing breast cancer. Women who had been diagnosed with breast cancer and who engaged in the equivalent of walking 3 to 5 hours per week, at an average pace, appeared to have the greatest benefits.[3] Physically active women have up to a 40 percent reduced risk of developing breast cancer.[4]

are not limited to any age or either sex, and may be achieved by all participants. Dubbert[5] suggests that people who are more active have lower levels of anxiety and depression. Hassmen, Koivula, and Uutela[6] found that individuals who exercised at least two times per week had less depression, anger, cynical distrust, and stress than individuals who exercised less often. The degree and extent to which these benefits are attained will vary depending on the participant and her dedication to a regular fitness activity.

Social benefits are certainly a part of the attractive package a fitness program can provide. These offer an opportunity to be a part of groups and organizations in which women not only enjoy the company of others but also gain a multitude of health benefits in the process. Health clubs offer a choice of activities, and often new friends with similar interests can be found. Community recreational programs often develop activity- related programs such as biking clubs; hiking, walking, or running groups; and tennis leagues in which one can find associates with mutual interests and lifestyles. Women can also associate with individuals having similar goals and interests by participating in special activities such as yoga, Tai Chi, meditation, and self-defense. (See *FYI:* "Mind–Body Exercise: Yoga.") The social benefits abound when participating in fitness-related activities whether in small- or large-group settings.

Achieving any one of these fitness benefits is a positive addition to our lifestyle. However, the good news is that we usually achieve many of them. Regardless of "why" you decide to participate in a fitness regimen, whether it is to reduce weight, relieve stress, or prevent bone-density loss, a woman still reaps a variety of the benefits. Fitness activities that improve your physical, psychological, and social well-being are worth your time, energy, and money.

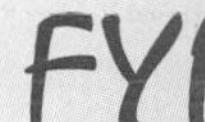

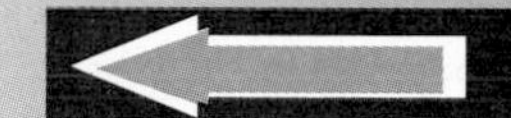

Mind–Body Exercise: Yoga

Yoga, either in mild and therapeutic form or in power form, can have multiple benefits for a woman's mind and body. This type of exercise has been practiced for centuries and supports a holistic approach to fitness, nutrition, and lifestyle. Research has revealed that yoga is a powerful method to reduce stress, lower blood pressure, improve concentration and balance, and increase muscular strength, endurance, and flexibility. Universities now offer yoga classes in physical fitness programs at various levels of difficulty. Women at any level of fitness can find and explore an appropriate style of yoga.[7]

HOW ACTIVE ARE TODAY'S WOMEN?

There is no doubt that physical inactivity contributes to the risks of developing diseases that are known to be the major killers of women. Women are more physically activity than in the past, and since Title IX was implemented

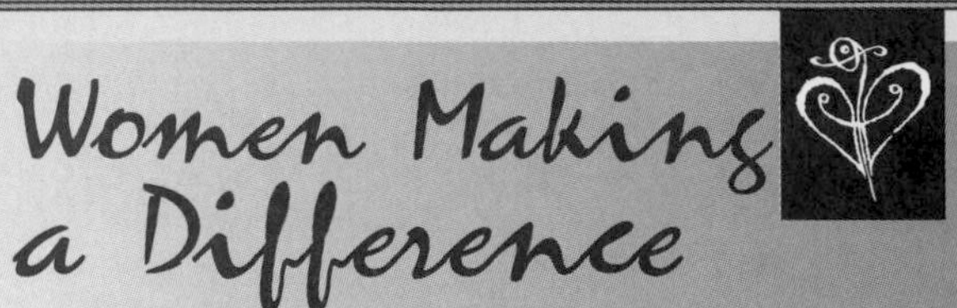

Melissa Johnson, M.S.: Executive Director, President's Council on Physical Fitness and Sport

Melissa Johnson is a nationally recognized leader in physical activity and fitness and health promotion. She was appointed, in 2002, by President Bush as Executive Director of the President's Council on Physical Fitness and Sports where she manages the activities and operations of the Washington, D.C.–based Council. The Council supports the President's HealthierUS initiative, designed to build a strong nation of healthy Americans through regular physical activity, sound nutrition, preventive screenings, and avoidance of risky behaviors.

Previously, Johnson was the Executive Director of the California Governor's Council on Physical Fitness and Sports, and Director of Operations for the National Fitness Leaders Association. She has also worked in corporate health promotion, designed wellness programs, and served as spokesperson for a variety of fundraising events for the American Heart Association and the American Cancer Society. She models fitness in her personal life and is a woman making a difference in the physical fitness for children, youth, and adults across the United States.

in 1972, more females have participated in organized sports. However, women still tend to be less physically active than men. Research conducted by Schoenborn and Barnes found the following:[8]

- Men (64.6 percent) were more likely than women (59.1 percent) to engage in at least some leisure-time physical activity.
- Men were slightly more likely than women to engage in light-moderate and/or vigorous physical activity at least five times per week.
- Men (34.4 percent) were more likely than women (27.3 percent) to engage in any regular physical activity.
- Men (27.2 percent) were more likely than women (18.7 percent) to engage in strengthening activities.

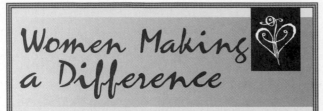

What do you think explains these findings? Why are women less active than men in leisure-time activities, fitness activity, and strengthening activities? (See *Women Making a Difference:* "Melissa Johnson" for an example of one woman who is actively promoting physical fitness.)

HEALTH-RELATED COMPONENTS OF FITNESS

Research firmly supports the concept of health promotion and disease prevention as a result of involvement in a regular fitness program. However, the fitness program must consist of several components. Do you have a friend who has no problem lifting, pushing, or carrying objects yet is out of breath after walking two flights of stairs? Well, your friend has developed one component of fitness (strength) but is lacking in another (endurance). A well-designed and comprehensive physical fitness program consists of four **health-related components of fitness:** cardiorespiratory endurance, flexibility, muscular strength and endurance, and body composition. Other components of fitness can also be an important part of a fitness program. However, these components—agility, balance, power, and speed—are performance-related fitness components and are outside the scope of this book. In creating your own personal fitness program, the four health-related components of fitness need to be included. A brief explanation of each component follows.

Cardiorespiratory Endurance

Cardiorespiratory fitness is considered to be the most important component of a physical fitness program because it affects vital organs of the body—the heart and lungs—and the arterial system, which deliver life-giving oxygen to every cell in the body. Their health and fitness are essential to the basic life support of our bodies. **Cardiorespiratory endurance** is the ability to perform prolonged, large-muscle, dynamic exercise at moderate to high levels of intensity.[9]

Activities that produce this outcome, called **aerobic activities,** include cycling, swimming, jumping rope, cross-country skiing, walking, running, aerobic dancing, roller blading, and jogging. Each of these calls for the use of large muscles and repetitive movements over a sustained period of time.

Principles of Conditioning To benefit from participation in cardiorespiratory endurance activities, you need to include the following principles of conditioning:

- *Intensity*. This is "how hard" you should engage in the aerobic activity. Intensity is determined by the number of times the heart beats (its pace) in 1 minute during any given activity. To determine the level of intensity, you must learn to calculate

Assess Yourself

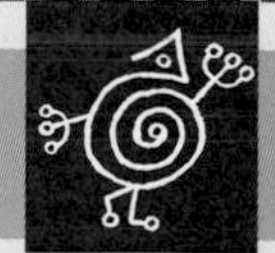

Calculate Your Target Heart Rate

To determine intensity during the aerobic phase of the physical activity workout, follow these simple instructions:

1. Measure your pulse rate at either the radial artery (on the thumb side of the wrist) or the carotid artery (found in the neck groove by the "Eve's" apple).
2. Use your index and middle finger to locate the pulse; do not press hard on these arteries or you will get an inaccurate measure.
3. Count your pulse for 30 seconds and multiply this by 2 to find your 1-minute pulse rate. During the workout, count your pulse for 10 seconds and multiply this by 6, which also gives you the 1-minute pulse rate.
4. To determine your target heart beat (the intensity at which you want to exercise to attain benefits), complete the following calculation:
   a. Find your maximal heart rate (MHR) by subtracting your age from 220. (For example, 220 minus 20 equals 200.) You now have your personal MHR.
   b. Now multiply your MHR by 60, 70, and 80 percent to determine the target heart rate (THR) that is less intense, moderately intense, or highly intense for you. Select one of these percentages depending on your initial physical condition, then increase the THR to 70 percent or 80 percent (or even 90 percent) as you become more fit.

Examples:

200	200	200
.60	.70	.80
120 beats/min	140 beats/min	160 beats/min

   c. As you increase your fitness level, you may want to increase your THR to continue to improve your physical fitness.

Note: Women who have not engaged in fitness activities for a period of time should begin at 60 percent or less of their MHR. Women over the age of 50 should seek a physician's clearance prior to engaging in a **comprehensive fitness program,** a fitness program that includes all components essential to fitness: cardiorespiratory endurance, flexibility, muscular strength and endurance, and body composition.

your target heart rate and then measure it during the activity. (See *Assess Yourself:* "Calculate Your Target Heart Rate.")

- *Duration.* This is "how long" you should spend in the aerobic phase of your fitness program. For minimal improvement, you should work continuously in the aerobic phase for 20 minutes at your target heart rate (THR). As your fitness level improves, increase the minutes engaged in activity at your THR per workout period. You will find that as you increase the duration of your workout, your cardiorespiratory endurance will improve.
- *Frequency.* This is "how often" you should engage in an aerobic workout. A minimum is considered to be three aerobic activity sessions per week; at this rate you will see slight improvement. The rate of five sessions per week provides greater and steadier improvement. It is not recommended to do seven sessions a week, but, instead, to "rest" at least 1 day between sessions so that the body can repair itself, and soreness, if any, can subside.

Flexibility

Flexibility allows an individual to use the full range of motion at a joint, which improves performance in fitness and recreational activities, and helps to reduce and prevent injuries and soreness. Flexibility has a genetic base; genetics determines how elastic the muscles and connective tissues will be and therefore makes individuals more or less flexible. This fitness component is joint specific and is affected by bulk and long arrangement of specific joints. Can you increase your flexibility? Absolutely! Stretching in one's exercise regimen helps reduce the rate that inflexibility occurs and reduces the shortening of muscles, tendons, and ligaments. At any age, flexibility can be greatly increased by using a variety of stretching exercises before and after fitness activities.

There are many stretching techniques that can improve one's flexibility. Following are four types of stretching techniques, with their specific benefits.[10]

- **Static stretching,** the safest way to stretch, involves stretching a specific muscle, usually for 10–30 seconds, until tension is felt. Remember, never "lock" a joint during stretching. It is believed that this activity will eventually produce a semipermanent change in muscle and tissue length. (See Figure 11.1.)
- Active isolated stretching involves the same muscles as in the static stretch, but the position is held only for 1–2 seconds and repeated eight to ten times.
- The positive aspects of this type of stretch are that the individual does not force the muscle to stay

FIGURE 11.1 Static stretch.

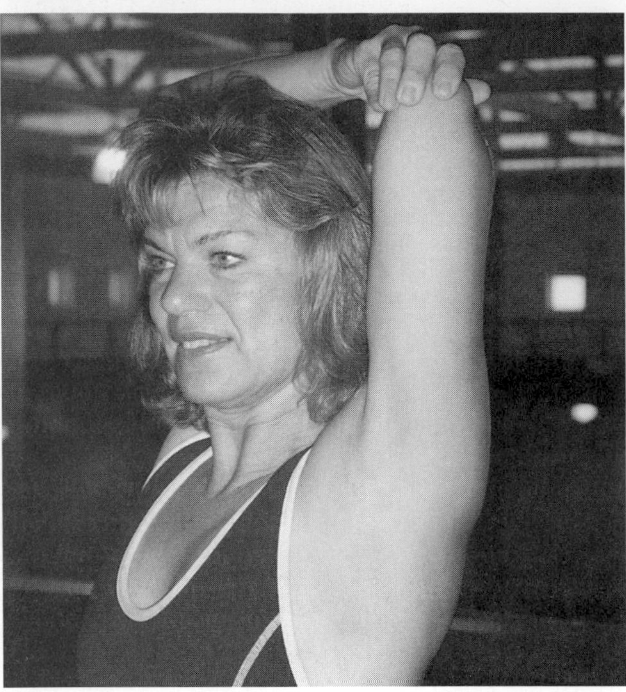

FIGURE 11.2 Isolated stretch.

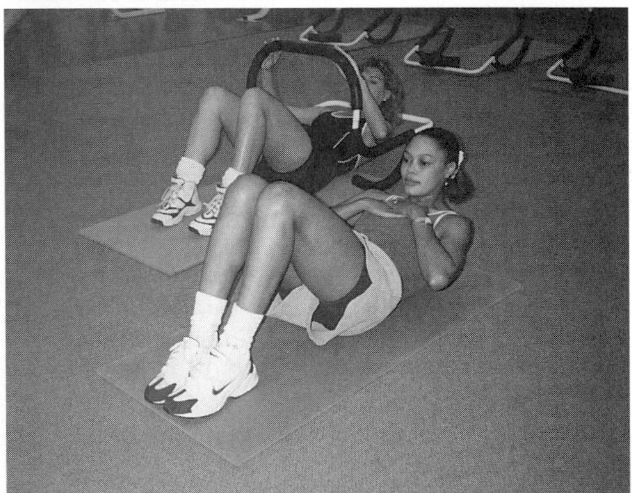

FIGURE 11.3 PNF stretch.

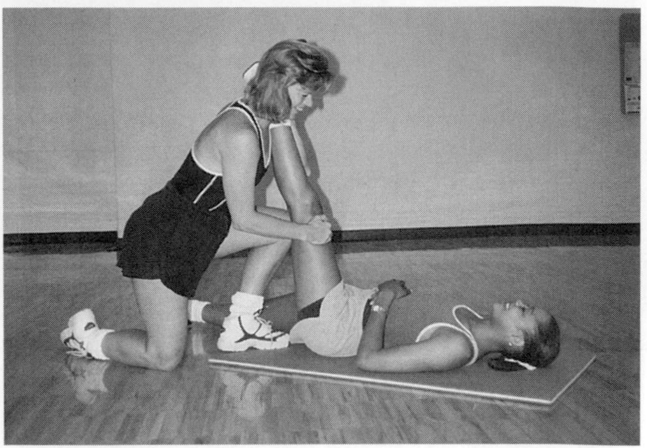

contracted and the muscle is relaxed between each stretch. (See Figure 11.2.)

- Proprioceptive neuromuscular facilitation **(PNF)** is often done with the help of a partner who helps the exerciser to contract, release, and then stretch a particular muscle or muscle group. When a muscle is contracted and released, the resistance is less and you will be able to stretch the muscle farther. (See Figure 11.3.)
- **Ballistic,** or dynamic, **stretching** is done by slowly moving into a particular stretch position, followed by a bouncing motion. This type of stretching, formerly used as the standard method of stretching, is believed to cause microscopic tears in muscles and connective tissues and is not recommended by exercise physiologists. (See *Health Tips:* "Tips for Safe and Effective Stretching" for proper stretching techniques.)

Passive stretching occurs when an external pressure, such as another person, assists in the movement of the

Health Tips

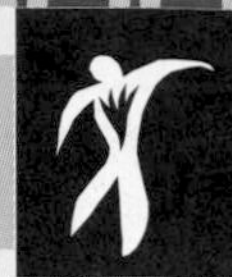

Tips for Safe and Effective Stretching[11]

- Prior to stretching, engage in a moderate activity, such as walking briskly, to initiate warming of muscles and joints.
- Stretch beyond your normal range, slightly beyond comfort, but not to the point of pain. (Pain is an indication that something is wrong and that injury has occurred or may occur in that area.)
- Hold the position for approximately 30 seconds, release, rest for 30–60 seconds, and stretch again. Try to make the stretch longer during successive stretches.
- Perform all stretches on both sides of the body.
- Increase intensity and duration of the stretching movements over several months.
- Use caution when stretching back and neck areas to avoid compressing the vertebrae and discs.
- Do not hold your breath during stretching; breathe normally.
- For maximum benefits, stretch five or six times per week; for minimal benefits, stretch three times per week.

joint that stretches the muscle. Active stretching consists of moving the joint and stretching the muscles as a result of the contraction of the opposing muscle, which is the muscle on the opposite side of the area being stretched.

Lack of flexibility reduces one's quality of life by limiting the enjoyable activities one can engage in as well as restricting the ability to carry out responsibilities. For example, Mary Jane, age 45, was restricted in her ability to play tennis with friends due to injuries to her skeletal system and subsequent weakening of the connective tissues. Additionally, not doing any flexibility exercises resulted in further weakening of connective tissues to her skeletal system. As a teacher, Mary Jane found that she had difficulty writing on the board and putting up classroom displays. Worse yet, she found it difficult to lift, carry, and play with her new grandchild. Upon consultation, Mary Jane's physician suggested a variety of stretching exercises to be done four or five times per week as well as simple muscle-strengthening activities. Mary Jane noticed an improvement after about 6 weeks and is determined to continue these activities to keep her connective tissue flexible and her muscles strengthened.

Flexibility training three to seven times per week improves physical performance; improves circulation as the temperature of the muscle tissue increases; improves posture through incorporating short, frequent stretch breaks throughout the day; and improves coordination and balance. Stretching has also been shown to provide relief from stress, improve mood, and increase alertness during the day.[12]

How many hours per day do you spend at a computer or sitting at a desk? Most of us spend several hours each day, which can lead to muscle tension and fatigue. By using a number of simple stretching exercises for 5 to 10 minutes, your entire body (and mind) can be revitalized and tension can be relieved. For computer and desk stretches you can use during the day to reduce tension and relieve muscle fatigue, go to the textbook Web site.

Keep these suggestions in mind as you go through the stretches:

- Only stretch to the limit where you feel mild tension and then hold according to the number of seconds suggested.
- Do not stretch to the point of feeling pain.
- Do not bounce into or during the stretch.
- Breathe in a low and rhythmic manner.
- When you have finished stretching, close your eyes and breathe slowly for about 10 seconds.

Muscular Strength and Endurance

Muscular strength is the ability of a muscle to generate force against some type of resistance; **muscular endurance** is the ability to continue to generate a force over a period of time or for a number of repetitions. As a result of muscular strength and endurance, a woman can improve her performance in physical activities, reduce the possibility of injury, improve physical appearance, and improve the ratio of lean body mass to fatty tissue. This is an essential component of effective weight-loss programs due to the "burning" of calories during weight training.

Increasing muscle strength can be achieved by participating in weight-bearing exercise such as free weights (barbells) and weight machines (such as Nautilus), performing exercises such as push-ups or pull-ups, or using fitness aids such as Thera-Bands. Classification of weight-training exercises includes isometric exercise, isotonic exercise, and isokinetic exercise. **Isometric** weight training applies force without movement such as applying force in the muscle and holding the force (for example, tightening the buttocks while sitting at your desk). Hold the isometric contraction for a maximum of 6 seconds; do this for 5 to 10 repetitions for best results. A form of **isotonic** weight training uses force with movement, such as use of a barbell; both the muscle and the weight move. Isotonic exercise is used more often than other forms of weight training because it better develops and utilizes strength in varied activities. Another type of weight training that can improve muscular strength is **isokinetic** weight training, an exertion of force (such as your leg) at a constant speed against an equal force exerted by a special strength-training machine. Although this type of exercise develops strength and endurance, strength-training machines are usually located in fitness facilities, which require that you be a member; the machinery is too expensive to purchase. (See Figure 11.4.)

You may need the help of an exercise professional in order to develop a strength- and endurance-training program that benefits all muscle groups. All areas of the body—calves, thighs, buttocks, abdomen, lower and upper back, arms, shoulders, and neck—should be included in a strength-enhancing workout. Determine your current level of fitness and the appropriate program needed to improve your strength and endurance. For example, lift approximately 80 percent of your maximum capacity to improve your strength. Choose less weight but increase repetitions to improve your endurance.[13]

Workouts to improve muscular strength and endurance should be done 2 to 4 days each week with rest between days to allow for recovery. However, you can train more than 4 days per week, if desired, by working out different muscle groups on different days. For example, work the lower-body muscles (legs, buttocks) one day, the upper-body muscles (upper back, arms, shoulders) on the next day, and then return to lower body on the third day. As you lift weights, select eight to ten exercises that focus on the muscle groups you

FIGURE 11.4 (*A*) Isometric exercise. (*B*) Isotonic exercise. (*C*) Isokinetic exercise.

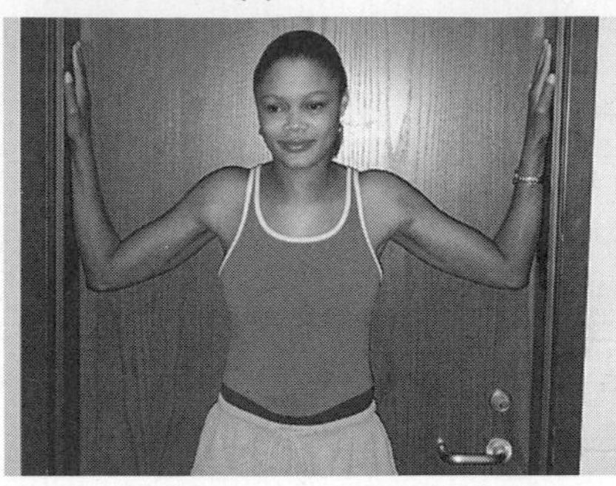

A

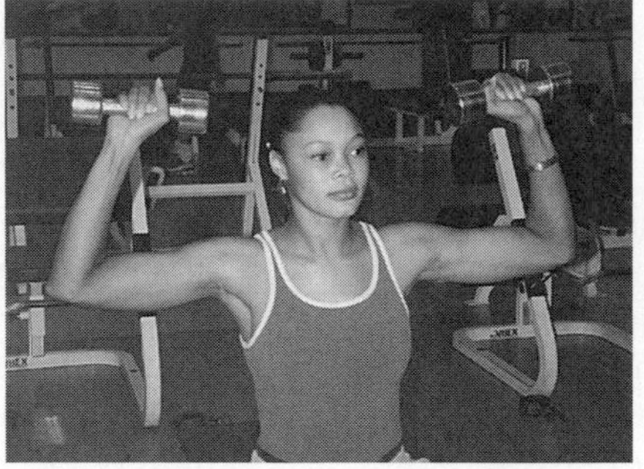

B

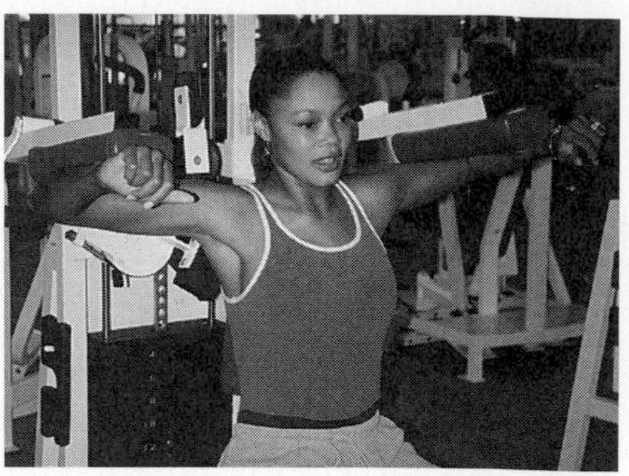

C

TABLE 11.2 Body Fat Standards for Women Recommended by Age Group[14]

CATEGORY	20–29	30–39	40–49	50–59	60+
Very low	<16%	<17%	<18%	<19%	<20%
Low	16–19%	17–20%	18–21%	19–22%	20–23%
Optimal	20–28%	21–29%	22–30%	23–31%	24–32%
Moderately high	29–31%	30–32%	31–33%	32–33%	33–35%
High	>31%	>32%	>33%	<34%	>35%

want to develop. Using heavier weights, according to your strength level, and performing fewer repetitions (between 1 and 5) will build muscle strength; using lighter weights but performing a higher number of repetitions (15 to 20) will build muscle endurance. For the exerciser who is interested in building both strength and endurance, include 8 to 12 repetitions for each strengthening exercise and use a weight that is heavy enough to create fatigue.[15] It is recommended that women over the age of 50 perform more repetitions (10 to 15 reps) but use lighter weights. This can reduce the chance of injury and rapid fatigue. Regardless of your age, be sure to include a warm-up stretch and a cool-down stretch routine with each weightlifting session.

Body Composition

Women with good to optimal body composition tend to be more active, healthier, and feel better about themselves. **Body composition** has two components: lean body mass that includes the muscles, bones, teeth, connective tissue, and organ tissue, and fat tissue that includes essential fat and nonessential fat. *Essential fat,* which makes up approximately 12 percent of total body fat in women, is just what the term implies—it is fatty tissue that is essential to normal, healthy functioning of the body. This particular type of fat is a component of our brain, nerves, mammary glands, and other important organs in the body and is necessary for proper body functioning. *Nonessential*, or storage, *fat* is located just below the skin within fat cells (adipose tissue) and around major organs. Although it offers cushioning for important body organs and stores energy for future needs, too much nonessential fat can be unhealthy and unsightly.

Measurement of body composition provides a better analysis of one's "body weight" than simply stepping on a scale and looking at the numbers. This measurement provides the weight for all the components of our body. The percentage of a woman's body weight that is fat, called percent body fat, is more important because too much fat is negatively associated with one's health status. Table 11.2 shows the range of percent body fat for women.

OTHER EXERCISE CONSIDERATIONS

A *warm-up* before engaging in the endurance component of a fitness program better prepares the body for a more effective workout and helps to reduce injury during the fitness activity.

As an individual begins the brief warm-up period (usually 5–10 minutes), the increase in body temperature produces a number of beneficial outcomes, including the fact that warm muscles and tendons are less prone to injury and produce improved performance.[16]

Health Tips

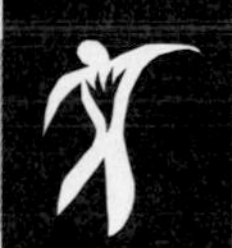

Putting Together a Physical Activity Program

The major components of a physical fitness program are included in the following example. Additionally, suggestions are provided for making your workout work better for you.

Warm-Up Phase

- Spend 10–15 minutes in the warm-up phase.
- Move slowly into an activity that is similar to what your aerobic activity will be (for example, walk, do slow dance movements, etc.) for about 5 minutes. This will start to cause an increase in heart rate.
- Following this, use long stretching movements that stretch the muscles and take the joints through their full range of motion for 5–10 minutes. Stretch all areas and joints of the body: neck, shoulder, arms, trunk, hips, legs, thighs, calves, knees, and ankles.

Workout Phase

- Spend 20–60 minutes, depending on your fitness level. Women who are less physically fit should begin working out 20 minutes three times per week and increase the number of minutes as fitness level allows.
- Include flexibility movements, muscle-strengthening exercises, and endurance activities.
- Remember to watch for the intensity, duration, and frequency of the activities you do (a minimum of 60 percent of your target heart rate for 20 minutes at least three times per week).
- Check your target heart rate; decrease or increase the intensity accordingly.
- Slow down and/or rest as needed.
- Remember that "no pain, no gain" is *not* a true statement.

Cool-Down Phase

- Ease into a reduced-intensity level of activity. This is a very important component of a fitness program.
- Spend 5–10 minutes reducing the heart rate and "coming down" from your workout.
- Slow your movements, and stretch each area of the body as well as all your joints.
- Do relaxing forms of activity to slow down your heart and breathing rates.
- Check your heart rate. It should be reduced from the level it was during the workout phase.

The warm-up period enables the person's body to receive sufficient blood and oxygen and prepares the muscle groups for more strenuous endurance activities.

The *cool-down* phase of the workout is similar to the warm-up period and is just as important. The major intent of the cool-down is to bring blood back to the heart for reoxygenation so that blood can supply essential oxygen to the brain, heart, and other major body organs, and not pool in major muscle groups. Additionally, during cool-down, the heart rate and breathing rate begin to return to normal and the body temperature begins to decrease. It aids the body in moving from an active state to a resting state. Engaging in a 5- to 10-minute cool-down stretching routine will reduce the probability of sore muscles and injury.

PERSONAL FITNESS PROGRAMMING

Having learned about the important components of a comprehensive fitness program, you can formulate a personal fitness program to meet your individual needs and interests. (See *Health Tips:* "Putting Together a Physical Activity Program.")

The Centers for Disease Control (CDC) and other agencies recommend focusing on the frequency, rather than the intensity, of physical activity. According to the CDC, women should accumulate 30 minutes or more at least 5 days each week by engaging in physical activity that involves body movements and energy expenditure. A well-designed and regular fitness program is desirable and will yield positive results. However, some activity is better than no activity, and many women who do not participate in *exercise* programs can still realize positive benefits by accumulating 30 minutes of physical activity (gardening, vacuuming, or walking) per day for 5 days each week.

Fitness Assessments

Deciding to participate in a fitness program is a major step, but designing a personal fitness program is quite another. It may call for some professional assistance, especially in the assessment area. (See *Her Story:* "LaToya: Designing a Fitness Program.")

Fitness assessments are designed to determine an individual's physical fitness condition as it relates to cardiorespiratory endurance, muscular strength and endurance, flexibility, and body composition. The following assessments can assist you in determining your

Her Story

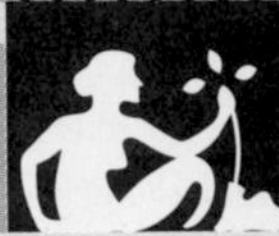

LaToya: Designing a Fitness Program

LaToya found that the responsibilities and stress that accompany a new job were beginning to be more than she could effectively handle. After discussing her concerns and symptoms with a number of friends, she concluded that participating in a physical activity program would be beneficial for her situation. She contacted an exercise specialist at a local health club. The exercise specialist gave LaToya fitness assessments to determine her endurance, strength, and flexibility, and then helped design a program to meet LaToya's needs.

- If LaToya had been unable to afford the advice of an exercise specialist at the fitness club, where else could she have found information about developing a personal fitness program?
- In addition to a regular exercise program, what other activities could LaToya integrate into her lifestyle to increase her daily activity level?

fitness level before engaging in a physical activity program.

1. *Cardiorespiratory endurance.* One easy and dependable method of determining your cardiorespiratory endurance capacity is to take the 3-minute step test. You will need only a stopwatch and a sturdy bench, block, or stepping tool that is 12 inches high. It will be easier and more accurate if you have a partner who monitors your time and counts your pulse upon completing the step test. You will start the stopwatch and begin your bench-stepping at the same time. As you proceed, be sure you place both feet on the bench and then both feet on the ground to the rhythm of 24 complete steps per minute for 3 minutes. It may be advantageous to say to yourself, "Up, up—down, down" as you step. Immediately upon completing the 3 minutes, sit down and have your partner count your pulse for 1 minute. The number of heartbeats counted in 1 minute is your heart rate. Compare it to the heart rates for your age in Table 11.3.[17]
2. *Muscular strength and endurance.* To assess muscular strength and endurance, complete the following two activities:
   a. *Modified push-ups.* Lie face down on a mat and with your knees bent, raise your upper body, supported by your arms. Your back and arms need to be straight. Lower your upper body until your chest is about 3 inches off the floor. Then return to the starting position. Count the number of push-ups you can perform within 1 minute. Refer to Table 11.4 to determine your strength level.
   b. *Abdominal muscle strength (curl-ups).* Lie flat on your back, cross your arms at the chest, and bend your knees at a 90-degree angle with your feet flat on the floor about 18 inches from the buttocks. If necessary, have someone hold your feet in place while you raise your head and chest off the floor or mat for 1 minute. Count the number of curl-ups you can do in 1 minute and compare this with Table 11.5. *Suggestion:* Keep your chin tucked in and sit up until your elbows touch your thighs.
3. *Flexibility.* Two ways to measure flexibility are
   a. *Shoulder flexibility.* Raise your left arm above your head and then bend it at the elbow and reach down your back as far as possible; at the same

TABLE 11.3 Scoring Standards for 3-Minute Step Test for Women (heart rate for 1 minute)[18]

CATEGORY	18–25	26–35	36–45
Excellent	72–83	72–86	74–87
Good	88–97	91–97	93–101
Average	110–116	112–118	111–117
Below average	118–124	121–127	120–127
Poor	128–137	129–135	130–152

TABLE 11.4 Test Standards for Modified Push-Ups for Women[19]

Excellent	24 or more push-ups
Good	14–23 push-ups
Average	8–13 push-ups
Fair	2–7 push-ups
Poor	1 or 0

TABLE 11.5 Canadian Trunk Strength Test for Women: Number of Trunk Curl-Ups Completed[20]

STRENGTH CATEGORY	<35	35–44	>45
Excellent	50	40	30
Good	40	25	15
Marginal	25	15	10
Needs work	10	6	4

TABLE 11.6 Sit and Reach Scoring for Women[21]

Excellent	9.0–10.5 inches
Good	6.0–7.5 inches
Average	3.0–5.0 inches
Fair	0.5–2.0 inches
Poor	−2.5–0.0 inches

FIGURE 11.5 Body fat determination using skinfold calipers.

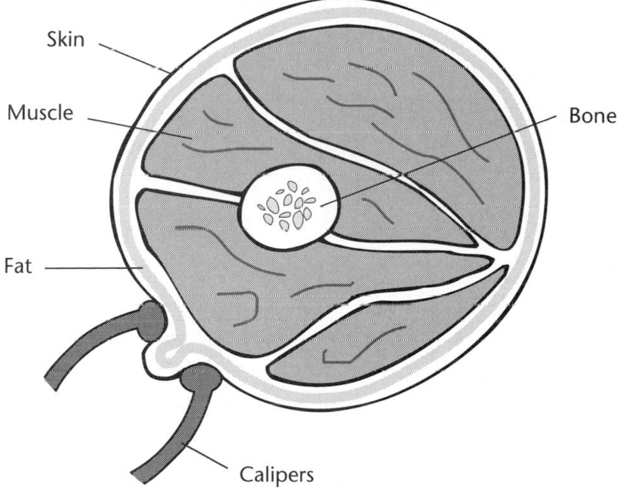

time, take your right arm and bend it behind your back and try to touch the fingers together from both arms. Finger overlap reflects fairly good flexibility; reverse the position and try to touch fingers again. You are usually more flexible on one side than the other.

b. *Sit and reach.* Using a box that is 8–12 inches high with a ruler taped on top and extending 6 inches in front of it, sit on the floor with legs outstretched and feet flat against the box. Slowly stretch your fingers across the ruler to determine how far you can reach. Make three attempts to stretch across the ruler. Be sure you warm up first! Compare your results with those in Table 11.6.

4. *Body composition.* Rather than "weighing in" each day to determine body weight, a much better measure is to determine healthy body weight by calculating body composition and comparing lean tissue to fat tissue. There are several methods of doing this, including skin-fold measurement and calculating body mass index (BMI).

   a. *Skin-fold measurement.* Using **calipers,** we can measure the thickness of skin at certain sites on the body and apply this measurement to a formula, which will give us the percentage of fat. (See Figure 11.5.) These skin-fold measurements have been compared to laboratory techniques that research studies have shown to be an accurate measure to determine body composition.

   b. *Bioelectrical impedance analysis (BIA).* This measures the electrical resistance of small currents directed through the body. Electrical impulses pass more freely through tissues containing water, such as muscle tissue. Fatty tissue, containing less water, is not a good conductor of electricity; therefore, the more resistance measured during BIA, the larger the percentage of fat in the body. To measure bioelectrical impedance, electrodes are attached to the body and then to a computer that provides feedback. The electrical current is harmless and painless, and the feedback regarding body composition is rapid. The accuracy of BIA is about the same as for skin-fold measurement.

   c. *Hydrostatic weighing.* Considered the "gold standard" of calculating body composition, this system measures the relative amount of fat and lean body mass while the person is submerged under water. Through the use of a special scale, a woman's underwater body weight is compared to her body weight out of the water, and then calculations are made to determine percentage of body fat. Some find this procedure uncomfortable because of the need to be submerged under water for a brief period of time.

   d. *The body pod.* The newest technology for measuring body composition, the body pod resembles a small chamber with computerized sensors. The procedure can be completed in 5 minutes. While the measurement principle is the same as for underwater weighing, this method uses air displacement rather than water displacement to determine the amount of air that is displaced by the person sitting in the chamber. The overall composition of the body can be measured by calculating the percentage of fat and lean tissue.

   e. *Body mass index (BMI)* is a method of expressing the relationship of body weight (expressed in kilograms) to height (expressed in meters) for men and women. Although the BMI does not determine body composition, it is quite accurate in determining healthy body weight. (See Figure 11.6 and Table 11.7.)

DESIGN YOUR PERSONAL FITNESS PROGRAM

Knowing the benefits and "how-to" of fitness workouts is one thing. We usually have a motivating factor (such as a wedding, spring break, or more energy) for beginning the program. However, keeping the program successful

FIGURE 11.6 Calculating BMI.

To determine your body mass index (BMI)

1. Divide your weight in pounds by 2.2 to convert it to kilograms.

   A = weight (kg) = your weight (lb) ÷ 2.2

2. Multiply your height in inches by 2.54 and divide by 100 to convert height to meters.

   B = height (m) = your height (inches) × 2.54 ÷ 100

3. Multiply B by B to get your height (in meters) squared.

   C = height (m) × height (m)

4. Divide A by C to determine BMI.

   BMI = weight (kg) ÷ height $(m)^2$

Example: 176-lb person, 72 inches (6 feet) tall

1. $A = 176 \div 2.2 = 80$
2. $B = \frac{72 \times 2.54}{100} = \frac{182.88}{100} = 1.83$
3. $C = 1.83 \times 1.83 = 3.35$
4. $BMI = \frac{80}{3.35} = 23.88$

TABLE 11.7 Desirable Body Mass Index in Relation to Age

AGE	BMI (kg/m²)
19–24	19–24
25–34	20–25
35–44	21–26
45–54	22–27
55–65	23–28
>65	24–29

enough to remain involved, called **exercise adherence,** creates a need for additional information and know-how.

Getting Started

How do you establish a fitness program that includes the necessary components, meets your needs, and safely helps you achieve the benefits you want to see? To answer this question, consider the following as an entry into a fitness program that can provide healthy and satisfactory rewards.

Should you get a physical checkup? Ask yourself the following questions to determine whether you should see a physician before embarking on your potential change of lifestyle program.

- Do I have any medical condition that might need special attention before starting a fitness program, such as heart problems, chest pains or pressure, dizziness or fainting spells, or high blood pressure?
- Have I experienced any shortness of breath after any type of exertion?
- Are my joints painful or my muscles overly sore following activity?
- Has my mother, father, brother, sister, or a grandparent had a heart attack before age 50?
- Have I had a physical exam within the past year, other than for an ailment (such as flu, cold, or other communicable disease)?
- Do I have any serious problems with my menstrual cycle?
- Am I bothered by breathing problems as a result of asthma or allergies?

If you answered "yes" to any of these questions, you should see your physician; if not, you are probably ready to engage in a sensible, fun, and comprehensive fitness program.

Another aspect of starting a fitness program is to assess your present physical condition to determine where you need to begin your program. The assessments found on pages 290–291 can assist you in this aspect of starting a fitness program.

The next step involves writing a personal contract about what you want to achieve as well as how and when you will carry out your plan. A contract not only will assist you in getting started but also will help you stay involved as well as achieve progress toward your objectives. *Journal Activity:* "My Personal Fitness Contract" provides an example of how to develop a fitness program contract.

Pacing yourself in the initial phase of your fitness program will allow you to build your fitness level gradually and avoid injury as well as burnout. Consider the information in the *Health Tips:* "Putting Together a Physical Activity Program" on page 289 and use this information to begin at the lower part of your target heart rate (around the 60 percent range). Over a period of several weeks, increase the intensity, duration, and perhaps frequency. After a month or so, you may want to change your routine as well as some of your goals. Consider a different environment, perhaps changing from an indoor facility like a health club to activities that take you outside and into a park or track facility, providing weather permits.

In summary, check with your physician, if necessary, then assess your current fitness level, develop a contract, and remember your personal goals of being involved in a fitness program (e.g., losing weight, looking better, having more energy, improving your mood, or preventing disease). Be sure to include the steps that assist you

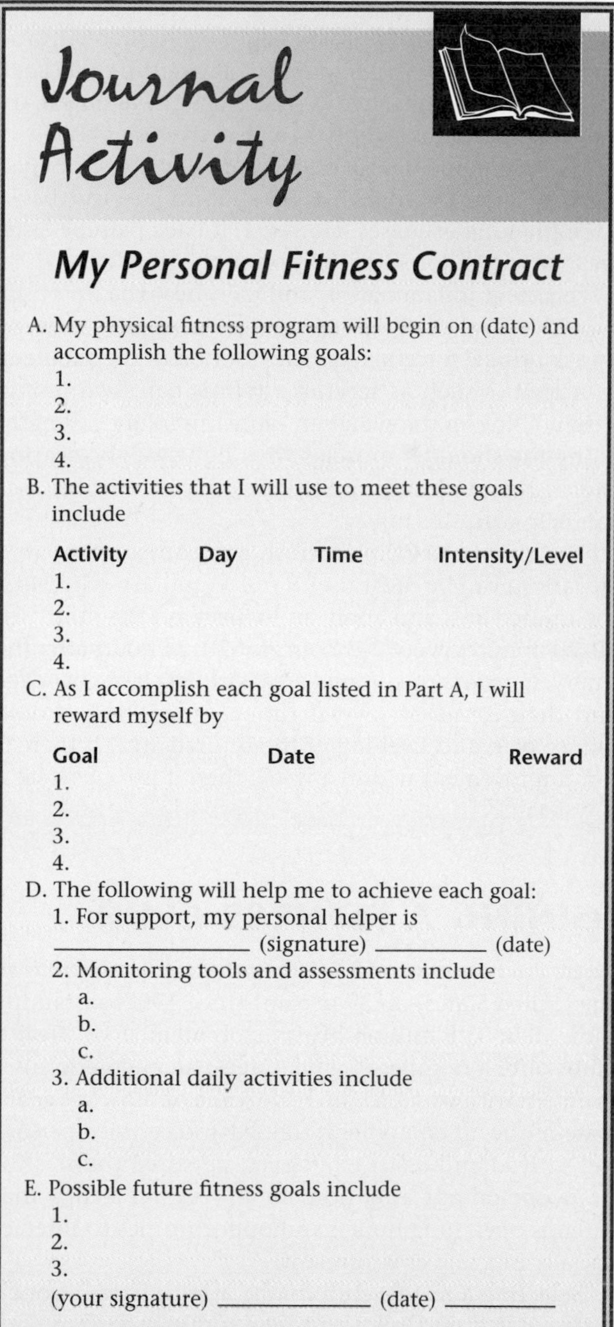
Journal Activity

My Personal Fitness Contract

A. My physical fitness program will begin on (date) and accomplish the following goals:
1.
2.
3.
4.

B. The activities that I will use to meet these goals include

Activity	Day	Time	Intensity/Level
1.			
2.			
3.			
4.			

C. As I accomplish each goal listed in Part A, I will reward myself by

Goal	Date	Reward
1.		
2.		
3.		
4.		

D. The following will help me to achieve each goal:
1. For support, my personal helper is ______________ (signature) __________ (date)
2. Monitoring tools and assessments include
   a.
   b.
   c.
3. Additional daily activities include
   a.
   b.
   c.

E. Possible future fitness goals include
1.
2.
3.

(your signature) ____________ (date) __________

in staying with your program: making a commitment, finding a partner, setting a schedule, checking your progress, varying your routine, and rewarding yourself.

Staying Involved

Starting a fitness program is usually easy to do because we have some knowledge of the benefits or have an impetus to begin a program. However, exercise adherence is often more of a challenge. Sometimes we don't have a structured program, or we engage in the wrong program for our personal needs, or perhaps we start at the wrong level and then proceed too fast or too slow. Usually, once our motivational factor has been achieved (such as losing weight, toning muscles, etc.), our activity regimen lessens or may stop altogether. What can you do to stay involved in a fitness program?

Dr. Jon Robison, a specialist in health promotion and health behavior, has developed a six-step program to promote adherence to fitness programs for clients at his preventive medicine center. These steps include writing a contract, charting your progress, working out with others, making your activity enjoyable, dealing with the details, and staying with your program.[22]

Following is a brief description of each of these suggestions:

1. *Develop a personal contract to reach an obtainable weekly or monthly fitness goal.* Be specific about what you want to achieve, when and how you will achieve this goal, and the reward (such as money) for attaining the goal. Have a support person sign the contract each time a goal is reached. Additionally, if you do not reach the goal, do not give yourself the reward.
2. *Keep track of your progress by knowing your starting physical levels and charting your progress each time you engage in a fitness activity.* Dr. Robison suggests giving yourself a "star" each time you participate. Place the "star" or sticker on an area where you can see the progress on a regular basis.
3. *Exercising with others holds you accountable to yourself and to at least one other person or group of people.* Find others at school or work who have similar fitness interests and goals, and share your activity time with them. We are all likely to have days when we just don't want to be active, but when others are counting on us, we tend to respond to the extra pressure. If necessary, place more pressure on yourself to be active by telling others your goals.
4. *An enjoyable fitness activity is more likely to be done than an unenjoyable one.* If you hate to run, don't run; if you hate to swim, don't swim! The best exercise is the one you like, whether it's walking, gardening, or a vigorous game of racquetball. Fitness activities should not feel like self-punishment, but more like a special time you give yourself. Not only should the activity be enjoyable, but you should also reward yourself with some self-indulgence after the week's fitness activities: a favorite movie, a massage, or a new CD.
5. *Plan for your fitness activity by taking care of the details.* After deciding which activity fits you, determine where and when to work out; what clothing, shoes, and equipment are needed; the time of day that is best for you and your activity partner(s); and

a contingency plan for unforeseen changes (weather or facility problems). Taking care of the details helps to eliminate excuses for not participating and lessens the perception of inconvenience.

6. *Staying with the program seems to be easier said than done.* Researchers contend that, if exercisers can stay with a fitness program for 6 months, the odds are they'll still be exercising after a year. It is important to see yourself as an active woman rather than someone who is temporarily involved in a fitness program to achieve a specific goal (for example, just to lose 5 or 10 pounds). This mindset usually happens after 6 months of being involved in a fitness activity. Just keep on plugging. After a few months, you will feel "unnatural" if you are not exercising.

Avoiding Injuries

Women who participate in sports and other fitness activities need to be aware of and take precautions to avoid injuries that hinder or suspend the continuation of their fitness program. Engaging in exercise too frequently or too intensely can result in a variety of injuries that are usually preventable. In general, most fitness-related injuries can be avoided simply by a warm-up and a cool-down stretching routine before and after every workout and by varying your fitness activities.

What are some of the more common injuries that women sustain during fitness activities, and what can be done about them? One of the more common and serious injuries is a tear of the **anterior cruciate ligament (ACL),** which is a major support structure of the knee. This injury occurs more often in active women than in active men and is usually an injury caused by contact of the knee with another object or when the leg is planted and then turned in another direction. If you experience swelling and pain of the knee, you should see a physician. This type of injury calls for rehabilitation exercises under the guidance of a physical therapist. Sometimes surgery is necessary. Another type of knee injury is called **patellofemoral knee pain,** which can result from, for example, repetitive jumping, improper stretching, or joint surface degeneration. Symptoms include inflammation with swelling, tenderness, and pain during movement.

Shin splints are recognized because of the pain that occurs in the shins and are usually caused by too much activity performed on hard surfaces such as gym floors or hard-surfaced roads. This may occur because of strains in the muscles that move the ankle and foot at the attachment points in the shin. Arch supports, either over-the-counter or, if needed, custom-made by a sports podiatrist, will usually cure the problem of shin splints. It may be necessary to reduce or temporarily discontinue your fitness activity until the injury is healed.

Low back pain can result from weak back or abdominal muscles, especially if you begin exercising with too much intensity or too frequently. Preventing low back pain can be accomplished in a number of ways: First, try reducing strenuous activity to a level that your body can safely accommodate. Second, improve your back muscles by carefully engaging in abdominal- and back-strengthening exercises. However, if back pain persists, see a physician for an evaluation of the problem.

Persistent inflammation and pain near the tip of the shoulder is called shoulder impingement and is caused by a continual forceful overhead motion of the shoulder.

Activities such as serving a tennis ball, swimming, weight lifting, or throwing can cause this injury. Strengthening the shoulder muscles with light weight-bearing exercises or eliminating activities that strain this area can help with this injury.

The simple **RICE** plan (rest, ice, compression, and elevation) can be most useful for temporary relief. *Rest* the injured area and apply an *ice* pack on the injury for 10–20 minutes every 2–3 hours for 20–24 hours after the injury. *Compress* the injured area with an elastic bandage and then *elevate* it several times a day. RICE should reduce pain and swelling of the injured area. If there is not improvement within a week, then it is time to see a physician.[23]

JOINING A FITNESS CLUB

There are more than 18,000 health and sports clubs in the United States, up 39 percent since 1997, sustaining more than 33.8 million health club members.[24] Health clubs offer a number of advantages: an energetic environment with women who have some of the same goals; state-of-the-art equipment; trained and certified personnel to lead and assist exercisers; personal trainers for more one-on-one attention; an all-weather facility that often is open long hours; and opportunities to interact socially in a safe environment.

Selecting a health club that is appropriate for one's fitness needs and goals can take some important consumer skills. If you choose to join a health club, *FYI:* "Choosing a Fitness Club" can be used in determining if the club is right for you.

Female-only clubs have become popular because they often provide an environment of reduced anxiety and intimidation and offer special classes that appeal to women, such as classes for pregnant women. Strength machines and other equipment are often sized for women clients, and facility hours accommodate the needs of women, with child care available during these periods. If you are considering joining a health club, it may be wise to consider women-only clubs for the programs and conveniences provided to members.

FYI

Choosing a Fitness Club[25]

Having structure and guidance in a personal fitness program is beneficial to many women. Health clubs with properly trained fitness instructors can be the answer. How do you know which health club to join? Use the following checklist to help you make this important choice.

Consider whether the club provides:	Yes	No
An attractive, safe, effective environment or facility	______	______
A clean and convenient facility	______	______
Certified staff current with CPR training	______	______
State-of-the-art exercise equipment that meets your needs	______	______
Individualized fitness and health assessments	______	______
Cost of membership within your budget	______	______
Contracts that are understandable/staff who provide explanations	______	______
Membership fees and services that are equivalent	______	______
Class size that is small enough for individual attention	______	______
Child care on the premises, if needed	______	______
Staff that is friendly and helpful and open to questions	______	______
Adequate parking for all members	______	______

SPECIAL CONSIDERATIONS

Exercise and the Menstrual Cycle

History tells us that women once went to bed during their menstrual period. In more recent years, menstruating women were told not to swim and not to participate in activity classes, and they were even excused from participation on sports teams. Today it is recognized that menstruation usually presents no problems to women who participate in active events.

However, a number of symptoms may interfere with a woman's participation in physical activities. Varying degrees of pain and cramping, which may be accompanied by pain in the lower back or legs, can curtail one's ability and desire to be physically active during the menstrual period. Painful menstrual periods, called **dysmenorrhea,** can be so severe that some women are incapacitated for several days. Certainly, women with this type of pain should seek and follow the advice of their physician.

Premenstrual syndrome (PMS) affects some women and is characterized by feelings of irritability, depression, bloating, headaches, tender breasts, and possible weight gain. Although most women who experience PMS can maintain normal functioning, some may need a variety of treatments and professional medical help. As a result of these monthly hormonal changes, a woman's motivation to continue her fitness activities may subside. Yet, engaging in a reduced-intensity level activity has been shown to reduce the symptoms of PMS and produce a feeling of well-being.

Amenorrhea, the cessation of the menstrual period, is related to overexercising, which can be the case with long-distance running, cycling, gymnastics, or swimming. When a woman's body fat drops below 12 percent, which often occurs in highly fit female athletes, irregular or absent menstrual periods often are the result.

If discomfort during the menstrual period is a problem for you, consider reducing the frequency, duration, and intensity of your fitness activity rather than eliminating it. Pamper yourself after a workout by enjoying a soothing, warm shower or time in a hot tub or briefly relaxing to pleasant music. It is also beneficial during the menstrual period to incorporate relaxing activities that promote a good night's sleep.

Exercise and Pregnancy

Pregnancy may be compared to preparing for and running a marathon, as far as the physical stress it can have on a woman's body is concerned. Therefore, a woman needs to prepare her muscles, increase her stamina, and boost the immune system in case of infection as she moves toward the big finish line: the birthing process. If a woman is exercising prior to pregnancy, then it is usually healthy to continue exercising during pregnancy, with her physician's approval, though perhaps with some modifications.

What are the benefits of exercising during pregnancy? Through research studies, numerous benefits have been determined for women who exercise during pregnancy. Appropriate exercise can relieve back pain and help improve posture by strengthening and toning

Viewpoint

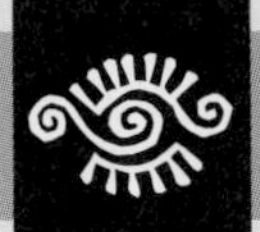

Should I Continue My Usual Exercise Level during Pregnancy?

Janene has been involved in an intense aerobic exercise routine throughout college. She married and became pregnant during her senior year. The energy, stress relief, and weight management that her aerobic running produced was something Janene wanted to continue to experience. She consulted her physician, who suggested reducing the frequency and intensity of her workout and changing the running to a walking program. Janene was not happy with that idea and discussed this suggestion with the members of her running club, many of whom were knowledgeable in the area of exercise physiology. Their opinion was that because Janene had been in excellent aerobic condition before the pregnancy, she would not have problems maintaining her previous fitness activities.

Consider the following:

- The fetus is in a "built-in" safe environment, surrounded by amniotic fluid that serves as a shock absorber.
- Exercise causes an increase in body temperature that results in an increase of temperature in the fetal environment that may not be safe for the fetus.
- A reduced sense of balance and coordination following the seventh month may increase the chances for accidents during activity.
- Aerobic activity such as bouncing, running, and step aerobics should not be undertaken during the third trimester.
- The heart rate should not exceed 140 beats per minute, depending on one's fitness level.
- After the fourth month of pregnancy, exercises that require lying flat on the back should be avoided.

What would you recommend that Janene do about her level of fitness and her fitness activities during her pregnancy? Who should she consult to make a decision about how much to exercise during pregnancy?

muscles; prevent joint injury by activating the lubricating synovial fluid in the joints; and ease labor because of stronger muscles, healthier heart, and increased endurance.[26] Pregnant women who exercise are also less likely to have hemorrhoids, low back pain, fatigue, or varicose veins than those who don't exercise.

The cardiovascular system must circulate about 30 percent more blood during the 267+ days of pregnancy. Exercise can aid in increased and more efficient circulation and can reduce the likelihood of swelling in the feet and legs. Controlling weight gain, avoiding low back pain, and improving the efficiency of the cardiorespiratory system can lead to an important psychological benefit during pregnancy. Exercise can give pregnant women a measure of control over their expanding bodies and enhance their chances to feel good, look good, and have a positive self-image.

The American College of Obstetricians and Gynecologists (ACOG)[27] offers exercise guidelines for pregnant women. This organization suggests that women should not exercise if they are at risk for pregnancy-induced hypertension, preterm membrane rupture, or persistent second- and third-trimester bleeding. Additionally, women who have an incomplete cervix, have had fetal growth retardation, or have experienced premature labor during a previous or current pregnancy should not exercise while pregnant.

However, women who have none of these risks are encouraged to exercise in moderation, with the supervision of their physician. ACOG offers the following suggestions to help pregnant women exercise safely: monitor your heart rate during exercise and do not allow it to go over 140 beats per minute; do not exercise at a strenuous level for more than 15 minutes; avoid twisting, jarring, jumping, and rapid change-of-direction motions; drink plenty of liquids throughout the workout period; do not exercise during hot, humid weather to avoid overheating; and after the fourth month, avoid exercises that require lying on the back to perform. (See *Viewpoint:* "Should I Continue My Usual Exercise Level during Pregnancy?")

If you want to exercise during pregnancy, you may want to use less strenuous exercises, which can achieve positive results. Your fitness level before becoming pregnant will dictate to a major degree the intensity, frequency, and duration of your exercise program. (*Do not* exercise during pregnancy without the consent of your physician.) Here are two less strenuous exercises:

- Swimming, one of the best exercises for pregnant women because swimming in a prone position promotes optimum blood flow. The water acts as a support cushion for both mother and fetus. The pressure of the water also encourages water loss, which can prevent edema, and does not place extra strain on joints and ligaments for women in their third trimester.

- Walking, maintaining a heart rate of under 140 beats per minute for approximately 15 minutes at least three times per week. If you exercised before pregnancy, you may increase the duration up to 30 minutes with physician approval. Supportive shoes and a pleasant and safe area in which to walk are additional benefits of this exercise.

Kegel exercises are movements that help strengthen the muscles of the pelvic floor, aiding in support of the extra weight of the baby. Conditioned muscles will make birth easier, and the perineum will more likely remain intact, with fewer tears and reduced need for an episiotomy, during childbirth. Kegels are performed by contracting and releasing muscles that are the same as the muscles that stop the flow of urine. Strengthening these muscles also helps stop urine leakage during a cough or sneeze and can also increase sexual pleasure during intercourse.

Here is how to perform Kegel exercises:[28]

- Empty your bladder.
- Either sitting or standing, tighten the pelvic floor muscles and hold for 10 counts.
- Relax muscles completely for 10 counts.
- Suggestion: perform about ten times, three times per day.

COMPULSIVE EXERCISE

Too often, women incorporate health-diminishing behaviors into their lifestyles to attain an ideal image—an image that is usually dictated through external influences. Whereas too little exercise will not produce positive results, too much can be detrimental to your health. Ironically, exercise can be overused by women to reach an unnatural and unhealthy thin appearance. It is possible to exercise too much, too often. When we have a distorted view of ourselves (a perception of oneself that does not match society's or the media's portrayal of the desirable body), we tend to adopt measures, regardless of the health consequences, to achieve this ideal. As a result, we can become an appearance junkie and a fitness zealot. **Compulsive exercising** is the need to engage in fitness activities beyond the normal standards for good health and despite potentially negative consequences. Edward J. Cumella, an expert in eating disorders and compulsive behavior, equates compulsive exercising to *exercise addiction (EA),* and states that EA can lead to medical complications such as stress factures, osteoporosis, cessation of menstruation, heart arrhythmias, and disturbances in the electrical conduction of the heart that could lead to sudden death.[29]

Despite injury, neglect of other responsibilities, or inconvenience, a woman with an addiction to exercise will continue at an intensity that is considered excessive. Symptoms indicative of overtraining, as described by John Draeger, include chronic fatique, decreased appetite, impaired concentration, apathy, and mood changes.[30] There is an apparent correlation between addictive behavior and poor self-concept, depression, stress, and eating disorders.

Researchers still do not understand all the factors that lead to addiction to exercise. What is the margin between gaining the benefits of a comprehensive fitness program and overdoing it? An exercise level equivalent to running 20 hours a week for 6 months appears to cause a stress response in our bodies. Feeling challenged, the body goes on the defensive and a number of negative physiological responses occur:[31]

- The levels of reproductive hormones, such as estrogen, progesterone, gonadotropin-releasing hormone, luteinizing hormone, and follicle-stimulating hormone, decrease, and cortisol, a hormone that regulates a number of body functions, increases. This new mix of hormones can have serious effects on the body.
  - The menstrual cycle and fertility can be affected due to excessive exercise. Ovulation and menstruation can stop or diminish.
  - Increased production of cortisol, which can suppress the immune system, causes an increased susceptibility to infections.
  - An energy imbalance caused by increased amounts of cortisol levels in the body can lead to the loss of lean body mass and fat cells. This can result in a form of malnutrition and fatigue.
  - Increased levels of cortisol and decreased levels of estrogen rob bone of minerals and can cause a reduction in bone density. Young female athletes may never reach their peak bone mass, and older women may increase the acceleration of bone loss.
- Excessive exercising can cause a decline in mood as well as in the ability to reason and concentrate.
- Increased numbers of injuries develop because of overuse of the body. These result in knee, joint, and bone problems.

Ironically, many of the physical and psychological benefits that we gain from a well-designed and moderate fitness program are the ones we lose when we exercise to excess. Compulsive or addictive exercise patterns harm the health of a woman and eradicate any benefits that are intended to be gained through fitness activities. Professional medical help is usually needed to deal with compulsive behavior of any type. When it may be life-threatening, as excessive exercising can be, especially in combination with eating disorders, it is imperative that a woman seek professional help. (See *Her Story:* "Averica: Battling Compulsive Exercise.")

Her Story

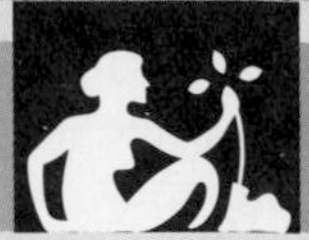

Averica: Battling Compulsive Exercise

Averica, while loving and admiring her sisters, also felt less attractive and less popular than both of them. She worked hard at proving herself at everything she tried. Discovering that she excelled in her physical education classes in high school, Averica began to spend more and more time and effort at running and swimming activities. She increased her distance, her intensity level, and the amount of time she spent running during the weekdays. But it was during the weekends that she ran really long distances. Her mother was concerned about this intense drive that Averica had to continually be so physically active. Her mother noticed a decline in Averica's weight and an increase in the number of colds and other minor infections that she continually contracted. But of greatest concern was the loss of Averica's monthly menstrual period. Her mother asked Averica to reduce the time she spent running and swimming. When Averica did this, she was irritable, restless, and unable to sleep, and she resented her mother for interfering with the activities in which she did so well. Averica decided to return to her former level of activities, and then sustained a knee injury. When Averica saw a physician for the injury, the doctor recognized signs that indicated the compulsive nature of Averica's running. The physician recommended a counselor who specialized in sport-related therapies. Averica, with the encouragement of her mother, is presently in counseling to find a way to engage in a running program without physically harming herself. Equally important, she is working on the emotional issues that pushed her to exercise compulsively in the first place.

- What are the detrimental health-related concerns that resulted from Averica's compulsive exercise habits?
- What other negative consequences could result from compulsive exercising?
- If you know someone who exercises compulsively, what physical, emotional, and social consequences do you see?

MANAGING WEIGHT THROUGH EXERCISE

Why do we all expect to look as if our bodies are ready for the fashion runway when, in reality, most of us can never achieve that physique? Nor is it necessarily healthy to achieve that look. Certainly, our concept of the ideal female body has changed over the decades. In one research study, Finnish researchers at University Central Hospital in Helsinki gathered department-store mannequins representing the fashionable female figure from the 1920s to 1990. The researchers worked out theoretical body fat percentages to determine body composition and size. Between 1920 and 1950, the mannequins representing women of those eras looked more like "real," robust women. However, after 1950, the mannequins tended to become taller and thinner; hip size went from about 34 inches to 31 inches, yet the average hip size of women today is about 37 inches.[32] Another study found that between 1959 and 1979, the idealized female physique, as portrayed in popular "male" magazines and by contestants in beauty contests, grew taller and thinner. Although a trend continues toward thin as the ideal image, this ideal is contradicted by reality; the reality is that the average college-age female is becoming heavier.

Despite the fact that the average female is heavier than in the past, many women still want to lose weight. Maintaining proper weight for a woman's body type and activity level can be achieved by participating in a comprehensive exercise program. A woman needs to expend at least the number of calories ingested with food intake each day so that caloric balance can be achieved. A recent research study determined that increasing exercise without nutritional changes did not result in effective weight loss. After a 16-month study, women who increased their exercise, but did not monitor dietary practices, experienced no change in weight. This study was compared to women in other studies who had increased exercise and monitored dietary practices, which resulted in an average weight loss of 13 pounds after 12 weeks.[33]

More than half of all ingested calories are used to keep our bodies and minds functioning. As we engage in fitness activities, not only do we expend additional calories at the time of the activity, but exercise increases our basal metabolic rate (the amount of energy needed to maintain normal body functions while at rest) even after the activity is over. Usually exercise alone (without dieting) will produce a weight loss; but even if you don't lose weight, it often helps you become thinner. The reason? A pound of muscle tissue will take up less space in your body than a pound of fat tissue. Building muscle and losing fat can cause a loss of inches without even losing a pound. The result is looking better and feeling better.

Once a woman has achieved the weight loss she desires, maintaining the new and healthy body then becomes the challenge. Successful long-term weight loss, defined as losing 10 percent of initial body weight and maintaining the loss for at least 1 year, was researched by Wing and Hill.[34] Common behavioral strategies of persons who maintained their weight loss included eating a low-fat diet, monitoring their own body weight and food intake, and engaging in high levels of regular physical activity. As these behaviors were continued and weight loss was maintained for 2 to 5 years, the chances increased for continued maintenance.

EXERCISING DURING THE LATER YEARS

Successful aging, rather than being determined by genetic factors, is largely shaped by individual lifestyle choices. Certainly a leading factor in successful aging is engaging in a physically active lifestyle. Research supports the multiple benefits of older women who participate in regular physical activity:

- Inactive, nonsmoking women, at age 65 have 12.7 years of active life expectancy, compared to highly active, nonsmoking women, who have 18.4 years of active life expectancy.[35]
- Exercise, in conjunction with commonsense interventions, reduced falls among older people by 44%.[36]
- Older adults have improved quality of sleep and reduced stress when participating in regular physical activity.[37]
- Older exercisers, compared to the sedentary elderly, are more likely to live to an advanced age and remain independent.[38]
- Midlife to elderly women who participate in moderate aerobic activities have significant improvements in stress-induced blood pressure levels and improved quality of sleep.[39]

Evidence continues to mount that women who engage in regular physical activity have an improved quality of life, have the energy and strength to meet the demands of busy lifestyles, and have reduced costs of medical care compared to inactive women.[40] As the number of older adults is projected to increase from 13 percent of the population in 2000 to 20 percent in 2030, promoting long-term health and well-being in older women is a national health priority. To assist with this priority, fifty organizations developed the *National Blueprint: Increasing Physical Activity among Adults Age 50 and Older,* which provides sixty specific recommendations to achieve a more physically active older population. This document can be accessed at the Robert Wood Johnson Foundation Web site at www.rwjf.org.

Health Tips

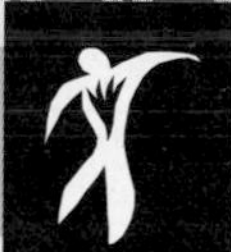

Make Exercise Fun!

Take the "work" out of workout and make exercise an enjoyable experience rather than an essential but unpleasant part of your day. As one excellent speaker attests, we are never too old for recess. So, how do we make exercise fun? Here are a few suggestions:[42]

- Select fitness activities that are fun: dancing, hiking, biking, sports, and active games.
- Develop hobbies that keep you moving: gardening, building, bird-watching, and participation in active organizations.
- Be creative while exercising: listen to music, talk to your exercise partner, or even make plans for the coming week.
- Vary your exercise routine with whom, what, when, and where you exercise, as well as varying the intensity of your activity.
- Give yourself fun and nonfattening rewards.

Midlife to older women engaging in regular physical activities should consider the following guidelines for safer and more effective outcomes.[41]

1. Engage in endurance, resistance, and flexibility exercises for better overall fitness.
2. Avoid extremes in temperatures and drink plenty of water.
3. Wear appropriate clothing for hot and cold environments.
4. Gradually increase intensity and duration over time and as condition permits.
5. Cool down slowly, do static stretching, and reduce heart rate to below 100 before stopping the cool-down/stretching segment of the exercise.

Of course, all exercise programs for older women should be started only after a physical exam and clearance from a physician. Plan to engage in lifelong physical activities; your quality and enjoyment of life will benefit from it as well as that of your family.

As with many other health-related behaviors, knowing is not the same as doing. We have presented information in this chapter that will help you develop a comprehensive and effective fitness program. That's the easy part. Engaging in the program and, more important, staying with it will be the challenge. Look at the suggestions for success with your fitness program in *Health Tips:* "Make Exercise Fun!" Establish your goals, make a commitment, find yourself a partner, and begin to realize all the positive results from this type of program. And good luck!

Chapter Summary

- Participating in a comprehensive fitness program provides a multitude of physiological, psychological, and social benefits.
- A comprehensive physical fitness program consists of four major components: cardiorespiratory fitness, flexibility, muscular strength and endurance, and body composition.
- When developing a fitness program, warming up and cooling down should be included as essential components.
- Developing an exercise program to meet your individual fitness needs includes assessments conducted to determine your cardiorespiratory endurance, flexibility, muscular strength and endurance, and body composition.
- Determining what you want to achieve from your fitness program, developing a personal contract with a built-in incentive, and taking measures to stay involved will help your program to be more successful.
- Injuries related to knees and joints, shin splints, back pain, and inflammation can often be prevented through use of proper equipment, effective stretching, and a commonsense approach to personal workouts. Treatment of these injuries can be helped by using the RICE method (rest, ice, compression, and elevation).
- Exercising during pregnancy can be beneficial for women, but only when done under the supervision of a physician.
- Weight management can be best achieved through having sensible eating habits and engaging in a comprehensive fitness program.
- Addiction to exercise can be detrimental to a woman's well-being. Professional counseling may be needed for recovery from this compulsion.
- Exercising throughout the life span produces multiple benefits for midlife and older women.
- One of the most effective weight-control methods is participation in a comprehensive fitness program.

Review Questions

1. In what ways does a physical fitness program benefit someone physically, psychologically, and socially?
2. What are the components of a comprehensive physical fitness program?
3. What are the differences between isometric, isotonic, and isokinetic weight training?
4. Why is it important to include the warm-up and cool-down phases of a workout session?
5. What methods can help to make your fitness program successful? What are some strategies for staying involved with your program?
6. What are four types of physical fitness injuries? What are the methods to avoid or reduce injuries?
7. What are the benefits and precautions a woman should consider if she chooses to exercise during pregnancy?
8. What are the potential negative consequences of compulsive exercise?
9. Why is exercise a positive and effective method of managing weight?
10. What precautions should older women take as they begin an exercise program?
11. What are methods that help make exercise more fun?

Resources

Organizations, Hotlines, and Web Sites

American Alliance for Health, Physical Education, Recreation and Dance
703-476-3400
www.aahperd.org

American College of Sports Medicine
317-637-9200
www.acsm.org

American Council on Exercise
800-825-3636
www.acefitness.org

American Volkssport Association
800-830–WALK
www.ava.org

National Association for Girls' and Women's Sports
800-213-7193
www.aahperd.org/nagws

President's Council on Physical Fitness and Sport
202-690-9000
www.fitness.gov

Women's Sport Foundation
800-227-3988
www.womenssportsfoundation.org

Suggested Readings

Coopersmith, G. 2006. *Fit & Feminine: The Perfect Fitness & Nutrition Game Plan for Your Unique Body Type.* Hoboken, NJ: John Wiley & Sons.

Cowlin, A. F. 2002. *Women's Fitness Program Development.* Champaign, IL: Human Kinetics Publishers.

Crawford, C., and P. Peeke. 2005. *Body for Life for Women: A Woman's Plan for Physical & Mental Transformation.* New York: Holtzbrinck Publishers.

Fahey, T. D., P. M. Insel, and W. T. Roth. 2007. *Fit & Well.* 7th ed., brief ed. New York: McGraw-Hill.

Goodman, W. C. 2002. *The Invisible Woman: Confronting Weight Prejudice in America.* Carlsbad, CA: Gurze Books.

Irwin, M. L., et al. 2003. Effect of exercise on total and intra-abdominal body fat in postmenopausal women. *Journal of the American Medical Association* 289 (3): 323–30.

Kettles, M., C. C. Cole, and B. S. Wright. 2006. *Women's Health & Fitness Guide.* Champaign, IL: Human Kinetics Publishers.

Nelson, M. 2005. *Strong Women, Strong Bones.* New York: Holtzbrinck Publishers.

Nordahl, K., C. Peterson, and R. M. Jeffreys. 2005. *Fit to Deliver: An Innovative Prenatal & Postpartum Fitness Program: Safe & Fun Exercises Tailored by Professionals to Benefit Both You and Your Baby.* Point Roberts, WA: Hartley & Marks Publishers.

Weeks, M. 2005. *The BalleCore Workout: Integrating Pilates, Hatha Yoga, & Ballet in an Innovative Exercise Routine for All Fitness Levels.* New York: Random House.

Wing, R. R., and J. O. Hill. 2001. Successful Weight Loss Maintenance. *Annual Reviews Nutrition* 21: 323–41.

References

1. Hu, F. B., et al. 2000. Physical activity and risk of stroke in women. *Journal of the American Medical Association* 283 (22): 2961–67.
2. Hu, F. B., et al. 1999. Walking compared with vigorous physical activity and risk of type 2 diabetes in women. *Journal of the American Medical Association* 282 (15): 1433–39.
3. Holmes, M. D., W. Y. Chen, D. Feskanich, C. H. Kroenke, and G. A. Colditz. 2005. Physical activity and survival after breast cancer diagnosis. *Journal of the American Medical Association* 293 (20): 2479–86.
4. The Scientific Program Committee. 2002. Physical activity across the cancer continuum: report of a workshop. *Cancer* 95: 100–17.
5. Dubbert, P. M. 2001. Physical activity and exercise: Recent advances and current challenges. *Journal of Counseling and Clinical Psychology* 70 (3): 526–36.
6. Hassmen, P., N. Koivula, and A. Uutela. 2000. Physical exercise and psychological well-being. *Preventative Medicine* 30 (1): 17–25.
7. American College of Sports Medicine. 2005. Mind–body exercise: Yoga and pilates. *Fit Society Page: Quarterly Report of the American College of Sports Medicine* (Spring): 3.
8. Schoenborn, C. A., and P. M. Barnes. 2002. Leisure-time physical activity among adults: United States, 1997–98. Department of Health and Human Services, CDC. Advanced data from *Vital and Health Statistics* 325 (April 7).
9. Fahey T. D., P. M. Insel, and W. T. Roth. 2007. *Fit & well.* 7th ed., brief ed. New York: McGraw-Hill, p. 30.
10. Sullivan, D. 1995. Stretching the truth. *Women's Sports and Fitness* 17:56–60.
11. Modified from: Prentice, W. E. 1997. *Fitness for college and life.* St. Louis: Mosby-Year Book; and Fahey, T. D., P. M. Insel, and W. T. Roth. 1997. *Fit & well: Core concepts and labs in physical fitness and wellness.* Mountain View, CA: Mayfield.
12. Luebbers, P. 2002. Enhancing your flexibility. *Fit Society Page: Quarterly Report of the American College of Sports Medicine,* Spring, p. 5.
13. Fahey et al., *Fit & well,* p. 86.
14. From *The Active Woman's Health and Fitness Handbook* by Nadya Swedan, Copyright © 2003 by Nadya Swedan. Used by permission of Perigree Books, an imprint of Penguin Group (USA) Inc.
15. Fahey et al., *Fit & well,* p. 86–87.
16. American College of Sports Medicine. 2005. Exercise right: Proper warm-up and cool down. *Fit Society Page: Quarterly Report of the American College of Sports Medicine* (Winter): 4.
17. Payne, W., D. Hahn, and E. Lucas. 2007. *Understanding your health.* 9th ed. New York: McGraw-Hill, p. 115.
18. Anspaugh, D. J., M. H. Hamrick, and F. D. Rosato. 2006. *Wellness: Concepts and applications.* 6th ed. New York: McGraw-Hill, p. 97.
19. Ibid., p. 137.
20. Anspaugh et al., *Wellness: Concepts and applications,* p. 133
21. Assessment activities: Physical activity labs—sit and reach test. 2003. *Health & human performance online assessments.* McGraw-Hill. www.mhhe.com/catalogs/sem/hhp/faculty/labs/index.mhtml (retrieved October 2, 2006).
22. Sharp, D. 1994. The quitter's exercise plan. *Health* 8 (3): 68–71, 75, 76.
23. *How to treat overuse injuries.* Melpomene Institute. www.melpomene.org/girlwise/Safety/Howtotreatoverusei njuries.htm (retrieved October 2, 2006).
24. Health club members log more time at the gym. 2002. *IHRSA Trend Report: International Health, Racquet & Sportsclub Association* 9 (4): 1, 4.
25. American College of Sports Medicine. 2005. Selecting and effectively using a health/fitness facility. *Fit Society Page: Quarterly Report of the American College of Sports Medicine* (Spring): 9.
26. KidsHealth. 2004. *Exercising during pregnancy.* kidshealth.org/parent/pregnancy_newborn/pregnancy/exercising_pregnancy.html (retrieved October 2, 2006).
27. Wang, T. W., and B. S. Apgar. 1998. Exercise during pregnancy. *American Family Physician* 57 (8): 1846–56.
28. Kegel exercises. 2001. *Medline encyclopedia,* www.nlm.nih.gov/medlineplus/ency/article/003975.htm (retrieved October 2, 2006).
29. Cumella, E. J. 2005. The heavy weight of exercise addiction. *Behavioral Health Management* 25 (5): 26–31.
30. Draeger, J. 2005. The obligatory exerciser. *Physician and Sportsmedicine* 33 (6): 13–23.
31. Overdoing it. 1996. *Harvard Women's Health Watch* 111 (12): 6.
32. The new American body. 1993. *University of California at Berkeley Wellness Letter* 10 (3): 1–2.

33. Donnelly, J., and B. Smith. 2005. Energy balance, compensation, and gender differences. Is exercise for weight loss with ad libitum diet? *Exercise and Sport Science Reviews* 33 (4): 169–74.
34. Wing, R. R., and J. O. Hill. 2001. Successful weight loss maintenance. *Annual Reviews Nutrition* 21:323–41.
35. Ferucchi, L., B. W. Henninx, S. C. Leveille, M. C. Corti, M. Pahor, R. Wallace, et al. 2000. Characteristics of nondisabled older persons who perform poorly in objective tests of lower extremity function. *Journal of the American Geriatric Society* 48 (9): 1102–10.
36. Salerno, J. A. 2003. Statement before the U.S. Senate, Special Committee on Aging. *Fitness and nutrition: The prescription for healthy aging.* www.nia.nih.gov/AboutNIA/BudgetRequests/FitnessNutrition.htm (retrieved October 2, 2006).
37. Ibid.
38. Ibid.
39. Schmitz, K. H., M. D. Jensen, K. C. Kugler, R. W. Jeffery, and A. S. Leon. 2003. Strength training for obesity prevention in midlife women. *International Journal of Obesity* 27:326–33.
40. Pratt, M., C. A. Macera, and G. Wang. 2000. Higher direct medical costs associated with physical inactivity. *Physician Sportsmedicine* 28 (10): 63–70.
41. Fahey et al., *Fit & Well*, p. 188.
42. How to make exercise fun. 1997. *Consumer Reports on Health* 9 (4): 37, 39–40.

Chapter Twelve

Using Alcohol Responsibly

CHAPTER OBJECTIVES

When you complete this chapter, you will be able to do the following:

- Explain the relationship between women, especially college women, and their use of alcohol
- Identify and describe the various types of alcohol
- Identify negative effects that the abuse of alcohol can produce upon the physical, behavioral, psychological, and societal aspects as well as upon relationships in the lives of women
- Describe the serious consequences between the use of alcohol during pregnancy and the negative effects on the fetus and infant
- Explain the process of addiction and alcoholism in women
- Identify the appropriate resources to assist alcoholic women and their families
- Suggest guidelines that can be used by colleges and universities to reduce alcohol abuse among college women

WOMEN AND ALCOHOL

Humans have been consuming alcohol, an intoxicating and toxic chemical, for thousands of years. Early writings about alcohol use are found in Hebrew script, Egyptian tablets, and Chinese laws in which the use of wine was either allowed or disallowed between 1100 B.C. and A.D. 1400.[1] Used for many purposes and reasons, alcohol is a drug of choice for present-day Americans, and in purely economic terms, alcohol-related problems cost society approximately $186 billion each year, but in human terms, the costs are incalculable.[2]

Societal attitudes regarding women's use of alcohol have been inconsistent and ambivalent. Roman laws did not allow women to drink alcoholic beverages because it was thought to make women aggressive and promiscuous; the Talmud denounced the overconsumption of alcohol by women, stating,

> One cup of wine is good for a woman;
> Two are degrading;
> Three induce her to act like an immoral woman;
> And four cause her to lose all self-respect and sense of shame.[3]

However, in ancient Babylon, women were temple priestesses who brewed beer. In Greco-Roman cults, women were a part of ceremonies in which alcohol was consumed. Through the centuries, alcoholic beverages were used medicinally and ceremoniously, but usually not in recreational circumstances, as they are presently used. In early America, women played a significant role in the control of alcohol use as participants of the temperance movement, which was an attempt to "temper" or curtail the use of hard liquor (distilled spirits).

The Women's Christian Temperance Union was formed in the late 1800s in Cleveland, Ohio, and Carrie Nation, Mary H. Hunt, and Frances Willard were actively involved with this movement. In fact, Carrie Nation, with fervent activities, was arrested more than thirty times. Rather than advocating temperance, these women promoted complete prohibition—no sale or consumption of alcohol. In 1920 prohibition became law with the ratification of the Eighteenth Amendment to the U.S. Constitution prohibiting the manufacture, sale, and transportation of "intoxicating liquors." However, this law was difficult to enforce as even former abstainers, in rebellion, began to drink; personal freedom was lost and alcohol use became a "smart thing" to do. Alcohol was manufactured and provided outside the law, and bootlegging became big business. By 1931 the Commission of Law Enforcement branded prohibition as a failure, and in 1933, after 13 years of attempting to enforce prohibition, the Twenty-First Amendment was passed, which repealed the Eighteenth Amendment. Today, alcohol is a legal substance with certain restrictions and is regulated by state governments.

Alcohol: The Beverage

Wine, beer, and distilled spirits contain **ethyl alcohol** or ethanol, a clear, somewhat tasteless, toxic liquid that initially causes a slight burning sensation when ingested and creates an intoxicating effect. It is produced through a process called **fermentation,** a chemical reaction between a mixture of yeast, sugar, and water. An average serving of wine (about 3½ oz), distilled spirits (1-oz shot), and beer (12-oz mug) each contain approximately one-half ounce of pure ethyl alcohol and therefore produce similar effects on blood alcohol levels.

The alcohol content of a beverage varies in the percentage of alcohol contained in it. Beer has about 4 percent alcohol content unless the beverage is labeled low-alcohol beer, which is then about 1.5 percent alcohol. Wine has about 12 percent alcohol content; however, fortified wine, such as port, contains 18 percent alcohol. Champagne is about 12 percent, and wine coolers are approximately 6 percent alcohol. The percentage of ethyl alcohol in distilled spirits (gin, rum, or scotch, for example) is stated in terms of **proof,** usually ranging from 80 to 190. In distilled spirits, proof is twice the percentage of alcohol by concentration (e.g., 100 proof would be 50 percent pure ethyl alcohol). The remaining ingredients in distilled spirits consist of *congeners,* which are by-products of distillation such as other types of alcohol, oils, and organic matter and other liquids that influence the taste and color of the beverage. (See *FYI:* "What Is a Hangover?")

FYI

What Is a Hangover?

Have you ever heard someone say, "I'll never drink again, I feel like I have the drum section of a marching band in my head." They probably were experiencing a hangover caused by overindulging in alcoholic beverages. Hangovers are believed to be the symptoms of withdrawal from alcohol and may include a headache, nausea, diarrhea, thirst, anxiety, depression, and general discomfort. Hangovers not only are caused by overconsumption of pure ethyl alcohol, but also are believed to be caused by congeners. Congeners, which are products of fermentation and the preparation process, provide the variety of taste, color, and smell in alcoholic beverages. What helps stop the distress associated with a hangover? A cold shower? another drink? coffee? Unfortunately, the "cure" is not quite that simple. Usually a painkiller for the headache and an antacid for the nausea will provide some relief. However, rest and time are the only "treatments" that will eventually eliminate the hangover. Perhaps you should decide if there is any "good time" for overconsumption of alcohol and whether it is worth the resulting misery of a hangover and the loss of a day in your life often needed to recover.

Alcohol, although providing calories in a person's diet, is not a good source of nutrition. A fluid ounce of distilled spirits will yield about 100 calories, and 12 ounces of beer about 150 calories. The nutrient density, however, is virtually nonexistent. These beverages contain no vitamins, minerals, fat, or protein, and only a small amount of carbohydrates. This is an example of what is meant by "empty calories," meaning calories consumed from a food source lacking important nutrients. If consumed in excess, alcohol can cause diseases by interfering with the nutritional status of the drinker.[4] As people have become more calorie-conscious, "light", or "lite" beer and wine have been introduced. The calorie content of these beverages has been reduced, but the alcohol content has *not* been reduced.

Alcohol is a simple chemical and does not need to be digested to move into the bloodstream. Following ingestion, 5 percent of alcohol leaves the body through sweat, urine, or breath unchanged by any chemical reaction. For the remaining 95 percent to be removed from the body, it must be metabolized, or chemically changed. To do this the body begins to break down ingested alcohol as soon as it reaches the liver through a process called **oxidation.**

FIGURE 12.1 BAC is the level of alcohol contained in a person's blood volume. For example, a woman with a BAC of 0.10 percent has one part of alcohol for every 1,000 parts of blood. A BAC of 0.08 and above is considered drunk in all states. However, a BAC as low as 0.05 percent can impair function enough to cause a serious accident.

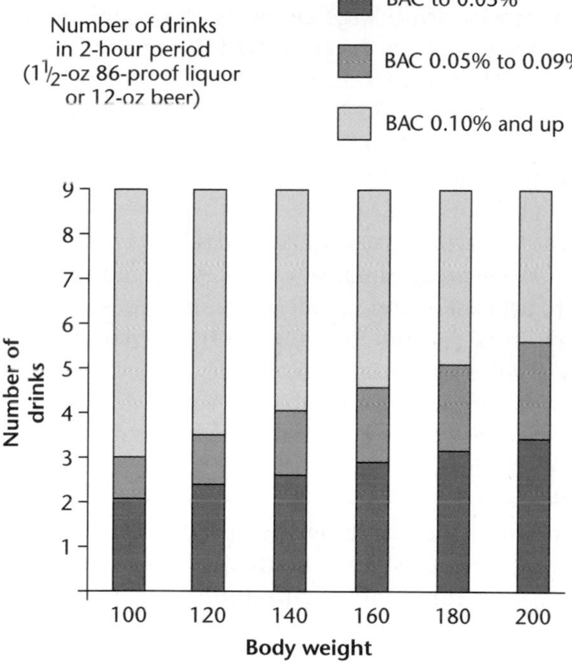

Absorption of alcohol takes place through the stomach, where about 20 percent is absorbed directly into the bloodstream, and from the small intestine where 80 percent is absorbed and moves into the bloodstream and to all parts of the body.[5] The absorption of alcohol in the body is determined by a number of factors. These include

- *Number of drinks consumed.* The greater the number of alcoholic beverages consumed by a female, the faster the alcohol will be absorbed into the bloodstream.
- *Strength of alcoholic beverage.* Beverages with higher concentrations of alcohol will increase the blood alcohol concentration (BAC). (See Figure 12.1.)
- *Rate of drinking.* Faster consumption of drinks will usually result in a higher blood alcohol level because more alcohol is absorbed into the system.
- *Mixture with other beverages.* Alcohol mixed with fruit juices or plain water will be absorbed at a slower rate; "straight" alcohol or alcohol mixed with carbonated beverages will be absorbed at a faster rate.
- *Foods in the stomach.* Foods with higher fat content will slow absorption of alcohol because there is less stomach area exposed and protein in the food retains the alcohol.

TABLE 12.1 Types of Alcohol

Ethyl (Ethanol)	Alcohol beverages Over-the-counter drugs
Methyl (Methanol)	Antifreeze, solvents
Isopropyl	Disinfectant in rubbing alcohol
Butyl	Industrial and medical applications found in anesthesia

- *Emotional factors.* Absorption of alcohol into the bloodstream can be affected by such factors as emotions (jealousy, anger, fear), illness, stress, and expectations of how it will make you feel (e.g., relaxed, high, sociable).
- *Blood chemistry.* Each of us is a biochemical individual; absorption may be quickened or slowed due to an individual's blood chemistry.
- *Body weight.* The more body weight a woman has, the lower will be the blood alcohol concentration.

Three additional types of alcohol are *methanol, isopropyl,* and *butyl,* each of which is toxic to human beings. (See Table 12.1.) Methyl alcohol, also called "wood alcohol," is an ingredient in such products as glass cleaners, turpentine, solvents, and antifreeze. Isopropyl, a clear, colorless, bitter liquid, is a disinfectant used in rubbing alcohol. Butyl alcohol, obtained from petroleum, is used in industrial and medication applications and may be found in anesthesia. *None* of these should be ingested because doing so could cause serious illness or death.

Why Liquor Is Quicker for Women

The absorption of alcohol in the body influences to an extent the physical and behavioral effects experienced by the person ingesting it. An enzyme, **alcohol dehydrogenase (ADH),** in the liver and in the stomach (gastric) lining helps to break down the alcohol before it enters the bloodstream. The ADH activity in the stomach is lower in women than in men. As a result, about 30 percent more alcohol enters the female bloodstream, thus causing more alcohol to reach the female brain at a faster rate, creating an intoxicating effect; therefore, higher blood alcohol concentration (BAC) is reached by women at a faster rate than for men. Over years of drinking, as frequency and consumption of alcohol increase the liver starts to fail, hence producing less ADH, causing the effectiveness of this enzyme to be impaired. Consequently, women who have been drinking heavily for many years will absorb almost all alcohol consumed without breaking it down, and the effect will be similar to alcohol being injected intravenously.

Drinking equivalent amounts of ethyl alcohol per pound of body weight will produce a higher peak of alcohol level for women than for men. This may be due to the higher percentage of body water in men (55–65 percent) than in women (45–55 percent), causing alcohol to be less diluted in women than in men. Ethyl alcohol is highly water- and fat-soluble. Because women have more body fat than men of the same weight and because alcohol is not diffused rapidly into body fat, females will have a higher amount of alcohol concentration in the blood than men. Considering each of these factors, a woman's ability to perform certain tasks (e.g., driving, speaking, decision making) will be impaired at a faster rate than a man's.

During the premenstrual stage of the menstrual cycle, alcohol is absorbed more quickly into the bloodstream. However, because of fluid retention during the premenstrual cycle, alcohol in the blood is more diluted and will have a reduced effect on the central nervous system, so a woman will not become intoxicated as quickly as at other stages of her cycle.

WOMEN AND ALCOHOL: A UNIQUE RELATIONSHIP

In the past, women have used alcohol medicinally to reduce menstrual cramps, to lessen pain associated with childbirth, and for fortification while breast-feeding.[6] It has been used in recreational settings to promote the "time away" environment and as a "social lubricant" to ease social interactions. Table 12.2 helps to explain the various classifications of alcohol consumers. This should provide you with what is meant by small, moderate, and heavy use of alcohol and foster a better perspective for alcohol use and its consequences.

Are there special concerns for use of this chemical by women? How much is too much? Alcohol, a depressant *psychoactive drug,* produces a number of unique qualities that are of special interest and concern for women. For example, a daily glass of wine with dinner can add as much as 10 pounds of body fat a year; it can increase the risk of developing breast cancer and osteoporosis. Women who drink large amounts of alcohol are more likely than men to develop cirrhosis of the liver and other alcohol-related diseases. The Centers for Disease Control analyzed alcohol-related health impacts and estimated the number of alcohol-attributable deaths and potential years of life lost: Annually, 10,395 females die from chronic conditions related to alcohol abuse and, on the average, 23 years of potential life per woman are lost.[8] Women who are heavy drinkers are more susceptible to depression and suicide attempts than women who don't drink or drink in moderation. Overconsumption of alcohol is less socially acceptable for women than for men. Society often considers women who drink too much more likely to engage in sexual activity. (Compare the differences between men's and women's drinking preferences during the college years in Table 12.3.)

Are women more vulnerable to alcohol's effects than men are? The physiological differences and effects from alcohol consumption discussed previously have some profound consequences for women. Consider the following:[9]

- *Liver damage.* Compared to men, women develop alcohol-induced liver disease over a shorter period of time and after consuming less alcohol and are more likely to die from cirrhosis.
- *Brain damage.* Brain images of the region involved in multiple brain functions are significantly smaller among alcoholic women compared to non-alcoholic women and alcoholic men.

TABLE 12.2 Drinking Classifications[7]

CLASSIFICATION	ALCOHOL-RELATED BEHAVIOR
Abstainers	Do not drink at all or drink less often than once a year.
Light drinkers	Per drinking occasion, may drink once a month in small to medium amounts or drink small amounts no more than three or four times a month.
Moderate drinkers	Per drinking occasion, drink small amounts at least once a week or drink medium amounts three or four times a month or large amounts no more than once a month.
Moderate/heavy drinkers	Per drinking occasion, drink medium amounts at least once a week or large amounts three or four times a month.
Heavy drinkers	Per drinking occasion, drink large amounts at least once a week.

NOTE: Small amounts = One drink or less per drinking occasion
Medium amounts = Two to four drinks per drinking occasion
Large amounts = Five or more drinks per drinking occasion
One drink = 12 fluid oz of beer, 4 fluid oz of wine, or 1 fluid oz of distilled spirits

- *Breast cancer.* Many studies have found that moderate to heavy alcohol consumption increases the risk for breast cancer.
- *Violent victimization.* Studies have shown a significant relationship between the amount of alcohol women reported drinking and their experiences of sexual victimization; female high school students who drank alcohol were more likely than nondrinking students to be victims of dating violence; problem drinking by wives has been linked to husband-to-wife aggression regardless of the husband's drinking levels.
- *Traffic crashes.* Women are less likely to drive after drinking and less likely to be in fatal alcohol-related crashes, but women have a higher relative risk of driver fatality than men at similar blood alcohol concentrations, and the proportion of female drivers involved in fatal crashes is increasing.

Alcohol Consumption

Approximately two-thirds of the adult population drink alcoholic beverages; however, according to the National Institute on Alcohol Abuse and Alcoholism, 81 percent of college students drink alcoholic beverages, which is down from 85 percent in the early 1990s.[10] People who choose to drink have varied drinking patterns and consumption levels. Only 20 percent of all alcohol beverages are consumed by approximately 70 percent of the drinking public. The remaining 80 percent of alcohol beverages are consumed by 30 percent of people who drink and they can be categorized as heavy drinkers or even alcoholics. This information was explained in an interesting and understandable way by Kinney:

> Ten beers shared among ten individuals who follow adult drinking patterns would likely be divided in this way:
>
> 3 persons abstain—representing the one-third who choose not to drink
>
> 5 persons share 2 beers—70 percent of drinkers drink 20 percent of the alcohol
>
> 2 persons share 8 beers—30 percent of drinkers drink 80 percent of the alcohol. Of these 2 drinkers, one drinks 2 beers and the other drinks 6 beers.[11]

See Table 12.4 for the drinking practices of Americans. Drinking patterns of American women reveal that the majority of women abstain from alcohol or are light drinkers. Drinkers may move from one type of drinking pattern to another during their lifetime. (To check your own drinking pattern, complete *Journal Activity:* "Alcohol Consumption Record.")

TABLE 12.3 What's the Difference in Drinking Preferences?[12]

ALCOHOL USE	WOMEN	MEN
Frequency	Less often	More often
Consumption amounts	Smaller amounts	Greater amounts
Beverage preference	Spirits, beer, and wine	Beer, spirits, and wine
Drinking locations	Restaurants, clubs	At games, dorms, and concerts
Drinking companions	Mixed groups	Male groups
Intoxication levels	Usually not to get drunk	Drink to get drunk
Effects of alcohol problems	Academics and relationships	Creates more problems (accidents, difficulties with family and school)

TABLE 12.4 Drinking Patterns of American Women (Percent)[13]

AGE	ABSTAINER	LIGHT DRINKER	MODERATE DRINKER	HEAVIER DRINKER
18–24	47.5	40.2	7.5	4.8
25–34	38.9	50.9	7.0	3.2
35–44	38.2	50.2	7.2	4.4
45–54	40.1	48.0	7.6	4.3
55–64	46.1	42.5	8.2	3.2
65+	63.1	28.4	6.4	2.1

Journal Activity

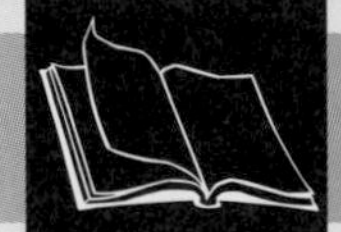

Alcohol Consumption Record

If you make the choice to drink, it is a wise idea to monitor your consumption. Below is a chart you can use to determine when, where, with whom, and how much you are drinking. If you find that you are experiencing problems as a result of alcohol consumption, it is important to seek professional help. The information recorded on this chart can help you determine if you do or do not have a drinking problem.

Date	Time	Where	With Whom	Number of Drinks

College-Age Women and Alcohol

Today, more than in the past, college females are more often engaging in violations of university policies and are experiencing greater negative health, academic, and social consequences. Why? Alcohol is a factor. A survey conducted by the Harvard School of Public Health revealed that in 2001, 81.3 percent of college women reported drinking within the previous year, with 18.7 percent abstaining from drinking alcohol.[14] Of concern is the increased practice of **binge drinking** among all college students, typically defined as consuming five or more drinks within 2 or 3 hours for men and four or more drinks within 2 or 3 hours for women. The same survey found that 40.9 percent of female college students engaged in binge drinking episodes in 2001.[15] However, colleges vary widely in binge drinking rates, from 1 percent on some campuses to more than 70 percent on others. The U.S. Surgeon General and the U.S. Department of Health and Human Services identified binge drinking among college students as a major public health problem, stating that "the perception that alcohol use is socially acceptable correlates with the fact that more than 80 percent of American youth consume alcohol before their 21st birthday, whereas the lack of social acceptance of other drugs correlates with comparatively lower rates of use.[16] According to *Women's Health, USA 2005,* alcohol misuse begins in adolescence and then rises significantly and peaks in the 18–25 age group. Among these young women, 31.8 percent reported binge drinking and 9.0 percent reported heavy drinking in the past month.[17] (See Figure 12.2.)

With the knowledge that abuse of alcohol certainly has serious consequences for some, women still feel the need to overconsume a chemical that can be a destructive force in their lives. (See *Her Story:* "Jessica: Driving under the Influence." Then read *Women Making a Difference:* "Candace Lightner and Cindi Lamb: Founders of Mothers Against Drunk Driving.")

If you choose to drink, for what reasons do you drink? How do your reasons compare with those of other college women, listed below?

- To relieve stress and anxiety
- To feel more sociable
- To decrease inhibitions
- For the "high" that results
- To be part of the group
- To lessen sexual inhibitions
- To escape
- To relieve worrying
- To become less self-conscious
- To reduce depression

Colleges and universities are taking a closer look at the serious consequences that result from overconsumption of alcohol on campuses. *FYI:* "Reducing Alcohol

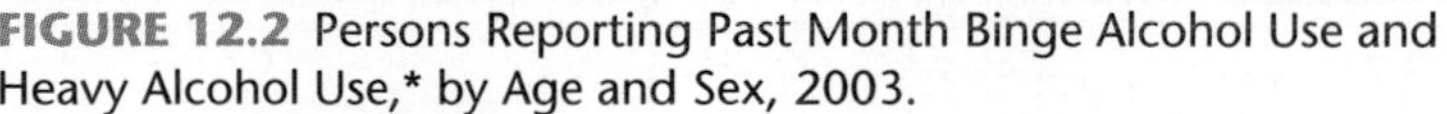

FIGURE 12.2 Persons Reporting Past Month Binge Alcohol Use and Heavy Alcohol Use,* by Age and Sex, 2003.

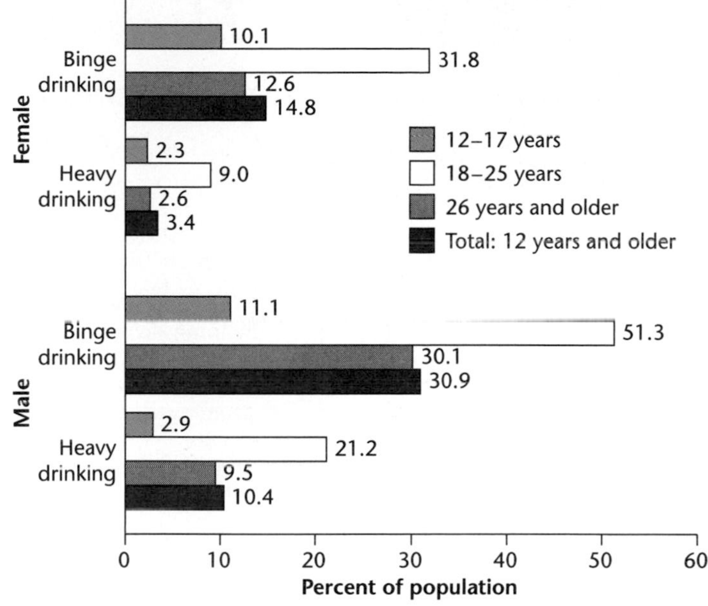

* "Binge" alcohol use was defined as drinking five or more drinks on the same occasion on at least 1 day in the past 30 days. "Occasion" means at the same time or within a few hours of each other. "Heavy" alcohol use is defined as drinking five or more drinks on the same occasion on each of 5 or more days in the past 30 days; all "heavy" alcohol users are also "binge" alcohol users.

SOURCE: Substance Abuse and Mental Health Services Administration, National Survey on Drug Use and Health.

Her Story

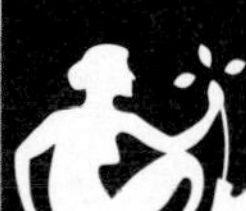

Jessica: Driving under the Influence

Jessica arrived for her freshman year in college and settled into her high-rise dorm room. She was invited by her roommates to go to the "Rooster House," a local bar frequented by college students. As a nondrinker, Jessica felt uneasy about this invitation, yet she also wanted to meet other students and become a part of the social scene. After deciding to join her new friends one evening, Jessica drove her own car to the bar so that she could leave when she chose. Having no former drinking experience, she began to feel the results of too many "drink specials" and decided it was time to go home. She drove back to the dorm under the influence, and was stopped and given a Breathalyzer test. Having a BAC of 0.13, she was arrested and convicted of DUI. This became a part of her driving record for many years and resulted in an increase in her car insurance rates.

- How could Jessica have met people in her new college environment other than going to a bar?
- Why did Jessica feel the effects of alcohol so quickly?
- What is the legal limit of alcohol consumption in your state?

Abuse on Campus" lists a number of measures that are being adopted on numerous campuses to curb the use of alcohol and the resulting consequences.

Health Tips: "Drinking Alcohol Responsibly" provides suggestions you can use as guidelines for drinking alcohol responsibly.

Associated Effects

Have you ever experienced negative consequences as the result of alcohol abuse? Overconsumption of alcohol can produce immediate and long-term negative physical, behavioral, psychological, social, and relational consequences. Although many of these negative outcomes are the result of chronic alcohol abuse, undesirable consequences can also result from occasional overconsumption of alcohol.

Hormonal Effects Physical effects resulting from alcohol consumption, especially long-term abuse of alcohol, can be serious and in some instances life-threatening. Serious consequences, for example, include the impairment of proper functioning of essential hormones, briefly defined as chemical messengers that control and coordinate the operation of all tissues and organs. Hormone impairment results in a number of significant and severe medical consequences. One significant hormonal consequence of alcohol abuse causes low blood sugar levels, called hypoglycemia, and prevents an

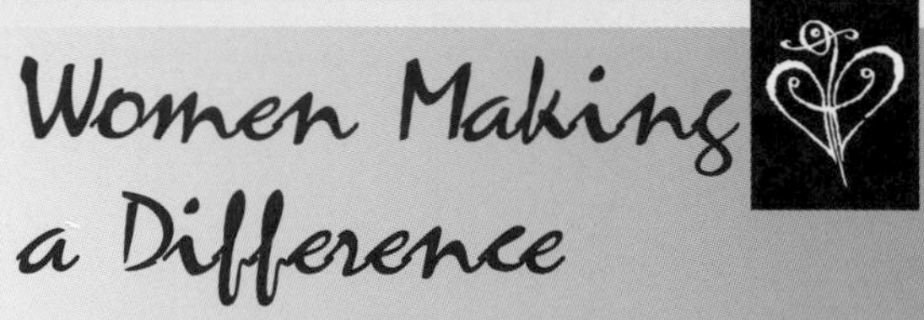

Candace Lightner and Cindi Lamb: Founders of Mothers Against Drunk Driving (MADD)

The death of Candy Lightner's 13-year-old daughter, Cari, in 1980, and the crippling of Cindi Lamb's 5½-month-old daughter, Laura, in 1979, both as a result of repeat drunk drivers, spurred these women to form the organization Mothers Against Drunk Drivers (MADD). This organization eventually was renamed Mothers Against Drunk Driving. From the time it was formed in 1981, MADD received donations from victims and concerned citizens, as well as grant funding, enabling it to expand to eleven chapters in four states. As a result of increased media attention, MADD began to develop in more states and to increase in the number of chapters across the United States. By its tenth anniversary in 1991, MADD had grown to 407 chapters, 53 community action teams, and 32 state offices with affiliates in Canada, England, New Zealand, and Australia. MADD's mission statement is "To stop drunk driving, support victims of this violent crime and prevent underage drinking."

Since MADD's inception, alcohol-related traffic fatalities have declined 43 percent. Due in large part to MADD's efforts, more than an estimated 138,000 people are alive today and an untold number have received comfort, support, and assistance in dealing with the consequences of drunk driving. Candace Lightner and Cindi Lamb and other dedicated and action-oriented mothers across the United States are truly women who make a difference.

effective hormonal response to this condition. When blood sugar levels are too low to provide enough energy for the body's activities, symptoms such as hunger, shakiness, confusion, and/or weakness may occur.

Chronic heavy alcohol consumption can hamper a female's reproductive hormone functioning leading to a number of serious health issues. For example, breast development, distribution of body hair, regulation of the menstrual cycle, and disruption of a pregnancy can be the results of impaired hormone functioning caused by alcohol abuse. Long-term consequences include serious hormonal deficiencies, sexual dysfunction, and infertility. A study of healthy nonalcoholic women found that even in females who were just "social drinkers," small amounts of alcohol stopped normal menstrual cycling and they became temporarily infertile.[18]

Chronic heavy drinking in college-age women can lead to menstruation cessation, menstrual cycle irregularities, failure to ovulate, and infertility. During pregnancy, alcohol use can increase the likelihood of spontaneous abortion (miscarriage). Studies indicate a relationship between

FYI

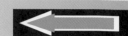

Reducing Alcohol Abuse on Campus

Colleges and universities across the nation are working to reduce alcohol abuse on campus. Here are some of the ways they are trying to achieve this:

- Banning alcohol from campus pubs.
- Banning alcohol from college-sponsored activities (among sororities, in residence halls, and at sporting events)
- Avoiding social and commercial promotion of alcohol
- Consistently enforcing alcohol-related laws and policies
- Conducting student orientation about alcohol abuse
- Conducting seminars for women concerning alcohol and other drugs
- Training female resident hall advisors in alcohol abuse awareness
- Training university counselors about women who have alcohol-related problems

Health Tips

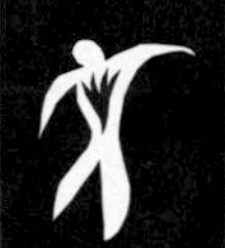

Drinking Alcohol Responsibly

- Drink no more than one drink per hour.
- Allow time to elapse between drinks.
- Intersperse alcoholic beverages with nonalcoholic drinks.
- Sip drinks; do not gulp them.
- Eat before drinking alcohol.
- Know your limits.
- Be comfortable choosing not to drink.
- Never encourage another woman to drink.
- Know when to say "no" when someone offers you a drink, and say it!

female alcoholism and sexual dysfunction, especially **anorgasmia.** The majority of female reproductive irregularities were found in studies of alcoholic women; however, a number of problems were also found in women who drank approximately three drinks per day.

Women, in general, are at increased risk for developing calcium-deficiency disorders, especially osteoporosis. However, alcohol consumption exacerbates this problem by causing hormone imbalances that reduce calcium absorption, excretion, and distribution. As a result, calcium metabolism is impaired and bone density is reduced. Additionally, an immediate effect of drinking alcohol is the prevention of proper utilization of calcium and a resultant increase in urinary calcium excretion. Because chronic drinking can disturb vitamin D metabolism, there is an increased risk of osteoporosis due to inadequate absorption of dietary calcium.

Studies have revealed a distinct link between alcohol intake and breast cancer. One recent study indicated that daily consumption of 1 ounce of pure ethyl alcohol (about two drinks) produced higher levels of estrogen in the body than when no alcohol was consumed. Increased production of estrogen has been linked to developing breast cancer. Dorgan[19] studied 51 postmenopausal women who were not taking hormone replacement therapy and followed them over three 8-week periods while they consumed 15 or 30 grams (½ to 1 ounce) of alcohol per day. The study found that even one drink per day increased the risk of developing breast cancer. Another study found that breast cancer was elevated by 9 percent for each 10-gram-per-day increase in alcohol intake.[20] To help explain this, if the risk for a female developing breast cancer is 1 in 10, the risk for a female drinker would be 1.5 in 10. In other words, 10 out of 100 nondrinkers might get breast cancer, whereas 15 out of 100 drinkers may develop breast cancer.

On a more positive note, postmenopausal women who ingested alcohol in moderation (three to six drinks per week) raised their estrogen levels and reduced the risk of developing cardiovascular diseases. This was accomplished without significantly reducing bone quality or increasing the risk of liver disease or breast cancer.

The effects of alcohol on hormone levels in women are important to know. For example, what effects do hormone levels and alcohol have on the progression of diseases such as osteoporosis and heart disease and the development of alcohol-induced liver disease in postmenopausal women who are heavier drinkers?[21,22] Additional concerns related to alcohol and medications containing hormones include the possibility of impairment of reproductive functioning, suppression of the immune system, the development of cancer,[23] adverse effects on the menstrual cycle, and potential for early menopause.[24]

FYI

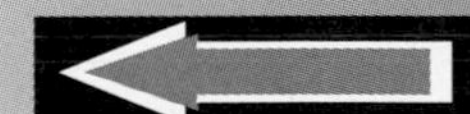

Are There Any Benefits to Drinking Alcohol?

Although the use and abuse of alcohol result in many negative consequences, studies have also determined that there are also a number of benefits from the *moderate* use of alcohol. Remember, moderate use of alcohol for women is one drink per day. (See Table 12.2.) These benefits include

- Decreased risk of heart attack.
- Increases in high-density lipoprotein (HDL), the "good cholesterol."
- Decreased risk of coronary artery disease.
- Decreased anxiety.
- Relaxation.
- Increased ease during social situations.
- Increased life expectancy.

Although these benefits have been reported in professional literature, it must also be noted that there are additional methods by which you can gain these benefits without using a potentially addicting and toxic drug. This is one of the many lifestyle decisions we must make by considering all potential alternatives and consequences.

Medications containing estrogen, such as birth control pills and hormone replacement drugs, affect a woman's reaction to alcohol. Approximately one in four postmenopausal women is on hormone replacement therapy.[25] Drinking alcohol in moderate amounts increases the estrogen levels in postmenopausal women. Light to moderate alcohol consumption may increase blood concentration of estrogen and the by-products of estrogen metabolism, and the results can increase the risk of serious diseases for women.[26] (See *FYI:* "Are There Any Benefits to Drinking Alcohol?")

What should you do? Consultation with a physician should help you weigh the benefits versus the risks of taking medications with estrogen. Consider your family medical history related to cancer, heart disease, and osteoporosis, and your lifestyle as it relates to alcohol consumption, exercise, diet, and other health promotion or health risk behaviors. (See Table 12.5.)

Dieting One interesting study revealed that college females who were dieting were more likely to drink alcohol than females who were not dieting.[27] In fact, there was a strong relationship between the impulsiveness of dieting and the serious consumption of alcohol. The study revealed that females who were not dieting

TABLE 12.5 The Physical Consequences of Alcohol Abuse[28]

Reproductive system	Early menopause, amenorrhea, infertility, miscarriage, fetal alcohol syndrome.
Sexuality	Reduced physiological arousal, decreased orgasmic intensity, sexual dysfunction.
Endocrine system	Increased possibility of osteoporosis, nutritional and metabolic disorders, poor absorption and utilization of essential nutrients.
Cardiovascular system	Hypertension, cardiomyopathy, dysrhythmias, coronary artery disease; slows manufacture of red blood cells; degenerates blood clotting ability.
Liver	Chemical imbalance: accumulation of fat in the liver, blood sugar imbalance, and altered protein production. Inflammation: impaired circulation, scar tissue formation, and alcohol-related hepatitis. Cirrhosis: poor circulation, kidney failure, and possibly death.
Digestive system	Oral: promotes possibility of cancer of the mouth, tongue, and throat. Esophagus: impaired swallowing. Stomach: irritation, gastritis, and ulceration. Pancreas: inflammation. Digestion: impaired absorption and possible malnutrition. Nausea: diarrhea and vomiting.

consumed less alcohol than females who were dieting. Additionally, dieting females who also drank alcohol experienced more harmful consequences, such as blackouts, unintended sex, and sexually transmitted diseases, than nondrinking dieters. Another interesting aspect of this study was that females who stopped dieting did not decrease their intake of alcohol.

Disease When compared to men, women with alcohol-related problems are disabled more frequently and for longer periods of time. Alcohol-related liver damage in women develops after shorter periods of alcohol use and lower levels of consumption than it does in men. Studies have shown that alcohol-related diseases in women were comparable to those in men, even when the women had been drinking to excess for a significantly shorter period of time than had the men (14.2 years for women versus 20.2 years for men). Such diseases and disorders as pancreatitis, hepatitis, cardiomyopathy (degeneration of the heart muscle), and myopathy (a degenerative disease of the skeletal muscles) developed in a briefer period of time for alcohol-abusing women than alcohol-abusing men.[29]

Ethnicity The drinking pattern of women can be influenced by cultural norms and practices of the ethnic groups to which they belong. A study by the Alcohol Policies Project revealed that 78 percent of women aged 12 and older reported ever using alcohol; 60 percent reported using in the past year, and 45 percent reported using in the month prior to the survey.[30] The ethnic breakdown of this information is as follows:

- 83 percent of white women reported ever using alcohol, and 49.7 percent reported using during the past month.
- 67.9 percent of African American women reported ever using alcohol, and 32.3 percent reported using in the past month.
- 60.8 percent of Hispanic women reported ever using alcohol, and 33.6 percent reported using in the last month.

The National Institute on Alcohol Abuse and Alcoholism has reported the drinking levels of females according to selected characteristics. These data reveal the following among female ethnic groups: 62.6 percent of Hispanic women are light drinkers and 1.3 percent report heavy drinking; 39.1 percent of non-Hispanic white women report being light drinkers, with 4.4 percent reporting heavy drinking; among non-Hispanic black women, 59.2 percent are light drinkers, with 2.3 percent reporting heavy use of alcohol.[31] For both men and women, genetic heritage, occupational and social roles, and social class contribute to their drinking patterns. Women's greater propensity to have negative affective states, such as depression, and to experience negative life events, including childhood or adulthood victimization, increases women's risk for developing alcohol problems.

Collins and McNair examined the drinking behavior of women from the four largest non-European ethnic groups in the United States.[32] Specific variables included religious activity among African American women, facial flushing response in Asian American women, the level of acculturation to U.S. society among Latinas, and historical, social, and policy variables unique to American Indian women. The level of religious participation of African American women tended to serve a protective function and shielded them from higher rates of alcohol use. Drinking patterns among Asian women in the United States were influenced by their ethnic communities and by a biological factor, manifested as facial flushing, which affects their ability to metabolize alcohol. A gene, inactive aldehyde dehydrogenase 2 (ALDH2-2), leads to slower than normal oxidation of acetaldehyde, resulting in higher levels of this chemical in the blood and producing numerous physical reactions: perspiration, headache, nausea, rapid heartbeat, and facial flushing. It is believed that the flushing response serves as a deterrent to drinking and results in lower rates of drinking and alcohol dependence in Asian women. In the Latina population, Mexican women who had immigrated to the United States reported higher levels of nondrinking than the general population of U.S. women. However, within three generations, Latinas adopt the drinking patterns of the general population of U.S. women. Therefore, acculturation is believed to cause increases in drinking patterns of Latinas because of changes in income, education, and professional occupation. American Indian women who lived on reservations where social norms did not promote drinking or tribal policies forbid it reported less drinking than American Indian women who lived in tribal communities where there were relatively high rates of drinking by American Indian men and the tribal policy did not prohibit drinking.

It appears that women's drinking patterns among the four largest non-European ethnic groups in the United States display some similarity due to biological characteristics, social roles, and lower social status relative to men. Drinking patterns, however, differ within and among the ethnic groups due to differences in ethnic norms.

Behavioral Effects Although long-term chronic alcohol abuse can cause a variety of negative physical consequences, a number of severe behavioral consequences can result from short-term or binge drinking. Alcohol-related behavior pertains not only to what women themselves do, but also to what women may allow others to do to them. Because alcohol reduces a woman's inhibitions, or concerns about "what may happen if," she is more likely to act upon the immediate circumstances rather than considering the consequences of her actions. Examples include making a decision to leave a party or club or have sexual relations with some person she just met, driving after drinking, or being verbally abusive to friends or family. The more heavily a woman drinks, the greater the potential for problems at home, at work, with friends, and even with strangers.[33] Each of these situations can lead to negative societal and relationship-related consequences. In each instance, a woman would probably make a different decision if she were not disinhibited by alcohol consumption.

A number of research studies have investigated the long-term behavioral effects of alcohol abuse in regard to women. One study determined that women who abuse alcohol often develop impaired ability to function in the social world, asocial behavior, and antisocial behavior.[34] Indicators of impaired functioning in the social world include such effects as financial irresponsibility, unusual accidents such as falling down stairs, impulsiveness, dysfunctional relationships, and poor parenting skills. Asocial behavior indicators include poor communication skills, irresponsibility regarding appointments or commitments, relinquishing former hobbies or activities, and even discarding friendships. Shoplifting and stealing from family or friends were cited as indicators of antisocial behavior of female alcohol abusers.

Psychological effects related to alcohol abuse can be serious. Women may experience anxiety, guilt, and stress; lose their inhibitions; display aggressiveness and other strong emotions; or have strong dependency needs. Women may become suspicious of others, grow defensive, or even demonstrate obsessive-compulsive behaviors such as being a "super student" or compulsively perfectionistic. Compared to male drinkers, female drinkers who chronically abuse alcohol are more likely to experience bouts of depression.

Social Effects Social consequences related to alcohol use and abuse are many. Alcohol often fosters relaxing effects that enable women to feel more confident, relaxed, and less inhibited in social situations. Although this may be perceived as a positive result of alcohol consumption, certainly being able to experience these qualities in social settings without the use of an intoxicating beverage would be an important skill to possess. In some instances, abuse of alcohol may become detrimental to our social well-being and to society at large. Negative situations can range from arguments to violent acts, from loss of a job to career destruction, from delinquent bills to financial ruin, from minor accidents in the home to deadly vehicular collisions, or from lousy dates to dysfunctional relationships. Alcohol can be seriously detrimental to our personal, familial, and professional quality of life.

Economic Effects Economic issues related to alcohol consumption reveal the financial burden and costs to society. Alcohol consumption costs you $683 each year, and that's only if you did *not* buy any alcohol. The cost related to alcohol abuse and dependence in the United States was estimated at $185 billion for 1998.[35] Fueling these costs were incidents related to crime, violence, vehicle crashes, and suicide, as well as employment issues such as lost work time, lower productivity, and higher health care costs. More than 70 percent of alcohol abuse costs ($134.2 billion) are attributed to lost productivity.

FYI 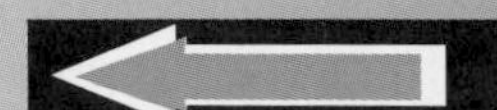

Alcohol-Related Consequences for College Students[36]

- 1,700 college students aged 18 to 24 die each year from alcohol-related unintentional injuries, including motor vehicle crashes.
- 599,000 college students aged 18 to 24 are unintentionally injured under the influence of alcohol.
- More than 696,000 college students are assaulted each year by another student who has been drinking.
- About 25 percent of college students report academic consequences of their drinking including missing classes, falling behind, failing exams and papers, and getting lower grades.
- About 11 percent of college students who drink report that they have damaged property while under the influence of alcohol.

Health Tips 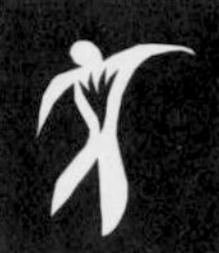

Alcohol and Dating: Safety Skills[40]

Drinking alcohol lessens your ability to be safe in many situations, including your intimate relationships with men. Remember the following tips to improve your safety when drinking alcohol while on a date. Remember the acronym RAPE!

R ealize what situations can place you in danger of being a victim of a rape.
A void and manage conflicts with partners and intimates, and ask female friends for help.
P erceive clearly what others are doing, or saying, or where they are going.
E stablish and communicate your desires and limits about sex.

Alcohol and crime seem to have a kinship to one another because criminals often have problems with alcohol abuse. Studies have determined that in the majority of crimes, such as assault, robbery, homicide, or rape, alcohol is a factor. Prisoners frequently are alcoholics or have other drug problems. About 40 percent of all crimes (violent and nonviolent) are committed under the influence of alcohol. Approximately 72 percent of rapes reported on college campuses occur when victims are so intoxicated they are unable to consent or refuse.[37] The four leading causes of accidental deaths in this country are (1) transportation accidents, (2) falls, (3) drowning, and (4) fires and burns, and alcohol is known to be a significant contributing factor to each. (*FYI:* "Alcohol-Related Consequences" lists percentages of alcohol-related accidents.)

Women who commit suicide often have abused alcohol prior to the act. According to one study, 40 percent of alcoholic women attempted suicide, compared to 8.8 percent of nonalcoholic women.[38] Another study revealed that 23 percent of suicide deaths are attributable to alcohol.[39] Suicides tend to be more impulsive and more violent when alcohol is involved.

Effects on Relationships Relationship failure can be related to the abuse of alcohol in the partnership or family. Conflicts often arise from the consequences associated with the time, money, and energy spent on alcohol consumption. Because alcohol affects a person's ability to think rationally and respond appropriately, spouses, children, other family members, or friends can be neglected, abused, or abandoned. Nurturing, intimate relationships of all types often degenerate as a result of excessive alcohol consumption. Social occasions with friends, holidays or vacations with families, and special times such as birthdays or anniversaries can be sabotaged because of alcohol abuse.

Most people will admit that their thinking ability becomes distorted when they are drinking alcohol. Drinking by both men and women greatly increases the chance that sexual relations will occur. When this sexual encounter is forced on a woman by her date or an acquaintance while under the influence of alcohol, it is called date or acquaintance rape. Approximately 72 percent of campus rapes are alcohol-related and usually result in long-lasting negative consequences.[41] A number of factors contribute to the increased likelihood of experiencing acquaintance/date rape while drinking alcohol: the decision-making abilities of both men and women are impaired; a man may be more aggressive, more insistent if under the influence; a woman may be fearful of angering her date by saying no or unable to refuse due to loss of consciousness. *Health Tips:* "Alcohol and Dating: Safety Skills" can aid you in avoiding situations involving alcohol and potentially dangerous relationship behaviors. (See *FYI:* "What's That in My Drink?")

For a more detailed discussion of alcohol and acquaintance rape, see Chapter 6.

FYI

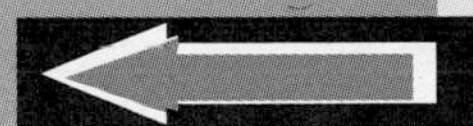

What's That in My Drink?[42]

The Drug Induced Rape Prevention and Punishment Act of 1996 states that it is a crime to give a controlled substance to anyone without his or her knowledge with the intent to commit a violent crime (such as rape). The punishment is severe, up to 20 years in prison and a fine of $250,000. Date rape drugs are sometimes used in sexual assault of women or in other types of sexual activity not agreed to by a woman. When ingested, these drugs produce helplessness, inability to refuse sex, and lack of memory of the event.

- *Rohypnol* (roofies) is NOT legal in the United States. It is legal in other countries and is even prescribed for sleep problems in Europe and Mexico. It is sold illegally in the U.S. Initially, Rohypnol causes mild relaxation, slows psychomotor responses, and lowers inhibitions. Blackout periods may last from 8 to 12 hours during which time the victim may or may not appear "awake." Usually the potential rapist puts the small pill into the victim's drink. New Rohypnol pills turn blue when added to liquids; they are odorless, tasteless, and easily dissolve in alcoholic or nonalcoholic beverages.
- *Gamma hydroxy butyrate acid* (GHB) is a fast-acting central nervous system depressant, similar to Rohypnol. GHB is an odorless, colorless substance that is most often in liquid form, but it is also available in powder capsules. As with Rohypnol, the potential rapist puts the GHB into the victim's drink. Effects of GHB include an initial feeling of euphoria and calmness followed by drowsiness, respiratory distress, dizziness, seizures, and amnesia. It can also intensify the effects of alcohol and may increase sexual feelings. Unlike Rohypnol, GHB is legal in the United States.
- *Ketamine* (known as "Special K"), used as an anesthetic in veterinary practices, is a legal drug that blocks nerve paths and depresses the respiratory and circulatory functions. Ketamine is a popular substance in rave clubs and can create a hallucinogenic effect as well as increase sexual desires. Amnesic dreamlike memories make it difficult to remember if a sexual assault occurred. Ketamine is usually available in liquid form, easily slipped in someone's drink, and can cause the heart to stop.

To prevent becoming a victim of one of these drugs:

- Never leave a drink unattended or accept a drink from a stranger.
- Watch the behavior of your friends; anyone acting too drunk in relation to the amount of alcohol consumed may be in danger.

If you think you may have ingested any of these drugs, ask someone to take you to the emergency room or call 911. Try to keep a sample of the beverage for analysis.

Alcohol and Pregnancy

Would you, as a mother, get your baby drunk after she was born? Would you deliberately attempt to sabotage your baby's opportunity to have a healthy productive life? Of course not! However, women who use alcohol, as well as other drugs, during pregnancy place their unborn child, and themselves, at risk for a reduced quality of life and reduced life expectancy. Pregnant women who consume alcohol are at greater risk for miscarriages. As a result of alcohol use during pregnancy, women may impair their personal health and increase the risk of the infant developing multiple problems related to **fetal alcohol syndrome (FAS).**

Scientists suspected a correlation between alcohol use and pregnancy complications as early as 1899, but it was not until 1973 that FAS was officially described in medical literature. FAS is a completely preventable cluster of birth defects including irreversible mental and physical disabilities that may develop as a result of expectant mothers consuming excessive amounts of alcohol. Characteristics of FAS include, but are not limited to, the following:

- Prenatal and postnatal growth deficiency. Additionally, most of these children do not attain normal size throughout their lives.
- Central nervous system dysfunction. Many children with FAS are jittery and poorly coordinated and have short attention spans and behavioral problems.
- A pattern of deformed facial characteristics such as flat face (the zone between the eyes and mouth), narrow eyes, short nose, thin upper lip, no upper lip crease, or underdeveloped jaws.
- Major organ system malformations such as heart defects.

FAS is considered the leading cause of developmental disabilities and birth defects in the United States, and each FAS child has one thing in common: a mother who

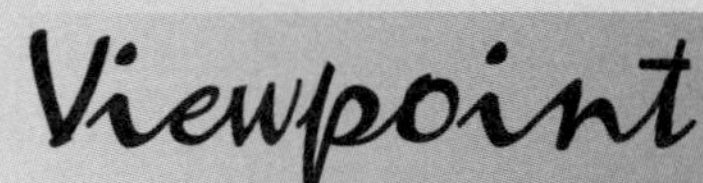
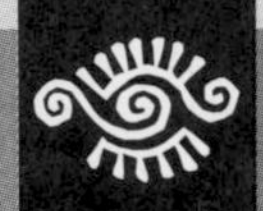

What Should Be Done about Pregnant Women Who Drink?

With all the information now available concerning fetal alcohol syndrome, what should be the legal consequences for women who consume alcohol during pregnancy and, as a result, have children with FAS? Does a woman have the right to choose unhealthy behaviors while pregnant with another human being? Should she be allowed to have more children and risk causing severe birth defects? Does the "right" to harm the fetus by drinking alcohol during pregnancy have any moral and legal ramifications?

consumed too much alcohol while pregnant. The 2002 Behavioral Risk Factor Surveillance System Survey, a study conducted by the CDC, indicated that approximately 10 percent of pregnant women used alcohol and approximately 2 percent engaged in binge drinking or frequent alcohol use.[43]

What does research reveal about the relationship between pregnancy and alcohol use? Alcohol crosses the placental barrier and decreases the amount of glucose and oxygen that get to the fetal brain. The fetus may be more severely affected than the expectant mother because the fetus is unable to break down the alcohol as fast and efficiently as the mother. The fetus is most vulnerable during the first trimester of pregnancy. How much alcohol consumption do physicians and researchers recommend for pregnant females? *NONE!* Correct: not any! Research hasn't established a "safe" level of alcohol use during pregnancy; therefore, there is no way to know if the fetus will be affected by any alcohol consumption during pregnancy. Even women who drink "moderately" may have children with **fetal alcohol effects (FAE),** a variety of less severe birth defects including below-average IQ, learning disabilities, hyperactivity, short attention span, and often physical malformations that are similar to FAS. Unfortunately, too many women do not appear to get the message. that drinking alcohol during pre gnancy is dangerous. (See *Viewpoint:* "What Should Be Done?")

Aren't you glad your mother took care of herself while she was pregnant with you? Do the same for your own children and return this morally and ethically correct courtesy should you ever become pregnant.

Research concerning paternal abuse of alcohol and resulting birth defects continues to be done. It is known that chronic alcohol abuse produces sexual dysfunction and impairs sperm production in both humans and animals. It appears that alcohol has a damaging effect on reproduction in males at all three levels of the male reproductive unit: the hypothalamus, pituitary, and testes.[44] Additionally, alcohol-related research using male rats indicates that paternal exposure to alcohol prior to mating has an adverse effect on normal development and behavior of their offspring. A possible explanation is that alcohol is toxic to the gonads and can have an adverse effect on synthesis and secretion of testosterone. Alcohol can cause significant deterioration in sperm concentration, output, and motility.[45] Although research is inconclusive to some degree, it does indicate that paternal alcohol use must be researched to create a complete picture of alcohol abuse and fetal consequences.

ADDICTION AND DEPENDENCY

Addiction to alcohol, or any other drug, is a compulsive, uncontrollable dependence on a substance, habit, or practice to such a degree that cessation causes severe emotional, mental, or physiological reactions.[46] Components of addiction include tolerance, physical dependence, and psychological dependence.

Dependency: What Is It?

Pharmacologically, alcohol is a depressant drug. With long-term continual use, it is capable of creating a physical and psychological dependence. **Physical dependency** means that body cells have come to depend on the presence of this depressant to maintain **homeostasis** (or balance). Once physically dependent, if the body is deprived of alcohol, an addict will experience **withdrawal symptoms.** Withdrawal symptoms can be extremely uncomfortable and even fatal. (See *FYI:* "Stages of Withdrawal from Alcohol.") Fatalities may be as high as one in seven. During the initial phase of withdrawal, called **detoxification,** or ridding the body of alcohol, women who have abused alcohol for a number of years may need to be hospitalized. Medically, withdrawal from alcohol is more severe and more likely to be fatal than is withdrawal from narcotic drugs.

Delirium tremens (DTs) are usually experienced in Stage 3 of alcohol withdrawal and are found mostly in serious cases of alcohol dependency. Although they often are manifested with shaking hands and jerky movements, DTs also produce vivid hallucinations and

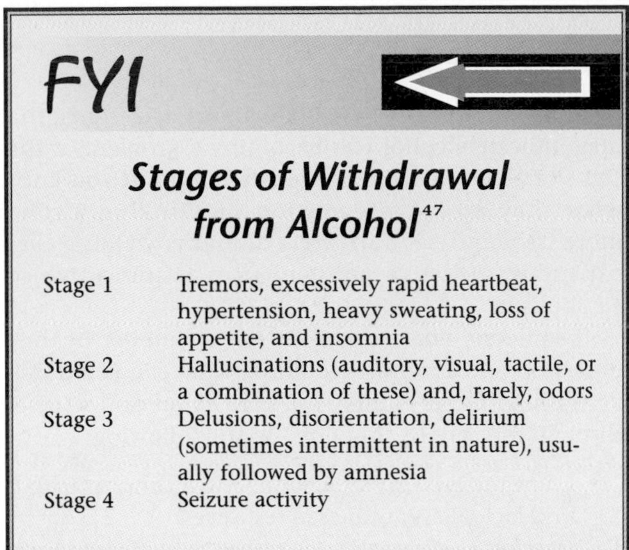

FYI

Stages of Withdrawal from Alcohol[47]

Stage 1	Tremors, excessively rapid heartbeat, hypertension, heavy sweating, loss of appetite, and insomnia
Stage 2	Hallucinations (auditory, visual, tactile, or a combination of these) and, rarely, odors
Stage 3	Delusions, disorientation, delirium (sometimes intermittent in nature), usually followed by amnesia
Stage 4	Seizure activity

nausea. Withdrawal symptoms such as insomnia, panic attacks, irregular breathing, abnormal blood pressure, and/or anxiety may last for weeks, and the woman can feel an intense craving for alcohol. Aftercare programs, discussed later in this chapter, are important during this time to prevent the woman from returning to use of alcohol.

Psychological dependence, a learned process affecting the behavior of a long-term drinker, occurs when the drinker strongly desires, or craves, the feeling alcohol provides. Like the mother of a newborn infant who learns to function with less sleep, alcohol drinkers learn to function with the effects of alcohol. Learning what to expect from alcohol intake in varying circumstances, the woman learns to control her behavior and act accordingly. Psychological tolerance deceives a woman into believing she can perform certain tasks under the influence of alcohol. In reality, she will not be able to determine to what extent the alcohol affects her abilities. Even if she looks and acts sober, it does not mean that she is capable of skilled performance such as driving a car, using sharp instruments, or operating mechanical devices. Because of the psychological feelings (e.g., temporary escape, mood swings, relaxation, euphoria) sometimes resulting from the use of alcohol, the ability to recover from this type of dependency may be more difficult to achieve than recovery from physical dependency.

ALCOHOLISM

> When a woman is unconscious about her starvation, about the consequences of using death-dealing vehicles and substances, she is dancing, she is dancing. Whether these are such things as chronic negative thinking, poor relationships, abusive situations, drugs, or alcohol—they are like the red shoes: hard to pry a person away from once they've taken hold.[48]

Demographics

Addiction to alcohol crosses all gender, economic, political, and social boundaries and generally is a well-established pattern of abuse by the time a male reaches his mid to late thirties or early forties, whereas women, if they develop alcoholism, generally do so at a later age and develop complications more easily and at a faster rate than males. **Alcoholism** is a chronic, progressive, and potentially fatal disease characterized by tolerance and by physical and psychological dependency; genetic, environmental, and psychosocial factors contribute to its development and progression. This disease is a direct or indirect result of ingesting alcohol and varies in the time it takes to develop. For some women the development can be somewhat rapid; for others, alcoholism may be years in the making. However long it takes to develop, this disease shortens life expectancy by an estimated 10 to 15 years. The number of female alcoholics in the United States is estimated at between 4 million and 7 million.[49]

A myth about alcoholism is that a person has to be drinking or drunk all the time to be considered an alcoholic. The truth is that patterns of alcohol abuse vary. Regular daily intake of large amounts of alcohol, regular heavy drinking that is limited to weekends, or long periods of not drinking interspersed with binge drinking that can last from days to several weeks can each be typical of alcoholic drinking patterns. Another myth regarding alcoholism is that an alcoholic can resume drinking after remaining sober for a number of years without her drinking getting out of control. Although some researchers have tried to prove this is the case, no one in recovery from alcoholism would agree. Once a woman has developed the disease of alcoholism, she will always have the disease. She may not always be a drinking alcoholic, but she will be unable to ever control her drinking again; therefore, abstaining from any drinking is imperative. (Read *Her Story:* "Amanda: Portrait of an Alcoholic?" to see what you think.)

Is Alcoholism a Disease?

There is an ongoing controversy about whether alcoholism is truly a "disease" or if it is a willful abuse of a harmful and intoxicating substance. The American Medical Association classifies it as a disease, as does Alcoholics Anonymous, with millions of members whose "only requirement for membership is the desire to stop drinking." However, some professionals and

Her Story

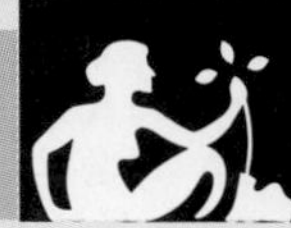

Amanda: Portrait of an Alcoholic?

Amanda, a 22-year-old mother of one and a community college nursing major, maintains above-average grades. She rarely misses class and is a responsible parent Sunday through Thursday nights. However, after class is over each Friday, she takes Alissa, her 2-year-old daughter, to stay with her grandmother. Amanda spends the remainder of the weekend drinking with friends and out of control: partying, driving while drunk, engaging in sexual activity, and disregarding any responsibilities related to school or her daughter. Amanda refuses to stop spending her weekends in a drunken stupor and feels that as long as she is taking care of her responsibilities during the week, she can do as she pleases on the weekends.

- Does Amanda meet some of the criteria in the definition of alcoholism?
- Is she creating present or future problems as a result of continual overconsumption of alcohol?
- What consequences could result from her continual abuse of an addicting, toxic substance?

researchers believe individuals should be responsible for their behavior under all circumstances and that it is wrong to "hide" behind the facade of disease to excuse any violent, antisocial, or illegal behavior because of alcohol abuse.

The cause of alcoholism is basically unknown, but studies have discovered that some of the following circumstances are revealed in the background of alcoholic women:

- Having an alcoholic parent or parents, which could mean that they have a genetic susceptibility or environmental influence to alcohol abuse; at least 60 percent of all alcoholics have at least one alcoholic parent.
- Childhood abuse, of which almost half is the result of parental alcohol abuse. It may contribute to the abuse of a child and, as a result of this experience, the abused child may become an alcoholic as well as a future child abuser.
- Excessive drinking as teens establishes the habit and social patterns, or even dependency.
- Social factors such as disappearance of the extended family, mobility of families, slackened family ties, and decline of religious affiliations.

Indicators of Alcoholism, and How to Help

If someone were to ask you about the signs that may indicate alcohol was becoming a problem or that signs of alcoholism were prevalent, would you know what they are? A progression of drinking alcohol more frequently and in larger amounts yielding ever-expanding negative consequences is indicative of alcoholism.

If someone you care about has a number of these indicators and continues to drink, what can you do? To better help the person(s) you care about and yourself through this serious situation, do the following:

- Learn the facts about alcohol and alcoholism, and find factual and unbiased resources.
- Develop a factual attitude rather than an emotional attitude toward the person and her drinking; avoid ridicule, criticism, and disgust.
- Don't use home remedies such as lecturing, hiding the liquor, soliciting promises the drinker won't or can't keep, saying, "If you loved me . . . ," or using a "holier than thou attitude."
- Find assistance for yourself and, if possible, the alcoholic such as your family doctor, minister, counselors, county agencies, and support groups (AA and Al-Anon).
- Talk with people who understand the illness, not just to friends and family.
- Allow the alcoholic to be responsible for her own behavior and the consequences of her drinking.
- Expect relapses and difficult days after recovery begins; immediate recovery will not happen.
- When protection from situations in which alcohol is present is not possible, the alcoholic has to learn to say "no, thanks" on her own.

Then complete *Assess Yourself:* "Do You Have a Drinking Problem?" to determine if you have a problem with alcohol.

A Family Disease

Growing up in a family in which alcohol was abused by one or both parents can produce lifelong negative consequences. Which would be a more difficult plight to endure: to be the daughter of alcoholic parents, to be the wife of an alcoholic, to be the mother of an alcoholic and having to see your child deal with alcoholism, or to be an alcoholic yourself? Each is hurtful, and many women experience all four circumstances. The physical and financial toll of alcoholism can to some degree be objectively calculated. However, the human loss to individuals, their families, communities, and society is incalculable. It is estimated that for every alcoholic,

Assess Yourself

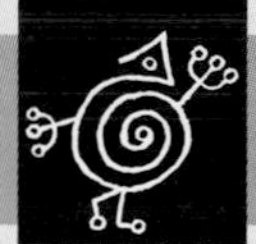

Do You Have a Drinking Problem?

Use the following questions to determine if alcohol is a problem in your life. Check "yes" if the statement is true or "no" if the statement is not true about your drinking behaviors and patterns. Then consult the suggestions at the end of this survey.

Yes	No	Question
______	______	1. Do you drink more than three times a week?
______	______	2. Do you drink more than three drinks each time?
______	______	3. When everyone else is drinking, do you feel you should be drinking also?
______	______	4. Do you think it is acceptable for people to get drunk once in a while?
______	______	5. Do you find it difficult to say "no" when someone offers you an alcoholic drink even when you don't really want it?

Suggestions: If you answered "yes" more than "no" to these questions, it would be a good idea not only to reduce the amount and frequency of drinking, if you can, but also to talk with a counselor who specializes in alcohol treatment. If you suspect a friend or relative has a problem, encourage that person to take the assessment too.

another four people are directly affected. The ripple effects from those four people then extend to numerous others.

Codependency Preoccupation with a particular individual and her or his problems to the point of self-neglect is an example of **codependency.** Eventually, the codependent's relationship with all others is affected. This results from prolonged association with the alcoholic and from the practice of oppressive "rules" that prevent the open expression of feelings, concerns, and problems. These rules, often developed subconsciously, include such things as it's not okay to talk about a problem; it's not okay to talk about feelings; do as I say, not as I do; don't rock the boat; it's not okay to play or be playful; be the best, but don't enjoy it! Codependent women often take care of their family's needs and wants. They tend to worry a lot; check on people; lose sleep over family problems; abandon their routine due to upset feelings about somebody or something; try to catch people in acts of misbehavior; control family members' behavior; think they know what is best for others; and try to control events and people through helplessness, guilt, coercion, threats, advice giving, manipulation, and/or domination. Codependency is unhealthy because the codependent woman tends to allow her physical, emotional, social, and mental quality of life to be dependent upon the quality of life of other people. Therefore, she feels as if she has little control over her own well-being. She is likely to develop stress-related disorders such as migraines, ulcers, arthritis, even heart disease and cancer. Women with codependent traits can obtain help through individual or family counseling with the alcoholic and other family members, involvement in twelve-step programs such as Al-Anon and Codependency Anonymous, and by reading the plethora of self-help material related to codependency and alcoholism.

Adult Children of Alcoholics *Adult children of alcoholics* (ACAs) grow up in a group of related people in which one or more members are continually unmanageable or stressful conditions, such as alcoholism, continually create a dysfunctional environment. The family is the most significant social unit in our society and is responsible for the development of habits and beliefs that influence members' decisions throughout the life span. Yet children in the dysfunctional family often do not have role models that exhibit good habits or profess beliefs that help children develop important systems that can enhance their life. The dysfunctional home environment places *children of alcoholics* (COAs) at risk for early alcohol and drug dependence, underachievement or unhealthy overachievement, inappropriate classroom or social behaviors, lying, delinquency, unhealthy relationships with peers and adults, and emotional distress that can manifest itself in withdrawal, depression, or suicide attempts. As COAs become ACAs, unless they receive help, many continue to have these risk factors. Three rules, although not written, are learned by COAs: don't talk or tell (don't discuss the problem; pretend it doesn't exist); don't trust (nothing is consistent or predictable);

and don't feel (numb out the anger and the pain; it hurts too much to feel). These rules lead to some serious consequences for ACAs. It sets the stage for shame and doubt, isolation, distrust of self and others, and uncertainty or numbing of feelings. Thus, there is no pain but, also, there is no joy.

Strategies for overcoming the effects that are experienced by ACAs include

- going to ACA meetings,
- reading about the ACA experiences of others and writing about their own,
- using and incorporating information about methods and techniques of recovery,
- defining and enforcing boundaries, and
- building a personal support network.[50]

Effects of Growing Up in an Alcoholic Family

Surviving difficult family circumstances often means that family members develop coping mechanisms and roles that help them momentarily deal with the chaos of living in an alcoholic family. Four roles, identified by treatment providers, that COAs often develop to help them cope with problems related to parental alcoholism are the hero, the scapegoat, the lost child, and the mascot. The hero is the super-kid, caretaker, the "type E" female: everything to everybody; she is the cheerleader, honor student, and president of the class. Often irresponsible, disruptive, or antisocial, the scapegoat may become defiant and delinquent; she is vulnerable to unwholesome peer groups and drug abuse. The lost child (the loner) has her own private world of reading, television, computer, music, or any other refuge she can find that enables her to escape from the family chaos; she is at risk for poor health choices (e.g., smoking, drinking), early natural death, or suicide. Seemingly carefree, funny, the center of attention, the mascot (or clown) deals with the dysfunctional family by denying there is a problem. She diverts attention from the painful family situation by offering comic relief; she is at risk for physical and emotional problems and drug abuse. These roles help children (and often adults) survive the dysfunctional family situation. Their development may be thwarted without help, and these coping roles may prevent them from leading fulfilling lives outside the family system. Many of these behaviors do not serve them well as adults when they use the behaviors on the job or when interacting with family or friends. ACAs must be taught the four Cs of a dysfunctional family: You didn't *cause* it, you can't *control* it, you can't *cure* it, you *can help yourself*.

Fortunately, as alcoholics are being assisted in overcoming their disease and dysfunctions, the family members can also be assisted in overcoming risk factors generated by growing up in an alcoholic family. Twelve-step programs, such as Al-Anon, ACA meetings, Codependency Anonymous groups, as well as individual and group therapy have been successful in overcoming negative behaviors associated with alcoholic families, and moving ahead to productive and positive lives. Schools also have developed support programs for COAs that include such activities as building self-esteem, establishing consistency, providing a safe environment for expressing feelings openly, and learning to trust. This is an attempt to reduce risk factors that could lead to development of alcohol and drug abuse among children of alcoholics and to build protective factors that are traits or conditions intended to assist COAs in the development of healthy and productive lifestyles. (See *Journal Activity:* "Who and What Does Alcohol Affect?")

WHAT CAN BE DONE?

No one approach seems to be successful for recovery from alcoholism. Instead, greater success is found by utilizing a combination of treatment approaches. It is important to remember that the alcoholic will rarely move to "treat" herself and may need assistance in seeking help. However, no one can force another adult into treatment unless the legal system intercedes, and this happens only after some crime has been committed because of alcohol abuse.

Resources

Locating resources for the alcoholic and yourself is an important first step toward resolving this problem. Who, what, where, how, and how much are all questions that need to have answers prior to movement toward assisting the alcoholic.

Intervention

Intervention is a process by which the alcoholic is confronted by a person or persons each describing the "facts" associated with their concern for the alcoholic's drinking problem. Individuals close to the alcoholic (e.g., child, parent, sibling, spouse, friends, employer) can share in this calm, yet truthful process that is intended to assure the alcoholic of their concern for her, but also assertively express the situation as it is. If the intervention is successful, the alcoholic should be willing to move into inpatient or outpatient treatment. Betty Ford states that when her family intervened because of her abuse of prescription drugs and alcohol, she became angry and hurt. But, as she

Journal Activity

Who and What Does Alcohol Affect?

As you read the various events listed below, determine the area of greatest impact on one of the following: (a) the drinker (health effect), (b) the family (social effect), (c) or society (economic effect). For each event write the effect in the "Who or What?" column, and in the last column, explain why this effect has such a great impact. (Hint: It may affect more than one area!)

Event	Who or What?	Why?
1. Court system	____________	____________
2. Auto death while DUI	____________	____________
3. Increased welfare costs	____________	____________
4. Injuring oneself in a fall	____________	____________
5. Job loss	____________	____________
6. Divorce	____________	____________
7. Cirrhosis of the liver	____________	____________
8. Neglect of one's children	____________	____________
9. Heart disease	____________	____________
10. Decreased work productivity	____________	____________
11. Spousal abuse	____________	____________
12. Passing out or vomiting at a party	____________	____________
13. Increased medical costs	____________	____________
14. Sexually transmitted diseases	____________	____________
15. Abusing a child	____________	____________
16. Depression	____________	____________
17. Fighting at a sporting event	____________	____________
18. Killing someone when driving drunk	____________	____________

listened, she heard the love that came through their comments to her, and she realized they loved her too much to ignore the problem any longer. She decided to seek treatment and continues in recovery, which she says will be ongoing as long as she lives. The Betty Ford Center in Rancho Mirage, California, was created as a result of her efforts and continues to treat thousands of individuals in need of alcohol and other drug therapy.

Intervention actions include developing individual action plans, selecting treatment centers, facilitating an intervention meeting, and facilitating pre-interaction, family, and follow-up meetings.[51]

Types of Treatment

Various approaches are used in the treatment of alcoholism and include not only what precipitated the originating use but also the complex consequences of the disease. Women comprise about one-third of the population with alcohol problems and slightly less than half of those who have problems with other drugs.[52] Lifestyle behavior change, stress management programs, individual counseling, spiritual renewal, hospitalization, drug therapy, support groups, and other therapies are often used in treatment for alcoholism.

Lifestyle Behavior Changes Lifestyle behavior changes include improved nutrition, engaging in exercise programs, developing stress management strategies, enhancement of self-worth, and recognizing a higher power. Treatment attempts to focus on making positive changes in one's life in addition to cessation of alcohol abuse.

Counseling Individual and/or group counseling assists the alcoholic in looking at issues related to the abusive behavior. It is important to determine whether alcohol abuse is the result of a variety of negative situations in one's life or the negative situations are the consequences of alcohol abuse. The counselor needs to be specifically trained in working with alcohol-dependent individuals as well as their families. Group therapy can provide an environment in which women feel safe discussing their alcohol-related problems and receive support from other women who understand and can relate to them. Realization that others have experienced the same pain, humiliation, or shame seems to bring relief because each woman no longer feels she is the only one.

Treatment Centers Use of hospitals or drug treatment centers has been beneficial for some women. In this environment women can go through detoxification under medical supervision, remove themselves from the surroundings in which they've had problems with alcohol, and begin to resolve the problems that caused this disease to develop. Treatment centers usually have a structured routine revolving around household duties, individual and group therapy, recreation, nutritious meals, and support group meetings, all of which help to reestablish routine, responsibility, and health. Many insurance companies provide for alcoholism treatment on both an inpatient and outpatient basis. Women in treatment often have different needs than men. Care of small children, finances, transportation, and even distrustfulness of male professionals hinder a woman's ability to engage in treatment programs. To promote recovery for women with these needs, treatment should include child care, female counselors, transportation, reduced fees, and women-only therapies.

Chemical Treatment Chemical treatment (drug therapy) occasionally becomes necessary if a woman cannot refrain from abusing alcohol through inpatient or outpatient treatment. Antabuse is a drug that inhibits an enzyme (acetaldehyde dehydrogenase) from breaking down acetaldehyde. As a result, a toxic effect to alcohol is created; therefore, if a woman who has taken Antabuse then drinks, extremely uncomfortable effects such as nausea, weakness, blurred vision, heart palpitations, and vomiting occur. These consequences are intended to impede the consumption of alcohol. Two drugs, nalmefene and naltrexone, both of which are opiate antagonists, block the brain's pleasurable response to drinking and help alcohol abusers to stop drinking compulsively. One research study discovered that only 15 percent of physicians, even among addiction specialists, prescribe naltrexone for alcohol abuse treatment.[53] Clinicians need to be better informed about drugs such as naltrexone so that patients can be prescribed the drugs and experience their positive effects. Drugs such as these can be beneficial in reducing a person's desire to drink and therefore decrease the high rates of alcoholics' relapse to heavy drinking, which occurs at a rate of about 80 percent.

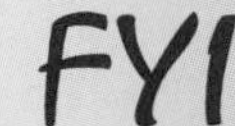

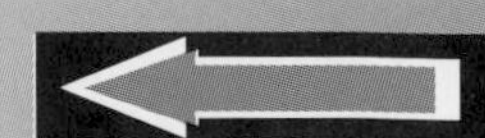

Facts about Alcoholics Anonymous[54]

- There are more than 100,000 AA groups worldwide in 150 countries.
- 35 percent of AA members are female.
- Approximately 36 percent of the members have been sober over 10 years; 14 percent have been sober between 1 and 5 years.
- About 66 percent of AA members are between the ages of 21 and 50.
- Average member attends two meetings per week.
- Average age of members is 48 years.
- Other treatment programs follow the AA model (for example, Codependency Anonymous and Cocaine Anonymous).

Aftercare Aftercare, continuing care following treatment for alcohol or other drug abuse, needs to be comprehensive as well as attentive to individual needs. Provision of support groups and varied services can enable women to live drug-free lives and foster development of skills and abilities leading to self-confidence and independence. What services and support structures are most beneficial following treatment? Contact with other recovering women, recovery and personal growth literature, personal and family therapy sessions, life skills and job training, vocational training and job placement are all beneficial as women seek to move ahead to a healthy, productive lifestyle. Support and self-help groups such as twelve-step organizations, including *Alcoholics Anonymous (AA), Al-Anon (AA), Adult Children of Alcoholics (ACA), Codependency Anonymous (CODA), and Women for Sobriety,* offer emotional support and social interaction among women who can share experiences and solutions for a disease that is known best by individuals who have shared in its devastating effects. (See *FYI:* "Facts about Alcoholics Anonymous.")

Involving cultural and geographic community support, such as phone chains, hotlines, and recovery group gatherings, can keep recovering women in contact with one another so that the healing process will continue. Women who have just come out of treatment programs need to have follow-up contact for as long as the woman and her counselor and/or case manager deem it important and necessary. (See the resources and suggested readings at the end of the chapter.)

PREVENTION

Of course, the most effective way to prevent problems associated with alcohol abuse and the disease of alcoholism is to abstain from alcohol consumption. Because there are millions of women who drink, and many of them do develop alcohol dependency problems, it is important to look at how those problems can be avoided.

Primary prevention programs are aimed at women, especially young women, who have not begun to use alcohol, and they focus on reducing the rate of new alcohol users. This type of prevention program attempts to provide and promote activities that reduce the factors related to early use of alcohol. These factors include lack of awareness in school and community of alcohol-related problems, insufficient knowledge about alcohol and other drugs, lack of understanding about negative effects of alcohol abuse, students' need for life skills training, infrequent involvement of parents in their children's schools, lack of awareness of positive alternatives to using alcohol. Insufficient knowledge about regulations and laws pertaining to alcohol use/abuse.

Activities can be developed to combat each one of these factors and thus reduce the possibility that young women will begin to use alcohol. Suggested activities pertaining to these contributing factors include, but are not limited to, some of the following:

- Raising awareness through involvement of community organizations, church groups, or parent groups by developing a media campaign using local newspaper, television, and radio; promoting a community alcohol awareness day designated by wearing certain colors or driving with headlights on; or proclamations by community officials. The more segments of community involvement, the greater the opportunity to enhance awareness in school and community of alcohol-related problems.
- Accurate, current, and age-appropriate information can affect good communication between parents, teachers, and their children/students. As part of a comprehensive approach to alcohol use prevention, purchasing materials and curricula and providing in-service programs for teachers, as well as providing opportunities for parents to become educated about alcohol use, can help to reduce the insufficient knowledge about alcohol and other drugs.

Young women often believe that alcohol use does not produce any negative consequences and therefore using this substance is okay. By developing strong anti-use policies in schools and communities and involving students in alcohol-free activities, young women are likely to behave accordingly and develop negative attitudes toward the use of alcohol.

Like all individuals, young women need life skills training. Activities and organizations that promote the resistance of peer influence enhance decision-making abilities, and aid young women in coping with personal and social issues, can provide a basis for choosing not to use alcohol. Developing leadership qualities and problem-solving skills can also reduce the likelihood of alcohol use by females.

Enhancing positive family influence and increasing involvement of parents and students in school can be accomplished by promoting parenting skills through parent-training programs in education systems or community organizations. More involvement in and allegiance to school means that students often adopt behaviors and values expounded by the school and have less time for alcohol-related activities or peers who may choose to drink. Club, sport, and other student–parent organizations not only involve the students but also provide reasons for parents to come to school events. Giving young women opportunities to engage in these activities can provide healthy alternatives to alcohol use. Youth centers, community and school recreation, and alcohol-free dances and parties can offer alternative activities to involvement with alcohol.

Regulations and laws can be useful in preventing abuse of alcohol and other drugs. Creating barriers to alcohol access and enforcing restrictions to curtail underage drinking and use of fake identification cards can be a deterrent to early use of alcohol. Increased supervision of youth and expanded security at places where young people congregate help prevent the influx of alcohol by underage consumers.

The majority of these suggestions are directed toward *young* women, because that is exactly when alcohol abuse prevention must begin. The younger the age at which females initially abuse alcohol, the greater the probability they will encounter negative consequences.

Prevention can yield the greatest benefit if initiated at an early age (e.g., preschool) and continued throughout the school years and into adulthood. During this process, many of the risk factors can be ameliorated and alcohol abuse prevented.

> Yes there is pain in being severed from the red shoes. But being cut away from the addiction all at once is our only hope. It is a severing that is filled with absolute blessing. The feet will grow back, we will find our way, we will recover, we will run and jump and skip again someday. By then our handmade life will be ready. We'll slip into it and marvel that we could be so lucky to have another chance.[55]

Chapter Summary

- Women and alcohol have a historical association that produced both positive and negative outcomes.
- Alcohol is the most commonly used psychoactive drug, and its use has a number of health benefits; the abuse of alcohol results in serious physical, psychological, social, and economic consequences.
- Women and men respond differently to alcohol both physically and behaviorally.
- Alcohol and pregnancy do not mix; there is no safe level of alcohol ingestion for pregnant women; fetal alcohol syndrome can result from drinking alcohol during pregnancy.
- Alcohol is an addicting, depressant drug that can cause the disease of alcoholism and result in serious consequences for the addict, her family, and other important components of her life.
- There are indicators that can be utilized as a means of informal assessment to determine if someone is alcohol dependent.
- Children of alcoholics (COAs) develop family roles that enable them to attempt to cope with the chronic distress and chaos present in an alcoholic's family. Without assistance, COAs may take these roles into adulthood.
- Finding resources, intervention, seeking treatment, and changing lifestyle behaviors can all be beneficial when recovering from alcohol addiction.
- Prevention of alcohol abuse is important if women are to avoid the possible devastation that can occur from alcohol abuse and addiction.

Review Questions

1. What attitudes toward women and alcohol were held by society at different times in history?
2. What are the four different types of alcohol? What does the term *proof* mean?
3. What is the process of alcohol absorption in a woman's body?
4. Why does alcohol affect women differently than it affects men?
5. What are the criteria used to classify different levels of drinkers?
6. What are the possible consequences for the mother and her fetus and infant if she drinks alcohol during pregnancy?
7. How does the addiction process relate to alcohol dependency?
8. If alcohol is a disease, why don't we know exactly what causes it, how to successfully treat it, and how to prevent it?
9. What indications may be displayed by a woman who either is developing or has developed an addiction to alcohol?
10. What is codependency? How does it relate to alcohol abuse?
11. What characteristics may develop in children who grow up in homes where either one parent or both parents are alcoholic?
12. What are some approaches that can be taken to assist a woman in overcoming alcohol dependency?
13. What are some of the methods that can be used to prevent alcohol abuse in women?
14. What is the difference between fetal alcohol syndrome and fetal alcohol effects?

Resources

Web Sites for Alcohol-Related Organizations

Addiction Intervention Resources
www.addictionintervention.com

Adult Children of Alcoholics (ACA)
www.adultchildren.org

Al-Anon Family Group Headquarters
www.al-anon.alateen.org

Alcoholics Anonymous (AA) World Services
www.alcoholics-anonymous.org

Alcohol and Drug Information, U.S. Department of Health and Human Services
http://ncadi.samhsa.gov/govpubs/rpo993

Alcohol Use and Aging
www.niapublications.org/engagepages/alcohol.asp

Higher Education Center for Alcohol and Other Drug Prevention
www.higheredcenter.org

Mothers Against Drunk Driving (MADD)
www.madd.org

National Clearinghouse for Alcohol and Drug Information (NCADI)
http://ncadi.samhsa.gov

National Council on Alcoholism and Drug Dependence (NCADD)
www.ncadd.org

National Institute on Alcohol Abuse and Alcoholism
www.niaaa.nih.gov

Videotapes

Date Rape Drugs: An Alert (1999)
Eat, Drink and Be Wary: Women and the Dangers of Alcohol (1999)
Women and Alcoholism(2003)
Facts on . . . Alcohol (2003)
Making of a Hangover (2002)
Films for the Humanities & Sciences, P.O. Box 2053, Princeton, NJ 08543-2053. Phone: 800-257-5126, Web site: www.films.com

Alcohol: A Women's Health Issue
Office of Research on Women's Health, OD, NIH, HHS, 1 Center Drive Building 1, Room 201, Bethesda, MD 20892. Phone: 301-402-1770

Spin the Bottle: Sex, Lies and Alcohol (2004)
DVD about the complex relationship between alcohol use, media influence, and personal responsibility. To order, go to www.mediaed.org or call 800-897-0089.

Educational Brochures

Alcohol ABC's
Binge Drinking
Drinking: What's Normal, What's Not
5 Smart Steps to Safer Drinking
Getting What You Want from Drinking
21st Century Drinking
(Many are available in bilingual format.)
Films for the Humanities & Sciences, Box 2053, Princeton, NH 08543-2053. Phone: 800-257-5126, Web site: www.films.com

Suggested Readings

A Call to Action: Changing the Culture of Drinking at U.S. Colleges. 2002. Final Report of the Task Force on College Drinking. NIH Publication No. 02-5010. Washington, DC: National Institutes of Health, U.S. Department of Health and Human Services.

Ettorre, E. 1998. *Women & Alcohol: A Private Pleasure or a Public Problem.* London: Women's Press Limited.

Gilson, C., and V. Bennett. 2002. *Alcohol and Women: Creating a Safer Lifestyle.* Dallas, TX: Authorlink.

High-Risk Drinking in College: What We Know and What We Need to Learn. 2002. Final Report of the Panel on Contexts and Consequences. Washington, DC: Task Force of the National Advisory Council on Alcohol Abuse and Alcoholism, National Institutes of Health, U. S. Department of Health and Human Services.

Jersild, D. 2002. *Happy Hour: Alcohol in a Woman's Life.* New York: HarperCollins.

Kirkpatrick, J. 2003. *Goodbye Hangovers, Hello Life: Self Help for Women.* Fort Lee, NJ: Barricade Books.

Robbins, A. 2004. *Pledged: The Secret Life of Sororities.* New York: Hyperion Press.

The National Center on Addiction and Substance Abuse at Columbia University. 2006. *Women Under the Influence.* Baltimore, MD: Johns Hopkins Press.

Wilson, T. M., ed. 2005. *Drinking Culture: Alcohol & Identity.* Gordonsville, VA: Palgrave Macmillan/Berg Publishers.

Woititz, J. G., and R. J. Ackerman. 2002. *Complete ACOA Source Book: Adult Children of Alcoholics at Home, Work and in Love.* Deerfield Beach, FL: Health Communications.

Zailekas, K. 2005. *Smashed: Story of a Drunken Childhood.* New York: Penguin Group.

Brochures from the National Institute on Alcohol Abuse and Alcoholism:
Alcoholism: Getting the Facts, NIH Publication No. 96-4153
Drinking and Your Pregnancy, NIH Publication No. 96-4101
How to Cut Down on Your Drinking, NIH Publication No. 96-3770
Frequently Asked Questions About Alcoholism & Alcohol, NIH Publication No. 01-4735
Make a Difference: Talk to Your Child About Alcohol, NIH Publication No. 00-4314

These are free and can be ordered at the following address: National Institute on Alcohol Abuse and Alcoholism, Publications Distribution Center, P.O. Box 10686, Rockville, MD 20849-0686.

References

1. Blume, S. 1990. Chemical dependency in women: Important issues. *American Journal of Drug and Alcohol Abuse* 16 (3&4): 297–307.
2. National Institute on Alcohol Abuse and Alcoholism. 2004. *Alcoholism: Getting the facts.* NIH Publication No. 96-4153. Bethesda, MD: National Institutes of Health.
3. Blume, Chemical dependency in women: Important issues.
4. Lieber, C. S. 2003. Relationships between nutrition, alcohol use and liver disease. *Alcohol Research & Health* 27 (3): 220–31.
5. Alcohol intoxication definition and causes. 2006. *eMedicine Health.* www.emedicinehealth.com/script/main/art.asp?articlekey=58696&pf=3&page=1 (retrieved October 3, 2006).
6. Engs, R., and D. Hanson. 1990. Gender differences in drinking patterns and problems among college students: A review of literature. *Journal of Alcohol and Drug Education* 35 (1): 36–47.
7. Ibid.
8. Centers for Disease Control and Prevention. 2004. *Alcohol-attributable deaths and years of potential life lost—United States, 2001.* http://jama.ama-assn.org/cgi/content/ full/292/23/2831 (retrieved October 3, 2006).
9. National Institute on Alcohol Abuse and Alcoholism. 1999. Are women more vulnerable to alcohol's effects? *Alcohol Alert* 46. Bethesda, MD: NIAAA.
10. Wechsler, H., J. E. Lee, M. Kuo, and H. Lee. 2000. College binge drinking in the 1990's: A continuing problem

Results of the Harvard School of Public Health 1999 College Alcohol Survey. *Journal of American College Health* 48 (5): 199–210.

11. Kinney, J. 2006. *Loosening the grip: A handbook of alcohol information.* 8th ed. New York: McGraw-Hill.
12. Pinger, R., W. Payne, D. Hahn, and E. Hahn. 1998. *Drugs: Issues for today.* 3rd ed. New York: McGraw-Hill.
13. National Institutes of Health, National Institute on Alcohol Abuse and Alcoholism. 2004. *Percent distribution of the drinking levels of females 18 years of age and older according to selected characteristics: United States, NHIS, 1997–2004.* www.niaaa.nih.gov/NR/rdonlyres/A0E61C3F-5BA5-4129-8D11-16EEBA37438E/0/dkpat27.txt (retrieved October 3, 2006).
14. Wechsler, H., J. E. Lee, M. Kuo, M. Seibring, T. F. Nelson, and H. Lee. 2002. Trends in college binge drinking during a period of increased prevention efforts. *Journal of American College Health* 50 (5): 203–17.
15. Ibid.
16. U.S. Department of Health and Human Services. 2000. *Healthy People 2010, conference edition* 11: 26–29. Washington, DC: Author.
17. U.S. Department of Health and Human Services, Health Resources and Services Administration. 2005. *Women's health USA 2005.* Rockville, MD: U.S. Department of Health and Human Services.
18. Emanuele, M. A., F. Wezeman, and N. V. Emanuele. 2002. Alcohol's effects on female reproductive function. *Alcohol Research & Health* 26 (4): 274–81.
19. Dorgan, J., et al. 2001. Alcohol increases hormone levels raising breast cancer risk. *Journal of the National Cancer Institute* 93 (9): 710–15.
20. Smith-Warner, S. A., D. Spiegelman, S. S. Yaun, et al. 1998. Alcohol and breast cancer in women: A pooled analysis of cohort studies. *Journal of the American Medical Association* 279 (7): 535–40.
21. Register, T. C., M. Cline, and C. A. Shively. 2002. Health issues in postmenopausal women who drink. *Alcohol Research & Health* 26 (4): 299–307.
22. Sampson, H. W. 2002. Alcohol and other factors affecting osteoporosis risk in women. *Alcohol Research & Health* 26 (4): 292–98.
23. Ksir, C., C. L. Hart, and O. Ray. 2006. *Drugs, society, and human behavior.* 11th ed. New York: McGraw-Hill.
24. National Institute on Alcohol Abuse and Alcoholism. 2002. Alcohol's effect on females' reproductive function. *Alcohol and Research & Health: Women and Alcohol, An Update* 26 (4): 274–81.
25. Smith-Warner, Spiegelman, and Yaun, Alcohol and breast cancer in women.
26. Register, Cline, and Shively, Health issues in postmenopausal women who drink.
27. Dieting coeds more likely to drink. 1992. *USA Today,* December, p. 11.
28. Adapted from: Payne, W. A., D. B. Hahn, and E. Lucas. 2007. *Understanding your Health.* 9th ed. New York: McGraw-Hill.
29. Center for Science in the Public Interest. 2000. *Alcohol Policies Project: Advocacy for the prevention of alcohol problems.* www.cspinet.org/booze/women.htm (retrieved October 3, 2006).
30. Ibid.
31. National Institutes of Health, National Institute on Alcohol Abuse and Alcoholism, *Percent distribution of the drinking levels of females 18 years of age and older according to selected characteristics: United States, NHIS, 1997–2004.*
32. Collins, R. L., and L. D. McNair. 2003. *Minority women and alcohol use.* National Institute in Alcohol Abuse and Alcoholism. http://pubs.niaaa.nih.gov/publications/arh26-4/251-256.htm (retrieved October 3, 2006).
33. National Institutes of Health, National Institute on Alcohol Abuse and Alcoholism. 2002. *Alcohol: What you don't know can harm you.* NIH Publication No. 99-4323.
34. Klee, L., C. Schmidt, and G. Ames. 1991. Indicators of women's alcohol problems. *International Journal of the Addictions* 26 (8): 879–95.
35. Harwood, H. 2000. *Updating estimates of the economic costs of alcohol abuse in the United States.* Report prepared by the Lewin Group for the National Institute on Alcohol Abuse and Alcoholism.
36. National Institute on Alcohol Abuse and Alcoholism. 2005. *A snapshot of annual high-risk college drinking consequences.* www.collegedrinkingprevention.gov/StatsSummaries/snapshot.aspx (retrieved October 3, 2006).
37. U.S. Department of Health and Human Services, Centers for Disease Control and Prevention. 2005. *Measures of alcohol consumption and alcohol-related health effects from excessive consumption.* www.cdc.gov/alcohol/factsheets/general_information.htm. (retrieved October 3, 2006).
38. Lisansky-Gomberg, E. S. 1989. Suicide risk among women with alcohol problems. *American Journal of Public Health* 79 (10): 1363–65.
39. Smith, G. S., C. C., Branas, and T. R. Miller. 1999. Fatal non-traffic injuries involving alcohol: A meta-analysis. *Annual Emergency Medicine* 33:659–68.
40. Alcohol and acquaintance rape: Strategies to protect yourself & others. 1996. www.edc.org/HHD/HEC/pubs/rapefly.htm (retrieved on October 3, 2006).
41. Wechsler, H., M. Mohler-Kuo, B. Dowdall, and M. Koss. 2004. Correlates of rape while intoxicated in a national sample of college women. *Journal Studies Alcohol* 65:37–45.
42. U.S. Department of Health and Human Services, Office on Women's Health. 2004. *Date rape drugs.* www.4woman.gov/faq/rohypnol.pdf (retrieved October 3, 2006).
43. Centers for Disease Control and Prevention. 2004. Alcohol consumption among women who are pregnant or who might become pregnant. *Morbidity and Mortality Weekly Report* 53 (50): 1178–81.
44. Emanuele, M. A., and N. Emanuele. 2001. Alcohol and the male reproductive system. *Alcohol Research and Health* 25 (4): 282–87.
45. Tuormaa, T. E. 1996. The adverse effects of alcohol on production. *Journal of Nutritional and Environmental Medicine* 6 (4): 379–91.
46. Anderson, K. N. 1994. *Mosby's medical, nursing, and allied health dictionary.* 4th ed. St. Louis: Mosby-Year Book.
47. Ksir, Hart, and Ray. *Drugs, society, and human behavior,* p. 259.

48. Estes, C. P. 1995. *Women who run with the wolves*. New York: Ballantine, p. 248.
49. van der Walde, H., F. T. Urgenson, S. H. Weltz, and F. J. Hanna. 2002. Women and alcoholism: A biopsychosocial perspective and treatment approaches. *Journal of Counseling and Development* 80:145–53.
50. *Adult children of alcoholics*. 2003. www.adultchildren.org/lit/Handbook.s (retrieved October 3, 2006).
51. *Addiction intervention resources*. 2006. www.addictionintervention.com/intervention/10_steps_fa.asp (retrieved October 3, 2006).
52. Greenfield, S. F., D. E. Sugarman, L. R. Muenz, et al. 2003. Epidemiology of substance use disorders in women. *Obstetrics & Gynecology Clinics in North America* 30:413–46.
53. Thomas, C. P., et al. 2003. Research to practice: Adoption of naltrexone in alcoholism treatment. *Journal of Substance Abuse Treatment* 24:1–11.
54. Alcoholics Anonymous Worldwide. 2006. www.alcoholics-anonymous.org/en_press.cfm?PressType=GENR (retrieved October 3, 2006).
55. Estes, *Women who run with the wolves,* p. 251.

Chapter Thirteen

Making Wise Decisions about Tobacco, Caffeine, and Drugs

CHAPTER OBJECTIVES

When you complete this chapter, you will be able to do the following:

- Explain why smoking-related deaths are the most preventable causes of death to women in this country
- Describe the role of women in the history of tobacco
- Identify the substances in tobacco and the role each plays in the development of smoking-related diseases
- Analyze the available methods that can be used for smoking cessation
- Clarify the relationship between the use of tobacco and the effects on reproduction in women
- Explain the importance of a smoke-free environment in the home, the workplace, and recreational facilities
- Describe the physiological effects of caffeine on women's health
- Explain the interaction between caffeine and pregnancy
- Discuss illegal drugs and their characteristics
- Determine the consequences of illegal drug use and its impact on a woman's lifestyle, health, and pregnancy
- Describe the social problems that women encounter as a result of illegal drug use

The chains of habit are too weak to be felt until they are too strong to be broken.

SAMUEL JOHNSON

TOBACCO: LOOKING BACK

More deaths could be prevented if individuals stopped using tobacco than by changing any other lifestyle behavior. Despite the overwhelming amount of research linking tobacco use to *morbidity* (illness) and *mortality* (death), more than 6,000 persons under the age of 18 begin smoking every day in the United States.[1] The Food and Drug Administration (FDA) can restrict and regulate access to tobacco products and control the labeling on tobacco packaging. However, the advertising of various forms of tobacco cannot be regulated by the FDA. The federal government, to some degree, has been reluctant to place major constraints on tobacco products because of the possible economic impact on the production, manufacturing, and selling of this product.

Yet, as you will read in this chapter, the substances found in tobacco cause serious health consequences, resulting in high costs in terms of poor health and an increased need for health care. Both the home and the workplace are negatively impacted.

The history of the United States and the use of tobacco are intertwined. When Columbus discovered America, he also discovered Indians smoking pipes containing leaves and stems. Following his second trip, Columbus returned to Spain taking this substance, tobacco, with him. The smoking of tobacco, called "drinking," eventually became widespread throughout Europe and Asia. History notes that the English Queen Charlotte, wife of King George III (1760–1820), was highly addicted to powdered tobacco, called snuff, and as a result was nicknamed "Snuffy Charlotte."[2]

Tobacco, possibly named for a province in Mexico, was used medicinally for over 300 years, between A.D. 1500 and A.D. 1800, to treat ailments such as colds, headaches, and of all things, coughs. However, physicians and researchers ultimately determined that tobacco was not the wonder drug it was purported to be. In the United States, the substance ceased to be used medicinally in the late 1800s. Today tobacco is considered a drug that is associated with serious health-related consequences resulting from using tobacco products.

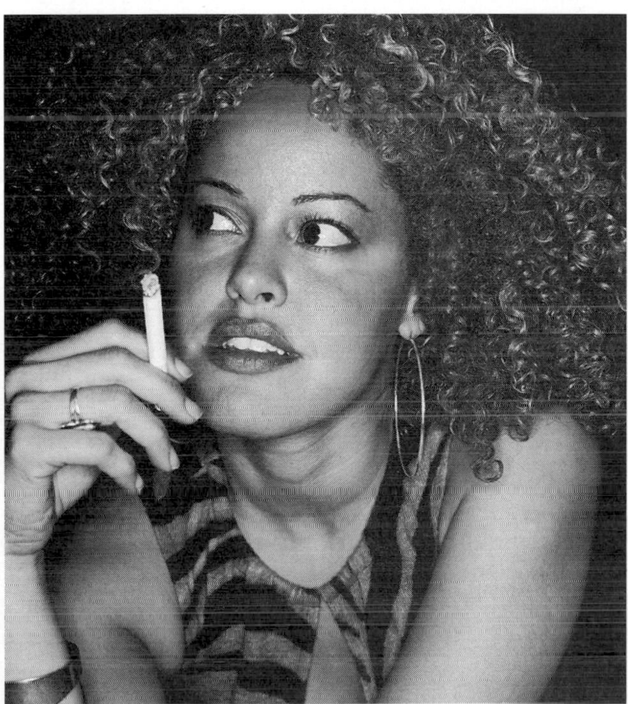

Unfortunately, the number of young women smokers is increasing.

WOMEN AND TOBACCO

Prevalence of Tobacco Use

The Centers for Disease Control and Prevention (CDC) states that 1 in 5 American women aged 18 or older (19 percent) smoke cigarettes. Women who smoke typically begin as teenagers. Among female high school students, approximately 22 percent reported smoking cigarettes within 30 days prior to a 2004 CDC survey.[3] Presently, there are 46 million smokers in the United States, and approximately 22 million of them are female;[4] at least 1.5 million are adolescent girls. One-half of all long-term smokers will die because they choose to smoke tobacco. These are alarming statistics, as former surgeon general David Satcher points out:

> When calling attention to public health problems, we must not misuse the word "epidemic." But there is no better word to describe the 600-percent increase since 1950 in women's death rates for lung cancer, a disease primarily caused by cigarette smoking. Clearly, smoking-related disease among women is a full-blown epidemic.[5]

Increased risks of heart and lung diseases, cancers, and reproductive disorders are much more prevalent in women smokers than in men smokers accounting for 39 percent of the 440,000 premature smoking-related deaths *each year.*[6] Since 1980, more than 3 million U.S. women have died prematurely as a result of choosing to smoke.[7] Adult women who smoke lose almost 15 years of life; it is the most preventable cause of premature death in this country. If women smoke, they usually initiate smoking as teenagers. As of 2001, 22 percent of high school students had smoked at least one cigarette prior to age 13; about 30 percent of ninth-grade girls and 40 percent of high school girls admitted smoking within 30 days prior to being interviewed.[8] Smoking rates for women who have less than a high school education are three times higher than for women who are college graduates.

Ethnicity is a factor in the prevalence of women who smoke. American Indian and Alaska Native women had the highest prevalence of smoking followed by white and African American women; the lowest prevalence was found among Hispanic, Asian, and Pacific Islander women.[9]

Each of these factors plays a significant role in the probability that a woman will die prematurely from the use of tobacco: the earlier the age at which a woman starts to smoke, the longer she smokes, the more she inhales, and the higher the level of tar and nicotine in the tobacco product.

Why Women Smoke

Media influence is pervasive, compelling, and influential. There are thousands of television stations, radio stations, daily newspapers, and magazines and billboards, all of which reach millions of women on a daily, even hourly basis. Many thousands of these media avenues promote the concept that smoking relates to a desired image and lifestyle, fun times, attraction to others, athleticism, and quiet moments in beautiful surroundings. Mass media has certainly been utilized by the tobacco companies to zealously promote their product. In fact, cigarettes are one of the most widely advertised consumer products in this country even though this commodity has been banned from television and radio advertising since 1971. Emerson Foote, who was a well-known president of two large advertising agencies, states: The cigarette industry has been artfully maintaining that cigarette advertising has nothing to do with total sales. This is complete and utter nonsense. . . . I am always amused by the suggestion that advertising, a function that has been shown to increase consumption of virtually every other product, somehow miraculously fails to work for tobacco products.[10] In 2002, the U.S. tobacco industry spent $12.47 billion advertising various tobacco products; this equates to $34 million each day.[11]

Through advertisements, the tobacco industry captured some of women's energy, perhaps unrest, and certainly their desire to make some of their own decisions. Using slogans, pictures, and scenarios, cigarette manufacturers promoted the idea of freedom, choice, and appeal. Female movie stars, music, and eventually television stars, all portrayed as desirable, attractive, modern, and sexy, were seen using tobacco—they "modeled" the woman who other women wanted to be. To the "common" woman, the women in tobacco advertisements personified confidence, a positive self-image, and appeal. Why not use a product that produces all of those benefits? The billions of dollars the tobacco industry has spent in promoting its products through the years has influenced women to embrace tobacco use and, in the process, negatively affected their environment, their health, and even the well-being of their children.

Maintaining weight may be another reason that women choose to smoke. Have you heard the comment that women experience weight gain once they quit smoking? There is an explanation for this. Nicotine decreases the strength of hunger contractions in the stomach (e.g., inhaling the smoke of one cigarette can reduce "hunger pains" for almost an hour), increases blood sugar level, and deadens taste buds. As an oral habit, smokers associate hand-to-mouth activity with pleasure (or relief from anxiety); therefore, when smoking stops, hand-to-mouth objects (food) substitute for the former hand-to-mouth smoking behavior. With cessation of smoking, the senses of taste and smell increase; therefore, food becomes more appealing. It is important to remember that the average weight gain following smoking cessation is only 5 pounds.[12] However, the amount of weight gain depends on the individual and her willingness to engage in behaviors that reduce the possibility of weight gain following the cessation of smoking. (See *Health Tips:* "Avoiding Weight Gain after Smoking Cessation" for suggestions to avoid weight gain.) There are far better ways to control eating than to engage in a behavior that is harmful and possibly lethal. Imagine this—a woman would need to gain between 50 and 100 pounds before she could come close to the equivalent health risks associated with tobacco smoking.

Other factors also influence women to use tobacco. As unbelievable as it may be, some women are unaware of the health risks that result from smoking tobacco; as you read this chapter you will gain a better understanding of these risks. Parental smoking influences children to adopt this behavior; children whose parents smoke (especially if *both* parents smoke) are much more likely to become smokers themselves than are children whose parents don't smoke. We are certainly influenced by our peers; almost 90 percent of teens who smoke have friends who also smoke, and young women who smoke are more likely to have boyfriends who are also smokers. Additionally, if "your group" is composed of numerous smokers, there is a much greater chance that you will also become a smoker. For example, associating with coworkers who smoke and friends who smoke at clubs and parties, or engaging in an activity at which participants smoke, such as bowling, may increase your chances of smoking. The environment in which we work and recreate plays a part in the choice to use tobacco. Take *Assess Yourself:* "Could You Become a Smoker?" to determine which factors could influence you to become a smoker.

Health Tips

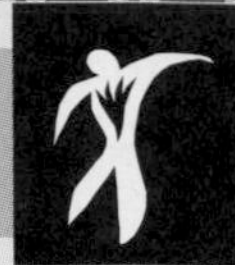

Avoiding Weight Gain after Smoking Cessation

If you are a former smoker and want to control the possibility of weight gain, consider the following suggestions. You may even want to incorporate these suggestions into your lifestyle as a matter of improving your overall good health habits.

- Have low-fat, nutritious snacks easily accessible to help satisfy the hand-to-mouth habit.
- Keep a straw or other harmless object handy to chew on or use with your hands.
- Enlist the help of a significant other and try new activities together.
- Walk, jog, bike, or swim at least three times per week.
- Include in your diet your very favorite food (in moderation) at least once each week.
- Reward yourself at designated intervals for remaining smoke-free.

Assess Yourself

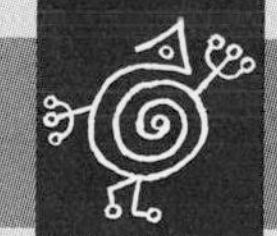

Could You Become a Smoker?

Listed below are a number of factors you may have encountered that may influence you to become a smoker. Check those that apply to you. Obviously, the more checkmarks you have, the greater the likelihood that you could become a smoker.

Factors	Yes	No
1. Mother smokes(ed)	_____	_____
2. Father smokes(ed)	_____	_____
3. Siblings smoke(d)	_____	_____
4. Friends smoke(d)	_____	_____
5. Coworkers smoke	_____	_____
6. Boyfriend or husband smokes	_____	_____
7. Believe smoking is okay	_____	_____
8. Know the health consequences of smoking	_____	_____
9. Like the way someone looks when smoking	_____	_____
10. Believe that you can relax by smoking	_____	_____
Total points	_____	_____

The best advice is that if you don't smoke, *don't start!* If you do smoke, *quit!*

SUBSTANCES IN TOBACCO

Over 4,800 chemical compounds are found in tobacco smoke, several thousands of which come from tobacco plants and derive from additives, pesticides, and a multitude of other compounds.[13] Approximately 60 of these are **carcinogenic,** or cancer-causing, compounds including tar, carbon monoxide, hydrogen cyanide, ammonia, formaldehyde, benzene, and nicotine.[14] Various compounds in tobacco smoke, such as carbon monoxide, are so potent that continual exposure would be lethal. There are numerous way that cigarette smoke does its damage. One is oxidation stress that mutates DNA, promotes atherosclerosis ("hardening of the arteries") and leads to chronic lung injury. Oxidative stress is thought to be the general mechanism behind the aging process, contributing to the development of cancer, cardiovascular disease, chronic obstructive pulmonary disease (COPD). and other diseases.[15]

An in-depth look at three major tobacco components—nicotine, poisonous gases, and particulate matter (tar)—will provide a better understanding of this drug. Each component has its unique set of consequences leading to serious illnesses and possible death.

Nicotine is a highly physically and psychologically addicting stimulant substance that has an accelerating effect on the central nervous system (CNS). The addictive property of nicotine, which acts on the dopamine neurotransmitter in the brain, provides insight into the reason so many women continue to smoke even with knowledge of multiple health risks. The immediate stimulation effect, produced by the release of adrenalin from the adrenal glands, causes an increase in heart rate, respiratory rate, and oxygen consumption, and a rise in blood pressure due to the constriction of peripheral blood vessels and bronchial tubes. As adrenalin increases the heart rate, there is an increased need for oxygen *by* the heart, but not an increased supply of oxygen *to* the heart, which can create serious consequences. Increased electrical activity of the CNS can induce arrhythmia (irregular heartbeat); increased platelet adhesives in the arteries can lead to possible blood clotting. As you might imagine, the body's immediate response to nicotine can seriously affect the entire cardiovascular system.

Once inhaled, nicotine enters the respiratory system and reaches the brain in a number of seconds. Intravenous nicotine takes about 13.5 seconds to travel from arm to brain; inhalation of nicotine is delivered to the brain in 7.5 seconds.[16] Nicotine acts as quickly as cyanide in delivering toxic chemical components to the body. Sixty milligrams of nicotine is a lethal dose in humans, causing death in only a few minutes. There is enough nicotine in one cigar for two lethal doses. An incredible 90 percent of the nicotine that reaches the lungs is absorbed into the bloodstream. Of the total amount of nicotine that enters the body, approximately 10 percent leaves the body chemically unchanged; the remaining 90 percent is metabolized by the liver and excreted in urine.

Over 270 *poisonous gases* are present in tobacco smoke, including carbon monoxide, nitrogen, carbon dioxide, hydrogen, and cyanide. Carbon monoxide, one of the best-known gases in tobacco smoke, increases the heart rate, elevates blood pressure, and impairs visual acuity. Carbon monoxide combines with oxygen to form *carboxyhemoglobin*. As a result, instead of oxygen being delivered to vital cells, tissues, and organs, a poisonous gas arrives and robs the body of life-giving oxygen. The blood of women who smoke today can have carbon monoxide levels far above the standards allowed for industry by the U.S. Air Quality Act.

Particulate matter, or **tar,** is a mixture of ingredients that are inhaled into the lungs when a person smokes and that inhibit effective functioning of the respiratory system. More than 90 percent of particulate matter remains in the smoker's lungs. Imagine your lungs coated with a sticky, yellow-brown substance that contains carcinogens. *Polycyclic aromatic hydrocarbons* are carcinogenic hydrocarbons, such as pyrenes, benzo(a)pyrenes, and chyrsenes, some of which have been linked to a gene that causes lung cancer.[17] Small particles of tar and gases move to air sacs in the lungs, called **alveoli,** and larger particles remain on the various passages that lead to the lungs.

Tar, as well as gases, creates another serious concern in the lungs. **Cilia,** hairlike structures that line the bronchi (the two primary divisions of the trachea that lead into the lungs), help to clear the lungs by sweeping debris, dust, and particles out of lung passages; then these are expelled through coughing or sputum. However, gases and particulate matter deposited by smoking damage the cilia, sometimes permanently, and therefore the cilia do not function to rid the lungs of tar and other debris. Therefore, the carcinogenic-laden tar stays in contact with the respiratory tract lining, which can lead to changes in cellular structure and to formation of cancerous tumors.

ADVERSE HEALTH EFFECTS

Smoking generates serious health problems for women just as it does for men, and long-term use of tobacco will cause various ill effects to become more discernible. Compared to nonsmokers, women who smoke more than double their annual risk of dying as a result of tobacco use.

Respiratory Concerns

Bronchiectasis is a condition that develops within the bronchial tree (the "branches" of the bronchi) and results in irreversible dilatation and destruction of the bronchial walls. Inflammation of airways and alveoli results in scarring and loss of elasticity in the airways of the lungs. Chronic bronchitis, characterized by long-term and persistent severe coughing, spitting, and excessive secretion of mucus, is a precursor to bronchiectasis. Smoking cigarettes causes the development of bronchitis or exacerbates the inflammation. This inflammation of the airways causes the passages to squeeze shut during exhalation, preventing the lungs from emptying completely.

Emphysema is a lung disease that occurs when tiny air sacs in the lungs are damaged, usually from long-term smoking. As airways lose their elasticity and trap unexpired air and toxins, the alveoli are destroyed and, thus, tear as a result of the pressure of inflation. Loss of alveoli will reduce the amount of surface area for gas exchange. This disease causes chronic shortness of breath due to the difficulty in exhaling and poor distribution of inhaled air in lungs. As a result, the heart must work harder to exchange and deliver oxygen-laden blood throughout the body. (See *FYI:* "The Reality of Emphysema" to learn more about emphysema.)

FYI

The Reality of Emphysema

Try this activity to have some realistic feeling of how the lack of the ability to breathe affects a woman physically, emotionally, and socially. Cut a small straw into about a 3-inch section. Place it between your lips, hold your nostrils closed and with lips closed tightly around the straw, breathe only through the straw for 1 minute. (Note: If you are unable to do this for 1 minute, stop any time you feel the need.) As you struggle to breathe through the straw, think of these questions:

- What is the most immediate physical need that you feel?
- Do you feel any dizziness?
- Is there a feeling of panic or wanting to gasp for breath?
- Could you walk up a flight of stairs breathing through the straw?
- With this limited air supply, could you engage in any recreational activity you enjoy (e.g., tennis, jogging, biking, swimming)?
- Would you be able to enjoy all the aspects of social or intimate relationships?
- In what other ways would difficulty in breathing affect your lifestyle?

Although the advertising media associates smoking with youth, vitality, and healthy appearance, the reality is the absolute opposite. Emphysema is only one disease that results from the use of tobacco; the only way to avoid the limitations that this disease creates is not to smoke.

Cardiovascular Diseases

Women who are smokers have a greater potential for developing heart disease and stroke than women who do not smoke. In fact, smoking is one major, if not *the* major, risk factor for the development of diseases of the cardiovascular system including hypertension, atherosclerosis, coronary heart disease, and aortic aneurysms. Smoking is linked to changes in blood chemistry. Cigarette smoking contributes to low levels of high-density lipoproteins (HDLs), which are considered to be beneficial components of the blood, and to an increase in low-density lipoproteins (LDLs). These two changes can lead to a buildup of plaque within the arterial system. The use of tobacco interferes with the production of red blood cells and reduces the blood's ability to clot, which can increase the possibility of hemorrhage during accidents or childbirth. Tobacco is a *vasoconstrictor,* and as such it can cause constriction of the coronary arteries. This condition is potentially dangerous because coronary arteries are the primary source of blood supply to the heart muscle; therefore, the reduction of blood supply to heart muscle tissue, even briefly, can at least damage the heart and at worst be fatal. Another detrimental effect of constricted blood vessels, combined with an increased heart rate, is the increase in blood pressure. The arterial system, therefore, endures more wear and tear as the heart works to force blood through smaller vessels creating high blood pressure. Smokers are more susceptible to cerebral infarction, or "stroke," due to the above-mentioned factors.

Taking oral contraceptives *and* smoking cigarettes increases the risk of heart attack, stroke, and blood clots in women over age 25. In fact, a woman is more likely to have a *fatal* heart attack if she smokes and uses oral contraceptives than if she only smokes.[18] The very serious likelihood of having a heart attack or stroke if you smoke and take birth control pills prompted the Food and Drug Administration to mandate that all oral contraceptives must include labeling that reads, "Women who use oral contraceptives should not smoke."[19]

Smoking and Cancer

There is a strong relationship between cigarette smoking and the development of the vast majority of cancers

Her Story

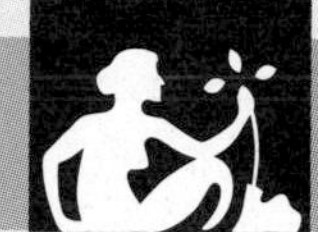

Sarah: Smoking and Lung Cancer

Sarah and her best friend, Betty, would sneak cigarettes from Sarah's mother's purse when they were very young. They pretended to smoke like her and the beautiful women they saw in their Saturday afternoon movie outings. In high school, Sarah smoked for real and developed an addiction to tobacco that she carried with her throughout college, marriage, and two pregnancies.

As Sarah "welcomed" her fortieth year, she began to experience a persistent cough and one respiratory infection after another. Her lack of energy, which she attributed to possible early menopause, curtailed her activity with her tennis group. She became frightened when she saw blood in her sputum. After a number of visits to her physician, she was advised to see her gynecologist. Then she went to see one medical specialist after another: a cardiologist, a respiratory therapist, and finally a pulmonary specialist who put Sarah through a series of tests that revealed shadows on her lungs. She was sent to an oncologist's office where, after X rays and **computerized tomography scans (CT scans),** she was diagnosed with lung cancer.

Not believing this could happen to her, Sarah sought the medical opinions of two other oncologists who confirmed the diagnosis of lung cancer. Anger, then rage filled Sarah's hours and days. Not to her, not to Sarah with the supportive, loving husband and family, the intelligent and well-liked children, the new house near friends and her tennis club! Yes, Sarah. Sarah of the 24-year smoking habit; the "I can quit when I want," Sarah.

Reality hit with the onset of her treatments: First, she received radiation to shrink the tumors, then surgery to remove all possible cancerous tissue, and then the series of chemotherapy treatments and the accompanying side effects. Amazingly, through all of this, Sarah still wanted a cigarette—she had a massive craving for nicotine and found the withdrawal from it one of the more difficult parts of the entire process.

Sarah's story does not end happily. She lost her battle against lung cancer 3 years after the original diagnosis. She lost the life she shared in her nice neighborhood with her loving husband and exceptional children. Sarah did quit smoking, but unfortunately she also quit everything else she loved and enjoyed.

- What symptoms did Sarah have that led her to the doctor?
- What suggestions do you have to prevent Sarah's tragedy from happening to other women?
- Have you ever thought that "this won't happen to me," and then lit up a cigarette and smoked anyway?
- What are your feelings about Sarah after reading her case study?

at sites located throughout the body. Smoking is associated with cancers of the oral cavity, larynx, pharynx, esophagus, lungs, stomach, uterus, and kidney. Risk of developing smoking-attributable cancers increases with the number of cigarettes smoked and the number of years of smoking.[20]

Smoking cigarettes accounts for 80 percent of the lung cancer deaths in women.[21] The 72,130 annual lung cancer deaths have replaced the 40,970 annual breast cancer deaths as the leading cause of cancer death in women.[22] Due to the continual exposure of body cells and tissues to carcinogens in tobacco smoke, women greatly increase the probability of developing many types of cancers if they choose to smoke. (See *Her Story:* "Sarah: Smoking and Lung Cancer.")

Other Physical Consequences

In addition to the health conditions already described, there are other health effects related to tobacco smoking. Research in many of these problem areas is ongoing. Cataract formation in the eyes of women has been researched; although the exact relationship between smoking and cataract formation is not known, smokers are two to three times more likely to develop cataracts than nonsmokers.[23] After surgery, smokers have more problems with wound healing and more respiratory complications.[24] Smoking causes peptic ulcers in smokers with *Helicobacter pylori* infections, and women smokers with ulcers usually develop complications of the ulcers.[25]

Conducting research on loss of bone density (e.g., osteoporosis) found that women who smoke have reduced bone density, which leads to an increased risk of hip fractures.[26] Female smokers often develop deeper facial wrinkles, sometimes called "smoker's face," at a faster rate than females who do not smoke. A possible explanation of this phenomenon may be the reduced amount of blood flow to the skin because of constricted blood vessels. Research in a multitude of areas continues; however, it seems clearly evident that women who smoke tobacco harm their bodies in many ways and increase their likelihood of premature death.

ADDICTION

Tobacco users develop a strong physical and psychological dependence on the product. A pack-a-day smoker has at least 50,000 hits of nicotine in a year; therefore, addiction and tolerance develop somewhat rapidly. Various studies have investigated the relationship between tobacco and addiction, and results indicate that between one-third and one-half of all individuals who experiment with smoking become addicted. According to one study, a large majority of people who smoke at least 100 cigarettes will ultimately become habitual smokers.[27] Does everyone who uses tobacco become addicted? No, in rare instances, 5–10 percent of individuals who smoke do not develop an addiction and do not experience withdrawal symptoms when they quit smoking.

Over 90 percent of women who smoke develop a dependence on nicotine, the major addicting agent in tobacco. Most women experience withdrawal symptoms such as irritability, lack of concentration, sleep disorders, anxiety, hunger, headache, and craving for nicotine if they stop smoking. A smoker's body cells adapt to a certain level of nicotine, and she is compelled to maintain that level. The half-life of nicotine, which is the time required for the body to eliminate one-half of the original drug dose, is about 100 minutes;[28] regular smokers seek to replenish nicotine as its level begins to drop following the initial peak concentration level.

Overcoming addiction is difficult, not only because of the physical and psychological dependency, but also because withdrawal symptoms are uncomfortable. Lifestyle rituals that accompany habitual smoking can also be difficult to change. Enjoying the morning cup of coffee, calling a friend, having a drink, riding in the car,

Viewpoint

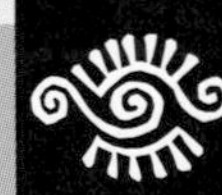

What Rights Does the Smoker Have?

As research continues to show that involuntary smoking is dangerous to women who breathe the chemical-laden smoke, more and more businesses, institutions, and schools are establishing a tobacco-free environment. Individuals spend the majority of their time indoors, which can lead to problems for smokers as well as nonsmokers. Designating smoking areas may not always protect the nonsmoker.

However, the individual who makes the choice to smoke does have a right to make that choice. Considering the rights of both smokers and nonsmokers creates a dilemma for businesses and institutions, as well as the personal environment of women in the home.

Consider the following questions and discuss the predicaments created by the situation:

- Does the person who smokes have a right to have a place to smoke?
- What can business and industry do to address the needs of both smokers and nonsmokers?
- If employers mandate a nonsmoking environment, should they pay for the assistance that the smoker may need to stop smoking?
- Where do individual rights and public rights begin and end in this situation?

or relaxing with a book may all be ritualistically tied to smoking a cigarette. Practices such as these bond the smoker to the substance and thus add to the difficulty of breaking the bonds between tobacco and user. (See *Viewpoint:* "What Rights Does the Smoker Have?")

ENVIRONMENTAL TOBACCO SMOKE

Environmental tobacco smoke (ETS), also referred to as *passive, involuntary,* or *secondhand* smoke, is inhaled from the surroundings in which we live and work. This smoke is discharged from the lighted end of the cigarette, called **side-stream smoke,** and accounts for about 85 percent of the smoke in a room where someone has a lighted cigarette. Side-stream smoke has two times as much tar and nicotine, three times as much carbon monoxide, and three times as much ammonia and benzopyrene as is found in **main-stream smoke,** which is the smoke drawn through the cigarette and inhaled and exhaled by the smoker. Side-stream smoke produces pollutants that, upon inhalation, lead to the creation of **free radicals** in the human body. Free radicals are toxic chemicals that cause damage to body cells and can lead to numerous ailments, including cancer. Remember, there is no filter for diluting the hazardous chemicals in side-stream smoke, so the smoke enters the person's environment with a higher concentration of unhealthy substances.

U.S. surgeon general Richard H. Carmona issued, in June 2006, a comprehensive scientific report which concludes that here is *no* risk-free level of exposure to secondhand smoke. The finding is a major public health concern due to the fact that nearly half of all nonsmoking Americans are still regularly exposed to secondhand smoke.[29]

The actual negative consequences from passive smoke are determined by the number of smokers in the room, as well as the number of cigarettes, ventilation, and amount of continual exposure. In the early 1990s, passive smoke was determined to present definite health risks to anyone who is exposed to it, especially on a long-term basis, such as smokers at home or at the workplace. A study of 1,906 women was conducted by medical center researchers to determine if there was a link between their exposure to side-stream smoke and the development of lung cancer. Of these women, 653 developed lung cancer. These researcher's found that women married to smokers were 30 percent more likely to develop lung cancer than those married to nonsmokers.[30] In this study, exposure to side-stream smoke was measured in environments outside the home. Passive smoke in the workplace produced a 39 percent increased risk of developing lung cancer, and women who were exposed to passive smoke for 2 hours a week for over 6 months in social settings had a 50 percent greater risk of developing lung cancer than non-exposed women. Women exposed to smoke both as a child and as an adult had almost twice the risk of developing lung cancer as women exposed only during the adult years.[31]

Is it any wonder that businesses, restaurants, schools and school events, airplanes, trains, and other entities have either banned smoking or segregated smokers into areas where nonsmokers will not be exposed to environmental tobacco smoke? As tobacco smoke adds significantly to indoor pollution, women usually experience watery, itchy eyes, coughing, wheezing, increased levels of stress, and unpleasant odors that often stay in clothes, skin, and hair long after the nonsmoker has left the smoking environment.

Children of smokers experience detrimental health effects from breathing air containing cigarette smoke. The more smoke a child is exposed to, the greater the child's health problems will be. Passive smoke increases the possibility of respiratory infections such as colds, bronchitis, and pneumonia, especially during the first 2 years of life. As children get older, if they continue to be exposed to passive smoke, they may develop a chronic cough and reduced lung function. The World Health Organization estimates that nearly 700 million—nearly half of the world's children—breathe air polluted by tobacco smoke.[32] Infants exposed to environmental tobacco smoke (ETS) have a reduced rate of lung growth.[33] Children exposed to ETS during childhood may have increased risks of developing cardiovascular disease in adulthood.[34] In addition to the physical

Journal Activity

A Bill of Rights

A "Bill of Rights" has been developed for nonsmokers. Briefly it includes guidelines related to the right to breathe clean air, to express one's discomfort around tobacco smoke, and to take legitimate action against tobacco pollution in one's personal environment. These are all fair and just ideas, as well as healthy suggestions. However, as discussed in the *Viewpoint:* "What Rights Does the Smoker Have?," there are also rights for people who choose to smoke. Even if you don't like the idea, write a "Bill of Rights for Smokers." Discuss these during a class period. Realistically, we must acknowledge that there are "rights" for both sides of this and many other issues.

consequences, the child of a smoker is more likely to become a smoker and to begin smoking at a young age.

Now that you have read about the effects of tobacco smoke, complete *Journal Activity:* "A Bill of Rights."

SMOKING AND PREGNANCY

Women who smoke while pregnant harm their babies in numerous ways, especially if they smoke throughout the gestation period. Despite knowledge that smoking during pregnancy has adverse health effects on the mother and the fetus, it is estimated that from 12 percent to 22 percent of pregnant women who smoke continue to do so *throughout* the pregnancy.[35] Negative consequences related to maternal smoking can be caused by nicotine's ability to constrict fetal blood vessels and breathing movements, and by carbon monoxide reducing the oxygen supply to fetal blood. Additionally, the ability of the fetus to metabolize vitamins is reduced. An increased risk of ectopic pregnancy has been shown to be related to maternal cigarette smoking during the time of conception, as well as almost two times the increased risk of spontaneous abortion (miscarriage). A research study conducted by Lieberman and colleagues found that maternal smoking during pregnancy, especially during the third trimester, produced reduced-weight babies.[36] A dose-related response has been found between smoking and infant birth weight: The more the mother smokes during pregnancy, the greater the infant weight reduction. Low birth weight is a leading cause of infant deaths, resulting in more than 300,000 deaths annually in the United States.[37] Children born to smoking mothers often will be shorter, have reduced reading and mathematical skills, exhibit hyperactivity, and have lessened social adjustment abilities than children born to nonsmoking mothers. Studies reveal that nicotine is found in breast milk; mothers who smoke while breast-feeding will transfer this drug and its potential effects to the infant.[38] As a result, the health and well-being of the newborn are placed in jeopardy. Smoking-related low birth weight and the requisite consequences to the baby are 100 percent preventable—don't smoke during pregnancy and avoid exposure to secondhand smoke!

Babies born to women who smoke during pregnancy have an increased likelihood of dying of **sudden infant death syndrome (SIDS).** This devastating death of an infant is generally unexplainable because the cause of death usually cannot be determined in a postmortem examination. This finding may be related to an environment in which the pregnant woman is exposed too often to passive smoke or due to the infant's exposure to environmental tobacco smoke. Studies have shown that one-half of women who quit smoking during pregnancy resume smoking once the baby is born.[39] Estimations are that 43 percent of all U.S. children between the ages of 2 months and 11 years live in an environment in which there is at least one smoker.[40]

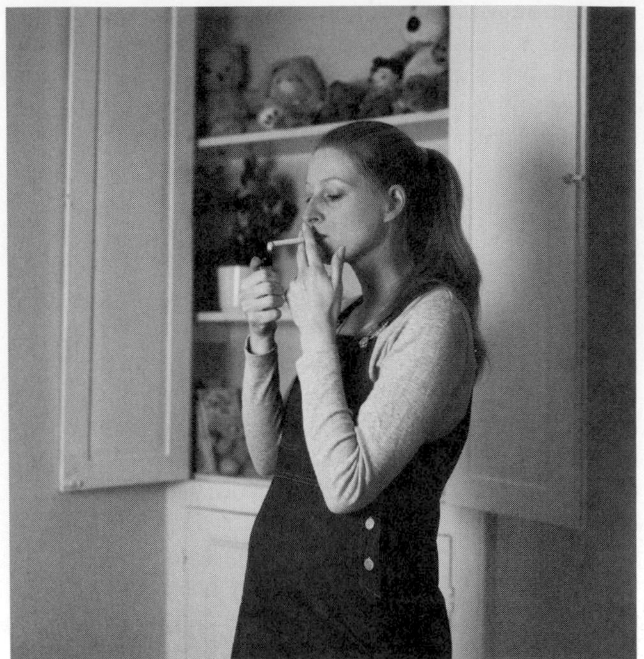

Pregnant women should avoid smoking as well as exposure to smoke to protect the health of the developing fetus.

During delivery, smoking mothers have an increased chance of hemorrhaging and an increased chance of delivering a stillborn infant or an infant that lives only for a brief time. Hospital stays are often longer for a smoking mother and her baby. Following delivery, smoking mothers heal slower and often must spend more time caring for newborns who have more difficulties with feeding, digestion, sleeping, and restlessness than newborns of nonsmoking mothers.

The bottom line is that there are serious health consequences for babies born to women who smoke during and after pregnancy. And there are also detrimental effects experienced by women who smoke during pregnancy. It is simple to avoid: do *not* smoke; if you smoke, it's time to quit.

SMOKING CESSATION

Why do women decide to quit smoking? According to one study, more than three-quarters of women who smoke want to quit, and almost one-half reported trying to quit.[41] Warnings of imminent health problems, becoming pregnant, having children, or working in a smoke-free environment can each provide the impetus to stop smoking. Smoking has become restricted in such areas as public buildings, domestic air flights, restaurants, and schools; the inconvenience of finding a place in which a person is allowed to smoke may lead to cessation of the habit. Most women quit several times before they are able to completely eliminate the habit. Each year, about 15 million smokers quit for at least one day, but fewer than 5 percent of them are able to stay tobacco-free for 3 to 12 months.[42] Therefore, smokers must be persistent in their attempts to stop. The benefits far outweigh the morbidity and mortality associated with smoking. Women may often need assistance in their attempts at smoking cessation, and a number of methods are available to assist women who want to quit.

Behavioral Changes

There appears to be no easy or right way to quit smoking, and those who have made the attempt, usually many times, will attest to that fact. Smoking cessation appears to be most successful for women who really want to quit and who consider all the beneficial reasons to quit and barriers that could make cessation unlikely.

Even though many women successfully quit on their own, **smoking cessation programs** that provide counseling and support groups may be more successful for women who smoke 25 or more cigarettes a day. Formal smoking cessation programs vary in their success rate, but, about one-third of smokers who quit for a year often start again.[43] Research reveals that success in smoking cessation is more likely when a woman has a readiness to quit and believes that she will be successful.

Nicotine Replacement Products

In recent years the FDA has approved several products that can help smokers quit. The products deliver small, steady doses of nicotine into the body to relieve some of the withdrawal symptoms and avoid the "high" that keeps the smoker addicted. There are a number of nicotine replacement products available, either by prescription or as over-the-counter products. These include two nicotine patches, nicotine gum, nicotine lozenges, nicotine nasal spray, and a nicotine inhaler.[44]

Nicotine chewing gum (Nicorette) contains 2–4 mg of nicotine. It has been on the market since 1984, first through prescription and since 1996 as an over-the-counter product. The dosage of nicotine in this product is intended to reduce the unpleasant effects associated with nicotine withdrawal, and it eliminates exposure to other harmful chemicals in tobacco. When a smoker craves a cigarette, she places a piece of gum in her mouth and chews very slowly. Nicotine gum is not designed to be chewed like normal gum. Persons who use this method intermittently chew and "park" the gum between the cheek and gums. A peppery taste or tingling sensation signals the smoker when to chew and when to "park" the gum. After 2 to 3 months the smoker is usually ready to reduce the use of the gum and eventually move toward the use of "sugarless" gum without nicotine. Usually chewing 9 to 12 pieces of gum per day controls the urge to smoke, but the maximum number should not exceed 24 pieces, depending on the type of Nicorette.[45] Caution: Do not continue to smoke when beginning nicotine gum therapy. Average cost is approximately $5 a day for average use for the first 6 weeks.

Nicotine replacement patches have been on the market since 1992, and in 1996 they became available as an over-the-counter product. Name brands for nicotine replacement patches are Nicoderm, Habitrol, Prostep, and Nicotrol; each resembles a small, thin bandage strip and delivers a continuous flow of nicotine through the skin. The patch, available in 21-, 14-, and 7-mg strengths, must be replaced daily and each time should be applied to a different area of dry, clean, nonhairy skin. It should be left on for the amount of time recommended in the package insert; some brands are to be worn all day, but one particular brand is worn only during the waking hours. The patch cannot be put on and removed as a substitute for a cigarette. Smokers usually start with a higher dosage of nicotine and after 1 to 2 months reduce the dosage, followed by another reduction within 2 to 4 weeks. The intent is eventually to eliminate all reliance on nicotine. Side effects exist from use of the patch, but they are usually minimal. The most common side effect is skin irritation in the area where the patch is placed, causing a mild itching, burning, or tingling. Important: Do *not* smoke *and* use the patch due to the potential of producing a heart attack. Pregnant or breast-feeding women should not use the patch, and people with angina, ulcers, or hypothyroidism should consult their physician before using this product. The average cost for over-the-counter nicotine replacement patches is about $4 per day.

The *nicotine lozenge* is the newest nicotine replacement product to be approved by the FDA. The nicotine lozenge resembles a piece of hard candy and slowly releases nicotine as the lozenge dissolves in the mouth. It is not recommended to bite and chew the lozenge as doing so could cause indigestion or heartburn. Available in 2 mg and 4 mg dosages, one lozenge is one dose and the dosage should not exceed 20 lozenges per day.[46] Avoid eating and drinking 15 minutes prior to using the lozenge and while it is in the mouth. Potential side-effects include soreness of teeth and gums, indigestion, and irritated throat. The cost is about $6 a day for average use (12 doses) up to $12 a day for maximum usage.

Nicotine nasal spray (Nicotrol NS) is a prescription-only nicotine replacement product approved in 1996 by the FDA. The method of delivery is inhalation through the nose from a pump bottle and then absorbed through the nasal lining into the bloodstream. Because nicotine is quickly absorbed through the nasal membranes, it reaches the bloodstream faster than any other nicotine replacement product and gives the user a quick "hit" of nicotine. While this is an effective delivery system, nasal and sinus irritation are common side effects of the nicotine nasal spray and, therefore, it is not recommended for people with nasal or sinus conditions, allergies, or asthma. The usual dosage is two sprays, one in each nostril, with a recommended maximum dose of 5 per hour or 40 per day. This product is intended for use for no more than 6 months with the idea that women will continue to reduce the number of times it is used during that time period. The average cost is about $5 per day for average use (13 doses), up to $15 per day for maximum usage (40 doses).[47]

The nicotine inhaler (Nicotrol) is a nicotine inhalation system, available only by prescription, that has been on the market since 1997. A mouthpiece attached to a plastic cartridge delivers nicotine inside the user's mouth. Nicotine is not delivered to the lungs, even though it is called an inhaler. Rather, it is delivered to the mouth and throat where it is absorbed through the mucous membranes. Each inhaler delivers up to 400 puffs of nicotine vapor, and it takes about 80 puffs to equal the nicotine in one cigarette. The maximum suggested dose is 16 cartridges per day. It is recommended for use for only 3 months. The Nicotrol inhaler can cause cough and throat irritation, and persons with a bronchospastic disease such as asthma should use it cautiously. The average retail cost of the nicotine inhaler is about $45/package, which contains 42 cartridges.[48]

Zyban (bupropion hydrochloride), approved in 1997 by the FDA, is a nicotine-free antismoking pill that reduces nicotine withdrawal symptoms and the urge to smoke. It is a prescription-only nicotine replacement product. Researchers are not sure exactly how the pill works, but it appears to affect the chemicals in the brain associated with nicotine addiction. Zyban can be used in combination with any of the previously mentioned nicotine replacement products under the supervision of a physician. Zyban use starts while the user is still smoking, 1 week before the quit date, and usually continues from 7 to 12 weeks. There should be at least 8 hours between doses, which is generally a total of 300 mg/day. Common side effects include dry mouth, sleep difficulties, shakiness, and skin rash; in rare cases (about 1 in 1,000) a person may have seizures. Women who have an eating disorder or epilepsy, or who are pregnant or breast-feeding, should not take Zyban. The average wholesale price of buproprion (generic Zyban) is $2.50 per day.

Chantix (varenicline), a new prescription medication approved for smoking cessation in May 2006, has the potential to be a significant therapeutic advance over existing therapies. This is the first new drug directed toward smoking cessation that the FDA has approved since 1997.

Chantix is unique because it is specifically designed to partially activate the nicotinic receptor and reduce the severity of the smoker's craving for, and the withdrawal symptoms from, nicotine. This new prescription drug, taken in a 1-mg dosage twice a day, is purported to nearly double the chance of quitting over Zyban and quadruples the chance of smoking cessation over placebos. Moreover, if a person smokes a cigarette while receiving treatment, Chantix has the potential to diminish the sense of satisfaction associated with smoking. This may help to prevent the cycle of nicotine addiction.[49]

Women must be aware of the serious consequences if they continue to smoke while using nicotine substitutes. Nicotine overdose symptoms include tremors, respiratory failure, low blood pressure, and fainting. Although these products provide a positive step toward smoking cessation, they are only one method. Drugs alone will not stop the smoker; a smoking cessation program needs to include support from family and friends and perhaps a formal stop-smoking program sponsored by the American Cancer Society or the American Heart Association. (See *Health Tips:* "Choosing a Smoking Cessation Program.")

How to Stop Smoking!

The American Cancer Society (ACS) has a variety of highly effective materials that individuals and groups can use to make the smart move and stop this life-destroying habit. The ACS suggests:[50]

- Make a decision to quit
- Set a quit date
- Make a plan
- Change smoking-related habits
- Deal with withdrawal
- Stay tobacco-free

Looking at each of these suggestions in more detail and following the steps suggested increases the smoker's understanding and chances of stopping this addiction.

In developing a plan to quit smoking, it is essential to determine the triggers that result in the use of tobacco, meaning the links between an event and smoking a cigarette. Discovering when and where you light up and what you are doing prior to lighting a cigarette can be a key component for successful smoking cessation. When

Health Tips 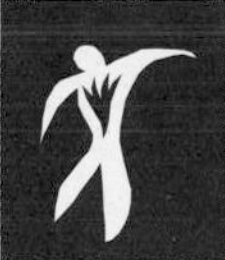

Choosing a Smoking Cessation Program

Formal smoking cessation programs can provide structure, suggestions, and support for women who need a specialized "tool in their stop-smoking tool box." They are intended to help women who smoke recognize and cope with problems that arise during their attempt to stop. Here are some tips to finding a program that can lead to successful smoking cessation. Effective smoking cessation programs

- Offer group or individual counseling.
- Have intense program counseling and goals.
- Have a leader who is trained in smoking cessation.
- Have sessions that are at least 20–30 minutes in length.
- Have at least four to seven sessions.
- Last for at least 2 weeks.

Avoid smoking cessation programs that

- Use pills, injections, or "special" or "secret" cures.
- Promise easy success with little effort from the smoker.
- Require a lot of money to participate.
- Cannot or will not provide references from previous attendees.

SOURCE: Adapted from American Cancer Society. 2006. *Guide to quitting smoking*. www.cancer.org (retrieved April 18, 2007).

the trigger occurs, find something else to do instead of smoking. Suggestions include take a walk, chew on a straw, have a glass of water, call someone, and chew sugarless gum.

Plan a "stop day" and complete and sign a "Stop Smoking Contract." Ask a friend to sign it as a means of support. Throw all cigarettes and related items away from your home, your car, and any other place where you may be tempted to smoke. You will feel a strong desire to smoke, but use the "Four D" technique to quell this feeling: delay, deep breathing, drink water, and do something else. Other suggestions include keeping objects such as gum, straws, and low-caloric snacks near when you need/want something in your mouth; utilizing nicotine chewing gum or patches, if needed; announcing that you are no longer going to smoke; placing "No Smoking" signs in important places; and treating yourself with something special when you stop.

Quitting smoking is one thing; remaining smoke-free may be more difficult. Some negative feelings may result within the first few days to weeks during withdrawal from nicotine. It is important to remember that these are normal and that they will go away. Find something else to do to cope with stressful situations other than falling back to a former bad habit—smoking! Include moderate exercise and nutritious, low-calorie food in your cessation program to avoid weight gain. Continue to remember all the very important reasons not to smoke. In fact, write them down often. Feel proud because, by quitting, you have done a healthy thing for yourself, for others, and for the future. Your life and the lives of people around you will be healthier and more enjoyable. If you remain smoke-free for 3 months, you will probably be able to enjoy the rest of your life as a nonsmoker.

It is clear that there are no positive outcomes from smoking, but there is an array of detrimental consequences. Prevention is essential because tobacco ingredients are highly addictive and smoking is difficult to quit. Because the vast majority of smokers start smoking before 18 years of age, educational systems must play a major part in prevention education. Schools and colleges should develop and enforce policies that prohibit tobacco use on the premises. Prevention education, beginning in kindergarten through grade 12, should include short- and long-term negative physiological, social, and financial consequences, as well as peer influence and refusal skills. Teachers need to be specifically trained to provide tobacco and other drug education, and families and the community need to be a part of the effort to prevent tobacco use.

BENEFITS OF SMOKING CESSATION

Quitting smoking makes a big difference—and quickly. Food begins to smell and taste better, and the smoker also smells better. The cough disappears, and energy begins to return. Women who have stopped smoking are sick less often, miss fewer days at work and play, and have fewer complaints about their general health than women who continue to smoke. Women increase their chance of quitting smoking when they have a low level of stress, a supportive nonsmoking partner, a high education level, and a positive sense of well-being.[51] (See *Women Making a Difference:* "Ann Richards: Former Governor of Texas.")

Incentives for smoking cessation can be enhanced when women realize that within a few minutes of quitting, their health can be affected in many positive ways. Table 13.1 summarizes the short- and long-term benefits that can be gained when a woman quits smoking.

Women Making a Difference

Ann Richards: Former Governor of Texas[52]

Ann Richards, governor of Texas from 1991 to 1995, was one of the most flamboyant and courageous political figures in Texas history. She held a number of political offices prior to her election as governor and made her mark as a woman of purpose and action regarding important state issues. Her tenure as governor was highlighted by appointing minorities and persons with disabilities to statewide offices, making institutional changes in the Texas prison system, reviving the state economy and creating the first Texas lottery, developing a statewide review of governmental agencies, and promoting meaningful evaluation of public schools.

Governor Richards, however, did not claim these accomplishments as her greatest achievements. Richards called "one of the great, great stories" of her life—her recovery from alcoholism and tobacco addiction and her nearly 26 years of sobriety—her best triumph. Entering a rehabilitation program in 1980, following a heartrending intervention by friends and family, she made this bold step in order to continue with her life and burgeoning political career. Ann Richards made the decision to be transparent about her alcoholism, stating that she liked to tell people that alcoholism was one of her greatest strengths. Not only did she support fellow alcoholics through notes and visits, but she started treatment programs in Texas prisons. Her strengths in recovery from alcoholism and addiction to tobacco were a source of inspiration for countless others.

Sadly, former Governor Richards succumbed to esophageal cancer on September 13, 2006, at the age of 73, leaving an exceptional legacy in Texas and national politics and a life of purpose and strength.

TABLE 13.1 Short- and Long-Term Benefits of Smoking Cessation

As soon as 20 minutes after your last cigarette, your body will begin to benefit from not smoking. These benefits will continue as long as you do not smoke. However, you will lose each of these benefits even if you smoke only one cigarette a day.[53]

TIME SINCE SMOKING LAST CIGARETTE	BENEFIT
20 minutes	Reduced blood pressure and pulse rate; body temperature becomes normal
8 hours	Normal carbon monoxide levels in blood; blood oxygen level increases to normal
24 hours	Chance of heart attack decreases
48 hours	Senses of smell and taste improve; nerve endings start regrowing
2 weeks to 3 months	Blood circulation improves; easier to engage in activities because lung function increases by 30 percent
1 to 9 months	Decrease in coughing, shortness of breath, fatigue; cilia regrow in lungs allowing cleansing dust and mucus from lungs; reduced chance of respiratory infection
1 year	Risk of coronary heart disease is half that of a smoker's
5 years	Lung cancer death rate for former one-pack-a-day smoker decreases by almost half; stroke risk is reduced to that of a nonsmoker 5–15 years after quitting; risk of cancer of throat, esophagus, and mouth is half that of a smoker
10 years	Death rate from lung cancer is half that of a continuing smoker; precancerous cells are replaced by healthy cells; decreased risk of developing cancer of the mouth, throat, esophagus, bladder, kidney, and pancreas
15 years	Risk of coronary heart disease is that of a nonsmoker

CAFFEINE

Because of the association of coffee and other caffeinated beverages with smoking, coverage of caffeine is discussed here. A variety of beverages containing caffeine have become popular drinks in this country. Teas of many types are served with meals or combined with a serene environment to provide a quiet, refreshing break from a stressful day. Cappuccino, latte, espresso, and cafe mocha are all flavorful specialty coffees that have gained widespread popularity, sometimes as a replacement for a high-calorie and fat-laden dessert. Nationwide, there are currently thousands of coffeehouses brewing all varieties of coffee. Coffee consumers in the United States number over 166.6 million and spend over $10 billion in retail sales and over $9 billion in the food service area each year.[54] With 54 percent of the U.S. adult population consuming coffee, the individual coffee drinker spends an average of $165 each year on this product.[55] Women consume an average of 1.4 cups of coffee daily.

What Is Caffeine?

Caffeine is among a family of chemical compounds called **methylxanthines,** which stimulate particular neurotransmitters in the central nervous system (CNS). Found in over 60 plants and trees, caffeine has a long history of use in many drinks such as colas, tea, coffee, and cocoa, as well as over-the-counter drugs. Legend has it that a third-century goat herder noticed his flock become more lively and animated when chewing berries from a particular plant. Monks, seeing the effects on the flock, began using the berries for a brew that helped them stay awake during evening prayers.[56]

Various types of coffee beans produce varying tastes and deliver different levels of caffeine. For example, high-quality arabica beans, which are often used in specialty coffees, have a stronger taste and less caffeine than robusta beans, which often are used in national name-brand coffees. The amount of caffeine in a drink is measured in milligrams, and the potency will vary according to the type of coffee bean used in the drink and the way the beverage is brewed.

Caffeine, taken into the body in a water-soluble form, is absorbed into the bloodstream principally through the small intestine. It takes about 30 minutes following ingestion for initial effects on the CNS to be felt; peak effects are felt within 2 hours.[57] Along with all other organs of the body, caffeine is distributed to the brain. It may also be passed from the mother's blood through the placenta and to the fetus of any woman who is pregnant.

Effects of Caffeine

Why is the use of products containing caffeine so prevalent? Perhaps it is due to the wide variety of possible stimulating effects that caffeine produces. Among other reasons, millions of women use this drug to wake up and feel more energized each morning. It has been demonstrated to increase alertness, produce quicker reaction time, and reduce drowsiness. Coffee or colas are often the beverages that college women drink to help "pull an all nighter." This is because studies have shown that caffeine can improve reading speed, produce better results on math and verbal tests, and increase the capacity for sustained intellectual activities. However, if one desires to sleep, caffeine, even in small amounts, can cause sleep disturbances and increase the amount of time it takes to go to sleep.

Some of the research on caffeine's effects is inconsistent. For example, some studies indicate that this drug may *not* improve verbal or math abilities or short-term memory. Caffeine purportedly enhances athletic performance by helping the body metabolize fats for use as energy, saving glycogen for long-term energy. Drinking caffeine also appears to delay the exhaustion that athletes feel following exertion. Yet other studies basically refute these findings because they found little or no link between caffeine consumption and enhanced performance.

Caffeine Products

Coffee was not always the popular beverage that it is in today's society. It has fallen in and out of favor with humans living throughout the world. English women, in 1674, published an anti-coffee pamphlet titled "The Women's Petition Against Coffee," because it was believed that men who drank too much coffee were "less lustful and more unfruitful."[58] Not true!

Coffee, in instant form, was introduced in the late 1800s and gained popularity during World War II. Instant coffee is less flavorful but more convenient in today's busy world. As women continue to take on more time-consuming responsibilities, a quicker avenue to an enjoyable product is most appealing. A healthier product appears to be appealing, as well, as evidenced by current widespread use of decaffeinated coffee. Americans today are consuming more decaffeinated coffee and less caffeinated coffee than ever before.

Tea in its early history was used medicinally but later came to be used more as a drink for social occasions. Pound for pound, tea has more caffeine than coffee, yet more cups of tea (about 200) are produced from a pound of dry tea leaves than cups of coffee (about 50–60) are made from a pound of coffee beans.[59] Therefore, less caffeine is found in an average cup of tea compared to an average cup of coffee. The caffeine content in a 5-ounce cup of tea can range from 18 mg to 107 mg, depending on the brand and the type of brew. As with coffee, flavored teas, instant tea, and herbal teas (some with artificial sweeteners) have gained greater popularity at home and in restaurants in this country.

Colas today contain less than 6 mg of caffeine for each ounce of cola. These types of beverages, both caffeinated and decaffeinated, are consumed increasingly worldwide. The history of colas is basically the history of the Coca-Cola Company, and most cola products are a replication of this product. Colas are considered to be refreshing, stimulating, and in sync with today's active lifestyle. Caffeine is an added ingredient in colas, whereas it is found naturally in coffee, tea, and chocolate. Although sugar-free and caffeine-free cola products are available and widely consumed, the well-known classic cola with sugar and caffeine is still the most widely sold. In the United States, the consumption of all colas averages approximately 50 gallons per person per year.[60]

Chocolate was introduced in Europe before coffee or tea, but its use grew slowly because the method of preparing it was not widely known. One of the women of history, Maria Theresa of France, wife of Louis XIV, thoroughly enjoyed chocolate and was instrumental in the promotion of its consumption. From chocolate beans, ground chocolate kernels, chocolate liquor, or cocoa butter to the Nestlé milk chocolate of today, this substance has become one of the most widely consumed forms of caffeine. Caffeine in chocolate, though not as strong as caffeine in coffee, has similar physical effects. A cup of chocolate milk has about 4 mg of caffeine whereas caffeine in denser baking chocolate ranges from 5 mg to 35 mg per ounce.

A number of over-the-counter (OTC) drugs containing caffeine produce a stimulating effect and suppress the appetite. They also may act as a stimulus for elimination of body fluids, called a diuretic. Products such as No Doz, Midol, Aqua-ban, and some cold remedies have from 30 to 200 mg of caffeine as an active ingredient. Although one product alone may not impact greatly on daily caffeine consumption, women often ingest beverages, food, and OTC drugs each containing varying amounts of caffeine, which, when added together, can cause a number of unwanted physiological effects. (See Table 13.2.)

Now complete *Journal Activity:* "Your Caffeine Consumption" to determine your daily caffeine intake.

TABLE 13.2 Comparison of Caffeine in Common Products

PRODUCT	CAFFEINE (MG)*
Coffee	
Starbucks coffee, grande (16 oz)	550
Starbucks, caffé latte (8 oz)	35
Starbucks coffee (8 oz)	250
Starbucks, caffé mocha (8 oz)	35
Maxwell House coffee (8 oz)	110
Decaf coffee (8 oz)	5
Medicine	
No Doz, max strength (1)	200
Excedrin (2)	130
Anacin (2)	65
Soft Drinks	
Cola (12 oz)	35
Mountain Dew (12 oz)	55
Cocoa or hot chocolate (8 oz)	5
Tea, leaf or bag (8 oz)	50

*The milligrams (mg) listed for these products are the average caffeine levels for drugs, foods, and beverages.

SOURCE: *The Caffeine Corner: Products ranked by amount. 1996. Nutrition Action Newsletter.* http://cspinet.org/nah/caffeine/caffeine_corner.htm (retrieved October 17, 2006).

Journal Activity

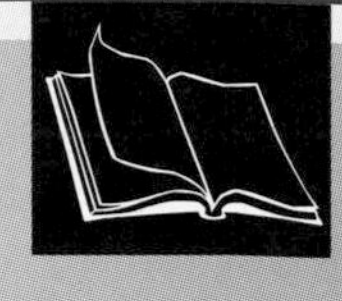

Your Caffeine Consumption

Over a 3-day period of time, record all intake of foods, drugs, and drinks you consume that contain caffeine. Determine your daily intake of milligrams of caffeine. The average intake of caffeine for a woman is 420 mg per day, about the equivalent of 4 to 5 cups of coffee. How does your consumption compare to this?

Effects of Caffeine on Health

Consumption of this psychoactive drug is widespread and acceptable; therefore, research studies regarding caffeine use are numerous, varied, and to a large degree inconclusive. Data have been collected researching caffeine and its relationship to cancer, osteoporosis, pregnancy, benign breast disease, heart disease, nutrient absorption, cholesterol, gastrointestinal problems, and others. Let's consider the results of some of the studies as they pertain to women.

Osteoporosis and Caffeine Osteoporosis is a loss of bone mass, especially in postmenopausal women, which can result in fractures and broken bones. A study reported by Bergman and colleagues found that women who consumed less than the recommended levels of calcium and who had a moderate intake of caffeine had decreased levels of calcium in the blood and increased bone tissue turnover.[61] More than two servings of foods or drinks with caffeine appear to increase the risk of having osteoporosis.[62] In this same report, researchers found a negative correlation between caffeine intake and dairy product intake, which magnifies the possibility of bone loss if a woman consumes low-calcium beverages in place of high-calcium beverages. The problem with loss of bone mass in women may not be due to consumption of caffeine-containing beverages, but drinking caffeine products instead of calcium-containing beverages. Women who do not consume calcium-rich foods throughout their life will increase their risk of osteoporosis, whether they drink caffeine or not.

Absorption of nutrients may be inhibited not by caffeine but by other substances in coffee, such as polyphenols. Important minerals, particularly calcium and iron, may not be utilized properly by the body as a result of drinking too many cups of caffeinated drinks each day. Because women are prone to develop osteoporosis, this information should create an awareness to be moderate in the consumption of caffeine-containing products.

Pregnancy and Caffeine Pregnancy and caffeine intake has been the subject of numerous studies. The American College of Obstetricians and Gynecologists recommends that pregnant women limit consumption of caffeine to one to two cups per day.[63] The intake of caffeine during pregnancy may cause slower growth rate for the fetus and therefore result in reduced birth weight.[64] Additional studies conclude that females who consume caffeine reduce their chance of conceiving and increase the risk of miscarriage even if caffeine is ingested a month prior to conception. Nursing mothers who consume high levels of caffeine every day report irritable and restless babies. Research is inconclusive about the levels of caffeine consumption that are safe. Because of this inconclusiveness, women should reduce or eliminate caffeine consumption if they are pregnant or are considering becoming pregnant.

Breast Health and Caffeine Fibrocystic breast disease consists of benign lumps that form in a woman's breast. Although these lumps are sometimes tender and painful, they are not cancerous. A plethora of research studies have found no relationship between caffeine intake and fibrocystic breast disease. However, some physicians advise women with benign breast lumps to eliminate caffeine consumption or at least to consume it moderately. However, there is little scientific evidence to suggest that elimination of caffeine from the diet will improve conditions associated with fibrocystic breast disease.

Caffeinism

Caffeinism is the result of continual and excessive use of caffeine products and may lead to a number of uncomfortable consequences. Women can develop a dependency and a tolerance to caffeine and, upon cessation of use, may experience headaches, nausea, irritability, depression, heart palpitations, insomnia, and reduced attention span. Although these symptoms are uncomfortable, they are short-lived and can usually be avoided by reducing caffeine consumption gradually.

Caffeine Research

As we have seen, caffeine research is largely inconclusive. Why is this so? Consider these variables: Each woman is biochemically different and the response to caffeine varies with each person; tolerance to caffeine may not be taken into account because studies often fail to isolate caffeine consumers from noncaffeine consumers; and the lifestyle of the research population may not be taken into account. For example, individuals who drink excessive amounts of coffee are sometimes more likely to smoke, have a high-fat diet, and not engage in exercise; therefore, negative health problems may be due to other lifestyle habits, not to caffeine consumption.

It appears that moderate use of caffeine-containing products produces no major detrimental effect, except for pregnant women. However, as with many other issues, it is best to check with your physician if there is a concern.

ILLEGAL DRUGS

Although both women and men use and abuse illegal drugs, women's abuse of drugs can yield more health problems than men's and these problems may progress differently in women than in men. In 2003, an estimated 12.5 million women used an illegal drug during the past year. Approximately 2 million women aged 18 or older met the criteria for abuse of or dependence on an illegal drug, including cocaine and marijuana.[65] In addition, hundreds of thousands of women have sniffed inhalants.

Many of today's illegal drugs were yesterday's legal drugs (such as cocaine and marijuana). Due to the potential for dependency and the devastating effects produced by using these drugs, the federal government declared them illegal substances. They cannot legally be bought, sold, used, or possessed in any state in the U.S.

Abuse of illicit drugs among women is of special concern. As women, we are responsible not only for our own personal health and well-being but also for the health and well-being of future generations. The discussion that follows explains how the abuse of drugs during pregnancy can produce devastating effects for both mother and fetus.

Drug Use and Pregnancy

Consequences to the fetus due to a woman's abuse of illegal drugs during pregnancy are of grave concern. Information about these consequences is not complete because of the ethics involved in conducting drug research on human babies. According to the combined 2003–2004 National Survey on Drug Use and Health data, an estimated 3.9 percent of pregnant women aged 15 to 44 used illicit drugs in the month preceding the survey.[66]

Research reveals that most drugs pass easily from the mother's blood through the placenta, the same route taken by oxygen and nutrients.[67] At least 90 percent of pregnant women take either prescription or nonprescription drugs, or use tobacco, alcohol, or illicit drugs sometime during their pregnancy. About 2 to 3 percent of all birth defects result from the use of drugs.[68] (See Table 13.3.) However, the time between drug intake and its transmission to the fetus varies with the type used. For example, marijuana can take hours to reach the fetal bloodstream, whereas opiates reach the fetus quickly. Data support the contention that alcohol causes fetal abnormalities, but research on the effects of various other illicit drugs on the fetus is inconclusive. Cocaine causes a decline in the delivery of oxygen and nutrients to the fetus because it is a *vasoconstrictor.* This results in an increase in blood pressure and heart rate. Marijuana increases the level of carbon monoxide in the blood, which decreases the amount of oxygen available to the fetus. Overall, drug use results in lower levels of oxygen and nutrients reaching the rapidly growing cells of the fetus.

Medical personnel should routinely ask pregnant women questions concerning their use of medications, alcohol, and other drugs. This information is important for administering proper medical care. Table 13.4 is an example of an indicator chart a physician might use to determine whether there is a need for urine and/or blood toxicology screening tests. Additional information regarding women and pregnancy can be found in Chapter 9.

If the outcome of the screening tests reveals that the woman is indeed using a particular drug, then immediate medical and antidrug treatment needs to be started. Additionally, drug therapy in the form of detoxification, support groups, and individual therapy should be sought. Upon delivery, the infant should be screened for drugs in the blood and, if the screening is positive, medical treatment as well as evaluation of the home environment is needed.

The following sections discuss the negative consequences of a woman's drug use on herself, her pregnancy, her fetus, and her newborn.

Cocaine and Crack

Cocaine is derived from a plant, *Erythroxylon coca,* which grows best in the mountains of South America. Substances in its leaves produce an exhilarating effect, providing quick energy, stimulation, and a sense of

TABLE 13.3 The Effects of Drugs on Mother and Baby[69]

ON MOTHER	ON BABY
Poor nutrition	Premature birth
High blood pressure	Low birth weight
Fast heart rate	Infections
Low weight gain	Small head size
Low self-esteem	Sudden infant death syndrome (SIDS)
Preterm labor	Birth defects
Sexually transmitted diseases	Stunted growth
Early delivery	Poor motor skills
HIV/AIDS	HIV/AIDS
Depression	Learning disabilities
Physical abuse	Neurological problems

TABLE 13.4 Indicators of Drug Abuse during Pregnancy[70]

INDICATOR	YES	NO
1. History of alcohol and other drug use?	____	____
2. Little or no prenatal care?	____	____
3. Mental condition such as incoherence or lethargy?	____	____
4. Lost custody of children?	____	____
5. Preterm delivery, labor, or membrane rupture in a previous pregnancy?	____	____
6. Third-trimester vaginal bleeding in a previous pregnancy?	____	____
7. Physical indicators of alcohol and/or drug use?	____	____
8. Symptoms of intoxication or withdrawal?	____	____

well-being. Early research in the 1800s led physicians to believe that cocaine was a new miracle drug. It appeared in patent medicines, tonics, and even leading soda drinks. Cocaine was found to be an effective topical anesthetic during surgery and beneficial for alleviating depression. As individuals became dependent on the products and medicines that contained this miracle drug, serious behavioral and health consequences resulted. Consequently, laws were enacted to put tight controls on the sale and use of cocaine. The Pure Food and Drugs Act in 1906 and the Harrison Act of 1914 reduced the legal availability of cocaine.

Crack is a rocklike substance that is the result of mixing cocaine with baking soda or ammonia. It is both easy to make and inexpensive to buy. Usually smoked in small pipes, it produces an almost immediate but brief high that is followed by depression and a strong longing for repeated use. Crack users quickly become dependent on the substance, often resulting in serious physical, legal, and financial consequences.

Consequences of Use The effects of cocaine on a woman's brain depend on the strength of the substance and the route of administration into the body. Cocaine can be inhaled by smoking, which requires only 8 seconds to reach the brain; absorbed by snorting, which requires 3 minutes to reach the brain; injected, which requires 14 seconds to reach the brain; or orally ingested, which requires 20 minutes to reach the brain.

Psychological and physical dependency develops with short- and long-term cocaine use. Research on both lab animals and humans reveals that the desire for cocaine effects is strong and that tolerance occurs with continual use. Tolerance is the capacity of the body to endure or become less responsive to a drug so that a larger amount is needed to obtain the same effect.

The short-term effects of cocaine use produce immediate bodily responses: increases in heart and respiratory rates and, coincidentally, an increase in blood pressure and elevated temperature. Appetite decreases, and the user feels more alert, excited, euphoric, and energized. The duration of cocaine's immediate effects depends on the manner in which it is taken. A faster route of administration, such as inhalation, will produce a more intense high and a shorter duration of action. However, due to lack of tolerance and experience and/or the high potency of cocaine, the user can also convulse, hemorrhage, or even experience heart failure.[71]

Long-time users of cocaine develop serious health consequences, including nasal inflammation, loss of appetite leading to malnourishment, a persistent cough, irregular heart rhythm, sleep disturbance, and even sexual dysfunction. Irritability, agitation, and paranoia can also result from continual use.[72] Psychological consequences can be as severe as paranoid psychosis. Fortunately, with the cessation of cocaine use, time seems to repair most of the physical and psychological damage.

Effects on Pregnancy Among pregnant women 15 to 44 years of age, 3.9 percent reported using illicit drugs in the month prior to the survey. However, over 9.9 percent of pregnant girls who are 15 to 17 years of age reported using illicit drugs in the month prior to the survey.[73] As a result, the effects on women and the number of cocaine and crack-exposed infants have also increased. Research has found a variety of consequences that occur from cocaine and crack use during pregnancy:

- **Intrauterine growth retardation,** which is delay in the development and maturation of the fetus, appears to be an outcome of cocaine use during pregnancy.
- Sudden and severe pregnancy complications such as premature separation of the placenta from the uterus, and even fetal and maternal death, can result.
- Premature labor and spontaneous abortion can result.

Consequences to the Fetus and Newborn The consequences of cocaine and crack use to the fetus and the newborn can be profound. While the full extent of the effects of pregnant women's cocaine use on their babies is not totally known, studies have determined that these babies are often born premature, have low birth weight, and have smaller head circumference. Fetal exposure to cocaine may lead to later deficits in cognitive performance and information processing and difficulty with attention to task, which reduces potential academic success.[74] Singer and Short studied the cognitive consequences of prenatal cocaine exposure to preschool children.[75] The research found that children scored significantly lower on some specific measures of intelligence; lower scores were especially significant in the areas of information, arithmetic, and reflecting visual-spatial skills. However, in examining the home environment of these children, these researchers determined that effective child-rearing strategies may result in more positive outcomes for children affected by prenatal cocaine exposure.

Marijuana

Resurging after a decade of decline, marijuana (*Cannabis sativa*) is now more potent and troublesome than when it was widely used in the 1960s and 1970s. The current trend can be attributed to references to the substance on popular television shows, in music and movies, and merchandising or marijuana symbols. Proponents of marijuana can be found on personal Internet home pages expounding its virtues and calling for decriminalization and legalization.

Cannabis is a unique and complex plant that contains over 400 chemicals, with the most active ingredients being the cannabinoids (of which THC is the most active). As a result of advances in plant genetics and growing methods, *Cannabis* growers have produced a more potent plant containing stronger substances, particularly the plant's active ingredient, **tetrahydrocannabinol (THC).** Drug products from *Cannabis sativa* include marijuana, which can be smoked in joints or pipes, or ingested in teas or other foods; hashish, which is the dried resin from the flowering and leafy parts of the plant; and hash oil, consisting of resins and other juices often spread onto tobacco cigarettes. Depending on the part of the plant used for consumption and its preparation, the percentage of THC can vary from 1 percent in the domestic *sativa* plant to 8–14 percent or more THC found in hashish. The higher the THC, the greater the consequences are to the marijuana user.

Marijuana can produce sedating, hallucinating, intoxicating, and/or analgesic effects. The effects of smoked marijuana are felt immediately after the drug enters the brain within a matter of seconds and usually last from 1 to 3 hours. If marijuana is used with food or drink, the short-term effects begin more slowly, usually in ½ to 1 hour, and last for as long as 4 hours. Smoking marijuana yields several times more THC in the blood than does eating or drinking the substance.[76] Use of marijuana at moderate doses produces feelings of euphoria, relaxation, and peacefulness. Individuals may experience mood swings and an altered sense of time, space, and distance. There appear to be few immediate negative effects from short-term moderate marijuana use, but because of the altered sense of time, space, and distance, it is wise not to drive or use any type of power tools or devices.

Consequences of Use After decades of research, we know that a multitude of negative consequences can result from chronic, long-term use of marijuana. Consider the following effects that are concerns for the body systems:

- *Central nervous system.* Reduces short-term memory, alters judgment, increases chances of developing mental illness, reduces cognitive skills, blurs and impairs vision perception, produces personality change, and alters motor coordination.
- *Respiratory system.* Can cause lung cancer, lung damage, pulmonary diseases, chronic bronchitis, and may cause trachea damage due to inhalation.
- *Cardiovascular system.* Produces tachycardia (rapid heartbeat), increases blood pressure and concerns related to angina and diabetes, and aggravates high blood pressure in women who already have angina and diabetes.
- *Reproductive system.* Disrupts the menstrual cycle, impairs ovulation and fertility, increases levels of testosterone in females, and may cause irreversible damage to the female ova.

Effects on Pregnancy Research on the effects of marijuana use on pregnancy and the fetus is lacking. However, once inhaled, THC easily crosses the placenta of the mother to the fetus and causes similar levels of THC in both mother and fetus. Studies have shown that infants born to women who smoked marijuana during pregnancy are likely to weigh less and are shorter in length than infants born to nonsmoking women. Other studies revealed that babies who were chronically exposed to marijuana chemicals in their environment had poor nervous system responses and less response to visual stimulation. Additionally, THC is transported to nursing babies through breast milk.

Heroin and Methadone

Originally marketed as a cough suppressant, heroin is a very addictive, semisynthetic narcotic produced from chemically changed morphine, a naturally occurring opiate derived from the opium poppy plant. In its early history, heroin was thought to be safe and a substance that would aid in recovery from morphine addiction. Interestingly, by producing this drug from morphine, chemists made a drug that is three times more addicting than morphine.[77] Heroin was declared illegal in 1924 by the U.S. government when the addictive properties and negative consequences became clear, and it became unlawful to manufacture, import, or possess heroin.

Consequences of Use *Heroin* is a fast-acting narcotic that is injected directly into a vein or under the skin ("skin poppers"), or snorted or smoked. It produces a dreamlike state and a feeling of euphoria in users, who often feel they have found the panacea for all their problems and a way to temporarily escape to paradise. Like most other narcotics, heroin creates a strong physical and psychological dependency. Addiction is fairly rapid; usually within just a few weeks the user feels the need to increase the amount used to achieve the "high" that she originally felt; thus tolerance is developed quickly. If the drug user stops taking heroin, she will experience unpleasant withdrawal symptoms—chills, nausea, tremors, diarrhea, and/or leg and abdominal pain—which can sometimes be severe and extremely uncomfortable though not life-threatening. Addiction to this chemical creates a situation in which women become so dependent on this drug that they may engage in life-threatening activities such as prostitution or stealing, in a never-ending pursuit to feed the addiction. As a result, their health and quality of life suffer as do those, especially children, who live with and around them.

Among the dangers associated with heroin use are factors related to the lifestyle of the user that result in accidents, injuries, diseases, infections, and sometimes death. The type of heroin, its potency, the contaminants in the heroin, the method of use (injection, smoking, snorting) and the risks of obtaining this illegal drug all contribute to its devastating effects. Adding to the concerns are the extended effects the use of this drug has on children, families, health care and judicial systems, the workforce, and the health of future generations.

Methadone is a synthetic narcotic that can be taken orally and provides a longer duration of its effects than heroin or morphine, usually lasting from 24 to 36 hours. It was developed during World War II as a substitute for morphine. Methadone can be used legally; with a doctor's prescription, to help avoid the negative effects of heroin and morphine withdrawal. It also produces physical and psychological dependency, as well as tolerance and withdrawal symptoms. Many of the same physical problems that result from the use of heroin and morphine can result from the use of methadone. However, because it is intended to be used as a legal, prescriptive replacement for heroin or morphine, the quality and dose of the drug are controlled.

Effects on Pregnancy A woman who uses heroin or methadone during pregnancy is putting herself and her fetus at risk for very serious consequences. **Toxemia,** also called blood poisoning, can occur in the blood of a pregnant woman, resulting in intrauterine growth retardation and even premature rupture of the amniotic membrane. Use of heroin or methadone can cause miscarriage and can also adversely affect delivery because these drugs may cause preterm labor or breech birth (delivery of the baby bottom-first). Of course, there also may be no effect from use of heroin or methadone during pregnancy. However, the risks are not worth the harmful effects the drugs *might* produce.

Newborns of heroin-addicted mothers tend to have low birth weight and smaller head circumference. These babies may be born either premature or stillborn and have a ten-fold increased risk of sudden infant death syndrome (SIDS). Infants born to methadone-addicted women may have normal birth weight but soon may experience weight loss due to lack of sleep and hyperactivity and may have to go through withdrawal. Complications such as poor fetal growth, premature rupture of the membranes, and placental abruption can occur.[78] During the newborn period, serious prematurity-related health problems, such as breathing problems and brain bleeds, which may lead to lifelong disabilities, have been found among infants exposed to heroin in utero.[79] Lower levels of learning, difficult behavior, and poor adaptation abilities were found in preschool children who were born to women addicted to methadone and heroin.

The harmful effects of drug use notwithstanding, this lifestyle often creates negative outcomes during pregnancy for mother and child. Lack of prenatal care, poor nutrition, and vitamin and mineral deficiencies can occur due to the time, energy, and money the mother must spend engaged in finding, obtaining, and using heroin. Consequences of using dirty needles include bacterial infections, sores, and hepatitis, as well as the risk of contracting HIV infection. There is also a greater likelihood of contracting other STIs such as chlamydia, herpes, and gonorrhea. Each of these, of course, can be passed on to the fetus in utero or during delivery.

Amphetamines and Methamphetamines

Stimulant drugs, which are completely synthetic, increase the activity of the central nervous system, resulting in increased alertness, euphoria, excitation, elevated blood pressure, insomnia, and loss of appetite. Amphetamines are used medically for weight reduction, narcolepsy, and attention deficit hyperactivity disorder (ADHD). Amphetamines used at low dosages produce increased energy, alertness, and elevated mood, but at higher dosages blood pressure and heart rate increase to near dangerous levels. Abuse of these drugs can yield strong psychological dependence, tolerance, and possible psychosis, with periods of depression following discontinuation of use.

Methamphetamines—street names include *speed, crank, meth,* and *crystal meth*—are illegal and are often produced in home drug laboratories. The most dangerous form is crystal methamphetamine, or *ice;* when it is smoked, the effects can be felt within 7 seconds, producing powerful physical and psychological feelings of exhilaration. While there are immediate "good" feelings, long-term users often experience multiple consequences such as weight loss, malnutrition, immune system deficiencies, and damage to body systems. Women who abuse amphetamines or use methamphetamines reduce their quality of life and the lives of their children and family.

Effects on Pregnancy As with other drugs, amphetamines and methamphetamines can have profound effects if used during pregnancy. Potential effects include damage to the liver, heart, and brain of the fetus and abnormal bone and organ development. There is a greater risk of miscarriage, stillbirth, and premature birth. Use of all types of illegal drugs during pregnancy results in devastating effects for the fetus and usually long-term reduced quality of life.

ILLEGAL DRUGS AND SOCIETAL PROBLEMS FOR WOMEN

Women, Drugs, and HIV Infection

Although men still have the greatest number of AIDS cases, the number of women who contract HIV is increasing at a rate almost four times faster than that of men. Additionally, there is a chance that women will pass the virus to their unborn children, thereby doubling the tragic consequences. HIV is transmitted through direct exposure to body fluids (such as blood, semen, vaginal fluids, and mother's milk). Women can contract HIV as a result of vaginal or anal intercourse with an infected partner and by injecting an illegal drug with a needle that contains HIV-infected blood. Among women, 26.9 percent of new AIDS cases were attributed to injection drug use (IDU). At the end of 2003, IDU was the method of contracting HIV in 35 percent of women living with AIDS.[80]

Researchers are looking at the use of psychoactive drugs that are not necessarily injected, such as alcohol, marijuana, and cocaine, but can cause activity that increases the risk of contracting HIV. Women are more likely to have unsafe sex while under the influence of alcohol and other drugs; therefore, women have an increased opportunity to contract or transmit HIV. For example, a past study revealed that female crack smokers were six times more likely than nonsmokers to have had twenty or more sexual partners, fifteen times more likely to be involved with prostitution, and four times more likely to have other sexually transmitted infections (STIs).[81] This extent of sexual activity increases the chances of contracting HIV and other pathogens that cause sexually transmitted infections.

The association between contracting or transmitting HIV as well as other STIs while under the influence of drugs is a serious concern. Wambach and colleagues conducted a study of 694 women and, among other concerns, examined the relationships between HIV-risk behaviors and substance use.[82]

The researchers found a significant relationship between using drugs, such as alcohol, cocaine, crack, and/or heroin, and having multiple sex partners. Women who abused drugs were more likely to have partners who were also drug abusers; were unaware of their main partner's sexual history, sexual orientation, or HIV status; were more likely to be involved in prostitution; and were less likely to use condoms. The women in this study tended to believe they were more at risk for HIV only if they *injected* drugs. However, this study found a strong link between uses of these drugs and poor decision making about the main sex partners and safer-sex practices of these women. The research suggests that it is of primary importance to address the use of all drugs, not just IV drugs, when attempting to educate high-risk women about HIV infection. Awareness, prevention, and support services are needed to help diminish the connection between women, drugs, and HIV. (See *FYI:* "What Are Designer Drugs?" to learn about other drugs that can cause problems for women.)

FYI

What Are Designer Drugs?

Designer drugs could be called *copycat drugs* because they are designed to mimic the effects of other illegal drugs but are different enough to avoid government control. You can imagine the risks involved in ingesting chemicals that are mixed and manufactured by persons using a clandestine drug lab such as a garage, a barn, or a basement where no regulations are required and ingredients are unknown and unclean. The potential for physical and psychological ill effects from using these designer drugs is enormous, creating the potential for injury and potential brain damage. Examples of designer drugs include

MDA (the "love drug"). This is a hallucinogenic amphetamine derivative that is slightly more potent than mescaline, a hallucinatory crystalline alkaloid that is the main active ingredient in peyote buttons.

DOM (STP). This is an amphetamine derivative with hallucinogenic effects that can sometimes be long-lasting.

MDMA ("ecstasy" or "XTC"). This drug produces hallucinogenic effects and strong psychological dependence; it can deplete serotonin levels, potentially leading to such concerns as depression, aggression, and anger.

Women, Drugs, and Homelessness

Use of drugs, including alcohol, is a major risk for women and children as it relates to homelessness. Seeking, buying, and consuming illegal drugs can interfere with a woman's ability to locate employment and purchase essential resources such as housing, food, and medical services necessary for her and her children's well-being. Homeless women comprise a subpopulation at-risk for substance abuse, and homeless substance-abusing women face severe barriers to drug abuse treatment.[83]

Even though homelessness is less prevalent among women than men, it is the woman who often has the responsibility for children. Therefore, if a mother is homeless, then her children are homeless as well. Although the effects of drugs themselves have serious consequences, abusing drugs has serious effects on the personal health of homeless women and children. In an attempt to "score" or purchase various drugs, women may engage in risky sexual activity that places them at risk for unintended pregnancy, STIs, including HIV, and street violence. Participating in criminal activities, such as prostitution, drug dealing, and theft, to buy drugs, or even basic necessities, increases the risk of jail, loss of work, and loss of her children.

Children of drug-abusing mothers also suffer greatly, sometimes even prior to birth due to the mother's drug abuse and illnesses. Substance-abusing women, especially homeless women, often have no prenatal care or postbirthing care and are prone to neglect, abuse, abandonment, and placing their children in dangerous circumstances and environments.

What barriers do these women face? Many! Too few substance-abuse treatment facilities to meet the special needs of addicted, homeless women is a serious problem, especially if they have children or are pregnant. Lack of money and insurance, often lack of family support, and inability to receive outpatient treatment because they don't have a place to live all present almost insurmountable barriers for homeless women and children.

Solving the complex issues related to drug abuse among homeless women with children is difficult. They need treatment programs that address a woman's drug addiction, her basic survival needs, health care, and care for her children.

Research indicates that up to 70 percent of drug-abusing women report histories of physical and sexual abuse, and they are more likely than men to report a parental history of alcohol and drug abuse. Many drug-abusing women refuse treatment because they are afraid of not being able to take care of or keep their children, fear reprisal from their partners, and fear punishment from authorities in the community.[84] Usually the model for drug treatment programs has been directed toward recovery for the male addict. However, treatment specific to women who abuse substances is needed. Research shows that women receive the most benefit from drug treatment programs that provide comprehensive services for meeting their basic needs and programs that help them sustain their recovery and rejoin the community.[85]

Chapter Summary

- Use of highly addictive tobacco products is a very serious health behavior among American women, and deaths related to tobacco use continue to increase.
- A number of factors influence women to begin and continue smoking. These include media advertising, parental and peer smoking habits, and the work and recreation environments.
- A number of substances in tobacco are toxic in the human body and cause morbidity and mortality in women. Types of morbidity include heart diseases, cancers, disease of the respiratory system, osteoporosis, and aging skin.
- Environmental tobacco smoke (ETS) produces an environment laden with toxic chemicals, and when breathed on a regular basis it can cause a number of very serious diseases in women and children.
- Pregnant women should not smoke because of the serious detrimental effects, not only to the woman but especially to the developing fetus. Young children exposed to ETS will suffer a number of negative consequences.
- Cessation of smoking is difficult because of the highly addictive nature of the substances in tobacco. However, there are a number of smoking cessation programs, prescriptive aids, and behavioral changes that can be beneficial in this endeavor.
- The benefits of smoking cessation are numerous, both for regaining one's physical health and for avoiding the high health care costs related to smoking.
- Caffeine is found in many popular and widely used products, and the health effects are still being researched.
- Caffeinated products such as colas, coffee, tea, and chocolate are sold all over the world and produce a number of concerns for the health of women.
- Women can develop a dependence upon caffeine.
- Caffeine can produce negative health consequences for women and their children.
- Illegal drugs such as cocaine, marijuana, and heroin can produce devastating results for women and their unborn fetus or newborn infant.
- Designer drugs have effects similar to those of illegal drugs but are different enough to fall outside the purview of federal regulation.
- Social problems such as homelessness and sexually transmitted diseases often result for women who abuse drugs.

Review Questions

1. What are mortality and morbidity? How has the number of women who smoke affected mortality and morbidity rates in recent years?
2. How many women are current smokers? In the past few decades, has there been an increase or a decrease in the use of smoking tobacco among women? Why?
3. What are four factors that influence women to smoke?
4. What effects do nicotine, carbon monoxide, and tar have on the body?
5. What are three diseases that result from smoking tobacco? How has smoking contributed to the development of these diseases?
6. What component in tobacco causes addiction? What types of addiction patterns occur because of tobacco use?
7. What effects does environmental tobacco smoke have on the health of women and children who are exposed to it?
8. What are the risks for the fetus and for infants born to mothers who smoke during pregnancy?
9. What methods can be used to assist with smoking cessation?
10. In what ways can the Food and Drug Administration regulate tobacco use in the United States?
11. What are the benefits of quitting smoking? What is the length of time before a smoker can expect to experience these benefits?
12. In what ways can women's use of caffeine interfere with reproduction?
13. Does caffeine increase the risk of developing breast cancer? Why or why not?
14. What are the physiological and behavioral effects associated with the consumption of excessive caffeine?
15. What is the difference between the amount of caffeine found in a 12-ounce can of Coca-Cola, one cup of brewed coffee, a bar of chocolate candy, and a cup of brewed tea?
16. What are the indications that a woman has developed a dependence upon caffeine, and what can she do to reverse the effects?

Resources

Web Sites

American Cancer Society
www.cancer.org

American Council for Drug Education
www.acde.org

American Lung Association
www.lungusa.org

ASH (Action on Smoking and Health)
www.ash.org/women.html

Caffeine Archives
www.caffeinearchive.com

Cocaine Anonymous
www.ca.org

Federal Trade Commission
www.ftc.gov/bcp/menu-tobac.htm

Narcotics Anonymous (NA)
www.na.org

National Alliance for Hispanic Health
www.hispanichealth.org

National Coffee Association of the U.S.A., Inc.
www.ncausa.org

National Institute on Drug Abuse
www.drugabuse.gov

Partnership for a Drug-Free America
www.drugfreeamerica.org

Substance Abuse & Mental Health Services Administration
National Treatment Hotline: 800-662-HELP
www.samhsa.gov

U.S. Drug Enforcement Administration
www.usdoj.gov/dea/index.htm

U.S. Library of Medicine: Medline Plus
www.nlm.nih.gov/medlineplus/smokingcessation.html

Web of Addictions
www.well.com/user/woa

Videotapes

Cigarettes: Who Profits, Who Dies?
Features stories of former cigarette models now dying of cancer, and tactics that tobacco companies to get people to start smoking and to keep smoking.
Films for the Humanities & Sciences, P.O. Box 2053, Princeton, NJ 08543-2053. Phone: 800-257-5126, Web site: www.films.com

The Feminine Mistake
Interviews with women smokers, cigarette advertising, and important messages.
Community Intervention, 529 South 7th St., Suite 570, Minneapolis, MN 55415. Phone: 800-328-0417, Web site: www.communityintervention.org

Scene Smoking: Cigarettes, Cinema, and the Myth of Cool (2001)
Interviews with big names in filmmaking, addressing the impact of movies and TV on viewers. Debates questions of artistic license and social responsibility and debunks the myth of smoking as a cool behavior.
Films for the Humanities & Sciences, P.O. Box 2053, Princeton, NJ 08543-2053. Phone: 800-257-5126, Web site: www.films.com

Smoking Out the Truth: Teens and Tobacco (2006)
Focus is on the illusions and misconceptions surrounding teen smoking, exposing faulty reasoning that leads young people to start or continue to smoke.
Films for the Humanities & Sciences, P.O. Box 2053, Princeton, NJ 08543-2053. Phone: 800-257-5126, Web site: www.films.com

Women and Cigarettes: A Fatal Attraction (2001)
Reports how tobacco industry targets women, how smoking endangers the fetus, and consequences of smoking in women.
Films for the Humanities & Sciences, P.O. Box 2053, Princeton, NJ 08543-2053. Phone: 800-257-5126, Web site: www.films.com

Suggested Readings

The American Lung Association. 2004. *How to Quit Smoking without Gaining Weight.* New York: Pocket Books.

Bryenton, B. B. 2006. *Playing with Fire: Wisdom for Women Who Smoke.* Victoria, BC: Trafford Publishing.

Durbin, R. J. 2002. *Tobacco's Deadly Secret: The Impact of Tobacco Marketing on Women and Girls.* Darby, PA: Diane Publishing Co.

Ettorre, E. 2006. *Revisioning Women and Drug Use.* New York: Palgrave Macmillan.

Gatley, I. 2001. *Tobacco: A Cultural History of How an Exotic Plant Seduced Civilization.* New York: Grove/Atlantic.

Kaur, N., and M. Kushner. 2006. *The Truth about Caffeine: How Companies That Promote It Deceive Us and What We Can Do About It.* Royersford, PA: SCR Books.

Kuhn, C., et al. 1998. *Buzzed: The Straight Facts about the Most Used and Abused Drugs from Alcohol to Ecstasy.* New York: Norton.

Murphy-Lawless, J. 2003. *Fighting Back: Women & the Impact of Drug Abuse on Families.* Chester Springs, PA: Liffey Press.

Oaks, L. 2001. *Smoking and Pregnancy: The Politics of Fetal Protection.* New Brunswick, NJ: Rutgers University Press.

Straussner, S. L. A., and S. Brown. 2002. *The Handbook of Addiction Treatment for Women: Theory and Practice.* San Francisco: Jossey-Bass.

Weinberg, B. A., and B. K. Bealer. 2001. *The World of Caffeine: The Science and Culture of the World's Most Popular Drug.* New York: Routledge.

References

1. Womenshealth.gov. 2005. *Steps to healthier women: Tobacco use.* www.womenshealth.gov/pub/steps/TobaccoUse.htm (retrieved October 5, 2006).
2. Ksir, C., C. L. Hart, and O. Ray. 2006. *Drugs, society, and human behavior.* 11th ed. New York: McGraw-Hill.
3. Centers for Disease Control and Prevention. 2005. Cigarette smoking among adults—United States, 2004. *Morbidity and Mortality Weekly Report* 54:1121–24. www.cdc.gov/mmwr//preview/mmwrhtml/mm5444a2.htm (retrieved April 18, 2007).
4. American Cancer Society. 2006. *Women and smoking.* www.cancer.org/docroot/PED/content/PED_10_2X_Women_and_Smoking.asp (retrieved October 5, 2006).
5. Centers for Disease Control and Prevention. 2001. *Surgeon general's report: Women and smoking 2001*, p. 2. www.4woman.org/quitsmoking/sgr/2001.cfm (retrieved October 7, 2006).
6. Womenshealth.gov.
7. Centers for Disease Control and Prevention, *Surgeon general's report: Women and smoking 2001.*
8. American Cancer Society, *Women and smoking.*
9. Ibid.
10. World Health Organization. 2000. *European Union directive banning tobacco advertising overturned: WHO urges concerted response.* Press release. www.who.int/inf-pr-2000/en/pr2000-64.html (retrieved October 5, 2006).
11. U.S. Federal Trade Commission. 2002. *Cigarette report for 2002.* www.ftc.gov/reports/cigarette/041022cigaretterpt.pdf (retrieved October 5, 2006).
12. Womenshealth.gov.
13. American Cancer Society. 2001. *Breathing easy: Create a smoke-free workplace.* www.cancer.org/downloads/COM/SmokefreeWorkplace.pdf (retrieved October 7, 2006).
14. Carroll, C. R. 2000. *Drugs in modern society.* 5th ed. New York: McGraw-Hill.
15. U.S. Department of Health and Human Services. 2004. *The health consequences of smoking. A report of the surgeon general.* Washington, DC: U.S. Department of Health and Human Services, Centers for Disease Control and Prevention, National Center for Chronic Disease Prevention and Health Promotion, Office on Smoking and Health, p. 619.
16. Carroll, *Drugs in modern society.*
17. Ibid., p. 170.
18. American Cancer Society, *Women and smoking.*
19. Food and Drug Administration. 2003, April 1. *Title 21: Food and drugs—patient inserts for oral contraceptives.* Code of Federal Regulations 21 (5): Sect. 310.501.
20. U.S. Department of Health and Human Services, *The health consequences of smoking*, pp. 39, 42.
21. Ibid., pp. 42, 62, 63, 116, 166.
22. American Cancer Society. 2006. *Estimated new cancer cases and deaths by sex for all sites, U.S. 2006.* www.cancer.org/downloads/stt/CAFF06EsCsMc.pdf (retrieved October 5, 2006).
23. U.S. Department of Health and Human Services, *The health consequences of smoking.*
24. Ibid.
25. Ibid.
26. American Cancer Society, *Women and smoking.*
27. Doweiko, H. 1996. *Concepts of chemical dependency.* Boston: Brooks/Cole.
28. Rustin, T. 1992. *Review of nicotine and its treatment.* LaCrosse, WI: Symposium at St. Francis Hospital.
29. U.S. Department of Health and Human Services. 2006. *The health consequences of involuntary exposure to tobacco smoke: A report by the surgeon general.* www.surgeongeneral.gov/library/secondhandsmoke/report/executivesummary.pdf (retrieved October 7, 2006).
30. University of Texas Health Science Center. 1997. *Passive smoking and lung cancer.* http://medic.med.uth.tmc.edu/ptnt/00000279.htm (retrieved October 5, 2006).
31. Ibid.
32. World Health Organization. 1999. *International consultation on environmental tobacco smoke (ETS) and child health.* January 11–14.
33. Ibid.
34. Ibid.
35. U.S. Department of Health and Human Services, *The health consequences of smoking*, p. 527.
36. Lieberman, E., I. Gremy, J. Land, and A. Cohen. 1994. Low birthweight at term and the timing of fetal exposure. *American Journal of Public Health* 84 (7): 1127–31.
37. U.S. Department of Health and Human Services, *The health consequences of smoking*, p. 555.

38. Ibid., p. 616.
39. Colman, G. J., and T. Joyce. 2003. Trends in smoking before, during, and after pregnancy in ten states. *American Journal of Preventative Medicine* 24 (1): 29–35.
40. Committee on Environmental Health. 1997. Environmental tobacco smoke: A hazard to children. *American Academy of Pediatrics* 99 (4): 639–42.
41. American Cancer Society, *Women and smoking*.
42. U.S. Department of Health and Human Services, *The health consequences of smoking*.
43. Ibid.
44. American Lung Association. 2004. *Nicotine replacement*. www.lungusa.org/site (retrieved April 14, 2006).
45. Ibid.
46. Ibid.
47. Ibid.
48. Ibid.
49. Pfizer, Inc. 2006. *Pfizer's smoking cessation medicine Chantix™ (varenicline)*. http://mediaroom.pfizer.com/index.php?s=press_releases&item=57 (retrieved October 7, 2006).
50. American Cancer Society. 1988. *Smart move*. Pamphlet no. 2515-LE; American Cancer Society. 2002. *Complete guide to quitting*. www.cancer.org/docroot/PED/content/PED_10_13X_Quitting_Smoking.asp#How_to_Quit (retrieved October 5, 2006).
51. Klesges, L. M., K. C. Johnson, K. D. Ward, and M. Barnard. 2001. Smoking cessation in pregnant women. *Obstetrics and Gynecology Clinics of North America* 28:269–82.
52. For an editorial on the special contributions of Ann Richards, see "Appreciations: Ann R., Alcoholic," by Maura J. Casey, *New York Times*, September 16, 2006, sec. A, p. 14.
53. American Cancer Society. 2003. *When smokers quit—the health benefits over time*. www.cancer.org/docroot/SPC/content/SPC_1_When_Smokers_Quit.asp?sitearea (retrieved October 5, 2006).
54. *U.S. coffee consumption shows impressive growth*. 2004. *Food & Drink Weekly*. www.findarticles.com/p/articles/mi_m0EUY/is_6_10/ai_113524726 (retrieved October 5, 2006.)
55. Coffeeresearch.org. *Coffee consumption in the United States of America*. www.coffeeresearch.org/market/usa.htm (retrieved October 5, 2006).
56. National Coffee Association of the U.S.A., Inc. 2003. *The history of coffee*. www.ncausa.org/i4a/pages/index.cfm?pageid=68 (retrieved October 7, 2006).
57. Ksir, Hart, and Ray, *Drugs, society, and human behavior*, p. 274.
58. Ibid., p. 264.
59. Ibid. p. 270.
60. Ibid., p. 273.
61. Bergman, E., M. L. Erickson, and J. C. Boyungs. 1992. Caffeine knowledge, attitudes, and consumption in adult women. *Journal of Nutrition Education* 24:179–84.
62. American College of Gastroenterology. 2006. *Osteoporosis: What you should know*. www.acg.gi.org/patients/women/osteo.asp (retrieved October 5, 2006).
63. International Food Information Council Foundation. 2002. *Caffeine & women's health*. http://ific.org/publications/brochures/caffwomenbroch.cfm (retrieved October 5, 2006).
64. UK Food Standards Agency. 2001. *Statement on the reproductive effects of caffeine*. www.food.gov.uk/science/ouradvisors/toxicity/statements/cotstatements2001/caffeine (retrieved October 5, 2006).
65. National Survey on Drug Use and Health. 2005. *Substance abuse and dependence among women*. www.oas.samhsa.gov/2k5/women/women.htm (retrieved October 5, 2006).
66. Substance Abuse and Mental Health Services Administration. 2005. *Results from the 2004 National Survey on Drug Use and Health: National findings*. Office of Applied Studies, NSDUH Series H-28, DHHS Publication No. SMA 05-4062. Rockville, MD: U.S. Department of Health and Human Services.
67. *Drug use during pregnancy*. 2003. Merck Manual Home Edition. www.merck.com/mmhe/print/sec22/ch259/ch259a.html (retrieved October 5, 2006).
68. Ibid.
69. National Institute of Drug Abuse. 1994. *Women and drug abuse*. Rockville, MD: U.S. Department of Health and Human Services.
70. Mitchell, J. L. (panel chair). 1993. *Pregnant, substance-abusing women*. DHHS Publication No. SMA 93-1998. Rockville, MD: U.S. Department of Health and Human Services.
71. NIDA Research Report Series. 2004. *Cocaine: Abuse and addiction*. NIH Publication No. 99-4342. Bethesda, MD: National Institutes of Health.
72. Ibid.
73. Substance Abuse and Mental Health Services Administration, *Results from the 2004 National Survey on Drug Use and Health*.
74. NIDA Research Report Series, *Cocaine: Abuse and addiction*.
75. National Institute of Drug Abuse. 2005. *Medical consequences of drug abuse: Prenatal effects*. www.nida.nih.gov/consequences/prenatal (retrieved October 5, 2006).
76. NIDA Research Report Series. 2005. *Marijuana abuse*. NIH Publication No. 05-3859. Bethesda, MD: National Institutes of Health.
77. Pinger, R. R., W. A. Payne, D. N. Hahn, and E. J. Hahn. 1998. *Drugs: Issues for Today*. 3rd ed. St. Louis: Mosby.
78. March of Dimes. 2006. *Illicit drug use during pregnancy*. www.marchofdimes.com/printableArticles/14332_1169.asp (retrieved October 5, 2006).
79. Ibid.
80. U.S. Department of Health and Human Services, Health Resources and Services Administration. 2005. *Substance abuse and HIV/AIDS*. HIV/AIDS Bureau. Rockville, MD.
81. Crack smokers pose high risk of contracting AIDS (particularly women). 1994. *Narcotics Demand Reduction Digest* (January): 6–7.
82. Wambach, K. G., J. B. Byers, D. F. Harrison, P. Levine, A. W. Imershein, D. M. Quadagno, and K. Maddox. 1990. Substance use among women at risk for HIV infection. *Journal of Drug Education* 22 (2): 131–46.
83. U.S. Department of Health and Human Services, Human Resources and Services Administration. 2000. *The health of homeless women*. www.med.jhu.edu/wchpc> (retrieved October 7, 2006).
84. National Institute of Drug Abuse. 2005. *NIDA InfoFacts: Treatment methods for women*. www.drugabuse.gov/InFofacts/treatwomen.html. (retrieved October 5, 2006).
85. Ibid.

Communicable and Chronic Conditions

Part Five

Chapter Fourteen

Preventing Sexually Transmitted Infections and Other Infectious Diseases

CHAPTER OBJECTIVES

When you complete this chapter, you will be able to do the following:

- Describe the consequences of untreated sexually transmitted infections (STIs) in women
- Compare and contrast the incidence and prevalence of various STIs
- Differentiate among the various forms of contraception that reduce the risk of transmitting STIs and HIV/AIDS
- Describe safer and riskier sexual behaviors
- Explain various ways to prevent the spread of STIs and HIV/AIDS among women and children
- Identify the highest risk groups for various STIs and HIV/AIDS
- Describe some strategies for preventing the spread of infectious diseases
- Identify signs and symptoms of some common infectious diseases
- Identify the trends in current infectious diseases

THE INCREASING THREAT POSED BY INFECTIOUS DISEASES

The significant advances in antibiotics and vaccines to fight infectious diseases during the twentieth century lulled many health officials and the public into thinking that the primary diseases of the twenty-first century would be chronic diseases caused primarily by lifestyle choices. The worldwide AIDS epidemic, the "bird flu," SARS, drug-resistant strains of tuberculosis, and the reemergence of many infectious diseases believed to be close to eradication have sparked renewed focus by health care researchers and providers. The Centers for Disease Control and Prevention (CDC) has developed a twenty-first-century century plan to prevent, contain, and research diseases that have the potential to impact huge numbers of persons worldwide. The CDC states that the emergence and reemergence of many infectious disease agents have been fueled by unprecedented worldwide population growth, increased international travel, increased transport of animals and food products, changes in food processing and handling, human encroachment on wilderness habitats, and microbial evolution with resistance to antibiotics and other antimicrobial drugs.[1]

The CDC has designated nearly fifty infectious diseases (including many STIs) as notifiable at the national level. The current infectious diseases that state departments, physicians, and clinics are asked to report to the CDC are listed in Table 14.1. The CDC tracks the incidence and prevalence of these diseases and provides weekly and annual reports. Some of these diseases and a few other common infectious diseases affecting college students will be discussed throughout this chapter. We begin with sexually transmitted infections and later address infectious

TABLE 14.1 Infectious Diseases Designated as Notifiable at the National Level, 2005[2]

- Acquired immunodeficiency syndrome (AIDS)
- Anthrax
- Botulism
- Brucellosis
- Chancroid
- *Chlamydia trachomatis,* genital infection
- Cholera
- Coccidioidomycosis
- Cryptosporidiosis
- Cyclosporiasis
- Diphtheria
- Domestic arboviral diseases, neuroinvasive and non-neuroinvasive
  - California serogroup
  - Eastern equine
  - Powassan
  - St. Louis
  - Western equine
  - West Nile
- Ehrlichiosis
  - Human granulocytic
  - Human monocytic
  - Human, other or unspecified agent
- Enterohemorrhagic *Escherichia coli* (EHEC), O157:H7
  - EHEC serogroup non-O157
  - EHEC, not serogrouped
- Giardiasis
- Gonorrhea
- *Haemophilus influenzae,* invasive disease
- Hansen disease (leprosy)
- Hantavirus pulmonary syndrome
- Hemolytic uremic syndrome, postdiarrheal
- Hepatitis A, acute, viral
- Hepatitis B, acute, viral
- Hepatitis B, chronic
- Hepatitis B, perinatal infection
- Hepatitis C, acute, viral
- Hepatitis C, infection (past or present)
- Human immunodeficiency virus (HIV) infection
  - Adult (>13 years of age)
  - Pediatric (<13 years of age)
- Influenza-associated pediatric mortality
- Legionellosis
- Listeriosis
- Lyme disease
- Malaria
- Measles
- Meningococcal disease, invasive
- Mumps
- Pertussis
- Plague
- Poliomyelitis, paralytic
- Psittacosis
- Q fever
- Rabies, animal
- Rabies, human
- Rocky Mountain spotted fever
- Rubella
- Rubella, congenital syndrome
- Salmonellosis
- Severe acute respiratory syndrome-associated coronavirus (SARS-CoV) disease
- Shigellosis
- Streptococcal disease, invasive, group A
- Streptococcal toxic-shock syndrome
- *Streptococcus pneumoniae,* Invasive disease,
  - drug resistant, all ages
  - age <5 years
- Syphilis
- Syphilis, congenital
- Tetanus
- Toxic-shock syndrome (other than streptococcal)
- Trichinellosis
- Tuberculosis
- Tularemia
- Vancomycin-intermediate *Staphylococcus aureus* infection (VISA)
- Vancomycin-resistant *Staphylococcus aureus* infection (VRSA)
- Varicella infection (morbidity)
- Varicella deaths
- Yellow fever

*Although varicella (chicken pox) is not a nationally notifiable disease, the Council of State and Territorial Epidemiologists recommends reporting cases of this disease to the CDC.

diseases such as mononucleosis, influenza, hepatitis, tuberculosis, and streptococcal diseases.

THE PRIMARY BURDEN OF SEXUALLY TRANSMITTED INFECTIONS

Sexually transmitted infections (STIs) can be physically, emotionally, and spiritually devastating for women The physical risks have potential serious and long-term complications such as pelvic inflammatory disease (PID), impaired fertility, ectopic pregnancies, chronic pain, cervical cancer, and chronic liver disease. The emotional and spiritual impact may range from feelings of shame to fear of reprisal and feelings of isolation to disconnection from others. Ignorance is not bliss when it comes to STIs since the consequences may be permanent injury or death.

The stigma attached to many STIs (particularly HIV/AIDS) can cause women to deny the possibility of having an STI, leading to a delay in testing and treatment. This stigma is perhaps more readily noticed in countries where women with STIs may be shunned, cast out, or physically harmed, but the United States also discriminates against women with these infections. Discrimination can be found in the form of laws and regulations, such as those in developing countries that deny women the right to protect themselves from infected husbands or from gender-based violence, as well as more explicitly at community and individual levels. In addition, stigma associated with addiction and illicit drug use, persistent social and institutional racism, and gender and economic inequities prevent many women from seeking the treatment they need.[3]

Until the 1980s, only five venereal diseases were regularly monitored. Today, nearly fifty different STI-related organisms and syndromes are recognized, and the complexity and scope of these STIs has changed drastically. The CDC requires that traditional sexually transmitted diseases, such as gonorrhea and syphilis, as well as other infectious diseases including vaginitis, human papilloma virus (genital warts), chlamydia, genital herpes, and hepatitis B be reported to the CDC.

Assess Yourself

Assess Your STI Risk

Answer the following questions by checking yes or no on the appropriate line.

Yes	No	
_____	_____	Are you sexually active?
_____	_____	Is it very important to you *not* to get pregnant in the near future?
_____	_____	Do you find it difficult to always use your current birth control method?
_____	_____	Has the recent change in a relationship caused a change in your method of birth control?
_____	_____	Do you wonder if your partner has ever had an STI?
_____	_____	Do you have difficulty discussing STIs with your partner?
_____	_____	Have you or your partner had sex with more than one person over the past several months?
_____	_____	Do you use alcohol or drugs?
_____	_____	Does it surprise you that some STIs have no symptoms?

Having unprotected sex, even once, can put you at risk for sexually transmitted infections or unintended pregnancy. If you are sexually active and answered yes to any of the previous questions, you may want to discuss prevention and protection with your health care provider.[4]

Women need to become knowledgeable about the most common STIs and infectious diseases. Asking questions and seeking information are not equated with being sexually active. In fact, when given a choice, women who know the risks may choose less risky sexual behaviors. Abstinence is the first line of protection against future sterility, PID, and ectopic pregnancies, and it is the only way to absolutely prevent all unintended pregnancies and STIs. However, when a woman becomes sexually active, she should choose to act responsibly and protect her body as much as possible. (See *Assess Yourself*: "Assess Your STI Risk.") A woman should know the risks associated with STIs and practice assertiveness skills to prevent unprotected sex.

COMMON BACTERIAL SEXUALLY TRANSMITTED INFECTIONS

Chlamydia

Chlamydia infection is the most common bacterial STI in the United States. The bacterium *Chlamydia trachomatis* causes chlamydial infection and can persist for long periods of time without causing symptoms. The exposure to chlamydia is usually sexual intercourse, and the site of infection is typically the cervix. Chlamydia infections range from lower genital tract infection and pelvic inflammatory disease (PID) in women to conjunctivitis and pneumonitis syndromes in newborns.[5] Approximately 75 percent of women with chlamydia are asymptomatic until they experience the fever and pain associated with pelvic inflammatory disease. Up to 40 percent of women infected with chlamydia develop PID if not adequately treated.[6] Twenty percent of women with PID become infertile; 18 percent experience severe, chronic pelvic pain; and nearly 9 percent experience ectopic pregnancies. Recent studies have suggested that women infected with chlamydia and exposed to HIV have a three- to five-fold increased risk of acquiring the virus.

Diagnosis Indicators such as nongonococcal **urethritis** (inflammation of the urethra), PID, and cervicitis are helpful in determining the incidence of chlamydia infections, but new diagnostic technology has allowed for more widespread screening. In the past, CDC used the incidence of nongonococcal urethritis (NGU) as an indicator of chlamydia infections. Today, a variety of tests, including cell culture, antigen detection tests, nucleic acid hybridization tests, and nucleic acid amplification tests, are used to diagnose chlamydia infection. Cell culture remains the gold standard for detecting chlamydia infection and is the diagnostic procedure of choice for women who have been raped or experienced incest. Many clinics routinely use nonculture tests because they are less expensive, provide quicker results, and have fewer handling requirements than cell cultures. However, these nonculture tests also have lower sensitivity for detecting chlamydia infections than cell cultures (40 percent versus 75 percent).[7]

A study of 2,607 women between the ages of 18 and 34 who belonged to a health maintenance organization concluded that routine screening significantly reduced the risk of PID.[8] These findings and other studies spurred the CDC to recommend annual screening of all sexually active women ages 25 or younger, and screening of older women with risk factors (e.g., a new sex partner or multiple sex partners). The CDC also recommends that all pregnant women with **cervicitis** be screened routinely because of the high rate of neonatal infection when chlamydia is left untreated. Symptomatic women may experience unexplained vaginal discharge, burning during urination, lower abdominal pain, bleeding between menstrual periods, fever, and nausea.[9]

Recurrence rates can be particularly disturbing. One study estimated that the rate of recurrence of chlamydia infection was 42 percent for girls aged 10 to 14 and 25 percent for young women aged 15 to 19. This study also found that the recurrence rate for African American young women was twice that for white women.[10] Recurrence increases the risk of infertility due to scarring of the fallopian tubes.

Asymptomatic women with chlamydia infections as well as their partners should be treated. If the partner's infection goes untreated, the risk of recurrence through a repeat transmission exists. If the woman's infection goes untreated, serious complications, including hospitalization for PID, may result. Complications associated with chlamydia infection include cervicitis, infertility, chronic pain, salpingitis (inflammation of the fallopian tubes), increased risk of ectopic pregnancy, stillbirth, reactive arthritis, and neonatal conjunctivitis and pneumonia.[11]

Treatment The treatment of chlamydia is relatively simple. Antibiotics are given to treat chlamydia, either in a 7-day or single-dose regimen, depending on the woman's compliance history and ability to pay. The single dose of azithromycin is three to five times more expensive than a 7-day regimen but has the advantage of one application. Many women who test positive for chlamydia infection do not comply with the treatment protocol. One research study found that between 25 and 50 percent of the women who tested positive did not seek adequate treatment.[12] Despite better screening procedures, treatment compliance is difficult to ensure.

Pregnancy The CDC now recommends that all pregnant women be screened for chlamydia and that women who test positive be treated with erythromycin (or amoxicillin for women with intolerance to erythromycin). Infants can be protected from contracting chlamyida if this treatment is completed before delivery.[13] A woman who tests positive for chlamydia infection risks severe complications if treatment isn't administered promptly. The CDC estimates that 30 percent of women without treatment will become sterile.[14]

Epidemiology Chlamydia affects an estimated 3 million to 5 million persons annually (nearly 485.0 per 100,000 women in the United States in 2004). Consistently, the reported rate of chlamydia for women substantially exceeds the rate for men, suggesting that many male partners are not screened or treated. Nearly one in ten adolescent girls tested for chlamydia is infected. (See Figure 14.1.)

Adolescent girls aged 15 to 19 represent over 45 percent of infections, and women aged 20 to 24 represent

FIGURE 14.1 Chlamydia: Age- and sex-specific rates, United States, 2004.

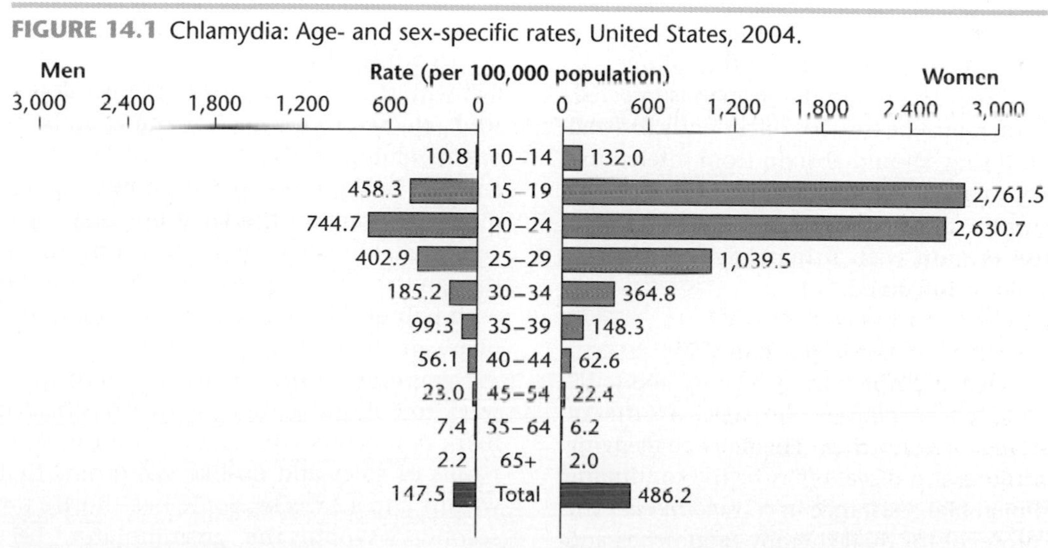

SOURCE: Centers for Disease Control and Prevention. 2004. *Sexually transmitted disease surveillance: Chlamydia.* www.cdc.gov/std/stats/chlamydia3.html (retrieved April 5, 2006).

another 30 percent.[15] The economic burden of genital chlamydia infections exceeds $3.5 billion annually, a cost that could be reduced substantially if proper screening of high-risk women was conducted annually. The CDC estimates that annual screening and treatment programs may cost $175 million, suggesting that $12 to $15 spent on complications from untreated chlamydia could be saved for every dollar spent on screening and treatment.

Gonorrhea

Gonorrhea is caused by the *Neisseria gonorrhoeae* bacterium. Gonorrhea can affect any of the mucous membranes, including the vagina, cervix, anus, throat, and eyes. Symptomatic women may experience a thick yellow or white vaginal discharge; burning during urination, intercourse, and bowel movements; and severe menstrual or abdominal cramps. The bacteria can move from the cervix, the site of first infection, into the uterus and fallopian tubes where they can remain indefinitely without causing symptoms and can begin to cause scarring and resultant chronic pain, ectopic pregnancy, or infertility. Nearly 50 percent of women who contract gonorrhea are initially asymptomatic. The first expressed symptoms may be those of pelvic inflammatory disease rather than gonorrhea. Ten to 40 percent of women infected with gonorrhea develop PID if inadequately treated.[16] Among women, the infection often remains asymptomatic until complications such as PID occur. Because women are often asymptomatic, prevention efforts must include screening of women who are deemed to be practicing high-risk behaviors. Many women who have gonorrhea are co-infected with chlamydia; thus routine dual therapy without testing for chlamydia infection is often conducted because the cost of therapy is less than the cost of testing.

Diagnosis A secretion is taken from the cervix, rectum, and throat for culturing to determine whether a person has been infected. Lab results of the culture take approximately a week to obtain. If a woman is infected, she and her partner must be treated concurrently to avoid re-infection, and they should abstain from intercourse during the treatment. Fortunately, most symptomatic men seek treatment quickly after gonococcal urethritis occurs because of pain with urination, and a man's partner(s) should be informed.

Treatment A large increase in resistant strains to first-line antibiotics such as ampicillin, penicillin, and tetracycline has caused a change in CDC treatment recommendations for gonorrhea. The most challenging aspect of controlling this disease may be the continuing spread of antimicrobial resistance in *N. gonorrhoeae*. The current U.S. protocol for dual therapy (gonorrhea and chlamydia) includes the administration of doxycycline, which may help prevent antimicrobial-resistant *N. gonorrhoeae*. Resistance of this bacterium is expected to continue to spread, necessitating that health care providers obtain a recent travel history from the infected person and her partner(s) to ensure that the appropriate therapy is administered. The only antimicrobial agents to which *N. gonorrhoeae* has not developed resistance are the broad-spectrum cephalosporins.[17] Untreated, acute gonorrhea can result in widespread, systemic, infection. Nearly 80 percent of gonococcal infection that has spread to other organs occurs in young women, with common features including arthritis, dermatitis, and inflammation of fluid surrounding tendons.[18]

Pregnancy and Infancy Gonorrhea results in adverse outcomes of pregnancy, including inflammation of the newborn's eyes. This disease can be prevented with topical treatment at delivery.

Epidemiology The incidence of gonorrhea continues to decline and the CDC reports rates of 113.5 per 100,000 persons annually. While the overall rate of gonorrhea infections has declined since the mid-1970s for all groups except teenagers and some minorities, minor increases have occurred in some instances. For example, between 2000 and 2004, the rate of gonorrhea reported among white women of all ages rose nearly 19 percent, from 33.6 per 100,000 to 40.0.per 100,000.[19]

Syphilis

Syphilis is caused by the spirochete *Treponema pallidum,* which spreads throughout the body within hours of infection. It is primarily transmitted through sexual contact, but it can also be passed from the infected mother to a fetus. Syphilis is characterized by active and latent phases, called primary, secondary, latent, and tertiary. The first symptom of primary syphilis, which occurs within 1 to 3 months (average 21 days) of contact with the infected partner, is a painless red or brown sore (chancre) or sores on the mouth, reproductive organs, or fingers. This chancre will last from 3 to 6 weeks and will heal on its own. In women, the chancre commonly appears on the labia but may develop on the cervix, making detection difficult or impossible. Even though the sore disappears, the person still has syphilis, with half of infected persons moving to the secondary phase and then the latent phase.[20]

Symptoms of the secondary phase appear within 1 week to 6 months after the sore has healed. The hallmark of this phase includes a rash that appears on the palms or soles and flu-like symptoms that disappear within 2 to 12 weeks. Some health care providers call secondary syphilis the "great imitator," because it may be mistaken for a rash from eczema, cutaneous drug reactions, psoriasis, measles, or even sunburn. The flu-like symptoms may be mistaken for influenza or infectious mononucleosis.[21]

Those who progress to the latent, hidden phases, the period of time between the secondary and tertiary phase, have no clinical signs or symptoms. They may remain asymptomatic, but they will still have syphilis unless they get treated. One-third will move to the tertiary phase. Today, few women progress to the tertiary phase due to penicillin therapy. The tertiary phase is characterized by destructive lesions, lymph node involvement, and organ destruction. The central nervous system may be involved, causing meningitis, spinal lesions, or cerebral vascular syphilis. Cardiac lesions may damage the cardiovascular system.[22]

Syphilis has also been linked to increased susceptibility to HIV infection because the open sores remove the virus barrier and carry mononuclear cells that easily draw HIV. The symptoms of syphilis may manifest differently for HIV-infected persons, so experts suggest that women who test positive for syphilis also get tested for HIV. They should also be counseled about their increased risk for HIV infection and the importance of condom use.[23]

Treatment Any woman with genital lesions should be tested for syphilis. Most primary, secondary, and early latent syphilis cases are treated with one injection of penicillin, which is the drug of choice. Women who are allergic to penicillin can be treated with alternative drugs. Those with tertiary syphilis will need a longer regimen of treatment. All persons must be monitored to determine the efficacy of the treatment.[24]

Infected persons receiving treatment must abstain from sexual contact until the syphilis sores are completely healed. Treated individuals may have a short period of protection from re-infection, but if they are exposed to syphilis sores, they may contract the disease again. Condoms are a good source of prevention; however, syphilis sores may occur outside the covered area, and a person may then become infected by coming in contact with the sores.[25]

Pregnancy Congenital syphilis is transmitted to the fetus during pregnancy and has a devastating impact on the newborn. It accounts for 40 percent of fetal and perinatal deaths in affected infants, and morbidity is even higher, with physical and mental developmental disabilities. Most cases of congenital syphilis are preventable if the pregnant woman is treated properly through early prenatal care. As syphilis rates decrease in women, the number of cases of congenital syphilis also decrease. The CDC recommends expanded screening to all women of childbearing age who live in cities with high incidence of syphilis and improving educational and service outreach for prenatal care to women in high-incidence environments.[26]

Epidemiology In 2000 the U.S. rate of primary and secondary syphilis was very low, 2.2 cases per 100,000. From 2001 to 2004, however, the rate of primary and secondary syphilis increased to 2.7 per 100,000, primarily resulting from an increase in cases among men who have sex with men (MSM). While syphilis continues to increase among this group, its rate among women remains low. Between 2000 and 2003, primary and secondary syphilis decreased from 1.7 to 0.8 women per 100,000 and remained at 0.8 in 2004. The year 2004 marked the first time since 1991 that the rate among women did not decrease.[27]

Serious racial and ethnic disparities persist in the number of reported cases of syphilis. Overall rates of primary and secondary syphilis for African Americans remain five to six times higher than the rates for whites, 9.0 cases per 100,000 versus 1.6 cases per 100,000. Between 2000 and 2004, the rate for African American men increased 23 percent and the rate for African American women increased 2 percent. Since 1991, syphilis among African American women has increased slightly, from 4.2 cases per 100,000 in 2003 to 4.3 cases per 100,000 in 2004.

Chancroid

Chancroid is caused by the bacterium *H. ducreyi*. It is characterized by a painful genital ulceration. This STI is most prevalent in Africa and Asia, although its prevalence in the United States is most likely underreported. It has been shown to be a risk factor for the transmission of HIV and is difficult to culture or test. In 1999 three states (Texas, New York, and South Carolina) accounted for approximately 72 percent of the 143 cases reported in the United States.[28]

COMMON VIRAL SEXUALLY TRANSMITTED INFECTIONS

Herpes Simplex Virus (HSV)

Herpes simplex is one of a family of common viruses including varicella zoster virus (chicken pox and shingles) and Epstein-Barr virus (mononucleosis). Herpes simplex virus (HSV) is a contagious infection that spreads from direct skin-to-skin contact of an infected partner to the other partner, particularly in the oral and genital areas. The two primary types of herpes simplex viruses are HSV-1 and HSV-2. HSV-1 usually manifests as cold sores or fever blisters, primarily around the mouth.

The symptoms of genital herpes vary from one individual to another. Most infected women may not recognize the signs of genital herpes, and many who experience an initial outbreak will never have additional outbreaks. Symptomatic persons may experience the first episode within 2 to 30 days of contact with an infected partner. The first symptoms of the active phase may include itching, burning, and swelling at the site of infection. A woman can experience symptoms common to all viral infections: fever, headaches, muscle aches, and chills. Eventually, small painful blisters (lesions) appear on the genitalia (sometimes the mouth), then rupture, form a scab, and heal. The blisters disappear within 1 to 3 weeks, but some of the herpes simplex virus remains. The virus travels along a nerve to the ganglia (a cluster of nerve cells) near the spine and remains dormant until another outbreak occurs. Then the virus travels along the nerve to the surface of the skin.[29]

Diagnosis Control efforts for HSV-2 are difficult because nearly 75 percent of individuals who transmit the virus are unaware of their infection. Often the infected person transmits the disease during periods of asymptomatic shedding of the virus. If a woman suspects that she has been exposed to HSV-2, she should consult a health care provider when she has lesions. The health care provider will take a sample from the lesions and request a culture to determine whether HSV-2 is present. New testing procedures may help providers with diagnosing and managing HSV-1 and HSV-2. A blood test can be conducted when a woman is concerned about herpes but has no visible symptoms.

Treatment There is no cure for herpes simplex, but the drug acyclovir (Zovirax) has effectively reduced the frequency and duration of recurrences in most people. Although acyclovir, an antiviral drug, prevents the herpes cells from replicating, it does not appear to reduce the transmission of the virus to one's partner. Acyclovir is available in pills, ointment, or injectable forms. The recommended regimen for the first episode of genital herpes is oral acyclovir taken five times a day for 7 to 10 days or until the active virus disappears. Valacyclovir (Valtrex) and famciclovir (Famvir) are two versions of acyclovir that absorb more readily and can also be prescribed.[30]

Prevention of Spread or Recurrence Prevention depends on the management of outbreaks and preventing the spread of the virus to a partner. (See *Her Story:* "Kristin: Herpes and Sexual Activity.")

A young woman with herpes can prevent recurrences by maintaining a healthy diet, exercising regularly, getting plenty of rest, and managing her stress level. Intimate contact remains the primary mode of transmission, and there is no way to ensure that a partner will remain unaffected because the virus can be present on the skin without recognizable symptoms. If the infected partner notices itching or tingling at the primary site of the infection or has blisters, she should avoid sexual contact or use additional precautionary measures. Sexual contact should also be avoided when sores are active (infected), during the healing process, and for several days after the healing has occurred. A woman has about a 75 percent chance of becoming infected if her partner is actively shedding the virus.

A woman can spread herpes to other parts of her body. This transfer is referred to as **autoinoculation** and occurs by touching or scratching an area of shedding active cells and then touching another susceptible area. To prevent autoinoculation, a woman should avoid touching active lesions or letting others touch the lesions. If her hands accidentally touch an active sore,

Her Story

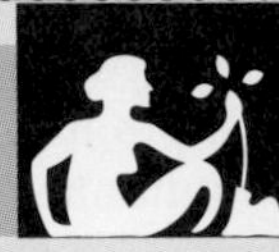

Kristin: Herpes and Sexual Activity

Kristin, a 19-year-old college sophomore, recently went to see Dr. Cox, a physician at the student health center. When Dr. Cox entered the room, she sat down and asked Kristin, "What brings you here today?" Kristin hesitated to answer, and Dr. Cox began to sense that something was bothering Kristin so she waited for her to speak. Finally, Kristin began, "Well, basically, I'm here to get some information from you. It is kind of hard to talk about it. I have been dating this really great guy for a long time now and, well, he is just so nice and considerate, and we really like each other. I have been thinking for a while that we might be ready to start getting sexually involved. I guessed he felt the same way so when we went out the other night I brought it up. Ben's reaction surprised me. He just looked down at the table and didn't say anything, and that is not like him, he usually is very willing to talk, even about hard things. I kept encouraging him to share his feelings. Finally, he did. And that is why I am here with you today. You see, Ben has herpes. I want to continue to be involved with Ben, but I am scared. Dr. Cox, I don't want to get herpes, and I don't want to overreact. So, what can I do?"

- Knowing the risks involved, is this a good time for Kristin to become sexually active?
- If Kristin chooses to become sexually active, what precautionary methods should she practice?

she should wash them immediately to avoid spreading the virus to other susceptible parts.[31]

Pregnancy A pregnant woman with recurrent HSV-2 diagnosed before pregnancy has a relatively low risk of transmitting the virus to her newborn. Pregnant women with undiagnosed primary HSV-2 have a higher risk of transmission to the newborn causing serious infections that can result in nerve damage and even death. Previously, cesarean sections were recommended for women with HSV-2 in an effort to prevent transmission of the virus to the newborn. Most women who had cesarean deliveries had recurrent lesions rather than primary lesions (a first or initial outbreak). Recently, some researchers have suggested that the rate of maternal morbidity and mortality from cesarean section may actually be higher than the rate of neonatal deaths that are prevented by this procedure. Cesarean deliveries increase the hospital stay, require longer recuperation, increase the number of follow-up visits, and greatly increase the delivery costs, and they are not completely effective in preventing transmission of HSV-2 to neonates. An analysis of cost effectiveness showed that for each case of HSV-2 prevented, $2.5 million was saved in lifetime costs for the newborn.[32] In another study evaluating the risk of pregnancy exposures to acyclovir, researchers found no increased risk for birth defects among infants exposed to acyclovir during pregnancy. However, the CDC recommends that acyclovir be administered intravenously only in life-threatening maternal infections and not systemically near term. The safety of acyclovir in human pregnancies has not been determined, and the risk with drug exposure to the fetus is unclear.[33]

Epidemiology HSV-1 affects four in five adults, or approximately 80 percent of all adults. HSV-2, commonly referred to as genital herpes, infects one in six adults, or nearly 45 million American men and women.[34] Nearly one in four U.S. women is infected with HSV-2. HSV-2 plays a major role in the transmission of heterosexual HIV, making the person infected with HSV-2 more susceptible and the HIV-infected person more infectious. HSV-1 and HSV-2 can manifest anywhere on the body, despite the common belief that HSV-1 is found only above the waist and that HSV-2 exists only below the waist.

Human Papilloma Virus

Human papilloma virus (HPV) refers to a group of more than one hundred viruses, one-third of which infect the genital mucosal sites. HPV is the most common STI and is nearly twice as high in women as in men. Genital warts, or condyloma, are usually spread by skin-to-skin contact with an infected person. The symptoms of genital warts include small, bumpy warts on the vaginal or anal area that vary from small to large, raised to flat, or single to clustered. Warts can appear several weeks to several months after contact with an infected person. They may remain undetected when located inside the vagina, on the cervix, or in the anus. Most warts are painless and flesh colored and will not disappear without medical attention. Some partners carry the virus without experiencing warts; others experience itching, pain, or bleeding.[36]

The relationship of genital HPV infection to cervical cancer is a significant concern for all women, particularly those infected with HPV and those who are sexually active and susceptible to HPV infection. In most cases, infected women do not know that they have HPV until an abnormal Pap smear is detected, and most of these women will not have experienced the external signs of genital warts. Genital HPV infections are generally characterized as either high-risk or low-risk types. High-risk types (e.g., HPV 16, 18, 31, 33, 35, 39, 45, 51, 52) are associated with low- and high-grade squamous intraepithelial lesions (LSIL and HSIL). Low-risk types (e.g., HPV 6, 11, 42, 43, 44) are associated with genital warts, LSIL, and recurrent respiratory papillomatosis.[37] Because genital HPV infection is not a reportable disease, estimates of its prevalence are difficult to ascertain. (See *Viewpoint: "HPV Vaccine."*)

Viewpoint

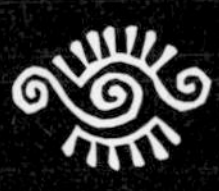

HPV Vaccine

In 2006, all members of the FDA advisory committee recommended that Gardisil, an HPV vaccine, be approved for distribution in the United States. The vaccine, developed by Merck and Co. is effective in preventing two types of HPV known to cause about 70 percent of all cervical cancer cases worldwide. The vaccine is being recommended as most effective when given to young girls between the ages of 11 and 12 years, and as young as 9. The vaccine is also recommended for 13- to 21-year-old females who have not been vaccinated. It is ideally given before girls and young women become sexually active.[35] A controversy has arisen around this vaccine. Is it appropriate for girls as young as 9 years old? Should girls be vaccinated to prevent possible transmission in situations of child abuse or rape? Should young men be vaccinated to prevent transmission to young women? Worldwide, 400,000 women are diagnosed with cervical cancer each year. The vaccine does not take the place of annual pelvic examinations because it does not prevent all types of HPV.

Diagnosis A woman should notify her health care provider if she detects any unusual growths, bumps, or skin changes in the vaginal or anal areas or if her partner has HPV. A health care provider diagnoses HPV by placing a drop of acetic acid on the infected area. This drop causes abnormal tissue to turn white and the HPV virus can then be detected through a colposcope, a magnifying lens.[38]

Treatment There is no cure for HPV although lesions can be removed with proper treatment and follow-up. Usually, several treatments are needed to remove visible warts. The type of treatment prescribed by the health care provider depends on the location and size of the warts and the woman's preference of treatment. Current treatments of HPV include a conservative approach using cryotherapy with liquid nitrogen or a cryoprobe. Other treatments include chemicals such as podophyllin or trichloracetic acid and laser surgery. Podofilox, an FDA-approved prescription solution or gel, has the advantage of being a topical application that can be administered at home.[39]

The decision to remove lesions located on the cervix depends on the severity and the risk of sexual transmission. They are usually removed by cryotherapy, laser, or excision. The goal of HPV treatment is the removal of external warts and the amelioration of signs and symptoms, not to cure the individual. Podophyllin and podofilox are not recommended treatment for pregnant women. Genital warts tend to proliferate during pregnancy, so experts recommend only the removal of visible warts.[40]

Prevention Most genital HPV infections are transmitted by sexual activity and are diagnosed on the basis of abnormal Pap smears. Studies have demonstrated that few (if any) cervical HPV infections have been found in females who have not yet been sexually active. The most commonly associated factors related to HPV infection are the number of sexual partners a woman has had and the number of sexual partners her partner has had. The most effective strategies to avoid HPV are abstinence or monogamy with a partner who is not infected. However, sexually active young women who do not have the HPV virus should consider the vaccine.

Risk of Cancer Approximately one-third of the estimated one hundred types of HPV are associated with infections of the genital area, and six are associated with cervical cancer. Some types of HPV, such as types 16, 18, 31, 33, and 35, cause cervical cancer or cervical dysplasia (precancerous changes in cell structure).[41] In fact, HPV type 16 accounts for nearly 50 percent of cervical cancer cases and high-grade dysplasia. HPV types 16, 18, 31, and 45 account for 80 percent of cervical cancer cases. These cervical cell changes must be monitored closely because they are linked to an increased risk of cervical cancer. The only effective treatment of cervical cancer is surgical removal of all or part of the cervix. In developing countries, cervical cancer surpasses breast cancer in mortality in women. The United States has reduced the mortality due to cervical cancer through early detection (Pap smear). It is recommended that women with HPV monitor their condition closely and have a Pap smear every 6 months. Other types of HPV, types 6 and 11, have been linked to cancers of the oral cavity, larynx, pharynx, and lungs.[42]

Pregnancy HPV types 6 and 11 not only increase a woman's risk of cancer but also are associated with potential disease in infants. An infant born to a woman with HPV type 6 or 11 can contract laryngeal papillomatosis (small tumors that grow on the voice box, vocal cords, or air passages).

Epidemiology Some studies have suggested that the annual incidence of genital HPV infection is 5.5 million and that 20 million infected persons are currently living in the United States. Population estimates suggest that more than "50% of sexually active women have been infected with one or more genital HPV types, 15% have evidence of current infection, 50–75% of which is with high-risk types, and 1% have genital warts."[43] Nearly 20 percent of sexually active women are estimated to have HPV type 16, which accounts for 50 percent of all cervical cancer cases.

Worldwide, estimates of cervical cancer (the number-one cancer killer of women in many developing countries) may be 400,000 to 500,000 cases annually. The prevalence of cervical cancer in the United States is approximately 14,000 cases with 5,000 deaths annually. This morbidity and mortality occurs despite nearly 50 million Pap smears a year. The annual Pap smear screenings detect an estimated 2.5 million low-grade abnormalities and 200,000 to 300,000 high-grade abnormalities. Most significantly, the annual estimated cost of treating HPV infection ranges from $1.6 billion to $6 billion a year, making genital HPV second only to HIV in total STI treatment costs.[44]

REPRODUCTIVE TRACT INFECTIONS

Vaginitis

One in ten women who visit their health care provider complains about vaginal discharge, a sign of **vaginitis,** or itching. Over 90 percent of vaginitis in women of reproductive age is classified as trichomoniasis, bacterial

FYI

What to Tell Your Health Care Provider

- When the symptoms started
- Texture, color, and odor of discharge
- Burning, itching, pain, or redness
- Change in bowel movements such as diarrhea
- Recent change in sexual partner or symptoms in current partner
- Problems in sexual intercourse such as pain with penetration during intercourse
- Anal intercourse
- Type of contraceptive used
- Use of home remedies or over-the-counter medications
- Number of pregnancies
- Previous pelvic infections, including during pregnancy

vaginosis (BV), or candidiasis. Nearly 45 percent have BV, 25 percent have trichomoniasis, and 25 percent have candidiasis.[45] Your health care provider will ask a number of questions to determine whether you have vaginitis or some other infection. The information provided in *FYI:* "What to Tell Your Health Care Provider" will help you prepare for the visit to your health care provider.

Bacterial Vaginosis (BV) Bacterial vaginosis, formerly called nonspecific vaginitis, *Gardnerella* -associated vaginitis, or *Haemophilus* -associated vaginitis, is the most common cause of abnormal vaginal discharge. BV occurs when bacteria usually found in the vagina multiply and replace the prevailing bacteria, changing the vaginal pH balance.[46] It frequently affects women with multiple sexual partners and is sexually associated, but not sexually transmitted. BV can also be caused by a chemical imbalance in the vagina. It is recognized by a homogeneous, white, non-inflammatory discharge with a fishy odor, either before or after a vaginal sample is examined with a drop of potassium hydroxide solution.

Bacterial vaginosis is associated with cervicitis, PID, and recurring urinary tract infections. In pregnant women, BV is associated with premature labor, lower birth weight, and postpartum endometritis. It can also increase the risk for HIV infections.

Treatment: Symptomatic women need treatment, but studies have not supported treating asymptomatic women. There is no recognized equivalent in male partners, and treatment appears contraindicated for preventing recurrences. The CDC recommends treating BV with a 7-day regimen or a single dose of antibiotics, or with one of two topical agents. The topical antimicrobial creams are more expensive but appear to be equally effective for treating BV. Some health care providers prefer the antimicrobial creams over oral antibiotics because of fewer possible side effects. Pregnant women are treated with topical agents because the oral antibiotic, metronidazole, is contraindicated.

Trichomoniasis *Trichomonas vaginalis (T. vaginalis),* the protozoan that causes trichomoniasis, is found in both men and women. It remains dormant in many asymptomatic women and causes vaginal irritation, itching, and diffuse, malodorous discharge in symptomatic women. The discharge varies but typically is thin, frothy, homogeneous, and yellow-green or gray. Most infected women experience red spots on the vaginal walls or uterus, whereas most infected men are asymptomatic.[47]

Treatment: Both partners need treatment for *T. vaginalis* to be effectively cured because *T. vaginalis* is sexually transmitted. **Trichomoniasis** is confirmed by the presence of trichomonads and a vaginal pH of 5 or higher. If confirmed, an oral antibiotic (metronidazole) is usually prescribed for the woman and her partner.[48] Clinical trials have resulted in cure rates of 90 to 95 percent.

Candidiasis Vulvovaginal candidiasis (VVC), commonly known as yeast infection, is not a sexually transmitted infection but may coexist with STIs. *Candida* is the name of a single-celled fungus often present in the human body. Symptomatic women will experience itching with vaginal discharge, burning, or irritation in the vulvovaginal area. Pregnant women and those who have significant changes in diet, have some type of immune suppression, and/or use broad-spectrum antibiotics commonly experience yeast infections. Nearly 75 percent of women will have one episode of VVC in their lifetime. Women with pelvic pain, a first-time yeast infection, multiple sexual partners, or unprotected sexual encounters and pregnant women should see a health care provider to get treatment.

Some women are more predisposed to recurrent yeast infections. The factors most often associated with repeat infections include diabetes, obesity, suppressed immunity, pregnancy, and using broad-spectrum antibiotics, corticosteroids, or birth control pills. Self-care is appropriate for women who have recurrent yeast infections.

Treatment: Candida and other yeasts are found in the vagina of nearly 20 percent of all women, many of whom are asymptomatic and do not need treatment. Most symptomatic cases are uncomplicated and easy to treat. FDA-approved over-the-counter (OTC) medications that cure yeast infections include vaginal topical creams, tablets, suppositories, and combination packs. Familiar trade names include Monistat 7, Gyne-Lotrimin, Mycelex-7, and Fem Care. Another choice of treatment is a single-dose tablet of fluconazole. Treatment of partners does not appear to reduce the incidence of yeast infections.

Unfortunately, some women who self-diagnose a yeast infection may actually experience BV or another infection that cannot be cured by OTC medications. If a self-diagnosed infection does not appear to respond to treatment, a health care provider should be consulted.[49] When yeast infections recur without one of the causes mentioned above, the health care provider should suspect or rule out HIV. (See *Health Tips:* "Preventing Recurring Yeast Infections.")

Pelvic Inflammatory Disease

Pelvic inflammatory disease (PID) has one of the most severe outcomes of sexually transmitted infections. PID is an infection of the upper portion of the female reproductive tract beyond the cervix. Common symptoms include severe pelvic pain, high fever, chills, nausea, and vomiting. Spotting or pelvic pain can occur between menstrual periods, and sometimes there is abnormal vaginal discharge.

Nearly 15 percent of women between ages 15 and 44 experience one incident of PID in their lifetime, and almost 1 million new cases of PID are diagnosed annually. Nearly 25 percent (250,000) of these women need costly hospitalization. Although the antibiotics used to treat PID cure most women, approximately 200,000 women will continue to experience chronic pelvic pain and 150,000 women will become infertile.

Accurate estimates of PID rates are difficult to obtain because complex and invasive procedures are needed to diagnose this disease correctly. Interpretations of clinical findings are often used when reporting PID, and these interpretations vary depending on the health care provider. The rate of PID-related hospitalizations of women 15 to 44 years of age has continued to decline over the past 20 years; however, the declines may be misleading because they may point to a change in treatment protocol from inpatient to outpatient and better screening for chlamydia infections.

PID is diagnosed by a health care provider through a pelvic examination or through analysis of cervical or vaginal secretions. If diagnosed, treatment includes antibiotics, rest, and sexual abstinence. Surgery may be required to remove any scars or abscesses or to repair injured reproductive organs. A single episode can damage the fallopian tubes. PID is the only cause of infertility that is preventable, accounting for as many as 30 percent of all infertility cases.[50]

Health Tips

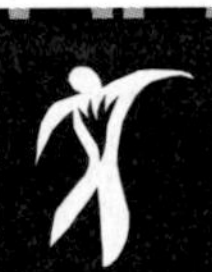

Preventing Recurring Yeast Infections

- Use mild soaps and perfumes.
- Use unscented toilet paper and sanitary pads rather than tampons.
- Do not use feminine hygiene sprays.
- Double-rinse undergarments washed in harsh irritants.
- Use 100 percent cotton undergarments to keep the genital area dry.
- Wear loose rather than restrictive clothing.
- Limit hot-tub episodes.
- Change swimsuits immediately after a hot tub or swim to reduce exposure of the genital area to moisture.
- Wipe from front to back after a bowel movement to reduce possible infections.
- Male partners must wash their penis or change condoms when moving from anal to vaginal intercourse.
- Avoid sugar binges.
- Avoid drastic changes in dietary patterns.

HIV/AIDS

Human immunodeficiency virus (HIV) is the organism that cause **acquired immune deficiency syndrome (AIDS)**, a group of signs or symptoms that causes the immune system to function improperly. The virus is transmitted from person to person through blood, semen, or vaginal secretions. It can be transferred through sexual contact with an infected person, by sharing injecting drug needles, from mother to infant before or during childbirth, through breast-feeding, and through receiving blood or blood products from someone infected with HIV. Persons receiving transfusions in the United States are virtually free from the possibility of blood or blood product transmission because all blood banks test for the virus.

Symptoms of AIDS may be similar to those of other diseases; however, they take longer to disappear and may recur. Some common early symptoms of AIDS are recurring fever including "night sweats"; rapid weight loss without diet or exercise; diarrhea lasting longer than several weeks; white, thick spots or coating in the mouth; a dry cough and shortness of breath; or purple bumps on the skin, inside the mouth, and in the rectum.

In the United States, the AIDS epidemic has increased most dramatically among women of color. (See Figure 14.2.) These increasing rates have placed an undue burden on an already impoverished group of women.

These women are faced with an array of psychosocial, economic, cultural, and relational issues. HIV/AIDS is indeed a family issue because many of these women are the primary care providers for their children and themselves. African American and Hispanic women account for 83 percent of AIDS cases reported among women, yet constitute only one-fourth of all U.S. women. In 2002, HIV/AIDS was the *leading cause of death* for African American women aged 25 to 34 years.

FIGURE 14.2 Race/ethnicity of women with HIV/AIDS diagnosed during 2001–2004.

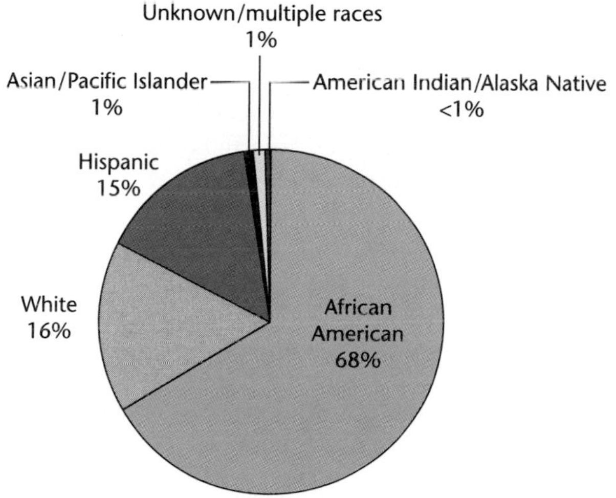

Total number=45,146

NOTE: Based on data from 33 states with long-term, confidential name-based HIV reporting.

SOURCE: Centers for Disease Control and Prevention. 2005. Trends in HIV/AIDS diagnoses—33 states, 2001–2004. *Morbidity and Mortality Weekly Report* 44:1149–53.

The most common methods for heterosexual women to contract HIV are through contact with bisexual or heterosexual men or by injected drug use. (See Figure 14.3.) Health care workers have been infected by a needle stick with HIV-contaminated blood or, less often, through contact with HIV-infected blood drops from a patient. Only one incident of infection of patients by an HIV-infected dentist has been documented. HIV has not been transmitted through casual contact, tears, or saliva. HIV does not survive well in the environment. In laboratory settings, CDC studies have found that drying a high concentration of HIV reduces the infectious virus by 90 to 99 percent within several hours. In addition, HIV cannot reproduce outside the living host. In family households with an HIV-infected person, transmission to other family members is rare. Transmission usually occurs when skin or mucous membranes are exposed to infected blood.

In the vast majority of full-blown AIDS cases, however, little is known about the mechanism by which the immune system breaks down. Scientists continue to study why exposure causes some individuals to become infected whereas others do not. It appears that the level of infection and the method of exposure both contribute to a woman's susceptibility.

Epidemiology

Nearly 95 percent of the global total of people with HIV live in developing countries. Women constitute nearly 46 percent of all people living with acquired immune deficiency syndrome (AIDS), further demonstrating that

FIGURE 14.3 AIDS in U.S. women by exposure category, 2001–2004.

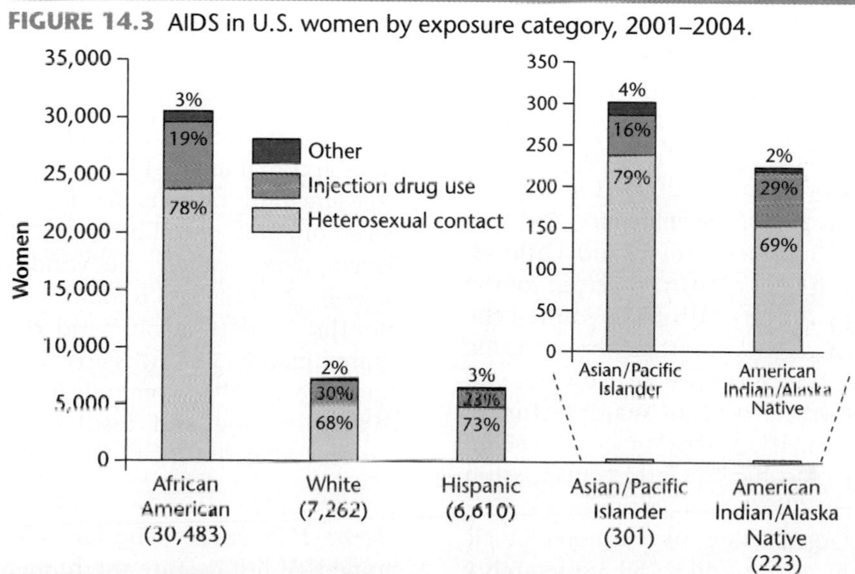

Note: Based on data from 33 States with long-term, confidential name-based HIV reporting.

SOURCE: Centers for Disease Control and Prevention. 2005. *Pelvic inflammatory disease—Fact Sheet*. www.cdc.gov/std/PID/STDFact-PID.htm (retrieved May 24, 2006).

Viewpoint 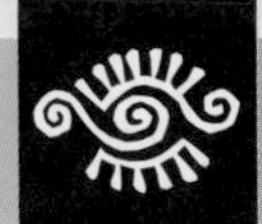

Seeking Solutions to Mother-to-Child Transmission of HIV

All women have the right to be treated for HIV infection. Here are some international problems and solutions.

- The Ministry of Public Health, Thailand, offers HIV-positive women AZT (azidothymidine) and free formula for their infants for 12 months.
- The Mulago Hospital postnatal clinic, Kampala, Uganda, began a "posttest club" that actively recruits husbands of HIV-positive women for voluntary HIV counseling and testing. The club has reduced subsequent pregnancies, marital breakups, and domestic violence.
- Zimbabwe is promoting self-reliance and economic self-sufficiency as a means to reducing HIV in women.
- Keeping young women HIV-negative will prevent HIV transmission to the next generation.
- Reducing the high prevalence of intergenerational sex and violence against young women by older men will help reduce the transmission of HIV.
- Improved treatment of HIV-positive women in the United States has reduced mother-to-child transmission by three hundred to four hundred cases per year.

How can better prevention efforts be directed worldwide? How can medical and technological advances be shared with underdeveloped countries?

AIDS is not a disease for men only! The Joint United Nations Programme on HIV/AIDS (UNAIDS) and the World Health Organization (WHO) estimate that more than 40.3 million women and children were living with HIV at the end of 2005. HIV/AIDS accounted for 3.1 million deaths worldwide in 2005, the highest number since the beginning of the epidemic.

In 2005, some 4.9 million women and children became infected with HIV. More than 90 percent of the children (age 14 and younger) with HIV acquired the virus at birth or through their mother's breast milk. Poverty, limited access to adequate health care, and lack of prevention efforts remain the major factors in the continued spread of HIV/AIDS.[51] (See *Viewpoint:* "Seeking Solutions to Mother-to-Child transmission of HIV.")

The World Health Organization suggests that biologic factors, epidemiologic factors, and social vulnerability cause women to be more susceptible to HIV than men. Women have increased biologic risk due to greater mucosal surface exposed during intercourse and high concentrations of HIV in seminal fluids. They have increased epidemiological risk because women date or marry older men who have often been with multiple partners. For instance, most teenage women date older males, many of whom have had several sexual partners. The more partners, the greater the risk of contracting HIV or another STI. Social vulnerability is an issue when women are forced to be sexual with a partner who refuses to use a condom or when women must rely on a partner's saying he is monogamous when in fact he is not. This male behavior or "assumed right" increases a woman's risk of contracting HIV and other STIs.

Diagnosis of HIV

If a woman believes she has been infected with or exposed to HIV through sex, injected drug use, or other contact with contaminated blood, she should request an HIV antibody test. Because women can be infected more easily than men, they should request testing if they have the slightest suspicion of exposure. The testing center should offer pre- and post-test counseling, as well as confidentiality from employers and health insurance. Some centers offer anonymous testing. Two tests are used for diagnosis: the **ELISA test** (enzyme-linked immunosorbent assay), a general screening test with high sensitivity, and the **Western blot test,** a less sensitive, more expensive but more specific test for the HIV antibody. If a person tests positive for the HIV antibody with the ELISA test, a second ELISA test is conducted on the same sample. If this test is positive, the Western blot test is conducted. If the Western blot test is positive, the person is said to be HIV-positive. Nearly 90 percent of low-risk persons who test positive on the ELISA test will test negative on the Western blot test. Results for each test often take up to a week for reporting.

A woman must wait nearly a month from the time of the suspected exposure before getting tested because it takes approximately 45 days from the time of initial exposure until the body develops enough antibodies for detection. This period between infection and antibody development, called the window period, can take between 2 weeks and 6 months but can take up to 18 months. Experts recommend that two sets of tests, approximately 6 months apart, be conducted for conclusive results. If a woman is unsure of where to go for HIV counseling and testing, she can contact the National AIDS Hotline (1-800-232-4636).

Home HIV Tests The FDA has approved only one home HIV test despite the numerous products advertised by companies on the Internet. Many people refuse to be tested at a health care facility because of concerns about breached confidentiality and potential loss of health insurance benefits. The home HIV test, Home Access Express, is marketed by Home Access Health Corporation and has been clinically proven to be 99.9 percent accurate. It is available for purchase through a toll-free number (1-800-HIV-TEST) and the Internet (www.homeaccess.com) and at pharmacies nationwide. The test kit includes detailed instructions on how to collect a blood sample, ship the product, and call for results. The sample is screened at a lab using the ELISA test. If this screen is positive, a more specific confirmatory test (immunofluorescence assay [IFA]) is used. An eleven-digit code (included in the kit) is all the individual needs to get the test results. The results are available within 3 days, and trained counselors at Home Access are available for confidential and anonymous support. If a woman does not have access to an anonymous testing site in her community, the FDA-approved home kit is beneficial. The earlier an HIV-positive woman knows her status, the earlier she can get treatment.

Use of non-FDA approved products is discouraged. The Federal Trade Commission tested a variety of home HIV products advertised and sold on the Internet by sending an HIV-positive sample to the companies. In all cases, the results came back indicating that the sample was HIV-negative.[52] Anyone relying on those results would have been misled! The FDA has issued numerous warnings to companies to take corrective action or there will be enforcement action if the violations continue. Warning letters had been sent to fourteen companies at the time of this writing.[53]

Rapid Testing for HIV/AIDS In 2004 the U.S. FDA approved another type of HIV test, the OraQuick Rapid HIV-1/2 Antibody Test, manufactured by OraSure Technologies. This is the first FDA-approved test for HIV in oral fluid samples instead of blood. When used correctly in an approved medical setting, OraQuick has a 99 percent accuracy rate. The advantage of rapid testing for HIV/AIDS is that the individual receives results in as little as 20 minutes. This is important because many persons who take HIV/AIDS tests through health departments and public clinics do not return to receive their results.

The OraQuick wand has an exposed absorbent pad on one end, which is swabbed once against both the upper and lower gums. When the swab is completed, the wand is placed into a vial containing a chemical solution. If the results indicate that antibodies to HIV/AIDS have been detected, a small window on the testing device will display two reddish purple lines. If a test result is positive, a second test using another method should be done to confirm the OraQuick results. Currently, OraQuick can be administered only by trained health care professionals and is not available for in-home use.

Journal Activity

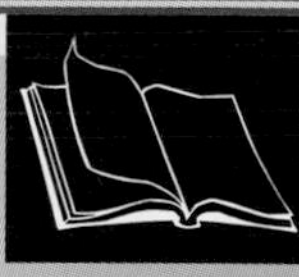

Browsing the Internet for AIDS Research

Browsing the Internet can be an effective way to keep updated on recent AIDS research advances. The National Institute for Allergies and Infectious Diseases has a Web page at www.niaid.nih.gov, which you can check for the most recent news releases. Which news release is of interest to you? Write a one-page summary of recent events. Share your findings with classmates.

No matter what type of test a woman chooses to confirm whether or not she is HIV-positive, it is important she receive test counseling throughout the procedure as a positive diagnosis for HIV/AIDS can be both frightening and life-changing.

Treatment of HIV

Drug treatment typically focuses on reducing the viral load or reinforcing the immune system. The viral load can be lowered or kept low by "blocking HIV attachment to the CDR cell, blocking antigens on the virus envelope, interfering with the uncoating of the virus as it enters the cell, disrupting the translation of virus RNA to cell DNA, and disrupting the assembly and maturation of virus particles in the CDR cell, and their release as a free-floating virus in the body."[54] Combinations of drugs are often used to impact the HIV virus at its various stages. Familiar drugs include Combivir, Atripla, Retrovir, and Videx and protease inhibitors such as Invirase and Viracept. Now, complete *Journal Activity:* "Browsing the Internet for AIDS Research" and then see *Viewpoint:* "Discrimination in AIDS Research."

HIV and Children

The number of cases of HIV in young children continues to rise worldwide as the rate of infection among heterosexual women of childbearing age rises. Most of these cases result from passing the HIV virus from HIV-infected mothers in utero or during childbirth and through breast-feeding. This rise in HIV in young children could be reduced dramatically, just as it has in the United States, by administering antiretroviral therapies

She has
her father's
eyes and her

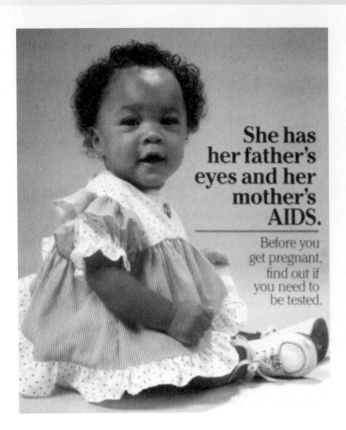

Before you
get pregnant,
find out if
you need to
be tested.

and earlier testing of pregnant women. The drop in HIV among children in the U.S. has been particularly significant for African American infants, who represent nearly two-thirds of all pediatric AIDS cases.

Determining an infant's HIV status after birth is difficult because a mother's antibodies may remain in the infant's system for several months. If a woman discovers her HIV-positive status upon becoming pregnant, she faces the shock of her own positive test concurrently with the possibility of transmitting the virus to her newborn. If the child tests negative, the mother still faces her own disease and the likelihood that she won't be able to raise her child without assistance. (See *Women Making a Difference:* "Clara M. Hale.")

Viewpoint

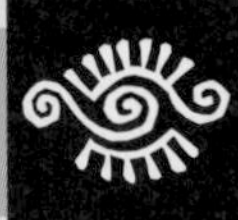

Discrimination in AIDS Research

Maureen Perry, in an issue of *Women Being Alive Newsletter,* wrote: "Fourteen of the 21 oncology/cancer trials currently in the ACTG [AIDS Clinical Trials Group] are studying treatments for Kaposi's Sarcoma, a cancer occurring almost exclusively in men. The exclusion of women from trial #216, though unethical, is not surprising. The ACTG has continuously ignored women in the epidemic, as well as minorities."[55]

The issue at hand was the handling of trial #216, a study originally designed to study the effects of the drugs isotretinoin and interferon in the prevention of anal and cervical neoplasia, precursors to cancer, related to anogenital human papilloma virus (HPV). The ACTG funded a project to address the drugs' potential to prevent recurrent anal intraepithelial neoplasia (AIN), ignoring the drugs' potential to prevent recurrent cervical intraepithelial neoplasia (CIN). Under public scrutiny, the ACTG funded a second study to address CIN. This is just one example of the limited (almost nonexistent) focus on women's symptoms of and treatment for HIV infections. In 2004 the adult AIDS Clinical Trials Group (AACTG) reported that a new study on the approaches used for preventing mother-to-child transmission of HIV in resource-limited settings had been initiated. It also highlighted ongoing efforts to enhance representation among women and other underrepresented minority populations in AIDS research.

What can you do to ensure that women receive fair and ethical treatment in medical research? What additional information do you need? What actions will you take?

STIs IN WOMEN WHO HAVE SEX WITH WOMEN (WSW)

Lesbians are at lower risk for STIs, but if the infections are left untreated, the risks are similar to those for heterosexual women. Yeast infections are the most common STIs in women who have sex with women (WSW) and can be passed from partner to partner. WSW are also susceptible to HPV, HSV, gonorrhea, chlamydia, and trichomoniasis. Female-to-female transmission of HIV is low, but some cases have been reported (CDC, unpublished data, 2006). This transmission indicates that vaginal secretions and menstrual blood are potentially infectious, and mucous membrane (e.g., oral, vaginal) exposure to these secretions has the potential to lead to HIV infection. Since the beginning of reported AIDS cases in the 1980s, only a small percentage of HIV-infected women have reported having sex with women; however, the vast majority had other risks (injected drug use, sex with high-risk men, and receipt of blood or blood products). It is difficult to know the actual transmission rate for WSW because many health care providers fail to ask whether a woman had sex with women or the HIV-positive woman did not volunteer the information.

Women Making a Difference

Clara M. Hale: Community Activist and Advocate for Families and Children

Clara McBride Hale was the founder of New York City's Hale House, one of the first private institutions dedicated to caring for babies and children born to alcohol and drug-addicted mothers. In the early 1980s, before HIV/AIDS garnered national attention, Hale House was among the first organizations offering care and services for children born positive for this devastating disease.

Hale House began unexpectedly in 1969 when Lorraine Hale, Clara's daughter, spotted a drug-addicted woman holding an infant on a city street corner. She spoke with the woman and encouraged her to seek help for her addiction, adding that her mother, then 63, would care for her child while she sought help. As news of Clara Hale's willingness and actions spread, other drug-addicted women, infants, and homeless children began arriving at her doorstep, many referred by city agencies and community groups or brought to her by police officers who had nowhere else to turn. In 1972, with help from members of New York City's government, Clara Hale purchased a brownstone at 122nd Street in Harlem, which grew to become the Hale House Center. Mrs. Hale's devotion to needy children eventually earned her the moniker "Mother Hale."

Before her death at age 87, Clara Hale received more than 370 awards and national recognition for her work, including mention by President Ronald Reagan in a 1985 State of the Union address. The work of the Hale House continues today, despite some legal and financial issues a few years ago.[56] Do you know of other women who are making a difference in helping mothers with AIDS or their children?

Regarding female-to-female transmission, WSW need to know the following:

- Exposure of a mucous membrane to vaginal secretions and menstrual blood is potentially infectious.
- Condoms (cut-open), dental dams, or plastic wrap can help protect them from body fluids during oral sex.
- Condoms should be used consistently and correctly when having sex with men or using sex toys.
- Bacteria in the rectum can cause infections in the vagina and urethra.
- Self-contact after touching a partner's genitals can transmit some STIs.
- STIs can be transmitted from vulva-to-vulva contact.
- A woman's own and her partner's HIV status can increase the risk of HIV infection.

PREVENTION STRATEGIES

STIs have special implications for women because women are less symptomatic, more difficult to diagnose, less frequently tested, and suffer more severe consequences then men. Also, the transmission of STIs is easier from men to women. These factors make prevention efforts extremely important. What prevention strategies are available for women? What sexual behaviors are considered safer?

Abstinence

Sexual abstinence is the only 100 percent effective method to prevent sexually transmitted infections. Abstinence means no exchange of body fluids and no skin-to-skin exposure of the genital areas. Young people need to understand that being physically developed does not necessarily equate with psychological readiness for a sexual relationship.

When is abstinence appropriate? *Anytime you choose!* Abstinence is certainly an appropriate choice for women when they are not psychologically ready to be sexually active, when they have been drinking, if they have had unprotected sex with a different partner without subsequent testing, or if they don't have adequate protection (condoms). Can you think of other times when a woman might choose abstinence?

Monogamy

More young women today are choosing to delay sexual intimacy until they have a committed relationship or until they are married. A committed relationship is not synonymous with "serial monogamy." Serial monogamy means having several relationships over time, with just

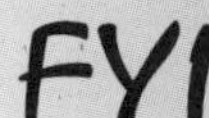

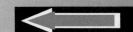

Playing It Safe with Sexual Behaviors[57]

Safe
Hugging
Dry kissing
Mutual masturbation on healthy skin
Oral sex with a latex barrier (condom, dams, gloves)
Touching, massage, fantasy

Less Safe
Vaginal intercourse or fingering with a latex condom or glove
Wet kissing
Anal intercourse or fingering with a latex condom or glove
Dildos with a condom

Risky
Oral sex without a latex barrier
Masturbation on skin that has cuts or abrasions
Exchanging sex toys without thorough cleaning
Anal-to-vaginal transmission

Dangerous
Vaginal intercourse without a condom
Anal intercourse without a condom
Sharing a needle or blood contact
Semen or urine in the mouth

Journal Activity

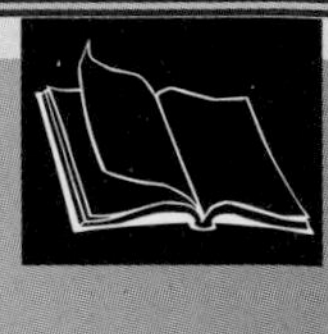

Reasons for Unprotected Sex

As a class assignment or an assignment with friends, brainstorm all the reasons that college women may give for putting themselves at risk for having unprotected sex with a partner. For each reason, write an alternative positive response in your journal.

Example
Reason: If I carry a condom with me, he could think that I'm planning to have sex.
Alternative response: I have a right to protect myself and the right to choose when and with whom I have sex.

one partner in each relationship. For teenagers, serial monogamy may mean having only one partner; however, the length of time for the relationship can vary from several days to several months. Reducing the number of sexual partners over one's lifetime and choosing a partner who has had fewer sexual partners translates into less exposure to the risk of contracting a STI.

Engaging in Less Risky Behaviors with Partners

Sexually transmitted infections are not dependent on who the person is but rather on what the person does. Sexual behaviors can be considered safe (dry kissing) to dangerous (unprotected vaginal or anal sex). Review the list provided in *FYI:* "Playing It Safe with Sexual Behaviors."

Are there other behaviors you would add to the list? Where would you place these behaviors? Then complete *Journal Activity:* "Reasons for Unprotected Sex."

Oral Contraceptives

Oral contraceptives are *not* effective in preventing STIs but may reduce the risk of PID. Most health care providers recommend using oral contraceptives and condoms to reduce the risk of unwanted pregnancies *and* STIs. However, recent studies have found that frequent use of **nonoxynol-9 (N-9)** can cause genital lesions in the vagina, which may increase the risk for HIV transmission. According to CDC guidelines, spermicides that contain N-9 should not be used for STI prevention and/or during anal intercourse.

Male Condoms

Male condoms are one of the most effective methods available for preventing STIs. Most viruses do not pass through the latex condom when properly used. The problem for many young women is their difficulty in insisting that their partner use a condom. If the partner refuses to use a condom, the woman is faced with additional decisions. If her partner consents to using a condom, she cannot ensure that he will use the condom properly, so she may want to consider not having sex with him.

In the past, STI prevention specialists recommended that condoms be latex with N-9. Those recommendations have changed. Condoms with N-9 have a shorter shelf life, cost more, and are associated with urinary tract infections in women. Males are still encouraged to use latex condoms consistently and correctly to significantly reduce the risk of HIV infection.

Female Condoms

The female condom offers a woman another alternative contraceptive method and allows her to have more control over the sexual experience. She can insert it before intercourse, unlike the male condom, which requires an erect penis before it can be put on. Also, the female condom protects the outer labia, thus offering better protection against HPV or HSV. The effectiveness of this method in preventing HIV or other STIs still remains uncertain.[58] Women have a variety of strategies available to prevent unwanted STIs and unintended pregnancies, from abstinence to proper protection. Keep informed! Stay assertive!

> **Health Tip**
>
> 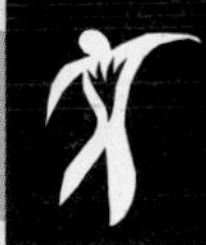
>
> **Adult Immunization Quiz**
>
> The Centers for Disease Control and Prevention provides an adult immunization quiz that allows you to determine the appropriate vaccinations for yourself. The quiz can be found at www2.cdc.gov/nip/adultImmSched. Questions are related to gender, pregnancy, birth year, lifestyle and work, and health status. Based upon your input, the CDC will provide a list of suggested vaccinations. Print the page for your health records.

OTHER INFECTIOUS DISEASES

Epstein-Barr Virus (EBV)

EBV is a member of the herpes virus family and is a common human virus. In the United States as many as 95 percent of adults between 35 and 40 years of age have been infected. When EBV occurs during adolescence or young adulthood, it causes infectious mononucleosis 35 to 50 percent of the time. Symptoms of mono include fever, sore throat, and swollen lymph glands. Although symptoms usually resolve in 1 or 2 months, the virus can reactivate (similar to other herpes viruses). Usually, laboratory tests are used to confirm mono, including an elevated white blood cell count, an increased total number of lymphocytes, and a positive reaction to a "mono spot" test. Bed rest and reduced physical activity are recommended to overcome the fatigue, fever, and other symptoms of the disease. While unusual, spleen, liver, heart, or central nervous system involvement can occur, indicating the importance of self-care during the time one is symptomatic. Transmission of mono occurs through intimate contact with saliva (found in the mouth) of an infected person, hence its name "the kissing disease." Transmission of the virus is virtually impossible to prevent, because 95 percent of healthy people have the virus in their saliva. These individuals are the primary reservoir for person-to-person transmission.[59]

Influenza (Flu)

The flu virus infects the respiratory tract (nose, throat, and lungs) and can cause mild symptoms to severe illness and life-threatening complications. Typical symptoms of influenza include high fever, headache, extreme tiredness, dry cough, sore throat, runny or stuffy nose, and muscle aches; children may experience stomach symptoms. The peak time for the "flu season" in the United States is late December through March, and the best way to prevent the illness is by getting a flu vaccination each fall. Transmission of the virus occurs person-to-person through respiratory droplets of coughs and sneezes. "Droplet spread" can be propelled up to 3 feet through the air and deposited in the nose or mouth of persons nearby. Hand washing is encouraged to prevent spread from respiratory droplets from one person to the nose or mouth of another person. A person with the virus is usually contagious for 1 day prior to and up to 5 days after the first symptoms. Once a person contracts the virus, she may develop some immunity to closely related viruses for one or more years. Persons with healthy immune systems have greater likelihood of immunity than persons with chronic diseases or weakened immune systems. Therefore, very young and elderly persons are at greatest risk for complications from the flu. The "flu shot" is an inactivated vaccine (containing killed virus) given by injection. It is approved for use in children older than 6 months and in adults, including healthy people and those with chronic medical conditions. The nasal-spray flu vaccine contains live, weakened flu virus and is approved for healthy children 5 years and older and for adults up to age 49 who are not pregnant. Each year, nearly 36,000 Americans die and more than 200,000 are hospitalized from complications of the flu. The premature deaths and hospitalizations could be greatly reduced by annual vaccinations. The CDC recommends that all persons who want to reduce their risk of complications from the flu be vaccinated.[60] (Now take the *Health Tips:* "Adult Immunization Quiz" to determine what vaccinations you should have. Then see *FYI:* "Who Should Consult a Physician Before Getting the Flu Vaccination.")

Hepatitis A

Hepatitis A virus (HAV) is a viral infection causing inflammation of the liver. Signs and symptoms may include jaundice, fatigue, abdominal pain, loss of appetite,

FYI

Who Should Consult a Physician Before Getting the Flu Vaccination?

- People who have a severe allergy to chicken eggs.
- People who have had a severe reaction to an influenza vaccination in the past.
- People who developed Guillain-Barre syndrome within 6 weeks of getting an influenza vaccination previously.
- Children less than 6 months of age (influenza vaccine is not approved for use in this age group).
- People who have a moderate or severe illness with a fever should wait to get vaccinated until their symptoms lessen.

nausea, diarrhea, and fever. Once a person has had HAV, she cannot get it again, and there is no long-term chronic infection. Transmission of HAV is usually spread person-to-person by putting something in the mouth that has been contaminated by the stool (feces) of a person with hepatitis A. Persons who are at risk for contracting HAV include those who have household contact with an infected person or sexual contact with an infected person; those who live in or travel to areas with increased rates of HAV; men who have sex with men; and injecting and non-injecting drug users. The best protection against HAV is vaccination. Short-term protection can happen with immune globulin if given before and within 2 weeks of coming in contact with HAV. Hand washing with soap is also a preventive measure.[61]

Nearly one-third of Americans have evidence of past infection (immunity). During epidemic years, the number of reported cases can reach 35,000, although HAV vaccine has greatly reduced the number of reported cases.[62]

Hepatitis B

Hepatitis B virus (HBV) is a viral infection causing inflammation of the liver. Transmission of HBV is similar to that of HIV, through exposure to infected blood and unprotected sexual intercourse, but HBV is more easily transmitted than HIV. In fact, HBV is a hundred times more contagious than HIV.[63] Persons at highest risk for contracting HBV include **hemodialysis** patients, injecting drug users, health care workers exposed to blood, infants born to HBV-positive women, gay men, and sexually active heterosexuals. Groups at highest risk for contracting HBV include Alaska Natives, Pacific Islanders, Asians, and others emigrating from high-incidence areas. International travelers to high-incidence areas may choose to receive the hepatitis B vaccine.[64] In women, heterosexual activity is the most common risk factor, followed by injected drug use. The modes of transmission often overlooked by individuals include tattoos, ear piercing, non-medication injections of vitamins, minerals, or steroids, and acupuncture treatments.[65] HBV can be transmitted through menstrual blood or the sharing of razors, toothbrushes, or other items with blood on them.

Recognizing the risk factors for HBV is important; however, more than one-third of adults with acute hepatitis B have no identified risk factors. Symptoms of acute hepatitis B include **jaundice** and a tender liver upon palpation. Hepatitis B follows a predictable course through four phases: incubation, prodrome, icteric, and convalescence. The prodome phase is characterized by generalized symptoms such as fever, fatigue, and discomfort. The icteric phase is recognized by jaundice and swelling of the liver, and the symptoms disappear during the convalescence phase.[66]

Nearly 95 percent of persons with hepatitis B recover, although a few persons develop fulminant hepatitis (acute liver failure) or experience persistent infections.

Diagnosis The type of hepatitis (whether A, B, or C) can be determined only through serologic testing. The hepatitis B virus is present in all body fluids.[67]

Treatment Persons with HBV should be evaluated for liver disease. Currently, five different drugs can be given to treat persons with chronic HBV. Drinking alcohol, because of its effect on the liver, can make the liver disease worse.

Vaccination for Hepatitis B College-age students continue to be a target for preventive vaccines; the American College Health Association recommends that all college students be vaccinated against HBV because HBV strikes healthy, young people. One-third of infected persons are college age, and more than one-third of infected persons do not have known risk factors. College women who are sexually active and have multiple partners, engage in any unprotected sex, have had another STI such as chlamydia or gonorrhea, or are studying for careers that involve exposure to blood should be vaccinated for HBV.[68] Sexually active women may reduce their risk of contracting HBV by using condoms and refraining from anal sex. The effectiveness of condoms in preventing the spread of HBV is unknown, but consistent and proper use is recommended.

Pregnancy and Infancy An estimated 22,000 infants are born to women with chronic HBV infection each year. These infants may not show early symptoms of infection, but they are at risk for developing chronic liver disease (hepatitis, cirrhosis, and carcinoma) as adults and even dying from it. This risk prompted the American College of Obstetrics and Gynecology, the American Academy of Pediatrics, and the American Academy of Family Practice to recommend screening for hepatitis B surface antigen in all pregnant women. They also recommended universal hepatitis B vaccination of infants.

Epidemiology An estimated 73,000 new cases of HBV are reported each year in the United States, and about 5,000 infected persons will die of HBV-related complications such as fulminant hepatitis, cirrhosis, or liver cancer. The greatest decline in HBV has been among children and adolescents because of the vaccine. Nearly 1.25 million Americans are chronically infected with HBV, and about one-third acquired the infection during childhood.

Hepatitis C

Hepatitis C virus (HCV) is a viral infection affecting the liver. Signs and symptoms include jaundice, fatigue, dark urine, abdominal pain, loss of appetite, and nausea. The virus is transmitted through blood from an infected person. HCV is spread through sharing needles, through needle sticks or sharps exposures at work, and from an infected mother to the infant during childbirth.

Persons at risk include injected drug users, hemodialysis patients, persons with undiagnosed liver problems, infants born to infected mothers, and health care/public safety workers. There is no vaccine for HCV, but at-risk persons should be vaccinated for HAV and HBV. Prevention includes not using someone else's personal care items that might have blood on them (razors, toothbrushes), avoiding tattoos and body piercing or at least ensuring that all instruments have been sterilized, and following routine barrier precautions if you are a health care or public safety worker. Persons with HCV should not donate blood, organs, or tissue. Current treatment includes interferon alone or in combination with ribavirin.

The annual number of HCV infections is approximately 30,000 and most are due to the sharing of needles. Transfusion-associated cases and perinatal transfusions are relatively low. Of the estimated 3.9 million Americans who have been infected with HCV, about 2.7 million are chronically infected.[69]

Tuberculosis (TB)

Tuberculosis is caused by the bacterium *Mycobacterium tuberculosis*, which usually attacks the lungs but can also attack other parts of the body such as the kidney, spine, and brain. TB, including resistant cases, is reported in every state in the U.S. An estimated 10 to 15 million Americans are infected with *M. tuberculosis,* and about 10 percent will develop TB if intervention doesn't occur. More than 14,000 cases are reported annually, so TB control remains an important endeavor. The TB bacterium is airborne, transmitted person-to-person by sneezing or coughing. It settles in the lungs, and when found in the lungs or throat, can be contagious. TB found in the kidneys, brain, or other parts of the body is usually not contagious. Latent TB infection occurs when a person has been infected, but the immune system is able to fight off the infection. The bacterium remains alive and can become active at a later time. A person with latent TB has no symptoms, is not infectious, and will usually have a positive skin test or serological test. This person will have a normal chest X ray and sputum test.

Active TB disease occurs then the immune system is unable to prevent the bacteria from multiplying. The bacteria attack and destroy tissue, and symptoms depend on where the bacteria are found. Symptoms of TB in the lungs may manifest as a bad cough that lasts 3 weeks or longer, pain in the chest, or coughing up blood or sputum. Other symptoms may include weakness and fatigue, weight loss, loss of appetite, fever, and night sweats. This person may spread TB to others, usually has a positive skin test or serological test, an abnormal chest X ray, or positive sputum smear or culture.[70]

Tuberculosis is a major, global public health problem, particularly in low-income countries. The United States is affected by the worldwide TB epidemic because nearly 40 percent of new U.S. cases occur in persons born in other countries, and soon there will be more cases among foreign-born persons than native-born persons. (See Figure 14.4.) The most effective control measure is curative treatment of patients with infectious pulmonary tuberculosis. In the United States, the most common medicines used to cure TB include isoniazid, rifampin, ethambutal, and pyrazinamide. BCG vaccine is a widely administered vaccine in many high-incidence countries, but wide variation in vaccine efficacy, ranging from 80 percent to zero, has been found. BCG does confer protection against serious forms of childhood TB (e.g., disseminated and meningeal TB) that are associated with high mortality rates. More recent studies have demonstrated that BCG vaccine also protects against the development of leprosy. However, because of questions about efficacy and skin hypersensitivity,

FIGURE 14.4 Number of TB cases in U.S.-born vs. foreign-born persons, United States, 1993–2003.

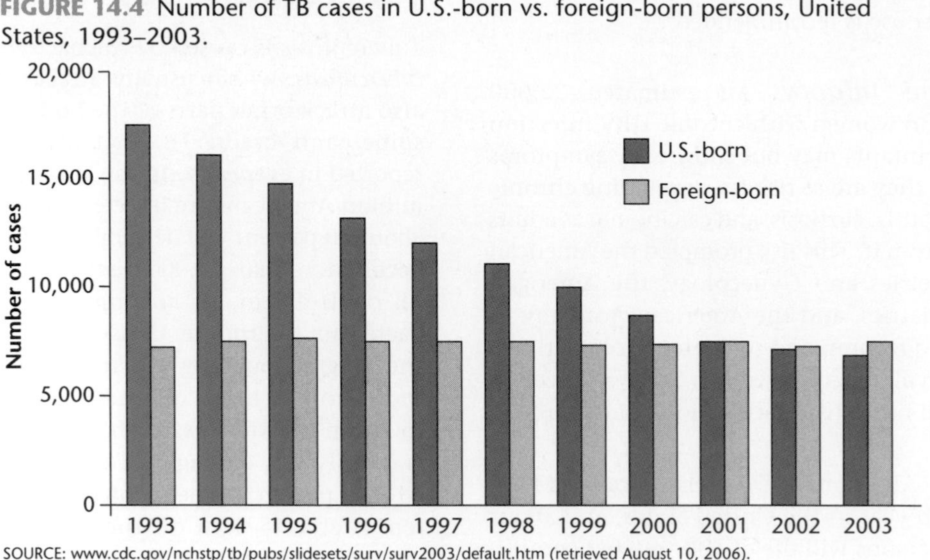

SOURCE: www.cdc.gov/nchstp/tb/pubs/slidesets/surv/surv2003/default.htm (retrieved August 10, 2006).

BCG is not routinely recommended for use in the United States.[71]

Streptococcal Disease

Group A streptococcus (GAS) is a bacterium found in the throat and on the skin. Most infections caused by GAS are relatively mild, such as "strep throat" or impetigo. Transmission is through direct contact with mucus or infected wounds or sores on the skin. Treatment with an antibiotic for 24 hours or longer will generally eliminate the spread of the bacteria in mild cases. In rare situations, the bacteria can get into the blood, muscle, or lungs and cause severe or life-threatening diseases such as necrotizing fasciitis or streptococcal toxic shock syndrome (STSS). Necrotizing fasciitis destroys muscle, fat, and skin tissue while STSS causes blood pressure to drop rapidly and organs to fail. Nearly 20 percent of persons with nectrotizing fasciitis and 50 percent of persons with STSS will die. STSS is not the same as toxic shock syndrome (from tampon use). Good hand washing is the best preventive measure against streptococcal disease, especially after coughing and sneezing and before food preparation and eating.[72]

One in five women carries group B streptococcal bacteria in her body, usually in the intestine, vagina, or rectum. While women who carry the bacteria are often asymptomatic, transmission through childbirth can cause sepsis of the bloodstream and meningitis in the newborn. CDC guidelines recommend that pregnant women be tested for group B strep at 35 to 37 weeks. Gynecologists now use this standardized protocol and have dramatically reduced the number of cases in newborns, by more than 50 percent in some places. Women who carry group B strep are given antibiotics intravenously at the time of labor and when their water breaks.[73]

Varicella (Chicken Pox and Shingles)

Varicella is an acute, contagious disease caused by varicella zoster virus, a member of the herpes virus group. Primary infection manifests as chicken pox, after an incubation period of around 14 to 21 days. Prior to the introduction of a vaccine in 1995, nearly 4 million cases of chicken pox were reported every year, with 4,000 to 9,000 hospitalizations and 100 deaths. Varicella vaccine is 85 percent effective in preventing disease; when vaccinated individuals contract the disease, the symptoms are usually quite mild. Immunity persists for more than 20 years. Vaccination is recommended for all children without an underlying condition or factor that increases the risk of complications. The vaccination protects not only the young child but also the adult who has not been vaccinated nor had chicken pox as a child. Maternal varicella from 5 days before to 2 days after delivery may result in a lethal infection of the newborn, a rate as high as 30 percent.[74]

Latent varicella infection, herpes zoster or shingles, occurs when the virus reactivates and causes a recurrent disease, usually in older adults. The risk of shingles is more common after age 50, with nearly 15 percent of persons having one episode by age 80. Shingles can cause numbness, itching, or severe pain followed by clusters of blister-like lesions. Pain can persist for weeks, months, or years, and persons with shingles can be contagious to others who have not had chicken pox.[75]

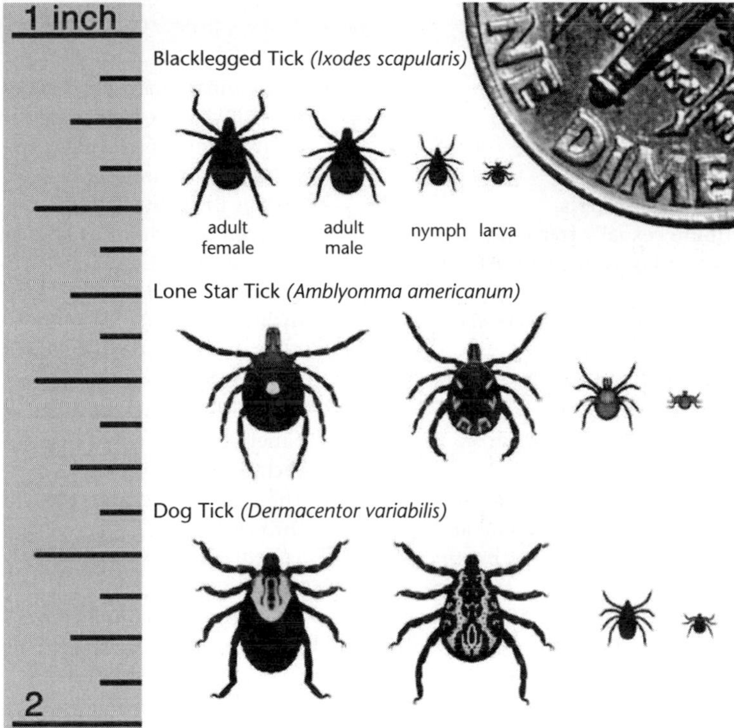

Comparison of ticks by appearance and relative size. Only deer ticks *(Ixodes scapularis)* are known to transmit Lyme disease.
SOURCE: www.cdc.gov/ncidod/dvbid/lyme/ld_transmission.htm (retrieved August 10, 2006).

Encephalitis and West Nile Virus

Arboviruses are a leading cause of viral encephalitis worldwide. In the United States, St. Louis encephalitis, eastern and western equine encephalitis, LaCrosse virus, and West Nile virus are transmitted by mosquitoes to humans. Fatality rates as high as 30 percent in eastern equine encephalitis and 5 percent in St. Louis encephalitis have been reported. Symptoms can range from fever with headaches to temporary paralysis, seizures that occur despite treatment, coma, and death depending upon the strain.

West Nile virus is a seasonal epidemic in the United States that occurs in the summer through fall months. One in 150 infected persons will develop severe illness, including high fever, headache, neck stiffness, coma, tremors, convulsions, muscle weakness, loss of vision, or paralysis. Nearly 20 percent of infected persons will have some symptoms, but nearly 80 percent will show no symptoms at all.

Mosquito control is the primary method of preventing the spread of encephalitis and West Nile virus. This involves avoiding outside activities at dawn and dusk, using insect repellant and wearing long sleeves and pants, draining areas where pooled water allows mosquito larvae to incubate, and keeping windows closed or ensuring that screens are free from tears or holes. Persons over age 50 are at greater risk for severe illness, and those who spend a lot of time outdoors have a greater chance of contracting the virus.[76]

Lyme Disease

Lyme disease is caused by a bacterium transmitted by the bite of infected blacklegged ticks, either the deer tick or the western blacklegged tick. Typical symptoms include fever, headache, and fatigue, and the first sign is usually a circular rash called erythema migrans at the site of the tick bite. The rash gradually expands over a period of several days, reaching up to 12 inches across. Untreated, the infection spreads to other body parts within a few days to weeks, producing a variety of symptoms. Later symptoms can include Bell's palsy (loss of muscle control in the face), shooting pains, heart palpitations, dizziness, and pain that moves from joint to joint. Many symptoms resolve, even without treatment, but for some people, chronic neurological complaints can persist. Early treatment is usually antibiotics, and most treatments are successful. Nearly 20,000 cases of Lyme disease were reported in 2004 in the United States, with the majority of cases on the East Coast and in the upper Midwest. Prevention of Lyme disease includes using insect repellant, removing ticks promptly, and avoiding unnecessary exposure to areas that are infested with ticks during late spring and summer.[77]

Chapter Summary

- Nearly fifty STI-related organisms and syndromes are recognized today.
- The United States has one of the highest STI rates of the industrialized countries.
- Teenagers account for 25 percent of all STIs.
- Chlamydia is the most common sexually transmitted infection in the United States and must be reported to the CDC by all fifty states.
- Chlamydia is treated with antibiotics, either in a 7-day or single-dose regimen.
- The number of cases of gonorrhea has declined since the 1970s except in teenagers and some minority groups. A large discrepancy in cases exists between African American and white teenagers.
- Syphilis is caused by the spirochete *Treponema pallidum.*
- Syphilis has four phases: primary, secondary, latent, and tertiary. Congenital syphilis is transmitted to the infant during pregnancy.
- Genital herpes is incurable and difficult to control. Autoinoculation is the self-spread of the virus from one body part to another. Acyclovir has some effectiveness in preventing a herpes outbreak.
- Several types of human papilloma viruses (genital warts) are associated with cancer.
- Hepatitis B is a viral infection causing inflammation of the liver. HBV is transmitted through exposure to infected blood and unprotected sexual intercourse. There is a vaccine to prevent HBV.
- Pelvic inflammatory disease causes chronic pelvic pain, infertility, and ectopic pregnancies.
- Most vaginitis is classified as trichomoniasis, bacterial vaginosis, or candidiasis.
- AIDS is the fifth leading cause of death in women between the ages of 25 and 44, and the third leading cause of death in African American women between the ages of 15 and 44.
- Invasive cervical cancer has been added to the list of AIDS-defining diseases. Invasive cervical cancer can be prevented with early detection.
- Epstein-Barr virus is a member of the herpes virus family.
- Ninety-five percent of healthy people carry the virus in their saliva.
- The peak flu season in the United States is late December through March.
- The flu shot and nasal-spray flu vaccine are available in the United States.
- Hepatitis causes inflammation of the liver.
- Hepatitis B vaccine is recommended for all college-age students.
- Strep A and strep B are bacterial infections that can have serious complications.
- West Nile virus and encephalitis are transmitted by mosquitoes to humans.
- Lyme disease is transmitted by the deer tick or western blacklegged tick.

Review Questions

1. Which STI has the highest incidence rate? What complications are associated with this STI?
2. Describe the four stages of syphilis.
3. What are the demographic characteristics that make a person more susceptible to STIs and/or HIV/AIDS?
4. Which individuals and groups are most susceptible to hepatitis B virus?
5. What complications can occur when pelvic inflammatory disease remains untreated?
6. What is the importance of the window period for determining the presence of HIV antibodies?
7. What are the known modes of transmission of HIV?
8. What measures can you take to prevent AIDS and other STIs?
9. Which STIs have vaccines available to prevent the disease?
10. Which STIs have antibiotics available to cure the disease?
11. Which infectious diseases have the most potential to lead to pandemics?
12. Which infectious diseases are most likely to impact college-age students?

Resources

Organizations and Hotlines

American Social Health Association
P.O. Box 13827
Research Triangle Park, NC 27709
919-361-8400
www.ashastd.org/index.cfm

CDC National Prevention Information Network (NPIN)
(Formerly the National AIDS Clearinghouse)
CDC NPIN
P.O. Box 6003
Rockville, MD 20849-6003
800-458-5231
www.cdcnpin.org

CDC National AIDS Clearinghouse
(Information and publication orders)
1-800-458-5231
TTY: 1-800-243-1098
International: 1-301-562-1098
International TTY: 1-301-588-1586
Monday–Friday, 9:00 A.M.–8:00 P.M. (Eastern)

CDC National STD Hotline
800-227-8922
Monday–Friday, 8 A.M.–11 P.M. (Eastern)
National Herpes Hotline
919-361-8488
Monday–Friday, 9 A.M.–7 P.M. (Eastern)
Sexuality Information and Education Council of the United States (SIECUS)
1706 R Street N.W.
Washington, DC 20009
202-265-2405
www.siecus.org
Vaccination Information for International Travelers
Centers for Disease Control and Prevention
404-332-4559

Web Sites

The Body: The Complete HIV/AIDS Resource
www.thebody.com
Centers for Disease Control and Prevention
www.cdc.gov
CDC Fact Sheet on Chlamydia
www.cdc.gov/std/chlamydia/STDFact-Chlamydia.htm
CDC Fact Sheet on Genital Herpes
www.cdc.gov/std/Herpes/STDFact-Herpes.htm
CDC Fact Sheet on Gonorrhea
www.cdc.gov/std/Gonorrhea
CDC Fact Sheet on HIV/AIDS & STDs
www.cdc.gov/std/hiv/default.htm
CDC Fact Sheet on Syphilis
www.cdc.gov/std/syphilis/default.htm
CDC HIV/AIDS Prevention
www.cdc.gov/hiv
Food and Drug Administration
www.fda.gov
Journal of the American Medical Association
www.jama.ama-assn.org
National Institute of Allergy and Infectious Diseases
www.niaid.nih.gov
Planned Parenthood Federation of America
www.ppfa.org
U.S. Department of Health and Human Services, National Institutes of Health
www.nih.gov

Suggested Readings

Baron-Faust, R., and J. P. Buyon. 2003. *The Autoimmune Connection.* New York: McGraw-Hill.

Bartlett, J. G., A. K. Finkbeiner, and Johns Hopkins AIDS Clinic. 2001. *Guide to Living with HIV Infection: Developed at the Johns Hopkins AIDS Clinic.* 5th ed. Baltimore, MD: Johns Hopkins University Press.

Becker, E., E. Rankin, and A. U. Rickel. 1998. *High-Risk Sexual Behavior: Intervention for the Vulnerable Populations.* New York: Kluwer Academic.

Handsfield, H. H. 2000. *Color Atlas and Synopsis of Sexually Transmitted Diseases.* 2nd ed. New York: McGraw-Hill.

Levine, P. 2003. *Prostitution, Race and Politics: Policing Venereal Disease in the British Empire.* London: Routledge.

Shilts, R. 1999. *And the Band Played On: Politics, People and the AIDS Epidemic.* New York: St. Martin's Press.

SIECUS Public Policy Office. *It Gets Worse: A Revamped Federal Abstinence-Only Program Goes Extreme.* (SIECUS Special Report). www.siecus.org/policy/Revamped_Abstinence-Only_Goes_Extreme.pdf (retrieved May 9, 2006.)

Wallman, S., and G. Bantebya-Kyomuhondo. 1996. *Kampala Women Getting By: Wellbeing in the Time of AIDS.* Athens: Ohio University Press.

References

1. Centers for Disease Control and Prevention. 2006. *NCID's strategy for the 21st century.* www.cdc.gov/ncidod/emergplan/summary/page_2.htm (retrieved May 14, 2006).
2. Centers for Disease Control and Prevention. 2007. Infectious diseases designated as notifiable at the national level during 2005. *Morbidity and Mortality Weekly Report* 54 (53): 2–92.
3. Centers for Disease Control and Prevention. 2006. *Elements of successful HIV/AIDS prevention programs.* www.cdcnpin.org/scripts/hiv/programs.asp (retrieved October 4, 2006).
4. U.S. Public Health Service. 1991. Curbing the increase in rates of STDs. *AIDS Weekly,* pp. 9–11.
5. Centers for Disease Control and Prevention, Division of AIDS, STD, and TB Laboratory Research. 2002. *Screening tests to detect* Chlamydia trachomatis *and* Neisseria gonorrhoeae *infections, 2002.* www.cdc.gov/STD/LabGuidelines/1-LG.htm#summary (retrieved September 28, 2006).
6. Division of STD Prevention. 1996, September. *Sexually transmitted diseases surveillance, 1995.* U.S. Department of Health and Human Services, Public Health Service. Atlanta: Centers for Disease Control and Prevention.
7. Hook, E. W., C. Spitter, C. A. Reichart, et al. 1994. Use of cell culture and a rapid diagnostic assay for *Chlamydia trachomatis* screening. *Journal of the American Medical Association* 272:867–70; S. D. Hillis, A. Nakashima, P. A. Marchbanks, et al. 1994. Risk factors for recurrent *Chlamydia trachomatis* infections in women. *American Journal of Obsterics and gynecology* 170:801–6.
8. Ibid.
9. Chlamydia prevalence and screening practices—San Diego County, California, 1993. 1994. *Morbidity and Mortality Weekly Report* 43(20):366–70; Update: New weapons in the war against chlamydia trachomatis infection. 1994. *Consultant* 34:103–5.
10. Hillis, Nakashima, Marchbanks, et al., Risk factors for recurrent *Chlamydia trachomatis* infections in women

11. Ibid.
12. Centers for Disease Control and Prevention, *Screening tests to detect* Chlamydia trachomatis *and* Neisseria gonorrhoeae *infections, 2002.*
13. Ibid.
14. Ibid.
15. Centers for Disease Control and Prevention. 2000. *Tracking the hidden epidemic: Trends in STDs in the United States.* www.wonder.cdc.gov/wonder/help/STD/Trends-Chlamydia.html (retrieved April 3, 2007).
16. Centers for Disease Control and Prevention. 2006. *Gonorrhea—Fact Sheet.* www.cdc.gov/STD/Gonorrhea/STDFact-gonorrhea.htm#What (retrieved September 28, 2006).
17. Centers for Disease Control and Prevention. 2002. *Sexually transmitted disease treatment guidelines, 2002.* www.cdc.gov/std/treatment/TOC2002TG.htm (retrieved September 28, 2004).
18. Kerle, K. K., J. R. Mascola, and T. A. Miller. 1992. Disseminated gonococcal infection. *American Family Physician* 45:209–14.
19. Centers for Disease Control and Prevention. 2005. *STD Surveillance 2004, national profile: Gonorrhea.* www.cdc.gov/std/stats/gonorrhea.htm. (retrieved May 15, 2006).
20. Goens, J. L., C. K. Janniger, and K. DeWolf. 1994. Dermatologic and systemic manifestations of syphilis. *American Family Physician* 50:1013–20; G. Bolan, C. Fontenot, et al. 1993. Syphilis: Are you missing it? *Patient Care* 27:126–42.
21. Centers for Disease Control and Prevention. 2004. *Syphilis—Fact Sheet.* www.cdc.gov/STD/syphilis/STDFact-Syphilis.htm (retrieved September 28, 2006).
22. Goens, Janniger, and DeWolf, Dermatologic and systemic manifestations of syphilis; Bolan, Fontenot, et al., Syphilis.
23. Goens, Janniger, and DeWolf, Dermatologic and systemic manifestations of syphilis; McCabe, E., L. R. Jaffe, and A. Diaz. 1993. Human immunodeficiency virus seropositivity in adolescents with syphilis. *AIDS Weekly* (December): 24.
24. CDC, Syphilis—Fact Sheet.
25. Holmes, K., P. Sparling, P. Mardh, et al., eds. 1999. *Sexually transmitted diseases.* 3rd ed. New York: McGraw-Hill, chap. 33–37.
26. CDC, Syphilis—Fact Sheet.
27. Centers for Disease Control and Prevention. 2006. Primary and secondary syphilis, United States, 2003–2004. *Morbility and Mortality Weekly Report.* www.cdc.gov/mmwr/preview/mmwrhtml/mm5510a1.htm (retrieved September 28, 2006).
28. Centers for Disease Control and Prevention. 2000. *Tracking the hidden epidemics: Trends in STDs in the United States, 2000.* www.cdc.gov/std/Trends2000/chancroid.htm (retrieved September 28, 2006).
29. Centers for Disease Control and Prevention. 2000. *Tracking the hidden epidemics: Trends in STDs in the United States, 2000.* www.cdc.gov/nchstp/dstd/ Stats_Trends/Trends2000.pdf (retrieved September 28, 2004).
30. Centers for Disease Control and Prevention. *Sexually transmitted disease treatment guidelines, 2002.*
31. Centers for Disease Control and Prevention. 2004. *Genital herpes—Fact Sheet.* www.cdc.gov/std/Herpes/STDFact-Herpes.htm (retrieved May 21, 2006).
32. Randolph, A. G., A. E. Washington, and C. G. Prober. 1993. Cesarean delivery for women presenting with genital herpes lesions: Efficacy, risks, and costs. *Journal of the American Medical Association* 270:77–82.
33. Centers for Disease Control and Prevention. Pregnancy outcomes following systemic prenatal acyclovir exposure—June 1, 1984–June 30, 1993. 1993. *Morbidity and Mortality Weekly Report* 42 (41): 806–9.
34. Centers for Disease Control and Prevention. 2004. *Tracking the hidden epidemic–Herpes.* www.cdc.gov/nchstp/od/news/RevBrochure1pdfHerpes.htm (retrieved May 10, 2006).
35. *HPV vaccine questions and answers.* www.cdc.gov/std/HPV/STDFact-HIV-vaccine.htm (retrieved September 29, 2006).
36. Centers for Disease Control and Prevention. 2004. *Genital HPV infection—Fact Sheet.* www.cdc.gov/std/HPV/STDFact-HPV.htm (retrieved September 28, 2006).
37. Ibid.
38. Centers for Disease Control and Prevention. 2002. *Sexually transmitted disease guidelines, 2002.* www.cdc.gov/STD/treatment/6-2002TG.htm #HumanPapillomavirusInfection (retrieved May 10, 2006).
39. Ibid.
40. Becker, T. M., C. M. Wheeler, et al. 1994. Sexually transmitted diseases and other risk factors for cervical dysplasia among southwestern Hispanic and non-Hispanic white women. *Journal of the American Medical Association* 271:1181–88.
41. Kozel, R., B. McGregor, and P. Manalo. 1993. Use of polymerase chain in detecting human papilloma virus in dual primary tumors of the upper aerodigestive tract. *Cancer Weekly* (February): 17–18.
42. Centers for Disease Control and Prevention, Division of STD Prevention. 1999, December. *Prevention of genital HPV infection and sequelae: Report of an external consultants' meeting.*
43. Centers for Disease Control and Prevention. 2002. *Sexually transmitted disease guidelines, 2002.* www.cdc.gov/STD/treatment/5-2002TG.htm#Trichomoniasis (retrieved September 28, 2006).
44. Ibid.
45. Deutchman, M. E., D. J. Leaman, and J. L. Thomason. 1994. Vaginitis: Diagnosis is the key. *Patient Care* 28:39–53.
46. Ibid.
47. Ibid.
48. Ibid.
49. Ibid.
50. Centers for Disease Control and Prevention. 2004. Pelvic inflammatory disease—Fact Sheet. www.cdc.gov/std/PID/STDFact-PID.htm (retrieved September 28, 2006).
51. National Institute of Allergy and Infectious Diseases. 2004. *Clinical alert: Important therapeutic information on the benefit of Zidovudine (AZT) for the prevention of the transmission of HIV from mother to infant.* www.niaid.nih.gov (retrieved October 4, 2006).
52. Federal Trade Commission. 1999. *Home-use tests for HIV can be inaccurate, FTC warns.* www.thebody.com/ftc/hometest699.html (retrieved October 4, 2006).

53. Food and Drug Administration. 2000. *Warning letters issued for unapproved HIV test kits*. www.fda.gov/oashi/aids/testwarn.html (retrieved October 4, 2006).
54. Media Guide: XI International Conference on AIDS, Vancouver, B.C. 1996.
55. Perry, M. 1994. AIDS clinical trials and tribulations: Research discriminates against women. *Women Being Alive Newsletter* (Spring).
56. Hale House Center: Biography of Mother Hale. www.halehouse.org/biography.html (retrieved September 28, 2006).
57. Adapted from American College Health Association. 2006. *Safer sex*. Brochure.
58. Planned Parenthood Federation of America. 2004. *The female condom*. www.plannedparenthood.org/birth-control-pregnancy/birth-control/female-condom.htm (retrieved September 28, 2006).
59. Centers for Disease Control and Prevention. 2006. *Epstein-Barr virus*. www.cdc.gov/ncidod/diseases/ebv.htm (retrieved September 28, 2006).
60. Centers for Disease Control and Prevention. 2006. *Who should get vaccinated?* www.cdc.gov/flu/keyfacts.htm (retrieved September 28, 2006).
61. Centers for Disease Control and Prevention. 2006. Viral *hepatitis A—Fact Sheet*. www.cdc.gov/ncidod/diseases/hepatitis/a/fact.htm (retrieved September 28, 2006).
62. Ibid.
63. Centers for Disease Control and Prevention. 2006. *Viral hepatitis B—Fact Sheet*. www.cdc.gov/ncidod/diseases/hepatitis/b/fact.htm (retrieved September 28, 2006).
64. Ibid.
65. Ibid.
66. Ibid.
67. Food and Drug Administration. 2006. *Donor screening assays for infectious agents and HIV diagnostic assays*. www.fda.gov/cber/products/testkits.htm (retrieved September 28, 2006).
68. Centers for Disease Control and Prevention, *Viral hepatitis B—Fact Sheet*.
69. Centers for Disease Control and Prevention. 2006. *Viral hepatitis C*. www.cdc.gov/ncidod/diseases/hepatitis/c/index.htm (retrieved September 28, 2006).
70. Centers for Disease Control and Prevention. *Questions and answers about TB*. 2005. www.cdc.gov/nchstp/tb/faqs/qa_introduction.htm (retrieved May 21, 2006).
71. Centers for Disease Control and Prevention. 1998. Development of new vaccines for tuberculosis: Recommendations of the Advisory Council for the Elimination of Tuberculosis (ACET). *Morbidity and Mortality Weekly Report* 47 (No. RR-13).
72. Centers for Disease Control and Prevention. 2005. *Frequently asked questions: What is group A streptococcus (GAS)?* www.cdc.gov/ncidod/dbmd/diseaseinfo/groupastreptococcal_g.htm#What%20is%20group%20A%20strep (retrieved September 28, 2006).
73. Morin, C. A., K. White, A. Schuchat, R. N. Danila, and R. Lynfield. 2005. *Perinatal group B streptococcal disease prevention, Minnesota*. www.cdc.gov/ncidod/EID/vol11no09/04-1109.htm (retrieved September 28, 2006).
74. Centers for Disease Control and Prevention. *Chickenpox: It's more serious than you think*. CDC, National Immunization Program, April 16–22, 2000. www.cdc.gov/nip/diseases/varicella/SampleOpEdchickenpox.rtf.
75. Centers for Disease Control and Prevention. *What is shingles?* www.cdc.gov/nip/diseases/varicella/faqs-gen-shingles.htm (retrieved on May 16, 2006).
76. Centers for Disease Control and Prevention. *West Nile virus—what you need to know*. www.cdc.gov/ncidod/dvbid/westnile/wnv_factsheet.htm (retrieved May 16, 2006); Centers for Disease Control and Prevention. *Arboviral encephalitis—Fact Sheet*. www.cdc.gov/ncidod/dvbid/arbor/arbofact.htm (retrieved May 16, 2006).
77. Centers for Disease Control and Prevention. *Learn about Lyme disease*. www.cdc.gov/ncidod/dvbid/lyme/index.htm (retrieved September 28, 2006).

Chapter Fifteen

Managing Cardiovascular Health and Chronic Health Conditions

CHAPTER OBJECTIVES

When you complete this chapter, you will be able to do the following:

- Describe how the cardiovascular system functions
- Differentiate among the types of heart disease
- Compare and contrast the various chronic conditions
- Determine risk factors for heart disease and other chronic conditions
- Describe ways to increase the protective factors that prevent heart disease and other chronic conditions
- Identify the early warning signals for heart disease and other chronic conditions
- Explain the current treatment protocols for heart disease and other chronic conditions

THE LEADING CAUSE OF DEATH IN WOMEN

Cardiovascular disease (CVD) is the single leading cause of death in U.S. females, killing more women than the next six causes of death combined and nearly twice as many women as all forms of cancer, including breast cancer. In 2003, cardiovascular disease claimed the lives of 483,800 women, a decrease from 1999 when CVD claimed the lives of 512,904 women. Since 1900, CVD has been the number-one killer in the United States, with the exception of 1918. Nearly 2600 Americans die of CVD each day, an average of 1 death every minute in women. The CDC/NCHS (National Center for Health Statistics) estimates that if all major forms of CVD were eliminated, life expectancy in the United States would increase by 7 years compared to 3 years if all forms of cancer were eliminated.[1]

One in four females has some form of heart or blood vessel disease. Although heart disease is more prevalent in men, it is infinitely more deadly in women. Thirty-eight percent of women who have heart attacks die within 1 year, whereas only 25 percent of men die within the same time frame. Within 6 years after a recognized heart attack, 35 percent of women will have another heart attack, 14 percent will develop angina, 11 percent will have a stroke, 6 percent will experience sudden cardiac death, and 46 percent will be disabled with heart failure.[2]

Public awareness has come a long way since the days when men received nearly all the media, medical, and research attention concerning heart disease. The

Framingham Heart Study, a landmark longitudinal study of heart disease that began in 1948, initially focused on premature heart disease and fatal heart attacks that occurred mainly in men. These researchers did not discover until decades later that, compared to men, women died in equal numbers from coronary heart disease (CHD); they just developed heart disease 10 or more years later then men! So, by age 65, the number of deaths from ischemic (restricted blood supply) heart disease is actually higher in women.

The first conference related to women's heart health, sponsored by the American Heart Association, was held in 1964. Its main focus was *how women could help protect their husbands' hearts*. It isn't surprising that the focus was on husbands because heart research often studied only male subjects, and when females were included, they were underrepresented. The findings and recommendations of heart research involving men were then projected to include women. Not recognizing the impact of heart disease in women was an unfortunate mistake. Still today, women's warning signs and symptoms are taken less seriously than men's, treatment is less aggressive, and research on heart disease is limited in number or excludes women altogether. Clinical trials often excluded women because researchers worried about conducting tests on women of childbearing age: They thought that hormonal fluctuations in these women might influence drug trials, and if they unknowingly became pregnant, drug exposure might harm the fetus. Women over age 65 with heart disease and other health problems were often excluded in clinical trials because of researchers' concerns that their illnesses might produce inaccurate results.

Research efforts to study the physiological differences between men and women have led to the new science of gender-specific medicine. Researchers have found that the specialized cells that make up the cardiac electrical system and the heart muscle itself are different in men and women, thus impacting the symptoms as well as the treatment. Women's electrocardiograph (EKG) patterns are influenced by hormonal fluctuations, with higher or lower levels of estrogen possibly causing the heart to be more susceptible to abnormal rhythms. EKG differences between males and females have been found to occur at the onset of puberty. Women are less likely to be diagnosed appropriately because of varying or unpredictable symptoms (e.g., arrhythmias, angina) or the health care provider's lack of knowledge. The time before seeking emergency treatment is greater in women than in men because women are less likely to recognize their own symptoms as being related to a heart attack. The treatment that women receive tends to be more conservative, with health care providers prescribing medications rather than aggressive interventions like clot-buster therapy (coronary thrombolysis), angioplasty, or coronary artery bypass surgery. Continued research will help reduce the gender discrepancy in diagnosis and treatment of CHD.

CARDIOVASCULAR DISEASES

Normal Cardiovascular Functioning

The **cardiovascular system** includes the heart and blood vessels. (See Color Plate 4.) The heart is a four-chamber pump composed of cardiac muscle. This muscular pump sends blood throughout the body from early conception until death. The heart is located in the middle of the chest, behind the sternum, and is about the size of a clenched fist. In general, a woman's heart is smaller than a man's because the size of the heart is proportional to the size of the body. The two upper chambers, called atria, receive blood. The right atrium receives deoxygenated blood from all parts of the body, and the left atrium receives oxygenated blood from the lungs. The two lower chambers, called ventricles, send blood. The right ventricle pumps deoxygenated blood into the lungs, and the left ventricle pumps oxygenated blood to the entire body. The blood in the heart passes through valves that separate these chambers. The opening and closing of the valves (tricuspid, pulmonic, mitral, and aortic) cause the familiar pumping sound heard in a stethoscope. If these valves fail to function properly, blood may flow back into a chamber and cause a murmur.

The Vascular System The vascular system is composed of arteries, veins, capillaries, arterioles, and venules. The **arteries** carry blood away from the heart and are larger closest to the heart. (See *FYI:* "Coronary Arteries.") As the arteries move farther from the heart, they become the arterioles that feed the **capillaries.** The capillaries filter the blood, taking food and oxygen from the arterioles and sending waste products and carbon dioxide to the venules. The venules carry blood into increasingly larger **veins** as blood flows to the heart.

Types of Heart Disease

The development of heart disease and the progression of atherosclerosis are influenced by a number of factors, including genetic predisposition, gender, race, advancing age, and lifestyle choices. Heart disease develops gradually as narrowing of the coronary vessels causes changes in the blood flow to the heart. The changes to the coronary vessels evolve into lesions that further obstruct blood flow. Initially, partial obstruction of a major vessel or its branches may occur. However, over time, a blood clot from somewhere above the obstruction may break free and lodge in the obstruction, thus causing a total blockage of the vessel.

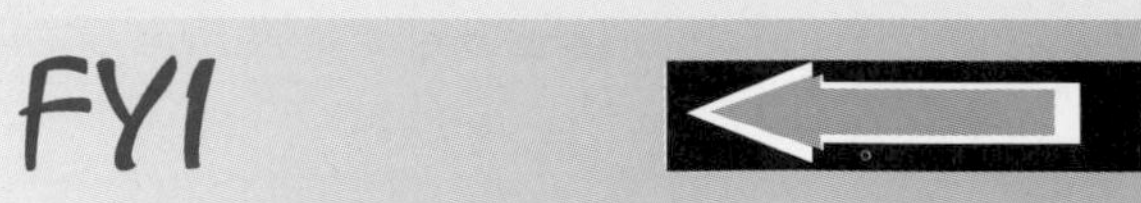

Coronary Arteries

The heart muscle has arteries to provide oxygen to itself. These arteries are the right coronary, the left anterior descending, and the left circumflex. The right coronary artery nourishes the back of the heart. The left anterior descending artery nourishes the front part of the heart. The left circumflex nourishes the side of the heart. Smaller coronary arteries called collateral arteries connect to larger arteries and help nourish the heart and may replace the function of larger arteries if they malfunction. Collateral vessels grow and enlarge in some individuals and act as alternative routes of blood flow when larger arteries are obstructed, causing myocardial ischemia (reduced blood flow to the muscular tissue of the heart). While women's hearts tend to be smaller than men's because of smaller body size, their coronary arteries may or may not be smaller than men's. The myth that coronary arteries are always smaller in women has resulted in some women not getting coronary bypass surgery when it was needed.

Atherosclerosis **Atherosclerosis** is a gradual thickening and hardening of artery walls caused by a complicated process starting in childhood. The process begins with inner vessel wall (endothelium) injury and ends with a buildup of fatty deposits that harden over time. Although heredity is often implicated, the primary factor is excess cholesterol circulating in the bloodstream. When excess cholesterol bombards the arteries over a prolonged period, several reactions may develop: fat permeates the tissue macrophages, artery walls break down, muscle tissue is replaced with less-elastic material, and plaque (accumulated fats, cholesterol, cellular debris, calcium, platelets, and other substances) forms and begins to block the artery.[3] (See Color Plate 5.) These plaques not only cause partial or total obstructions to blood flow but they also can rupture, causing a blood clot (thrombus) to break off and travel to other parts of the body. A traveling blood clot is known as an embolus and can cause a heart attack, stroke, pulmonary embolism, or gangrene, depending on where it lodges.

The primary risk factors for developing atherosclerosis are dietary intake of saturated fatty acids, elevation of systemic blood pressure, cigarette smoking, and glucose intolerance. Other factors include diabetes, obesity, sedentary lifestyle, stress, hormone therapy, and heavy alcohol consumption. Tobacco smoke, whether mainstream or secondary, greatly worsens and speeds up the process of atherosclerosis in coronary and other arteries of the body.

Angina Pectoris Chest pain is a common complaint heard by health care providers. **Angina,** from a Greek word that means "to strangle," describes a cluster of symptoms associated with oxygen deprivation. All attacks of angina begin as **ischemia** of the working heart muscle, forcing the heart to work in an anaerobic state (i.e., in the absence of oxygen). Chemical substances accumulate in the anaerobic state, and these substances are believed to initiate the pain associated with angina.

Older women in particular appear to have a higher incidence of angina than men, and for many, it may be the first warning sign of coronary heart disease (CHD). Stable angina (or chronic) is usually predictable and occurs when there is oxygen deprivation due to blockage or narrowing of one or more of the heart's arteries. It is initiated by physical exertion, strong emotions, or extreme temperatures. Normally, relief comes within minutes of rest or use of the drug nitroglycerin. Unstable angina results when the heart does not get enough oxygen, often because atherosclerosis blocks or constricts a portion of the artery. It usually occurs at rest, and the discomfort is usually more severe and prolonged. Prinzmetal's (variant) angina is a type of unstable angina caused by a coronary artery spasm near the atherosclerotic blockage. It usually occurs at rest and typically between midnight and 8 A.M.

Angina is *not* a heart attack, and once the pain passes (usually in less than a minute) blood returns to the heart muscle and the cells function normally. Angina manifests as a feeling of heaviness, squeezing, pressure, or burning in the chest, with pain radiating into the back, jaw, neck, and stomach and sometimes into the inner part of the left arm. Feelings of suffocation and impending death are quite common. Other symptoms include cold sweat, nausea, or light-headedness. Women who experience angina often exhibit signs dissimilar to typical angina symptoms. In fact, the signs are often more subtle in women than in men and can be very confusing. Women frequently experience inconsequential chest pains and fleeting rhythm disturbances when they are young. Therefore, they may be more likely to mistake angina for heartburn, gastric disorders, asthma, allergies, and bronchitis because they mimic the symptoms of angina. Some women describe a feeling of weakness and unusual fatigue. However angina manifests itself, women need to inform their health care provider when they experience chest pain.

A condition known as silent ischemia occurs when the heart is deprived of oxygen. A woman may not know she has this condition because she does not sense the typical symptoms of angina. Silent ischemia is most common in diabetics, particularly those who suffer from a sensory disturbance (not feeling body sensations). Silent ischemia that ends in tissue death is considered a silent myocardial infarction, or heart attack.

Angina is *not* a minor symptom and should be taken seriously by a woman and her health care provider. Although nearly 80 percent of angina pains will not develop into heart attacks, these pains may be a precursor to heart disease and may precede a full-blown heart attack. The factors that may reduce or control angina include quitting smoking; exercising regularly and managing weight; avoiding high altitudes and cold air; avoiding excessive alcohol, salt, or heavy meals; and decreasing emotional stress and physical exertion.[4]

Too often, women tend to ignore their chest pain and do not have it checked by the health care provider. The primary objectives for treatment of angina are to improve coronary blood flow and to reduce the amount of oxygen needed by the heart. Health care providers may prescribe nitroglycerin, beta blockers, calcium antagonists, or antiplatelet agents such as aspirin for ischemic heart disease.

Surgical procedures such as **coronary artery bypass grafting** (CABG) or percutaneous transluminal coronary **angioplasty** (PTCA) are designed to increase coronary blood flow. Previously, many women suffered complications during angioplasty from tears to the arteries caused by the large balloons used to expand the collapsed artery. Today's smaller and finer balloons have improved the prognosis for women. (See Color Plate 6.) Newer techniques include laser angioplasty, a procedure to vaporize the plaque, and atherectomy, a procedure to remove plaque from arteries by grinding it away. These procedures are typically followed by a stent procedure (use of a wire mesh tube, or stent, to prop open an artery) and can be done in conjunction with angioplasty. In CABG, the internal mammary artery or segments from the saphenous vein (leg) are used to bypass the obstructed coronary artery.[5] Transmyocardial revascularization has been used for those suffering from severe angina but who weren't candidates for bypass surgery or PTCA. This procedure involves exposing the heart through an incision on the left chest and using a laser to "drill" 20 to 40 holes from the outside of the heart into the ventricle.

Health Tips

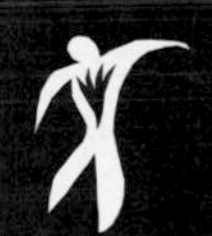

Warning Signs of a Heart Attack[6]

Women often experience more vague symptoms than men when it comes to heart attacks. Knowing the possible warning signs of a potential heart attack is important. Every minute counts. Remember: *Don't wait.* Women tend to delay seeking treatment, a dangerous choice.

- Chest pain or discomfort
- Uncomfortable pressure, fullness, squeezing in the center of the chest
- Shortness of breath
- Nausea or vomiting
- Unusual fatigue
- Spreading pain in the back, stomach, or abdomen
- Neck or jaw pain
- Cold sweats
- Light-headedness (feelings of fainting)

Myocardial Infarction When **myocardial infarction (MI)** occurs, blood flow to the affected heart area ceases. This condition is commonly created when a moving blood clot (embolus) lodges in a coronary vessel and causes complete occlusion of the vessel. Occlusion occurs at a point where the vessel is too small for the clot to pass through. The heart tissue normally served by this vessel begins to experience almost immediate ischemia, and tissue death occurs unless collateral vessels provide the needed oxygen.

Angina pain occurs immediately and intensely in most MI cases. The difference between angina and MI is that the pain with MI cannot be alleviated by drugs because the tissue is depleted of blood flow. Some tissue death occurs with all MIs, but the extent of damage is dependent on the size and location of the artery supplying oxygen and the degree to which the tissue area remains deprived of oxygen. If collateral arteries are present, they can aid in supplying oxygen to tissue after an MI, thus reducing infarct size.

Regardless of age and treatment, MI is often more lethal for women than for men. Women are more likely to die within a year of the first heart attack (1 in 3) or to have a second MI within 6 years. Among women, African Americans are 60 percent more likely to die of CHD than whites. Women experience more in-hospital mortality, more recurrent angina, and more congestive heart failure after discharge than men do.[7] (See *Health Tip:* "Warning Signs of a Heart Attack.")

Congenital Heart Disease Congenital heart disease describes a structural problem in the heart that occurs during the development of the baby's heart. Nearly fifteen types of congenital heart defects are recognized, including holes in the wall of the heart or blood vessels and problems with heart valves, the development of the heart, and the placement or development of the blood vessels near the heart.[8] According to the American Heart Association (AHA), at least 9 of every 1,000 infants born each year have a heart defect. In the United States, approximately 36,000 babies are born each year with cardiovascular defects, most of which can be helped by surgery even when the defect is severe.

Advances in medical treatment have dramatically altered the outlook for children with congenital heart disease. Many who previously would have died as children can expect to live a full adult life. About 1 million Americans alive today have congenital heart defects, and approximately 25 percent are children.[9] In the United States, the number of women living with congenital heart disease is growing. These women need health care providers who understand the nuances of this disease. Many had surgery as children but did not recover completely. Thus, as adults, they face the possibility of long-term medical surveillance and further treatment.

It is important for adults with congenital heart disease to seek medical professionals who specialize in the treatment of their disease because congenital heart defects in adults are not common. Increasing numbers of specialty centers are being formed as the need for them increases. Adolescents face problems such as scars and chronic illness and have to deal with questions about types of exercise, sexual activity, type of contraception, and so on. The levels of physical activity and exercise are individualized for people with heart defects. These levels are dependent on the type and severity of the heart defect and can be determined by a cardiologist with the aid of tests such as echocardiogram, Holter monitor, or exercise test. According to the AHA, most people with heart defects can work in virtually any occupation, but if a person's heart condition has a high risk for fainting or dizziness, safety may be a consideration when choosing an appropriate job.

Young women with congenital heart disease have further considerations. Menarche occurs slightly later in adolescents with congenital heart disease, especially in women who are cyanotic (blue) from insufficient oxygen. Women with cyanosis are also more likely to have irregular menstrual periods. If women with heart defects are considering whether to have children, they need adequate counseling for family planning. Although many women with heart defects can have successful pregnancies, they should still discuss this with their cardiologist before becoming pregnant. In some cases, pregnancy may not be recommended.

Pregnancy for women taking anticoagulants (drugs that prevent coagulation [clotting]) as a result of their heart disease will require special consideration from the health care provider. Adjustments in their medicication will probably need to be made during the pregnancy. The changes in a woman's body, especially in the second and third trimesters, can make symptoms of congenital heart disease worse. Even in women who have not had prior symptoms, these body changes can cause problems to develop. The mother's heart condition, as well as medications commonly prescribed for heart disease, can also pose added risks to the fetus. The AHA indicates that the risk of heart disease in the fetus is higher if either parent has a congenital heart defect. Whether the affected parent is the mother or father, the frequency of heart defects increases from less than 1 percent in the general population to 2 to 20 percent when the parent is affected. Having close family members with congenital heart disease further increases the risk of having a child with a heart defect.

Advancements in science and genetics are improving our ability to predict the presence of heart disease in some people. Genetic counseling should be considered for women with heart defects who want to become pregnant. A slight increase in the incidence of birth defects, including heart defects, has also been shown for children with mothers who have diabetes. An expectant mother's exposure to certain substances, including prescription medications, X rays, industrial chemicals or solvents, alcohol, viral infections, and recreational drugs, leads to a higher incidence of heart disease in her offspring.[10]

Women who have congenital heart disease should get regular medical care from their primary care provider and cardiologist. Regular dental care is also recommended to minimize the chance of oral infections that could affect the heart. In addition, antibiotics usually are recommended by the dentist prior to dental work for persons with congenital heart disease to prevent the occurrence of heart infection as a result of the dental care. A woman with heart disease needs to be cautious before taking any over-the-counter medications, vitamins, or herbal preparations and should discuss the potential for cardiac side effects or drug interactions with her health care provider or pharmacist.

A major dilemma for some young adults is the issue of health insurance. Parents need to be aware of the implications of health coverage when considering job changes. Some health plans have waiting periods, which may impact the child's quality of care. Once coverage under a parent's policy ends, adolescents need to make plans for their own coverage. The Americans with Disabilities Act and Work Incentives Improvement Act try to ensure equal hiring for all people, including those with congenital heart defects.[11]

Arrhythmia Arrhythmia refers to disturbances in the normal sequence of cardiac electrical activity that causes irregular or abnormal heart rhythms. The normal electrical conduction for heart rhythm is generated in the sinoatrial or sinus node ("natural pacemaker") found in the right atrium. The electrical impulse then travels through the heart's conduction pathway to cause synchronized contractions of the atria and ventricles. Arrhythmias include a variety of abnormal electrical disturbances, and their effects range from insignificant "skipped" beats to more serious, pump-impairing irregularities that can be life-threatening. Tachycardia refers to a fast heart rate of more than 100 beats per minute. Bradycardia is a slow heart rate of fewer than 60 beats per minute. No treatment is needed for many arrhythmias. Once an arrhythmia has been documented, it is important to determine where it originates. Some arrhythmias (such as "skipping a beat") are quite normal in children and adolescents. Others require regulation with medications, an implanted pacemaker, cardioversion (medically controlled electrical shock to the heart), ablative techniques using a radiofrequency or electrocautery approach, or an automatic implantable defibrillator.

Atrial fibrillation is the most common serious heart rhythm abnormality, and an estimated 2.2 million Americans live with this arrhythmia.[12] Atrial fibrillation is a result of uncoordinated electrical signals originating in the atria that cause fast, uneven contractions from the upper heart chambers. Symptoms from atrial arrhythmias may include dizziness, light-headedness, fainting or near fainting, palpitations (noticeable heart fluttering), shortness of breath, and chest pain. Heart disease can cause arrhythmias, but other causes include stress, caffeine, tobacco, alcohol, diet pills, electrolyte imbalance, and cough/cold medications. Atrial fibrillation may not be life-threatening, but it can lead to conditions that are, such as stroke. According to the AHA, a person with atrial fibrilliation has a five times greater chance of having a stroke than someone without this condition.[13]

An artificial **pacemaker** is a medical device implanted to treat slow heart rate (bradycardia). Many misconceptions exist about artificial pacemakers because older models had more potential problems than newer models. Women with pacemakers do *not* need to be concerned about microwave ovens, most home appliances, or tools, but they do need to be cautious with cell phones, traveling through airports, some dental equipment, diagnostic radiation, and surgery. Women with pacemakers should always carry their pacemaker identification cards and, in most cases, avoid standing near electronic article surveillance or metal detectors (including hand-held ones) for any length of time.[14] (See *Her Story:* "Mandi: From Pacemaker to Mother.")

Her Story

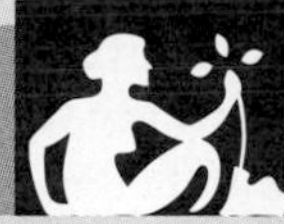

Mandi: From Pacemaker to Mother

Mandi experienced heart palpitations and fatigue from a young age. It seemed that every time she got up from a chair or cleaned up after a meal, she would feel lightheaded. She was always tired. But when she ran long distances on the track team, she didn't notice any symptoms. At age 16, she fainted while talking to friends in the school hallway. She went to her family health care provider who recommended further tests. The tests showed bradycardia and the cardiologist recommended a pacemaker. The cardiologist was not accustomed to implanting a pacemaker in a young, thin woman. After the surgery, Mandi felt like a new person. She had more energy and the symptoms had disappeared.

Last year, at the age of 23, Mandi gave birth to a healthy baby girl. Mother and baby experienced no problems through the natural birth process. Do you know someone with a pacemaker? What symptoms did they have before getting the pacemaker? How do they feel today?

Congestive Heart Failure (CHF) **Congestive heart failure** (or simply, heart failure or cardiac failure) occurs when the heart is too weak to pump blood adequately to the body. It is more common in women, particularly older women, and results from cumulative damage to the heart muscle. Overworked or damaged heart muscle results from a variety of possible factors: prior heart attacks, coronary artery disease, hypertension, heart valve disease, cardiomyopathy (a serious inflammation of heart muscle), congenital heart disease, or infection of the heart valves or muscle itself.[15] The best treatment is prevention of further damage. Gender differences in CHF are known to exist. While men tend to experience weakening of the heart muscle, women tend to experience stiffening and loss of elasticity of the heart muscle. Hormone deficiencies, such as occur with hypothyroidism, may accelerate the loss of elasticity. Women with hypothyroidism should seek medical attention and may need thyroid replacement therapy.[16]

Symptoms of CHF include shortness of breath, weight gain, and edema (swelling), especially of the lower extremities or abdomen. Women with CHF tire easily and have difficulty exerting effort. Various medications can be prescribed to decrease the workload of a weakened heart. These include ACE inhibitors (inhibitors of angiotensin converting enzyme), beta blockers, diuretics (water pills), digitalis, and vasodilators (blood vessel dilators). In addition, a fluid-restricted or salt-restricted diet (less than 1500 mg) may be recommended. Coronary artery bypass or PTCA may be needed to improve blood flow to the heart muscle itself, and in some cases a heart transplant may be considered. Statistics from the AHA for 2003 revealed that 61 percent of deaths from CHF were women; death rates were higher for African American women than for white women until the age of 85 when the death rate is higher in white women.

Endocarditis **Endocarditis** has also been called infective endocarditis and valve infection. It is an inflammation or infection of the inside lining of the heart chambers and heart valves that can damage or destroy the heart valves. Endocarditis occurs when certain organisms in the bloodstream lodge on preexisting abnormal heart valves or other damaged heart tissue, and it rarely occurs in people with normal hearts.

Bacterial infection is the most common source of endocarditis although other organisms such as fungi can be causative. Given that certain bacteria are "normal" inhibitors on parts of the body such as the mouth, upper respiratory system, skin, and intestinal and urinary tracts, some surgical and dental procedures cause a brief bacteremia (bacteria in the bloodstream). Bacteremia is common after many invasive procedures, but only certain bacteria can cause endocarditis. Procedures that create greater risk of endocarditis include professional teeth cleaning; tonsillectomy and adenoidectomy; rigid bronchoscopy (examination of respiratory airways with a scope); certain urinary and gastrointestinal tract procedures; injected drug use; prior valve, gallbladder, and prostate surgery, and the existence of central venous access lines.

Women with a known history of a heart condition, including congenital heart defects, a heart murmur, mitral valve prolapse, or other heart valve problems, should inform their health care provider and dentist of this condition. Preventive antibiotics are often prescribed prior to procedures that could predispose high-risk individuals to endocarditis. Women with existing heart conditions may consider carrying an endocarditis wallet card issued by the AHA that informs health care professionals of their particular condition. Good oral hygiene is important for all women but especially for those with heart conditions.

Symptoms of endocarditis may develop slowly or suddenly, and it is difficult to diagnose because multiple organ systems may become involved. A few symptoms include fever, chills, weakness, cardiac murmur, weight loss, and night sweats. Hospitalization with intravenous antibiotic administration often is required. Antibiotic therapy generally is given for 4 to 6 weeks. Complications from endocarditis can include **dysrhythmia** (abnormality of an otherwise normal rhythmic pattern), congestive heart failure, stroke, and other organ damage as a result of blood clots traveling from the infected valves.

Mitral Valve Prolapse **Mitral valve prolapse (MVP)** is a condition in which one or both flaps of the mitral valve are enlarged and fail to close properly as they prolapse or "flop" back into the left atrium during contraction of the left ventricle. MVP may or may not be accompanied by mitral regurgitation in which blood flows back into the left atrium causing an auditory "murmur." According to the National Heart, Lung, and Blood Institute (NHLBI), MVP can be present from birth or develop at any age and occurs equally in men and women, contrary to previous indications that it was more prevalent in women. Slightly more than 2 percent of adults have MPV. The cause is unknown although some studies suggest that MVP is an inherited disorder. The majority of individuals with MVP don't know they have the condition because they have no symptoms. Women who may have symptoms with MVP might experience palpitations, shortness of breath with exertion or lying flat, chest pain that comes and goes, dizziness, migraine headaches, or symptoms that mimic a panic attack.

All women with MVP should be under health care supervision because of the risk for bacterial endocarditis and should receive antibiotics prior to certain medical procedures, including dental work. Sometimes medications such as beta blockers may be required, and in more serious valve prolapse, surgery for valve replacement could be indicated. Women with MVP should have regular checkups with their cardiologist during pregnancy because the changes in and the stress of pregnancy place added strain on the heart. However, in most cases, the chances are good for an uncomplicated, successful pregnancy.

Children and Cardiovascular Disease

Cardiovascular disease in the number-two cause of death for children under the age of 15. Most CVD in children is related to congenital heart defects, but more children are developing many preventable risk factors for cardiovascular disease. High blood pressure, smoking, high blood cholesterol, physical inactivity, overweight and obesity, and metabolic syndrome are contributing to the rise in cardiovascular procedures in children and adolescents. Adolescents with metabolic syndrome are at increased risk for developing diabetes and CVD, as well as increased mortality from CVD.

Nearly 1 million adolescents between the ages of 12 and 19 have metabolic syndrome (MetS). In adolescents, MetS is defined as three or more of the following abnormalities:

- Waist circumference at or above the 90th percentile for age and sex
- Serum triglyceride level of 110 mg/dL or higher
- High-density lipoprotein (HDL) cholesterol level that is lower than 40 mg/dL

FYI

Risk Factors for Cardiovascular Disease

Unchangeable Risk Factors
- Family history
- Race
- Gender
- Increasing age

Risk Factors That Can Be Modified, Treated, or Controlled
- Tobacco smoke
- High blood pressure
- High blood cholesterol
- Physical inactivity
- Obesity and overweight
- Diabetes mellitus

Other Contributing Factors
- Menopause and estrogen loss
- Birth control pills
- High triglyceride levels
- Excessive alcohol intake
- Individual response to stress

SOURCE: American Heart Association, 2006.

- Blood pressure at or above the 90th percentile for age, sex, and height
- Elevated fasting glucose of 110 mg/dL or higher[17]

Risk Factors

The American Heart Association has identified several factors that increase the risk of heart disease and stroke. A woman's chance of having a heart attack or stroke increases when more risk factors are present. Some of the factors cannot be controlled, but most of them can be modified, treated, or controlled to reduce a woman's chances of developing heart disease or having a stroke. (See *FYI:* "Risk Factors for Cardiovascular Disease.")

Unchangeable risk factors for heart disease include increasing age, family health history, race, and gender. In addition, women with prior histories of heart attack or stroke are at higher risk for future CVD episodes. The risk factors that can be modified, treated, or controlled include tobacco smoke, high blood pressure, high blood cholesterol, physical inactivity, obesity and overweight, and diabetes. Other contributing factors for women include menopause and estrogen loss, oral contraceptives, high triglyceride levels, excessive alcohol consumption, and stress.

Unchangeable Risk Factors

Increasing age As women age, their risk of heart disease and stroke begins to increase. African American women aged 65 to 74 have a higher rate of new and recurrent heart attacks than other women but lower rates at age 75 and older than other women. In older ages, women who experience heart attacks are more likely than men to die within a few weeks.

Family health history A woman's chances of developing heart disease or having a stroke are increased if her close blood relatives have had a heart attack or stroke.

Race African American women have a greater risk of heart disease and stroke than white women, which is largely attributed to their higher average blood pressure levels. In comparison, African American women are also more likely to die of stroke than white women. Mexican Americans, American Indians, native Hawaiians, and some Asian Americans also have higher risk, most likely due to higher rates of obesity and diabetes.

Gender Men have a greater risk of heart attack than women, and they have attacks earlier in life. Although more than half of the total stroke deaths occur in women, there is an overall equal incidence of stroke for men and women. Heart disease is the leading cause of death in both men and women.

Risk Factors That Can Be Modified, Treated, or Controlled

Tobacco smoke The nicotine and carbon monoxide in tobacco smoke reduce the amount of oxygen in the blood and damage blood vessel walls, causing plaque to build up. Tobacco smoke worsens atherosclerosis and speeds its buildup in arteries. In addition, tobacco smoke can trigger the formation of blood clots, cause arrhythmias in persons with chest pain or previous heart attacks, and promote heart disease by reducing HDL ("good" cholesterol). Smokers have a two to four times greater risk for developing CHD, a ten times greater risk for developing peripheral vascular disease (PVD), and a two times greater risk of stroke, heart failure, or sudden cardiac death. Nearly 35,000 *nonsmokers* die each year from CHD resulting from exposure to environmental (secondhand or passive) tobacco smoke. Nearly 1,000 *infant deaths* also occur annually as a result of women smoking throughout the pregnancy. Use of oral contraceptives by women smokers is discouraged because of a higher risk for heart attack or stroke.

TABLE 15.1 Classification and Management of Blood Pressure for Adults*

BP CLASSIFICATION	SBP MMHG	DBP MMHG	LIFESTYLE MODIFICATION	INITIAL DRUG THERAPY: WITHOUT COMPELLING INDICATIONS	INITIAL DRUG THERAPY: WITH COMPELLING INDICATIONS
Normal	<120	and <80	Encourage		
Prehypertension	120–139	or 80–89	Yes	No antihypertensive drug indicated.	Drug(s) for compelling indications.‡
Stage 1 Hypertension	140–159	or 90–99	Yes	Thiazide-type diuretics for most. May consider ACEI, ARB, BB, CCB, or combination.	Drug(s) for the compelling indications.‡ Other antihypertensive drugs (diuretics, ACEI, ARB, BB, CCB) as needed.
Stage 2 Hypertension	≥160	or ≥100	Yes	Two-drug combination for most† (usually thiazide-type diuretic and ACEI or ARB or BB or CCB).	

*Treatment determined by highest BP category.
†Initial combined therapy should be used cautiously in those at risk for orthostatic hypotension.
‡Treat patients with chronic kidney disease or diabetes to BP goal of <130/80 mmHg.
NOTE: DBP, diastolic blood pressure; SBP, systolic blood pressure. Drug abbreviations: ACEI, anglotensin converting enzyme inhibitor; ARB, anglotensin receptor blocker; BB, beta blocker; CCB, calcium channel blocker.

Statistics from the AHA suggest that 20.4 percent of non-Hispanic white women, 20.2 percent of African American women, 10.9 percent of Mexican American women, and 40.8 percent of Native American/Alaska Native women are smokers. The prevalence of smoking is highest among women living below the poverty level and is three times greater among women with fewer years of education (9 to 11 years versus 16 years). An ongoing survey of young women in grades 9–12 shows that 24.6 percent of females report current tobacco use, a higher rate than for all age groups of women.[18]

High blood pressure **Hypertension,** often called the silent killer, remains a major risk factor in heart attack, stroke, congestive heart failure, blindness, and kidney failure. Essential or primary hypertension, the most common type, has no known underlying cause. Although the causes of hypertension in 90 percent of the cases are not known, the contributing factors of uncontrolled hypertension are understood. Secondary hypertension, caused by an underlying disease and less common overall, is more common in women than men.

Hypertension occurs when the heart is forced to exert more pressure to pump blood through the arteries to the body. This pressure not only overworks the heart but also contributes to atherosclerosis, hardening of the arteries. Blood pressure is, simply, the force of blood against artery walls. It is measured with a sphygmomanometer: A rubber cuff is wrapped around the arm, temporarily stopping blood flow to the brachial artery, and a stethoscope is used to listen for blood flow as it begins to flow through the brachial artery. **Systolic blood pressure** is the amount of pressure the blood exerts against the arteries while the heart is contracting. **Diastolic blood pressure** is the amount of pressure the blood exerts against the arteries while the heart is filling and resting between beats. When stating BP, systolic and then diastolic are given (e.g., 120/80). Normal blood pressure is below 120 mm Hg systolic and below 80 mm Hg diastolic. Prehypertension is 120–139 mm Hg systolic *or* 80–89 mm HG diastolic. Prehypertension means that there is a greater likelihood of developing hypertension later, but lifestyle changes may delay the onset. Nearly 90 percent of persons over the age of 55 are likely to experience hypertension in their lifetime. Stage 1 hypertension in adults has been defined as blood pressure between 140 and 159 mm Hg systolic *or* between 90 and 99 mm Hg diastolic. Stage 2 hypertension is a systolic reading equal to or greater than 160 mm Hg *or* a diastolic reading equal to or greater than 100 mm Hg.[19] Lifestyle changes are encouraged for persons with stage 1 and stage 2 hypertension, and drug therapy is usually prescribed. (See Table 15.1.)

Most American women will develop high blood pressure during their lifetime. Even slight elevations in blood pressure double the risk for the development of cardiovascular disease. High blood pressure is the most important risk factor for stroke. High blood pressure tends to run in families, but it has no known cause and appears without symptoms. Other uncontrollable factors include age, race, and gender. Obesity, diabetes, sleep apnea, and regular alcohol use increase the likelihood of developing high blood pressure. Oral contraceptive use can occasionally contribute to hypertension, and it may be necessary for hypertensive women to use other birth control methods. In one study, women aged 40 to 59 with high blood pressure were expected to encounter five times the normal rate of angina, heart attack, or sudden death. Losing weight, reducing sodium intake, exercising regularly, and taking medication can act as protective factors. However, hypertension controlled by drug therapy remains a risk factor because it does not decrease the risk of CHD.

Complications from high blood pressure during pregnancy are also possible. High blood pressure can be detrimental for both the mother and the fetus, potentially causing harm to the mother's kidneys and other organs, and low birth weight and early delivery of the infant. Preeclampsia, a toxic condition that typically starts after the 20th week of pregnancy, is associated with an increase in blood pressure, swelling of hands and feet, and protein in the urine. Preeclampsia has increased by nearly one-third in the past decade. When preeclampsia leads to eclampsia (preeclampsia with seizures), the condition becomes much more serious and is recognized as the second leading cause of maternal death in the United States.[20] (See Chapter 9.) All women with severe preeclampsia are given an anti-seizure medication to prevent eclampsia.

High blood cholesterol High blood cholesterol is a major risk factor for heart disease, with the risk increasing as the blood level rises. Cholesterol, a normal fatty substance of body cells, enters the blood in two ways: through absorption in the small intestine from animal products that are consumed and from its production in the body, mainly the liver. Since cholesterol and other fats cannot dissolve in the blood, cholesterol is transported through the blood on lipoproteins of varying densities. Low-density lipoprotein (LDL) has become known as the "bad" cholesterol because high levels of cholesterol in this lipoprotein increase a person's risk for coronary heart disease. Cholesterol carrying LDL can slowly build up in the inner walls of the arteries and, thus, narrow the lumen of the vessel. High levels of LDL are a better predictor of heart disease risk than total cholesterol levels. Lp(a) cholesterol is a genetic variation of plasma LDL and is an important risk factor for the development of premature atherosclerosis. Cholesterol in high-density lipoprotein (HDL) is commonly known as the "good" cholesterol because high levels of HDL *decrease* the risk of coronary heart disease. (See Table 15.2.)

TABLE 15.2 Healthy Levels of Cholesterol[21]

Your total blood cholesterol will fall into one of these categories:	
Desirable	Less than 200 mg/dl
Borderline high risk	200–239 mg/dl
High risk	240 mg/dl and over
Your LDL cholesterol level will fall into one of these categories:	
Optimal	Less than 100 mg/dl
Near optimal/above optimal*	100–129 mg/dl
Borderline high	130–159 mg/dl
High	160–189 mg/dl
Very high†	≥190 mg/dl
Your HDL cholesterol level will fall into one of these categories:	
Normal	50–60 mg/dl
Low	Less than 40 mg/dl
Your triglyceride level will fall into one of these categories:	
Normal	≤150 mg/dl
Borderline high	150–199 mg/dl
High	200–499 mg/dl
Very high	500 mg/dl or higher

*In coronary heart disease patients with LDL cholesterol levels of 100–129 mg/dL, the doctor should consider whether to initiate drug treatment in addition to recommending that the patient follow the American Heart Association Therapeutic Lifestyle Changes (TLD) diet.

†In men less than 35 years of age and premenopausal women with LDL cholesterol levels of 190–219 mg/dL, drug therapy should be delayed except in high-risk patients such as those with diabetes.

Young women appear to have higher HDL than men, particularly during childbearing years when estrogen levels are higher. However, by age 55, women tend to have higher *total* cholesterol as well, which decreases the protective advantage against coronary heart disease. The goals for reducing cholesterol in women are to lower total cholesterol and LDL levels and to raise HDL levels. The strongest predictors of heart disease death in women appear to be low blood levels of HDL and high levels of triglycerides.[22]

Total cholesterol and LDL cholesterol levels can be reduced by a diet low in saturated fat and cholesterol. Food products with monounsaturated and polyunsaturated fats should replace those with high saturated fats, trans fats, and triglycerides. High levels of trans-fatty acids in foods can raise a woman's cholesterol level. Food products containing hydrogenated oils are high in trans-fatty acids and should be avoided when trying to lower a cholesterol level. Reducing the amount of saturated fat and trans fats in the diet is more of a major factor in reducing blood cholesterol than is reducing the intake of cholesterol itself.

The average HDL cholesterol level for women is 50–60 mg/dL. Keeping HDL levels high (60 mg/dL or more) by quitting smoking, maintaining a healthy weight, and being physically active is important in fighting atherosclerosis. Women should be familiar with the absolute numbers of their total cholesterol and HDL because these levels are important in determining appropriate treatment by a health care provider.

While female sex hormones (estrogen) raise HDL cholesterol levels, male sex hormones (testosterone), progesterone, and certain steroids lower the HDL level. Hormone replacement therapy (HRT) is no longer recommended to prevent heart disease in postmenopausal women. Women whose blood cholesterol levels remain elevated despite dietary changes, regular physical activity, and weight loss may need to take cholesterol-lowering medications. The most effective and widely tested cholesterol-lowering drugs for women are called statins. These medications, like most medications, have potential side effects and should not be a substitute for healthy lifestyle changes. At times, cholesterol-lowering medications are used in combination with one another for more effectiveness.[23]

Physical inactivity Women who are inactive have twice the risk of heart disease as women who exercise regularly. This risk is comparable to high blood cholesterol, high blood pressure, or cigarette smoking. Exercise has many benefits, including decreasing levels of LDL and triglycerides and increasing levels of HDL. Although conflicting recommendations for physical activity exist, the NHLBI suggests that women should engage in moderate-intensity activity for 30 minutes per day daily, and an additional 30 minutes per day is recommended to prevent gradual weight gain. The physical activity does not require one duration, but can occur in short spurts, that is, 10 to 15 minutes of activity several times a day. Women with more education and higher incomes are more likely to exercise regularly, but overall, women are less likely than men to engage in some leisure-time physical activity.[24]

Obesity and overweight **Overweight** is defined as a body mass index (BMI) of 25 or greater. **Obesity** is considered to be a BMI of 30 or greater, and **extreme obesity** is a BMI greater than 39. You can determine your BMI and develop a meal plan by accessing the Web sites www.cdc.gov/dphp/dnpa/bmi and www.mypyramid.gov.

Estimates suggest that nearly 62 percent of American women (ages 20 to 74) are overweight, 34 percent are obese, and 6 percent are extremely obese. Obesity is the second leading preventable health problem in the United States, and among middle-aged women it has increased approximately 2 percent or more each year over a 40-year span. Obesity has a strong inverse relationship with socioeconomic status (that is, obesity increases as income level decreases) and is associated with large decreases in life expectancy.[25]

Non-Hispanic black women have the highest prevalence of overweight and obesity followed by Mexican American women. The risk of chronic disease such as heart disease increases with an increase in BMI. In fact, when BMI exceeds 30, the risk of death related to obesity increases by 50 percent. Women who have too much fat are at higher risk for multiple health problems, including premature death, type 2 diabetes, high blood pressure, gallbladder disease, respiratory dysfunction, gout, osteoarthritis, and dyslipidemia (a lipid disorder that results in increases in cholesterel and/or triglyceride levels). Stroke and heart disease are health problems that are significantly related to women who carry their weight around the waist. The waist-hip ratio is recognized as a more accurate indicator of risk for coronary artery disease (CAD) than BMI, with a recommended ratio of 0.8 or less.[26] (See *FYI:* "Countering the Myths of Some 'Protective Factors.'")

FYI

Countering the Myths of Some "Protective Factors"

Three previous factors that were believed to protect women from heart disease have now been found to show no benefit. First, hormone replacement therapy was believed to protect women from heart attacks. A study by the Women's Health Initiative found that HRT may *cause* heart attacks, stroke, or blood clots in *some* women. HRT is no longer recommended. Second, antioxidant supplements such as vitamin E and beta carotene were believed to reduce cardiovascular disease risk and have other health-promoting properties. Several clinical trials have shown no benefit, and in some studies, an increase in hemorrhagic strokes was found. Some antioxidant supplements may actually interfere with statin therapy. The role of antioxidants in stopping the progression of heart disease remains an area of study. Third, aspirin was believed to lower the risk of heart disease. However, potential benefits may be outweighed by risks such as stomach bleeding or ulcers in low-risk women. Aspirin therapy is recommended only for women at highest risk for heart attack (those who already have cardiovascular disease, diabetes, or chronic kidney disease), but regular use is contraindicated in this group if certain conditions exist.[27]

Diabetes Women with diabetes are at higher risk for multisystem diseases, especially cardiovascular disease than women without diabetes. Over the past 30 years, deaths from heart disease in women with diabetes have increased 23 percent compared to a 27 percent decrease in women without diabetes. Diabetic women are at greater risk for stroke, have three to seven times the risk for heart disease and heart attack, and have two times the chance of having a second heart attack.[28] Dyslipidemia, called diabetic dyslipidemia in people with diabetes, is a condition associated with insulin resistance. Dyslipidemia is characterized by high levels of LDL, high levels of triglycerides, and low levels of HDL. This lipid triad is associated with greater risk for atherosclerosis, a major contributor to coronary heart disease in women.[29]

Other Contributing Factors

Menopause and estrogen loss Although the evidence is not clear, it is believed that estrogen acts as a protective factor against heart disease. Due to the natural loss of estrogen after menopause or the surgical removal of the ovaries, evidence suggests that an increased risk of heart disease occurs. At one time it was believed that HRT was beneficial in decreasing this risk in menopausal women. In 2002, clinical trials showed that HRT did *not* reduce the risk of cardiovascular disease and stroke in postmenopausal women. In fact, the Women's Health Initiative discontinued its HRT study because of the undue risk of blood clots and stroke for women participating in the study. In 2004, the NIH discontinued the estrogen-only trial because of an apparent increased risk of stroke.

Oral contraceptives Women's risk of heart disease and stroke for those who take low-dose oral contraceptives has decreased over previous high-dose oral contraceptives. The risk still remains high for women who have high blood pressure or choose to smoke while taking oral contraceptives. Using oral contraceptives is contraindicated for women who smoke and are 35 years of age and older, and women who develop high blood pressure while taking oral contraceptives may be advised to stop taking them. Recent studies have shown that the risks of blood clots in legs and lungs are higher for women using Ortho Evra, the birth control patch, compared to women using birth control pills.

High triglyceride levels Triglycerides are a form of fat that comes from food and are also made in the body. Women with high triglyceride levels may need to modify their lifestyle by controlling weight, choosing foods low in saturated fats and cholesterol, increasing physical activity, not smoking, and in some cases, drinking less alcohol. Limiting the intake of carbohydrates to no more than 40–50 percent of total calories is sometimes encouraged. It is not clear whether high triglycerides alone are a risk factor for heart disease, but the AHA suggests that high triglyceride levels may increase the risk of heart disease more for women than for men. High triglyceride levels seem to be found along with high total cholesterol and LDL levels and low HDL levels.[30]

Excessive alcohol intake Women who drink moderate amounts (an average of one drink daily) have a lowered risk of heart disease than non-drinkers. Despite this finding, it is not recommended that non-drinkers start using alcohol or that drinkers increase their use of alcohol. Excessive alcohol intake can lead to high triglyceride levels, high blood pressure, heart failure, and stroke, and it can produce irregular heartbeats. Drinking too much alcohol also can contribute to obesity, alcoholism, unintended injuries, and suicide.

Stress A woman's individual response to stress can be a contributing factor to heart disease. Negative responses such as overeating, smoking, or excessive alcohol intake are examples of how one's response to stress can contribute to the risk for heart disease. Studies show that women who hold in anger are more susceptible to heart attacks than those who express their anger. The bleakest survival prognosis for women with CHD is for women who are divorced, work full-time, lack a college education, and earn less than $20,000 a year. These women tend to suppress anger, resentment, and loneliness.

The issue for women who work outside the home is the level of satisfaction with the job. According to one study, low job satisfaction, less perceived emotional reward, and lower perceived financial status were risk factors among employed women. The risk factors for women who did not work outside the home included symptoms of tension and anxiety, loneliness, difficulty sleeping, infrequent vacations, and perception of susceptibility to CHD. Low educational level, tension, and infrequent vacations, regardless of the woman's employment status, were risk factors for both groups.[31]

Screening and Diagnosis

Women who suspect they have heart disease should be assertive in getting a proper diagnosis. Many of the traditional tests used for screening for heart disease were developed for men. For example, women often have been falsely diagnosed with heart disease from the traditional stress test, which is a treadmill test. The stress test is not specific or sensitive enough for women. Women can receive better results from a stress echocardiogram, which is a noninvasive technique that uses a

Viewpoint

Gender Bias in Diagnosis and Treatment

Studies have found conflicting results regarding the effect of gender bias on the diagnosis and treatment of heart disease. Some studies showed that, compared to men, women received fewer diagnostic tests for heart disease, received fewer referrals for exercise rehabilitation, had a greater risk of death, cardiac distress, and reinfarction within 1 year of MI, and had treatment withheld or delayed.[32] Other studies found no bias in referral for cardiac catheterization and suggested that differential treatment resulted because women delayed medical care, were older when they developed heart disease, and had more complications at the time of diagnosis.[33] A review of current strategies for angioplasty and coronary artery bypass surgery suggested that the research remains ambiguous regarding gender bias in treatment and stressed the need for future randomized tests.[34] One recent study did find that women gain benefits similar to men from aggressive treatment. Mortality and heart attack rates 6 months later were similar in 2,200 women and men who underwent angioplasty (10.7 percent in women and 10.9 percent in men). Once a diagnosis of heart disease is made, women do equally well as men.[35]

Many family physicians remain unaware that diagnostic tests to determine heart disease differ for men and women. The most effective diagnostic tool for men is the treadmill test, but women need the treadmill combined with an echocardiogram or nuclear imaging. How can a woman determine if her health care provider is biased against women in diagnosing and aggressively treating heart disease?

treadmill test and ultrasound pictures of the heart. The ultrasound pictures allow the cardiologist to view the heart muscle contractions at peak exercise. Another test that uses radioactive tracers to assess blood flow during rest and exercise is equally accurate in women and men. (See *Viewpoint:* "Gender Bias in Diagnosis and Treatment.")

STROKE

Stroke is the third leading cause of death in women and the leading cause of adult disability, yet few women know the warning Symptoms. (See *Health Tips:* "Warning Symptoms of Stroke.")

Health Tips

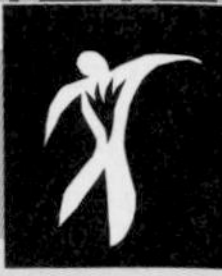

Warning Symptoms of Stroke[36]

Common stroke symptoms in both women and men:

- Sudden weakness or numbness on one side of the body, usually the face, arm, or leg
- Sudden blurred or dim vision, often on one side
- Sudden loss of speech or difficulty comprehending speech
- Sudden severe headaches with no known cause
- Sudden, unexplained falls with trouble walking, dizziness, or lack of balance
- Recurring TIAs, or mini-strokes that last several minutes

Unique stroke symptoms that women may report:

- Sudden face and limb pain
- Sudden hiccups
- Sudden nausea
- Sudden general weakness
- Sudden chest pain
- Sudden shortness of breath
- Sudden palpitations

Over 96,243 women died of stroke in 2003 (61.0 percent of the total stroke deaths). The disability and death rate for African American women is considerably higher than that for non-Hispanic white women (69.1 compared to 50.5).[37] Although stroke is more common in men in most age groups, more women die from stroke at all ages. Some evidence suggests that lower socioeconomic status and less education are related to higher risk for stroke.

Stroke is a form of vascular disease with many causes and levels of severity. An artery carrying oxygen-rich blood to the brain may suddenly become clogged or burst, preventing blood flow to the brain. The two primary types of stroke include hemorrhagic and ischemic stroke. Hemorrhagic strokes are further subdivided into subarachnoid stroke and intracerebral stroke, depending on the location in the brain of the burst blood vessel. Hemorrhagic strokes, about 12 percent of all strokes, are more common in young women, and 67 percent of all subarachnoid strokes occur in women. Ischemic stroke, which is about 88 percent of all strokes and is more common in older women, occurs when a blood vessel is blocked and oxygen is prevented from flowing to the brain. Ischemic stroke results from an embolism, large artery thrombosis, or small penetrating artery thrombosis.[38] (See Color Plate 7.)

Risk Factors for Stroke

The risk factors for stroke include those that cannot be changed, those that can be reduced with medical treatment, and those that can be reduced with lifestyle changes. The risk factors that cannot be altered include increasing age, race (African American and Hispanic women are at increased risk), heredity, gender, and the experience of a prior stroke or heart attack.

The risk factors that can be reduced with medical treatment include hypertension, tobacco use, heart disease, diabetes, high red blood cell count, atrial fibrillation, carotid or other artery disease, TIAs, sickle-cell anemia, high blood cholesterol, physical inactivity and obesity, excessive alcohol, and some illegal drugs.

Transient ischemic attacks (TIAs) are "mini" or small strokes that produce stroke-like symptoms but are only temporary. TIAs are strong predictors of stroke. A woman who has had a TIA is nearly ten times more likely to have a future stroke. Hypertension, or high blood pressure, is the most important risk factor for stroke. As a woman's blood pressure goes up, so does her risk of stroke. Treatment for high blood pressure (higher than 140/90) is the key to reducing the chances of future strokes. The use of anticoagulants (blood thinners) or antiplatelet medicines such as aspirin can be helpful in the prevention of ischemic strokes. These agents would probably not be recommended for a woman who has had or is at risk of hemorrhagic stroke.

Another risk factor that can be altered with medical treatment is atrial fibrillation, or irregular heartbeat. Atrial fibrillation increases the risk of a blood clot breaking free and moving to the brain. Women with atrial fibrillation are five times more at risk for stroke. Research suggests that blood thinners can dramatically reduce the risk of stroke from atrial fibrillation by preventing clots from forming.

The risk factors that can be modified with lifestyle changes include reducing blood cholesterol and lipids, quitting cigarette smoking, limiting alcohol intake, not abusing drugs, being physically active, practicing relaxation techniques, and maintaining a desirable weight.

Several studies may be of particular interest regarding risk factors in women. One study found a significant dose-response relationship between daily cigarette consumption and ischemic stroke. Women who smoked more cigarettes and for more years had a greater risk of stroke. Women who stopped smoking, regardless of their age at starting smoking or the number of cigarettes smoked, experienced significant reduction in stroke risk within 2 to 4 years.[39] Circulation improves within 2 weeks to 3 months of quitting, and stroke risk is reduced to that of a nonsmoker 5 to 15 years after quitting. As stated earlier, HRT increases the risk of blood clots. As a result of the Women's Health Initiative study, women were encouraged to visit their health care providers to discuss alternatives to HRT to treat postmenopausal symptoms. Women's health advocates suggest there is no reason to believe the results would be any different for other estrogen and/or progesterone drugs used for HRT and recommend against using HRT to control the symptoms of menopause.[40] Illegal drug abuse, in particular IV drug abuse and cocaine use, is also a risk factor. Cocaine use, even first-time use, has been closely associated with increased risk for strokes, heart attacks, and other cardiovascular complications.

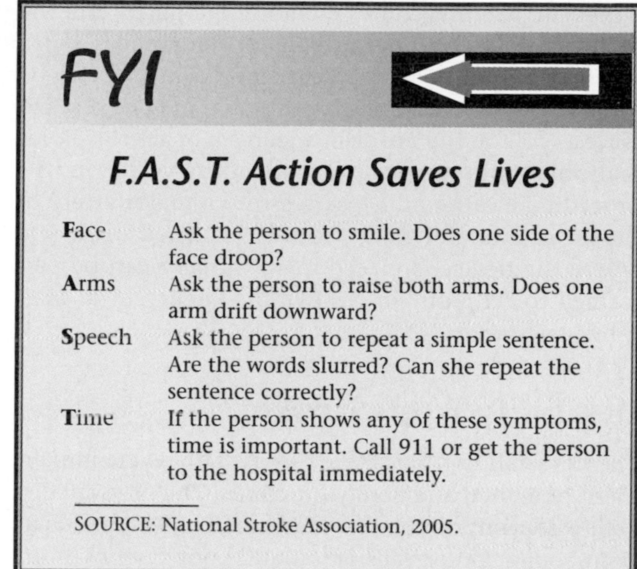

FYI

F.A.S.T. Action Saves Lives

Face	Ask the person to smile. Does one side of the face droop?
Arms	Ask the person to raise both arms. Does one arm drift downward?
Speech	Ask the person to repeat a simple sentence. Are the words slurred? Can she repeat the sentence correctly?
Time	If the person shows any of these symptoms, time is important. Call 911 or get the person to the hospital immediately.

SOURCE: National Stroke Association, 2005.

Treatment

Stroke should be treated as an emergency. Whenever a warning sign occurs, a woman should act F.A.S.T. (See *FYI:* "F.A.S.T. Action Saves Lives.")

Knowing the warning signs is important because new drugs (e.g., TPA, or tissue plasminogen activator) can break up clots and limit damage to the brain if administered within 3 hours of the start of symptoms. Treatment approaches differ depending on the type of stroke a woman experiences. Health care providers find it far easier to predict survival than functional outcome. Level of consciousness is the best predictor of short-term survival, whereas recovery during the first 30 to 60 days predicts potential functional outcome.

A surgical procedure, carotid endarterectomy, has prevented thousands of strokes. This surgery removes fatty buildup (atherosclerosis) in the carotid arteries (blood vessels in the neck that supply oxygen to the brain). This procedure was shown to be less beneficial for women, the elderly, and those with disabilities.

Other surgical procedures include angioplasty and the placement of stents (meshlike tubes), which help keep a carotid artery open and prevent reblockage.

For hemorrhagic stroke, a procedure may be done to place a "coil" at the site of an aneurysm or arteriovenous malformation to prevent rupture of the vessel. In this procedure a catheter is inserted into a major artery of the leg or arm and guided to the weakened vessel site where the device is placed. Also, surgery can be performed to "clip off" or remove the aneurysm or malformed vessels.

Disability from Stroke

The devastation from stroke can include severe impairment of mental and bodily functions. The physical disability depends on the area of the brain affected such as sight, sound, motor skills, autonomic body systems (heart rate, respiration, body temperature), or language. Physical changes (permanent paralysis, impaired speech or thought processes, and memory loss) and emotional changes (loss of sexual desire, poor body image, depression) are common. The rehabilitation of a stroke patient begins as soon as possible with health care staff and family members offering support and encouragement. The key to helping a woman recover from a stroke is access to rehabilitation. If she has private insurance to cover the cost of rehabilitation, her prognosis for recovery is better.

OSTEOPOROSIS

Osteoporosis (porous bone), a bone-weakening disease, results in bone mineral loss and increases the risk of skeletal frailty and fracturing. Although perceived as a disease of old age, osteoporosis starts in childhood. It has been described as a "pediatric disease with a geriatric outcome."[41] Genetics, age, menopausal status, diet, and exercise play major roles in determining peak bone mass, an indicator of future bone density. Primary prevention focuses on increasing peak bone mass, reached between the ages of 30 and 35 years, and reducing bone loss in later life. The greatest loss in bone density occurs in women during the first 5 to 10 years after menopause before leveling to approximately 1 percent a year. Osteoporosis is often called the "silent disease" because bone loss occurs without symptoms. Without early diagnosis, the first symptom in many cases is a bone fracture.

Osteoporosis threatens the bone health of 44 million Americans (55 percent of all persons over age 50). An estimated ten million Americans have osteoporosis, and an estimated 34 million have low bone mass, which puts them at increased risk for osteoporosis and fractures.[42] Eight million (80 percent) of those affected by osteoporosis are women, particularly postmenopausal women.

Women Making a Difference

Lillian Wald: Nurse, Suffragist, and Social Activist

Lillian Wald, best known as the founder of both the Henry Street Settlement and the Visiting Nurse's Service, was born in 1867 in Cincinnati, Ohio, to a wealthy German-Jewish family. In 1889, she enrolled in the nursing program at the New York Hospital Training School. After graduation, she began teaching classes in home nursing for poor and immigrant women on New York City's Lower East Side. She witnessed firsthand the high rates of contagious and chronic diseases endemic in the immigrant population, due in large part to poor or nonexistent sanitation and extreme overcrowding.

In 1895, Ms. Wald moved to 265 Henry Street, where, with a staff of six nurses, she founded the Henry Street Settlement. The Settlement was an organization devoted to providing nursing care and health and hygiene education to impoverished immigrants of Lower Manhattan. She led the Settlement until her retirement in 1930, having nurtured it into a major organization offering not only health care, but housing assistance, education and recreational activities to thousands of needy New Yorkers.

Recognized in 1922 by *The New York Times* as one of the twelve greatest living American women, Wald continued working tirelessly on behalf of the poor, the needy and the marginalized. Together with her work at the Henry Street Settlement, Wald championed women's suffrage, civil rights, and peace activism. She died in 1940 at the age of 73. Now, over 100 years later, Wald's legacy of the Henry Street Settlement continues to serve New York City.[43]

Twenty percent of non-Hispanic white and Asian women, 10 percent of Hispanic women, and 5 percent of African American women are estimated to have osteoporosis. Loss of height, spinal deformities such as kyphosis, and severe back pain, all resulting from collapsed vertebrae, are signs of advanced osteoporosis. Nearly half of all women over the age of 50 are predicted to have a bone fracture during their lifetime related to bone loss.

Some 1.5 million osteoporosis-related fractures occur yearly with 700,000 of these being vertebral fractures. Bones of the spine, hips, ribs, and wrists are especially susceptible to osteoporosis-related fractures. Of special concern are fractures of the hip and spine because these fractures can lead to prolonged or permanent disability

Assess Yourself

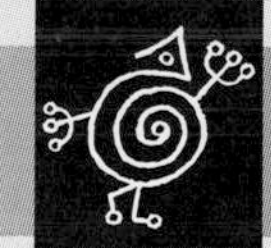

Determine Your Risk for Osteoporosis

Check the following risk factors that pertain to you.

_____ 1. A small, thin frame (low body mass index)
_____ 2. Caucasian or Asian
_____ 3. Family history of osteoporosis
_____ 4. Estrogen deficiency
  _____ Early or surgically induced menopause
  _____ Postmenopausal women
  _____ Hypogonadism in women and men
_____ 5. Excessive thyroid medication
_____ 6. Prolonged use of cortisone-like drugs for asthma, arthritis, or cancer
_____ 7. Low lifetime calcium intake
_____ 8. Sedentary lifestyle
_____ 9. Cigarette smoker
_____ 10. Excessive alcohol intake
_____ 11. Personal history of fractures after age 50
_____ 12. Current low bone mass
_____ 13. Being female
_____ 14. Anorexia nervosa
_____ 15. Amenorrhea
_____ 16. Vitamin D deficiency
_____ 17. Advanced age
_____ 18. History of fracture in primary relative
_____ 19. Gastrointestinal malabsorption syndromes

The more items you have checked, the greater your risk for developing osteoporosis. What can you do to increase your protective factors and reduce your risks?

or even death. Nearly 24 percent of hip fracture patients age 50 and over die in the year following their fractures. Although the rate of hip fractures is two to three times higher in women than in men, men have twice the mortality rate in the first year following a hip fracture. Twenty percent of persons who were able to walk prior to a hip fracture will require long-term care, and only 15 percent of long-term care persons will be able to walk unassisted 6 months after the fracture.[44]

Heredity also influences the risk of osteoporosis. Common genetic differences have been found to account for 7 to 10 percent of the difference in bone density, particularly at the hip and spine.

Young women who are at increased risk for osteoporosis include highly trained female athletes with amenorrhea and those suffering from anorexia nervosa. Complete *Assess Yourself:* "Determine Your Risk for Osteoporosis."

Hypogonadism (sex glands produce low levels of or no hormones) is a secondary outcome occurring with excessive exercise or anorexia nervosa. Exercise can be a risk factor for competitive female athletes, particularly distance runners, gymnasts, and dancers. These athletes commonly experience exercise-induced amenorrhea due to intense training regimens and extremely restricted calorie intake. Although the exact cause of amenorrhea is unknown, reduced body fat appears to be a major factor. These athletes, whether young girls or mature women, experience a reduction in bone density despite intense weight-bearing activity. The effects of short-term amenorrhea seem to be reversible; however, research has not determined the impact of long-term amenorrhea (2 to 3 years) on future bone density. If bone density loss is irreversible, the likelihood of osteoporosis increases.[45]

Exercise-induced amenorrhea is not a minor problem. Any female athlete who experiences more than 6 months of amenorrhea should be evaluated for loss of bone density and strongly encouraged to reduce training to a level at which menstruation resumes.[46] Health care providers may prescribe oral contraceptives to induce menstruation and increase estrogen levels.

Anorexia and bulimia nervosa can also contribute to rapid bone loss and fracture. Women who have these conditions may experience estrogen deficiency, malnutrition, and altered carbohydrate metabolism. One study found that calcium supplementation, resumed menstrual function, and exercise did not significantly restore skeletal mass within 2 years.[47] However, longitudinal studies suggest that bone mass may return within a longer time frame. Women who have exercise-induced amenorrhea or anorexia nervosa should be encouraged to gain weight to a level at which menstruation occurs naturally. Oral contraceptives can be prescribed for estrogen deficiency but are ineffective until weight gain and full endocrine function are restored.[48]

Smoking affects the processing of vitamin D and reduces the calcium absorption necessary for maintaining bone density. One study found that bone density in men and women over age 60 varied directly with the number of cigarettes smoked. Women were especially impacted by the number of cigarettes they smoked.[49] Thus, quitting smoking at any age may reduce bone loss. Results of studies related to excessive alcohol consumption, more than three drinks a day, and bone loss were mixed. Some studies suggested that excessive drinking interferes with calcium and vitamin D absorption, and others found no relationship between alcohol intake and osteoporosis. Some research implicates caffeine and high sodium intake as increasing the loss of calcium through the urine. Overall, women over the age of 65, younger postmenopausal women with one or more additional risk factors, and postmenopausal women who have a history of fractures should have a bone mass density (BMD) test.[50]

Protective Factors against Osteoporosis

Exercise Exercise, particularly weight-bearing activities, acts as a protective factor against bone loss and fracture. Weight-bearing activities such as running, brisk walking, hiking, weight lifting, and aerobics increase bone mineral density. Swimming, biking, and other weight-supported activities have less benefit. The greatest increase in density occurs at the site of maximum stress and repetition.[51] For instance, a tennis player's dominant arm is considerably larger than her nonplaying arm. Exercise provides the added benefit of muscle strength, tone, and balance, all important factors in reducing the likelihood of falls and fractures in older women.

Diet Calcium and vitamin D are two major nutrients needed to prevent osteoporosis. Studies have found that peak bone mass can be increased by drinking milk during childhood and adolescence and increasing calcium intake beyond the current Recommended Dietary Allowances. The most critical years for building bone mass are between preadolescence and age 30. (See *Health Tips:* "Recommended Calcium Intakes.")

Calcium plays a variety of roles in body functioning besides increasing bone density. When blood levels of calcium drop, the heart, muscles, and nerves deplete the calcium from bones to function properly. Surveys have shown that American women and girls are taking in less than half the amount of calcium recommended for growth and maintenance of bone tissue. Approximately 1,000 to 1,300 milligrams of calcium per day are recommended. Because the amount of calcium from food sources may not be adequate for some women, calcium supplements may be needed. It is important to recognize that a high calcium intake will not protect a woman against bone loss caused by estrogen deficiency, physical inactivity, smoking, alcohol abuse, and certain medical disorders and treatments.

Vitamin D, essential for building bone, must be present for calcium to be adequately absorbed through the small intestine. Vitamin D is synthesized by skin exposed to sunlight, and with aging, the skin seems to lose the ability to produce adequate amounts of vitamin D. Thus, milk and vitamin supplements are important sources of vitamin D in later years. Vitamin D also can be obtained from egg yolks, saltwater fish, and liver. The recommended intake is between 400 and 800 IU per day. Excessive amounts of vitamin D may be harmful; therefore, stay below 800 IU unless a high dose is prescribed by a health care provider.

Health Tips

Recommended Calcium Intakes[52]

Age	mg/day
Birth–6 months	210
6 months–1 year	270
1–3 years	500
4–8 years	800
9–13 years	1,300
14–18 years	1,300
19–30 years	1,000
31–50 years	1,000
51–70 years	1,200
70 or older	1,200
Pregnant and Lactating	
14–18 years	1,300
19–50 years	1,000

Measuring Bone Density

The bone density of female athletes, women with eating disorders, women 60 to 70 years of age with a history of fracture, and perimenopausal women should be assessed. A bone mineral density (BMD) test is the only way to diagnose osteoporosis and determine a woman's risk for future bone fracture. Early diagnosis is important because osteoporosis, a "silent disease," can go undetected for many years without symptoms. Multiple types of BMD tests exist, and they are painless and noninvasive.

Treatment

Osteoporosis has no cure, but it can be treated or prevented with different drug therapies. Antiresorptive drugs that are used to slow progressive thinning of bone include bisphosphonates such as Fosamax and Actonel, calcitonin, and estrogen analogs such as raloxifene. Bone forming drugs such as parathyroid hormone continue to be investigated and show encouraging results. Hormone replacement therapy (HRT) is no longer considered a treatment option because of the associated risks for stroke, thromboembolism, cancer, and other diseases.[53]

DIABETES MELLITUS

Diabetes mellitus, the sixth leading cause of death for women of all races, is a serious, costly, and near epidemic disease in the United States. In the 10-year span from 1990 to 2000, adults diagnosed with diabetes increased 49 percent. One in five adults over age 65 and approximately 8.8 percent of all women 20 years or older in the United States live with diabetes. Hispanics and non-Hispanic black women have higher rates than non-Hispanic white women for type 2 diabetes, but slightly lower rates for type 1 diabetes. Compared to non-Hispanic white women of the same age, non-Hispanic black women and Hispanic women have nearly a two times higher risk of diabetes and American Indian/Alaska Native women have a threefold higher risk of diabetes.

Diabetes is a chronic disorder of carbohydrate metabolism with a deficiency in insulin production, insulin action, or both. Normally, insulin allows glucose (a form of sugar) to enter the cells so that energy can be produced. The disruption of normal carbohydrate metabolism causes high levels of glucose in the blood, which results in damage to many of the body's systems, especially blood vessels and nerves. Complications associated with diabetes mellitus include diabetic retinopathy (a leading cause of blindness), kidney failure, heart disease, gum disease, diabetic neuropathy (sensory nerve damage to extremities), and diabetic foot disease, which can lead to amputation if left untreated. Cognitive decline and Alzheimer's disease have been found in some women with type 2 diabetes, particularly when blood-sugar levels are uncontrolled. Heredity and autoimmune and environmental factors have been found to be possible causes of type 1 diabetes. Obesity is the leading contributor to the exponential increase in type 2 diabetes. Ninety to ninety-five percent of all diagnosed diabetes is type 2, but type 1 and gestational diabetes are also significant. Prediabetes is a condition that increases the risk for type 2 diabetes, heart disease, and stroke and is receiving more attention from the medical profession. Persons with prediabetes have impaired fasting glucose and/or impaired glucose tolerance. Losing weight and increasing physical activity can prevent or delay the onset of diabetes.[54]

Type 1 Diabetes

Type 1 diabetes was once called insulin-dependent or juvenile-onset diabetes. This form develops most frequently in young children and adolescents, but its rate is increasing among adults. The American Diabetes Association (ADA) estimates that 500,000 to 1 million Americans and approximately 1 in every 400 to 600 children and adolescents have this form of diabetes. In type 1 diabetes, the pancreas produces little or no insulin and daily insulin injections or the use of insulin pumps is required to maintain normal blood-sugar levels and provide the body's cells with energy. Physical activity and healthy eating are also important in managing this disease. Researchers are experimenting with islet cell transplantation, pancreas transplantation, artificial pancreas development, and genetic manipulation to allow persons with diabetes to manufacture their own insulin.[55]

Type 2 Diabetes

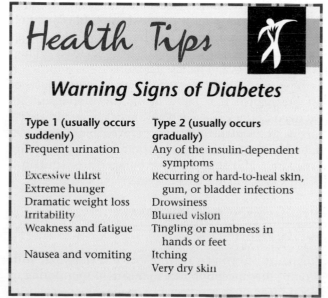

Type 2 diabetes was once known as non-insulin-dependent or adult-onset diabetes. In this form of diabetes, the pancreas produces insulin but for some reason the body is resistant to the insulin and is unable to use it properly. As the insulin level rises, the pancreas loses more of its ability to produce insulin. Type 2 diabetes is the most common form of diabetes and appears more frequently in adults over the age of 45, but it is increasingly being found in adolescents and children. This type of diabetes is linked to obesity and physical inactivity and can be controlled by a healthy diet, physical activity, and weight control, and by insulin injections and/or oral medications. In addition, some studies have found that women who smoke have a higher risk of developing type 2 diabetes than women who never smoked or who quit smoking. Also, the risk of developing type 2 diabetes appears to be dose related; that is, the more cigarettes a woman smokes, the greater her risk.[56] (See *Health Tips:* "Warning Signs of Diabetes.")

Gestational Diabetes

Gestational diabetes occurs in 2 to 5 percent of all pregnancies. A screening test that measures blood glucose level is usually done between the 24th and 28th weeks

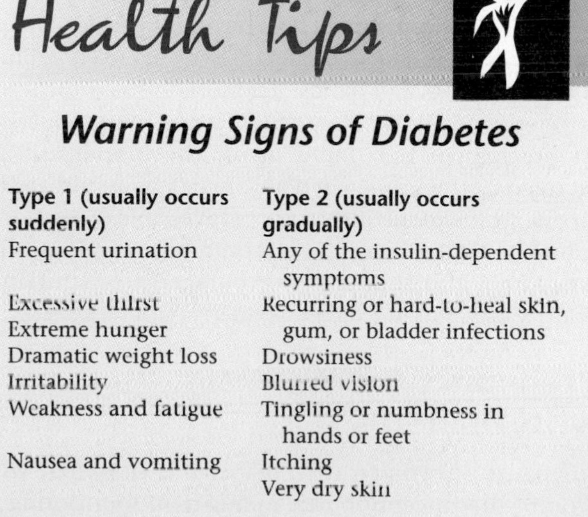

Health Tips

Warning Signs of Diabetes

Type 1 (usually occurs suddenly)	Type 2 (usually occurs gradually)
Frequent urination	Any of the insulin-dependent symptoms
Excessive thirst	Recurring or hard-to-heal skin, gum, or bladder infections
Extreme hunger	Drowsiness
Dramatic weight loss	Blurred vision
Irritability	Tingling or numbness in hands or feet
Weakness and fatigue	Itching
Nausea and vomiting	Very dry skin

of pregnancy. Pregnant women with high blood glucose levels during pregnancy who had no previous signs of diabetes are said to have gestational diabetes.

Gestational diabetes usually appears around the 24th week of pregnancy. Although the cause is unknown, it may be related to the large quantities of hormones that the placenta starts producing at that time. These hormones may block or cause an insulin resistance in the mother's body that lasts until the pregnancy is over.

Many women who experience gestational diabetes will experience a return to normal blood-sugar levels after the pregnancy. However, studies show that these women remain more susceptible to gestational diabetes in future pregnancies, and more than half of them will develop type 2 diabetes later in life. Approximately 20 to 50 percent of women who had gestational diabetes develop type 2 diabetes within 5 to 10 years. Also, older women who become pregnant have an increased risk of developing gestational diabetes.[57]

Although babies born to mothers with gestational diabetes do not have any greater risk for birth defects than those delivered from nongestational diabetic mothers, they are more at risk for other problems. These include macrosomia (large or fat bodies), hypoglycemia (low blood glucose) after delivery, jaundice, and respiratory distress syndrome (RDS). Macrosomic babies may need to be delivered by cesarean section if they are too large for vaginal delivery. Large babies can cause difficult deliveries for both the mother and baby, with the baby being at risk for arm and shoulder injuries or even oxygen deprivation for a period of time. If an ultrasound shows that a woman is carrying a macrosomic baby, an amniocentesis test may be recommended to determine the baby's risk for RDS because macrosomic babies are also at increased risk for premature birth.

Women with gestational diabetes are at higher risk for preeclampsia, urinary tract infections, and ketonuria. Preeclampsia is a potentially life-threatening condition in which a woman experiences pregnancy-induced high blood pressure usually accompanied by edema (swelling) of the lower legs and hands. Ketonuria is the presence of ketones in the urine. Ketones are acidic by-products of fat breakdown that build up in the blood and are excreted in the urine when a woman's body utilizes fat for energy when no other source is available. Gestational diabetic mothers should be monitored closely during pregnancy and should be encouraged to maintain a healthy diet and to exercise regularly.

Pregnancy for Women with Diabetes

Pregnancy in women with diabetes is risky, but with prompt preconception care and careful monitoring of blood sugar, these women will have healthy pregnancies and healthy babies. Women considering birth control methods should be aware that oral contraceptives can affect glucose levels and diabetes management and that IUD use can lead to infection. IUDs are typically contraindicated for women with diabetes because they already have a higher risk for infection.[58]

ASTHMA

Asthma is a chronic, incurable disease of the lungs, characterized by inflammation and narrowing of the air passageways leading from the mouth and nose into the lungs. Women and children with asthma suffer periodic episodes, or attacks, with mild to severe symptoms that may include shortness of breath, wheezing, coughing, chest pain or tightness, or any combination. In severe cases, an asthma attack can lead to the death of the individual.

Asthma rates in the United States have increased during the last 2 decades. Adult women outnumber adult men as sufferers, and women over 20 are more likely than men to develop asthma. Each year, more women than men die of asthma-related complications, and women account for 65 percent of deaths due to the condition. African American women have the highest mortality rate and are at least 2.5 times more likely to die from asthma than non-Hispanic white women.[59]

It is estimated that asthma costs Americans, directly or indirectly, nearly $18 billion per year. Nearly $10 billion accounts for the direct costs of hospitalization and $5 billion accounts for lost wages and earnings due to asthma-related sick days, disability, or death.[60] Nearly 15 million workdays are missed or lost per year due to this condition, while among school-aged children 5 to 17, asthma is the leading cause of school absences due to chronic illness.[61]

While the root causes of asthma remain unknown, heredity is believed to play a role. A child with one parent having asthma has a 1 in 3 chance of developing asthma, while a child with two parents with asthma has a 7 in 10 chance of developing the condition.[62] Currently, nearly 20 million Americans suffer from asthma.[63] While persons of any ethnic or socioeconomic group may develop asthma, living in poverty or with little access to health care on in urban areas where air quality is poor or working in occupations in which exposure to lung irritants is more likely, appears to account for more disparity in the disease than simply gender or ethnic differences.[64]

Types of Asthma

Asthma is divided into two types: allergic and nonallergic. *Allergic asthma* is most common, with nearly 50 percent of sufferers having this type. As its name implies, allergic asthma is triggered in susceptible individuals by exposure to common airborne pollutants and allergens, including mold spores, pollen, dust mites or roaches, animal dander, feather bedding, perfume, foods, tobacco smoke, or other environmental contaminants. *Non-allergic,* or *intrinsic,* asthma may be triggered by allergens but is often triggered by other factors including stress, anxiety, extreme weather changes, exercise, viruses, and bronchial illnesses including colds and flu, and lung infections. For women, monthly hormonal cycles or the hormonal changes that occur during pregnancy may trigger the onset of adult asthma. Menopausal women may also experience adult-onset asthma for the first time. For some patients, however, asthma symptoms may disappear or lessen in adulthood, as asthma is most often diagnosed during childhood.

Managing Your Asthma

If you have asthma, controlling the condition and your symptoms is important for your continuing health and quality of life. First, educate yourself about your asthma by staying current with new information and research. Checking your lungs for air flow on a daily basis with a device called a peak flow meter can help you detect potential changes in your condition that should be brought to the attention of your health care provider. If your asthma is triggered by food allergens, know which foods or food ingredients you are sensitive to and avoid them. Avoid exposure to fabrics or chemicals that are known irritants, and keep your living or work spaces as free of irritants and allergens as possible. During warm weather, when ozone or air particulates are at high levels, you may wish to stay away from outdoor activities, as poor air quality may also trigger attacks.

There are many effective medications which help control symptoms, including some that are available over-the-counter. It is important to take all your medications as prescribed. Any changes to your current drug regimen or additions of over-the-counter medications should not be attempted without first consulting your health care provider, as this could cause potentially harmful drug interactions. Let your health care provider know if, over time, your condition does not improve or your symptoms worsen.

Asthma and Pregnancy

When an asthmatic woman becomes pregnant, controlling her symptoms is vital for both her health and the health of her unborn baby. A developing fetus depends on its mother's blood for its oxygen needs, and frequent asthma attacks may lead to a lessening of the oxygen supply available to a fetus. Having a sufficient level of oxygen in the fetal blood is essential for its correct development, and inadequate oxygen at key times throughout this development could result in impaired growth or even in fetal death. As many as 3.7–8.4 percent of pregnant women may have asthma, making it one of the most common serious medical conditions affecting pregnancy.[65]

Uncontrolled asthma has been associated with a greater risk for a pregnant woman's developing hypertensive problems, including preeclampsia, a potentially serious or even life-threatening condition that affects some women. It may also cause other problems, including premature birth or having a low-birth-weight baby.[66] Because the risks of uncontrolled asthma on a pregnancy outweigh those of most asthma medications, a woman who is already on a prescribed drug regimen for this condition should not stop or change this regimen unless directed to do so by her physician or health care provider.

While some prenatal or postpartum problems are seen more frequently in women with uncontrolled asthma, medical experts are still uncertain as to the exact role asthma may play in causing these conditions. Until more is learned in this regard, keeping adequate medical control over her asthma is the best way for a woman to ensure both a healthy pregnancy and a healthy baby.

Asthma and Tobacco Smoke

Tobacco smoke may contain up to 4,000 trace chemicals, many of which are known toxins, including arsenic, formaldehyde, and cyanide. Secondhand smoke, the smoke that is emitted as a result of a lit cigarette, pipe, or cigar, has been rated as a Group A carcinogen by the U.S. Environmental Protection Agency, with Group A carcinogens ranked as the most serious.[67] As more is learned about the dangers from exposure to secondhand smoke (SHS), research indicates that children who are routinely exposed to SHS have a greater likelihood of developing asthma, allergies, and other serious lung conditions. The chance of a child dying from sudden infant death syndrome (SIDS) greatly increases if one or both parents are smokers.[68]

Because children's lungs are still maturing, they are more sensitive to the effects of tobacco smoke and the chemicals burned off in the process of smoking. Children exposed to these chemicals may experience impaired lung function, may have more infections of the respiratory tract, and may suffer from more allergies than children who are not exposed to tobacco smoke. Secondhand, or passive, smoking may worsen asthma in teens and may create up to 26,000 new cases of asthma each year.[69] Infants up to 18 months old who are exposed to secondhand smoke may be at greater risk for lung infections and infections of the lower respiratory tract, which incur high medical costs if the infant needs hospitalization.

If an adult must smoke, smoking should be done outside of a home and outside of areas such as cars, buildings, or play areas in which children are likely to spend time. In the long-term, ceasing the smoking habit, while difficult, remains the best strategy for adults to ensure not only their own lung and respiratory health, but that of their children as well.

EPILEPSY

Epilepsy, a chronic brain disorder characterized by recurrent seizures, is a general term for more than twenty different types of seizure disorders. It occurs when abnormal electrical activity in the brain causes an involuntary change in body movement or function, sensation, awareness, or behavior lasting from a few seconds to a few minutes. Any disturbance of the normal pattern of neuron (nerve cell) activity can lead to seizures. Epilepsy can result from abnormal electrical neuron activity, an imbalance of neurotransmitters, or a combination of these factors. Symptoms during a seizure will depend on the site of the electrical activity in the brain. A person experiencing a grand mal seizure may lose consciousness, fall to the ground, and have rigidity and muscle jerks. During a complex partial seizure, a woman may seem confused or dazed and won't be able to answer questions or follow directions. Absence (petit mal) seizures can go undetected as the person may experience only a short period of rapid blinking or staring into space.

Approximately 2.7 million Americans have some form of epilepsy. Although epiloptic seizures may be caused by lack of oxygen, head trauma, stroke, brain tumor, poisoning, infection/fever, inherited conditions, or fetal development complications, there is no known cause for the majority of them. According to the Centers for Diseare Control and Prevention, treatment can control seizures in about 80 percent of the people with epilepsy. Seizure-preventing drugs known as antiepileptic drugs are the most common form of treatment. Surgery, vagal nerve stimulation, and a special ketogenic diet are sometimes tried when drug therapies do not work. Various anticonvulsants can be used depending on the type of seizure experienced. If a woman has more than one type of seizure, it is possible that several medications will be prescribed. Surgery for epilepsy may be considered although there is no guarantee that the seizures will be reduced or eliminated. Vagal nerve stimulation is a form of electrical stimulation of the brain through the vagus nerve in the neck. With this procedure, a small battery is placed in the chest wall and programmed to deliver short bursts of electrical energy to the brain. The ketogenic diet is a strict high-fat, low-carbohydrate diet that is reemerging as a possible treatment for epilepsy, especially for children whose seizures are not controlled by other means. This diet is a serious treatment with potential side effects including vitamin deficiencies. Further research is needed to evaluate this method of treatment for children and adults. Women on this diet may experience menstrual irregularities, pancreatitis, vitamin deficiencies, dehydration, constipation, decreased bone density, eye problems, and kidney or gall stones.[70] Additional research is being conducted with stem cell transplants, neuron stimulation, and the development of a device to more readily predict seizures several minutes before they occur.

Photosensitivity epilepsy occurs in 5 percent of people with epilepsy, particularly in children and adolescents. With this condition, exposure to flashing lights of certain intensities or wavelengths can trigger seizures. Photosensitive epileptic seizures may be triggered by television, video games, computer monitors, fire alarms, strobe lights, or even natural sunlight when there is a flickering or rapid flashing effect from the light.[71] (See *Health Tips:* "First Aid for Seizures.")

Initially, controlling the seizures is the primary concern of health care providers and the person with epilepsy. However, it doesn't take long to realize that the social stigma connected with epilepsy is often more difficult to overcome.

Psychosocial and Economic Considerations

The person with epilepsy and her caregiver (if dealing with a child) may know a lot about the illness, including what seizures are, what to do when one occurs, what

Health Tips

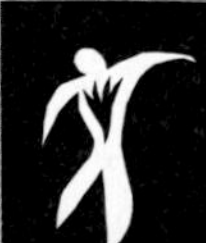

First Aid for Seizures

What to Do
- Look for medical identification.
- Loosen collars and ties.
- Protect the head from injury.
- Protect the person from nearby hazards.
- Turn person on side to keep airway clear.
- Call for aid.

What Not to Do
- Do not place anything in the mouth. (The tongue cannot be swallowed.)
- Do not provide any liquids during or immediately after the seizure.
- Do not give artificial respiration.
- Do not restrain the person.

medications do, how they should be taken, and their potential side effects. But what about the psychosocial, legal, and economic aspects of epilepsy? How are these addressed? Many questions arise: Should I tell my instructors? Is it safe to drive a car? Can I drink alcohol? What will my friends think, how will they act, if I tell them I have epilepsy? Is it safe to get pregnant? Educating the person with epilepsy and her caregiver is important, but so is educating the public. Education is the only way to reduce or eliminate the stigma associated with epilepsy. Employers, family, and friends of persons with epilepsy need to educate themselves about the disorder. Remember: Epilepsy is what a woman has, not what she is. She is a woman with epilepsy; not an epileptic woman.

Birth Control, Conception, and Pregnancy

Over one million girls and women in the United States live with a seizure disorder. Birth control, conception, and pregnancy create special circumstances and concerns for these women. Despite the special concerns, more than 90 percent of women with epilepsy who become pregnant give birth to normal, healthy infants.

Some antiepileptic medicines can lower estrogen concentrations by 40 to 50 percent, complicating the use of hormonal birth control methods. Women need to keep their health care provider informed when using these two medications concurrently because adjustments may need to be made if midcycle bleeding occurs, indicating poor birth control regulation. In addition, there is a 25 to 30 percent lower fertility rate for women with epilepsy. The reasons for the lower fertility rate are unknown but appear to range from genetic predisposition, seizure type and frequency, and side effects from antiepileptic medications to social pressures to refrain from having children.

Women with epilepsy should plan their pregnancies with a health care provider because medications will need to be monitored closely and adjusted before and throughout the pregnancy. The effects of medication on a developing fetus occur primarily in the first few weeks after conception. Women with epilepsy have a 4 to 6 percent higher risk of having a child with a birth defect when they take antiepileptic drugs during pregnancy. It is important for these women to take their prenatal vitamins, especially folic acid, before and during pregnancy to decrease the risk for brain and spinal abnormalities. Not only do the antiepileptic medications pose special concerns, but seizure activity itself during the pregnancy can be hazardous for both the mother and the fetus. Breast-feeding is considered safe for most women with epilepsy but should be discussed with the health care provider. Safety for infants and children should also be discussed because the mother with epilepsy could have unexpected seizures.[72]

Women with epilepsy may experience sexual difficulties because seizures and antiepileptic drugs may cause alterations in normal hormonal levels. Women may have a lack of sexual desire, experience painful intercourse due to vaginal dryness or spasms, or be afraid that seizures might occur during intercourse. Women with seizures that originate from the temporal lobe of the brain seem to be more susceptible to sexual difficulties. An endocrinologist may need to be consulted to assist in managing the complexities of hormones, seizures, and medications. Research has brought advances in diagnosis and treatment of epilepsy effectiveness of medications, and knowledge of pregnancy issues. Women with epilepsy can help control their own seizures by taking medications as prescribed, avoiding unusual stress, maintaining regular sleep cycles, and complying with the health care provider's treatment protocol.[73]

ARTHRITIS

Arthritis is an inflammatory condition of the joints, characterized by swelling, pain, and/or difficulty moving that persists for more than 2 weeks. (See *Health Tips:* "SERIOUS: The Warning Signs of Arthritis.")

Over a hundred types of arthritis and related diseases (known as rheumatic diseases) have been classified, with consequences ranging from mild to debilitating. The variety of arthritis and related diseases that women often encounter include osteoarthritis, rheumatoid arthritis, systemic lupus erythematosus, fibromyalgia, carpal tunnel syndrome, gout, Marfan syndrome, and scleroderma. If you experience arthritis, you need to know

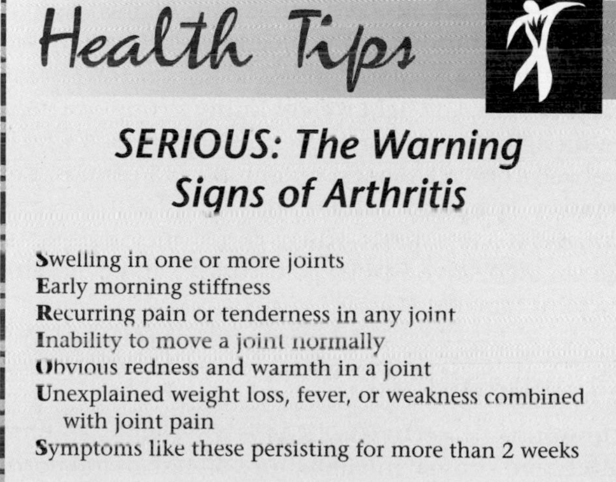

Health Tips

SERIOUS: The Warning Signs of Arthritis

Swelling in one or more joints
Early morning stiffness
Recurring pain or tenderness in any joint
Inability to move a joint normally
Obvious redness and warmth in a joint
Unexplained weight loss, fever, or weakness combined with joint pain
Symptoms like these persisting for more than 2 weeks

which type because treatment protocols vary. Arthritis or chronic joint symptoms affect approximately 66 million adults in the United States (1 in 3 adults). Women are more likely than men to have arthritis, and the prevalence of arthritis increases with age. Rates are similar in African American women and white women, but lower in Hispanic women.[74] Arthritis is a leading cause of work-related disability with nearly one-half of persons aged 65 and over reporting some degree of arthritis. The estimated prevalence of arthritis has risen over the past 10 years, along with reported activity limitation as those with arthritis get older.

Treatment can include rest, relaxation, weight control, physical activity, the use of heat or cold, medications for pain and inflammation, surgery, and use of assistive devices. Many traditional or alternative therapies exist that can be beneficial to a person suffering from arthritis, but as a consumer you need to be informed and watch carefully for quackery. Self-management programs that increase a person's ability to manage the chronic condition have also proven to be effective.

Osteoarthritis

Osteoarthritis (OA), or degenerative joint disease, occurs when cartilage that provides a smooth, gliding surface and cushion between the bones breaks down, resulting in pain, swelling, and altered joint function. It is the most common kind of arthritis and affects the weight-bearing joints, particularly the knees, hips, and ankles, but it can also affect the hands, lower spine, and neck. Osteoarthritis pain is often worse after overuse of the joint or periods of inactivity. Osteoarthritis is more common in women and people over age 45. The causes of OA are unknown, but factors such as heredity, aging, obesity, prior joint injury, muscle weakness, nerve injury, and overuse have been implicated in increased risk for the disease. Treatment focuses on minimizing the pain and improving joint movement. Management of the disease includes patient education, medications for inflammation and pain, weight control, heat/cold therapy, joint protection, physical activity to keep the joints flexible, and light weight lifting to improve muscle strength. Research indicates that in a person who is overweight even a modest weight loss (15 pounds) can improve symptoms of OA by almost 50 percent. Surgery is considered when other measures have proven ineffective against pain control and maintaining joint function.[75]

Rheumatoid Arthritis

Rheumatoid arthritis (RA) is a systemic, autoimmune, and chronic inflammatory disease of unknown cause that involves inflammation in the lining of the joints (synovium) and/or other internal organs. RA occurs two to three times more frequently in women than in men and is most prevalent in postmenopausal women. Symptoms often begin in women between the ages of 30 and 60. Research is being conducted to find the cause of RA so that better treatments might be found. Genetic and environmental factors, as well as endocrine, nerve, and immune system factors, are being studied. Research also is focused on the potential role of infectious agents as triggers of RA. The joints become swollen, red, and inflamed, and this condition lasts for an extended period of time. A pattern of flare-ups and remissions begins, and eventually the cartilage between the joints disappears and bone-to-bone irritation and pain ensue. RA can lead to long-term joint damage resulting in chronic pain, loss of function, and disability. Inflammation of RA most often affects joints in the hands and feet and is symmetrical (occurs equally on both sides of the body). This helps distinguish it from other forms of rheumatic (inflammatory) diseases.

Early diagnosis and treatment of RA are critical in preventing joint injury, thus limiting joint damage and loss of movement. The treatment approach to RA has changed dramatically over the past decade. The traditional pyramid approach to treatment involved a first-line therapy, consisting of non-steroidal anti-inflammatory drugs, bed rest, and physical therapy. As joint pain increased, second-line therapy was added. This approach has been replaced by a more aggressive intervention. Health care providers now begin treatment efforts aimed at preventing early joint injury. Second-line therapy, using a variety of drugs, begins at the first sign of clinical or functional deterioration.[76] Three classes of drugs are commonly used in the treatment of RA: non-steroidal anti-inflammatory agents (NSAIDS), corticosteroids, and disease-modifying anti-rheumatic drugs (DMARDS). DMARDS are being used more aggressively in the first 2 years to slow cartilage damage and bony erosions. In addition to drug therapy, physical activity, joint protection, and self-management techniques are used to improve the quality of life. Pregnancy creates a difficult situation because most of the medications used are not recommended during pregnancy and may need to be discontinued throughout the pregnancy.

Systemic Lupus Erythematosus (SLE)

Systemic lupus erythematosus (SLE) is the most common of three types of **lupus** and is recognized by the red, butterfly-shaped rash found across the bridge of the nose and cheeks. SLE is a chronic, autoimmune, rheumatic disease of connective tissue that causes inflammation affecting joints, muscles, and vital organs, especially the skin, kidneys, heart, lungs, and brain.

Lupus develops between the ages of 15 to 45 and affects nearly 1.5 million Americans; it is nearly ten to fifteen times more frequent in adult women than in men. SLE primarily affects women of childbearing age. For most women, lupus is a mild disease. Nearly 80 to 90 percent of women with SLE can expect to live a normal life span.

Lupus is three to four times more common in women of color, particularly African American, Hispanic, Asian, and Native American women. The cause of lupus is unknown; however, a combination of genetic, environmental, and hormonal factors have been implicated. Close to 37 percent of SLE deaths occur among young persons between 15 and 44 years of age. Death rates are three times greater for non-Hispanic black women than for non-Hispanic white women. While current rates indicate a significant increase in deaths, the reality may be that better reporting techniques have inflated the actual increase.[77]

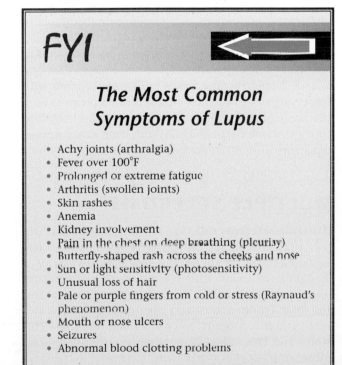

Signs and Symptoms The most commonly reported symptoms of SLE are found in *FYI:* "The Most Common Symptoms of Lupus."[78] The pattern of remission and flare-ups is common and can be fatal if left untreated. Flare-ups are often precipitated by exposure to sunlight, an infection, or a drug reaction. For some women, the use of estrogen may induce or trigger a lupus flare-up. The risk of blood clots is a real concern for women who are taking estrogen, and estrogen is contraindicated in women whose blood tests show a presence of antiphospholipid antibodies.[79] Women with lupus are much more likely than other women to suffer fractures due to osteoporosis. The bone loss associated with lupus is due to the use of certain medications, stress, and less physical activity.

Diagnosis and Treatment The immunofluorescent antinuclear antibody (ANA) test is a screening test for the presence of autoantibodies and is used to diagnose SLE. Determining whether a woman has SLE depends on the results of the ANA test and a minimum of four supporting symptoms. With fewer symptoms, additional laboratory tests will be conducted to diagnose SLE. Diagnosis of SLE can be difficult, and it may take some time to associate various symptoms of the past with newer symptoms in the present. There is no cure for SLE, but early treatment of symptoms is important for long-term management of this highly individualized disease. Treatment for SLE is symptom based, and the prognosis for women who follow treatment protocol is excellent.

Prevention of Flare-Ups Preventive measures are equally important, including avoidance of excessive sun exposure, use of sunscreens, regular exercise, stress management, no smoking, limited or no alcohol consumption, proper use of prescribed medications, prompt treatment of infections, and maintaining proper nutrition. Support from family and friends can help alleviate the effects of stress, especially when dealing with the unpredictable aspects of the disease.

Pregnancy and Lupus Health care providers suggest that women considering pregnancy try to time the pregnancy for a period when the disease is least active. For some women, the first symptoms of lupus may appear during pregnancy, and for others, they may occur immediately after childbirth. Careful monitoring is necessary to minimize harmful effects on the expectant mother or her fetus.

Fibromyalgia

Fibromyalgia is a common and chronic musculoskeletal syndrome characterized by fatigue; widespread pain in the muscles, ligaments, and tendons; and multiple "tender points" on the body where there is increased sensitivity to touch or slight pressure. Fibromyalgia is considered a rheumatic condition, but unlike arthritis, it does not cause inflammation or damage to the joints. The American College of Rheumatology (ACR) states that fibromyalgia affects 3 to 6 million Americans with 80 to 90 percent being women. Fibromyalgia is generally diagnosed during middle age (between ages 30 and 50), but the symptoms may exist much earlier. (See *FYI:* "Common Signs and Symptoms of Fibromyalgia.")

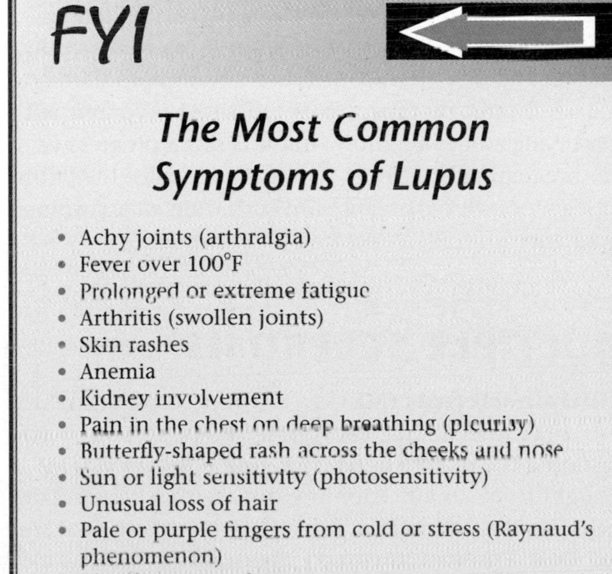

FYI

The Most Common Symptoms of Lupus

- Achy joints (arthralgia)
- Fever over 100°F
- Prolonged or extreme fatigue
- Arthritis (swollen joints)
- Skin rashes
- Anemia
- Kidney involvement
- Pain in the chest on deep breathing (pleurisy)
- Butterfly-shaped rash across the cheeks and nose
- Sun or light sensitivity (photosensitivity)
- Unusual loss of hair
- Pale or purple fingers from cold or stress (Raynaud's phenomenon)
- Mouth or nose ulcers
- Seizures
- Abnormal blood clotting problems

Common Signs and Symptoms of Fibromyalgia[80]

- Widespread muscle pain
- "Tender points" which are sensitive to touch or slight pressure
- Fatigue (mild to incapacitating)
- Sleep disturbance
- Chronic headaches
- Irritable bowel syndrome (IBS)
- Painful menstrual periods
- Numbness or tingling of the arms or legs
- Restless legs syndrome
- Temperature sensitivity (especially to cold)
- Cognitive or memory impairments ("fibro fog")
- Jaw-related facial and head pain (TMJ)
- Morning stiffness
- Sensitivity to odors, loud noises, or bright lights
- Muscle twitching
- Irritable bladder

FIGURE 15.1 The location of the eighteen tender points that comprise the criteria for fibromyalgia.

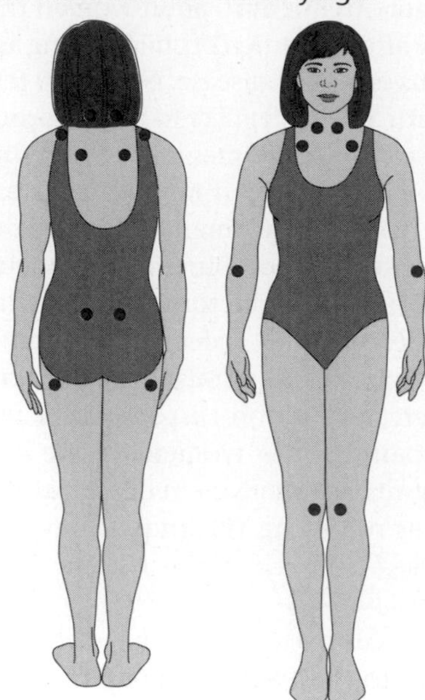

SOURCE: National Institute of Arthritis and Musculoskeletal and Skin Diseases, National Institutes of Health, Department of Health and Human Services. www.niams.nih.gov/hi/topics/fibromyalgia/fibrofs.htm (retrieved August 10, 2006).

The cause of fibromyalgia continues to be debated and researched. The multiple precipitating factors may include traumatic physical or emotional events, repetitive injuries, illnesses such as HIV infection, Lyme disease, or flu-like viral infection. Hereditary and environmental causes are being studied.[81] Women with certain rheumatic diseases such as rheumatoid arthritis (RA), lupus (SLE), and ankylosing spondylitis (spinal arthritis) have a greater likelihood of developing fibromyalgia.[82]

Fibromyalgia is difficult to diagnose because the main symptoms of pain and fatigue overlap with numerous other conditions. Diagnostic laboratory tests are unavailable for diagnosing the condition, so other potential causes must be ruled out prior to making a diagnosis of fibromyalgia. The ACR has set specific criteria for establishing a diagnosis, including eleven of eighteen designated "tender points" located on the body. (See Figure 15.1.)

Symptom-specific medications such as sleep medications, muscle relaxants, headache remedies, pain medications, and anti-inflammatory drugs may be used to treat the symptoms of fibromyalgia based on the woman's presenting complaints. Antidepressants that increase brain chemicals including serotonin and norepinephrine are the most useful in treating symptoms by modulating sleep, pain, and immune system function.[83]

Women with fibromyalgia may also benefit by reducing stressors in their lives and getting deep-level (stage 4) sleep at night. Practical suggestions for enhancing quality of sleep can be found in numerous publications. Women can learn to balance daily activities with rest periods; eat more healthy foods; avoid or limit alcohol and caffeine intake; exercise to improve muscular strength, flexibility, and aerobic endurance; and seek external support to deal with depression, anxiety, and stress. Changes in weather, cold or drafty environments, as well as infections and allergies, can contribute to symptom flare-ups, so care should be taken to avoid them. Women with fibromyalgia need to know that it is not a progressive or life-threatening condition. It does not damage the joints, muscles, or internal organs, and with time, many women experience improvements in their condition.

MULTIPLE SCLEROSIS

Multiple sclerosis (MS) is a chronic, debilitating disease that affects the central nervous system (CNS) including the brain, spinal cord, and optic nerves. MS is thought to be an autoimmune disease that causes damage to and loss of myelin, the fatty white tissue that surrounds and protects the nerve fibers of the CNS and aids in the smooth conduction of electrical impulses. This injury and loss, called demyelination, results in areas known as plaques and scar tissue (sclerosis) that disrupt the normal conduction of electrical impulses causing the various symptoms of MS. The exact cause of this disease is still unknown, but it is believed that there is an abnormal response of the body's immune system that causes it to attack its own myelin. The autoimmune response in MS is believed to be triggered by multiple factors including genetics, gender, and environment. Some possible environmental triggers being studied are trauma, viruses, and heavy metals (toxins). Although there is no evidence that MS is inherited, genetic factors may make certain people more susceptible to MS. The prevalence of MS is higher among persons who live in certain geographic regions farther from the equator that have cold, damp climates, particularly areas that are 40 degrees north in latitude.

The onset or diagnosis of MS is usually between the ages of 20 and 50 years and is two to three times higher in women than in men. MS is a leading cause of neurologic disability in early adulthood and is found more commonly in non-Hispanic whites and people of northern European ancestry. The National Multiple Sclerosis Society estimates that approximately 400,000 Americans have MS and 200 more people are being diagnosed weekly.[84] Studies have demonstrated high rates among identical twins. If one identical twin develops MS, the other twin has a one in three chance of developing the disease.[85]

Health Tips

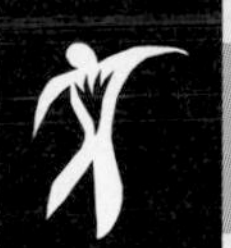

Possible Symptoms of Multiple Sclerosis[87]

- Gait (walking) disturbances
- Muscle weakness
- Spasticity and muscle rigidity
- Impairment of pain, temperature, and touch senses
- Pain (moderate to severe)
- Tremor
- Speech and swallowing disorders
- Vision disturbances (blurred or double vision, blindness in one eye, or green-red color distortion)
- Vertigo and dizziness
- Bladder, bowel, or sexual dysfunction
- Depression or emotional problems
- Cognitive abnormalities
- Headaches
- Fatigue
- Hearing loss
- Itching
- Numbness
- Seizures

Signs and Symptoms

Precipitating events such as infection, trauma, or pregnancy can bring on or exacerbate the symptoms of MS. Symptoms of MS are unpredictable and depend on the site(s) of demyelination in the CNS. Symptoms vary from person to person and can even vary within the same person. (See *Health Tips:* "Possible Symptoms of Multiple Sclerosis.")

The symptoms can be mild to severe, long or short in duration, and may appear in various combinations. Symptoms can worsen when women with MS are exposed to higher temperatures whether inside or outside the body. Environments or activities that raise a woman's core body temperature by one-quarter degree can cause to one-half temporary aggravation of MS symptoms.[86] The initial symptom of MS is often a visual disturbance that, inexplicably, has a tendency to clear up in the later stages of MS. Most people with MS experience muscle weakness of the extremities with impaired coordination and balance at some time during their lives. Nearly 50 percent of women with MS will have cognitive impairments of which they will not be aware. Cognitive disturbances may include problems with attention, concentration, memory, and good judgment. Cognitive impairments usually are mild and sometimes remain unnoticed. Although depression is a common symptom, other emotional changes can be experienced that cause a person with MS to have inappropriate emotional reactions or facial expressions such as the "laughing/weeping syndrome."

There are four major clinical courses that multiple sclerosis may follow.[88] Each form may vary from mild to moderate to severe. The relapsing-remitting form of MS is the most common (85 percent) and consists of clearly defined flare-ups of symptoms followed by partial or complete recovery periods. The primary-progressive form is a slow but nearly continuous worsening of the disease from the onset with no distinct relapses or remissions. A woman may experience varying rates of progression and temporary improvements. The secondary-progressive form includes an initial period of relapsing-remitting disease followed by a steady decline with or without flare-ups. Most persons with relapsing-remitting MS experience this form within 10 years of the initial diagnosis, but new drug therapies have slowed this tendency. The progressive-relapsing form is rare (5 percent) and includes flare-ups but does not have the recovery component. The disease progression is continuous. Twenty percent of the MS population has a benign form of the disease and shows little or no progression after the initial attack. MS is rarely fatal, and most individuals will have a normal life expectancy. Ongoing studies may lead to a redefinition of the course of this disease.

Diagnosis and Treatment

Overall, diagnosing MS by the presenting symptoms is difficult because of the unpredictable and varying nature of the disease. Many women endure years of tests before an accurate diagnosis is made. A diagnosis is made by reviewing a woman's history of symptoms, performing multiple tests and procedures, and evaluating the functioning of her present nervous system (e.g. reflexes and coordination). Diagnostic tests include magnetic resonance imaging (MRI), evoked potential tests, and a spinal tap. The MRI scan gives a more detailed view of the CNS, but other tests are needed for confirmation of MS. In addition, an injection of a contrast agent known as gadolinium can be given before the scan to help distinguish newer lesions from older ones. Evoked potential tests measure the speed and accuracy of a woman's nervous system in response to certain stimuli. A spinal tap allows for the observation and testing of the cerebrospinal fluid (CSF) for indicators of MS and for distinction from other diseases. A final confirmation of MS requires that a woman have signs of MS in different parts of the nervous system and two separate flare-up episodes (relapses).

There is no cure for MS, but fortunately many women with the disease do not need any treatment. The aim of treatment is to enhance quality of life by addressing the symptoms and improving functionality. Exercise has numerous benefits including better cardiovascular endurance, increased muscular strength and endurance, an enhanced mental outlook and participation in social activities, and better bladder and bowel control. Steroids, which have anti-inflammatory properties, can be used to reduce the duration and intensity of a flare-up, particularly in women with motor or movement symptoms. However, steroids have a multitude of side effects, so they usually are not recommended for long-term use. Newer treatments are being developed and studied. Different forms of naturally occurring antiviral proteins known as interferon are being used to treat MS. Beta-interferon injections have decreased the number of flare-ups and seem to slow the occurrence of physical disability. These medications also can have serious side effects. Immunosuppressive therapies are being used to inhibit the autoimmune nature of MS. The risk of this treatment is that it compromises the body's natural ability to fight off infection. Cost and side effects are the major issues that must be weighed by the health care provider and the person with MS.[89]

Pregnancy and MS

A woman's ability to become pregnant is not affected by MS, and the course of pregnancy, labor, and delivery is not adversely affected by MS. The symptoms of MS often remit or stabilize during pregnancy. This is thought to be related to normal changes in a pregnant woman's immune system that allow her to carry a fetus that is in essence partially foreign tissue to her since the fetus carries genes from the father. The downside to this temporary reprieve is that 20 to 40 percent of women with MS have a relapse within 3 months following delivery. A woman with MS who is considering becoming pregnant should also consider the potential side effects of MS drugs on the fetus and the physical limitations that may make it difficult to carry a fetus to term.

Support System

Multiple sclerosis can affect the entire family or immediate support network of a woman with MS. The financial, physical, and emotional stresses of MS may require support groups and possible counseling to assist a woman and her support network in coping with the disease.

ALZHEIMER'S DISEASE

Alzheimer's disease (AD), the most common form of dementia, causes a gradual, progressive loss of brain cells that eventually leads to death if death does not occur from another cause first (often from bronchiopneumonia). It is characterized by confusion, progressive memory loss, behavioral disturbances, loss of language skills, and decline in the ability to perform routine tasks. Alzheimer's affects the brain cells that control memory and cognitive thinking skills first and then progresses to other regions of the brain. AD advances at different rates and may last 3 to 20 years. The average life span is 8 to 10 years after diagnosis.

The exact cause of AD is unknown. A protein called apolipoprotein (apoE) is being investigated for its relationship to Alzheimer's disease. ApoE is a normal component in the body that helps carry cholesterol in the blood. The apoE gene has three forms, one of which seems to increase the likelihood of a person developing AD. Scientists know that AD involves the malfunction or death of nerve cells and believe the triggers begin damaging the brain years before symptoms appear. Abnormal brain tissue associated with AD, including "plaques" and "tangles" as markers of the disease, is being studied to determine the actual cause of death to the brain cells. Amyloid plaques are the clumped protein fragments that are found outside the AD brain cells, and neurofibrillary tangles are the clumped proteins found inside the cells.[90]

Increasing age is the leading risk for developing AD, with as many as 10 percent of all people 65 years and older having AD. Approximately half of all people 85

Health Tips 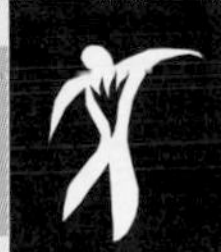

Ten Warning Signs to Recognize AD

- Memory loss that affects job performance and daily living
- Difficulty performing familiar tasks
- Problems with language such as forgetting simple words or using words inappropriately
- Time and space disorientation
- Poor judgment
- Problems with abstract thinking
- Misplacing items
- Changes in mood or behavior; rapid mood swings
- Changes in personality
- Loss of initiative

and older will have AD, but AD is not considered a normal part of aging. Having a parent or sibling with AD is another risk factor that increases a woman's risk of developing the disease. More familial AD means a higher risk for other family members. Researchers have strong evidence that high cholesterol, high blood pressure, and vascular disease elevate the risk of AD. The heart–head connection is important to recognize when looking at risks that might be controlled by diet, exercise, and maintaining good health behaviors. AD is a costly disease affecting nearly 4.5 million Americans, a doubling in cases since 1980. It is the eighth leading cause of death in America and kills nearly 55,000 people yearly.[91]

Signs and Symptoms

A key component of AD is memory loss, exhibited by forgetfulness. Actions such as missed appointments, unreturned telephone calls, trouble finding the right word, and difficulty understanding conversation may be signs to watch. Failing to recognize people, getting lost while alone, relinquishing important responsibilities (such as paying the bills), or reducing social circles may also be signs. The Alzheimer's Disease Association provides a list of ten warning signs to recognize AD.[92] (See *Health Tips:* "Ten Warning Signs to Recognize AD.")

Diagnosis

An early diagnosis is important for the person with AD and her family so that they can plan for the future and initiate early treatment of symptoms. Although a definitive diagnosis cannot be made until an autopsy of the brain tissue reveals the plaques and tangles, a diagnosis of "probable" or "possible" AD can be made with about 90 percent accuracy. A complete medical history is required to review past and present medical conditions as well as testing to determine current mental and physical functioning. A diagnosis is made after ruling out other potential causes through mental status evaluation, physical examination, neurological exams, laboratory tests, psychiatric and psychological evaluation, and various brain scans.

Treatment

No treatments can stop the progressive loss of brain cells in AD, but current drug treatments can help minimize or stabilize the symptoms for a period of time. Three medications known as cholinesterase inhibitors are commonly prescribed for the early treatment of AD (Aricept, Exelon, and Reminyl). They are designed to inhibit the breakdown of acetylcholine in the brain. Acetylcholine is a chemical messenger that is important for memory and other cognitive skills. Cholinesterase inhibitors keep the levels of acetylcholine high, helping to maintain cognitive functioning or improve cognitive symptoms. Memantine, a receptor antagonist, is now prescribed for moderate to severe AD. It appears to regulate the activity of glutamate, a chemical messenger that helps with learning and memory. Other medications may be necessary to help control behavioral symptoms such as agitation, wandering, depression, sleeplessness, and anxiety. Other substances, such as vitamin E, antidepressants, antianxiety medications, and antipsychotics, are being studied to determine their efficacy in slowing the progression of AD or to treat behavioral and psychiatric symptoms. Any supplement or medication used by an individual with AD should be discussed with a health care provider. For instance, vitamin E may not be recommended for persons taking "blood thinners."

Nondrug therapies include providing the AD patient with a stable and familiar environment. During the mild to moderate stages of AD, the family should encourage the person with AD to function independently, and the daily routine should become familiar. A consistent schedule for daily activities reduces agitation, and safety can be enhanced by placing locks on doors. Collecting and sharing personal items helps to stimulate the memory of persons with AD. Nursing homes that accept persons with AD often provide alarms and codes to secure doors, visual pictures for communicating and stimulating memory, and measures to prevent wandering.[93]

Role of Caregiver

AD seriously impacts caregivers as well as persons with AD. Caregivers suffer from anxiety, depression, and anger. They can receive needed assistance by joining a support group. These support groups offer emotional support and current information about additional home health services, the behavior of persons with AD, and help in nursing home placement. Recent studies suggest that a person with AD can remain at home nearly a year longer if caregivers have a support system that offers emotional and informational support. Most urban areas provide support groups for caregivers, and the national office of the Alzheimer's Association provides information regarding the location of your local chapter.

Now complete *Journal Activity:* "Your Family Tree and Chronic Disease."

Journal Activity

Your Family Tree and Chronic Disease

Now that you have finished this chapter, create a family tree that includes siblings, parents, grandparents, and great-grandparents. Under each name, include the diseases or conditions that each person has or had. Select one disease or condition and write all the protective factors that you can practice to reduce your risk of contracting this disease.

Chapter Summary

- More women die from cardiovascular disease than any other disease.
- African American women are at greater risk than white women for coronary artery disease.
- Atherosclerosis is a gradual process of artery breakdown that causes plaque to accumulate and form occlusions.
- Heart attacks are more lethal for women than men.
- High blood pressure is defined as a systolic pressure of 140 mm Hg and/or diastolic pressure of 90 mm Hg and/or taking antihypertensive medication.
- Stroke is the third leading cause of death and the leading cause of disability in women.
- Osteoporosis is a bone-weakening disorder causing bone mineral loss that can result in skeletal frailty and fractures.
- African American women compared to white women are 50 percent more likely to develop type 2 diabetes.
- The best way to overcome the stigma of epilepsy is by educating the public.
- Arthritis, an inflammatory condition of the joints, is the leading cause of work-related disability.
- Systemic lupus erythematosus affects primarily women of childbearing age.
- Multiple sclerosis affects primarily young white women, often between the ages of 30 and 40.
- Alzheimer's disease is the most common dementia, and a key component is memory loss.

Review Questions

1. What is the leading cause of death in women?
2. What is atherosclerosis?
3. What are the signs and symptoms of angina?
4. What is the difference between a heart attack and congestive heart failure?
5. What are the primary risk and protective factors for heart disease?
6. How can hypertension be controlled?
7. What are the warning signs of stroke? type 2 diabetes? arthritis?
8. What are the risk and protective factors for osteoporosis?
9. What causes lupus? multiple sclerosis? Alzheimer's disease?
10. What can you do to protect yourself against chronic conditions?

Resources

Organizations and Hotlines

Alzheimer's Association (National Office)
225 N. Michigan Avenue, Floor 17
Chicago, IL 60601
800-272-3900
www.alz.org

American Diabetes Association
ATTN: National Call Center
1701 North Beauregard Street
Alexandria, VA 22311
800-DIABETES (800-342-2383)
www.diabetes.org

American Heart Association
National Center
7272 Greenville Avenue
Dallas, TX 75231

800-AHA-USA (800-242-8721)
www.americanheart.org

American Stroke Association
(A division of the American Heart Association)
National Center
7272 Greenville Avenue
Dallas, TX 75231
888-4-STROKE (888-478-7653)
www.strokeassociation.org

Epilepsy Foundation
4351 Garden City Drive
Landover, MD 20785-7223
800-332-1000
www.efa.org

The Lupus Foundation of America, Inc.
2000 L Street N.W., Suite 710
Washington, DC 20036
202-349-1155
www.lupus.org

Multiple Sclerosis Foundation
6350 North Andrews Avenue
Fort Lauderdale, FL 33309-2130
800-225-6495
www.msfacts.org

National Heart, Lung, and Blood Institute
P.O. Box 30105
Bethesda, MD 20824-0105
301-592-8573
www.nhlbi.nih.gov

National Multiple Sclerosis Society
733 Third Avenue
New York, NY 10017
www.nationalmssociety.org

National Osteoporosis Foundation
1232 22nd Street N.W.
Washington, DC 20037-1292
202-223-2226
www.nof.org

National Stroke Association
9707 E. Easter Lane
Englewood, CO 80112
800-STROKES (800-787-6537)
www.stroke.org

Related Diseases Association, Inc.
(information on women and autoimmune diseases)
15475 Gratoit Avenue
Detroit, MI 48205
313-371-8600
www.aarda.org/women.html

Web Sites

American Lung Association
www.lungusa.org

Centers for Disease Control and Prevention (CDC)
www.cdc.gov

Diabetes Public Health Resource (CDC)
www.cdc.gov/diabetes

Fibromyalgia Network
www.fmnetnews.com

March of Dimes
www.marchofdimes.com

National Fibromyalgia Association
www.fmaware.org

National Institute of Arthritis and Musculoskeletal and Skin Diseases (NIAMS)
www.niams.nih.gov

National Institutes of Health
Osteoporosis and Related Bone Diseases
National Resource Center
www.osteo.org

WISEWOMAN (a CDC initiative)
(**W**ell-**I**ntegrated **S**creening and **E**valuation for **Wom**en **A**cross the **N**ation)
www.cdc.gov/wisewoman

Suggested Readings

Bohme, K., and F. Budden. 2001. *The Silent Thief: Osteoporosis, Exercises and Strategies for Prevention and Treatment.* Westport, CT: Firefly Books.

Gersh, B. J. 2000. *Mayo Clinic Heart Book.* New York: HarperCollins.

Greenberger, P., and J. Wider, eds. 2006. *The Savvy Woman Patient: How and Why Sex Differences Affect Your Health.* Society for Women's Health Research. Herndon, VA: Capital Books.

Hankinson, S. E., F. Speizer, G. A. Colditz, and J. E. Manson, eds. 2002. *Healthy Women, Healthy Lives: A Guide to Preventing Disease from the Landmark Nurses' Health Study.* New York: Simon & Schuster.

Lagato, M. J. 2002. *Eve's Rib: The Groundbreaking Guide to Women's Health.* New York: Three Rivers Press, Random House.

Morrell, M. J., and K. L. Flynn, eds. 2002. *Women with Epilepsy: A Handbook of Health and Treatment Issues.* New York: Cambridge University Press.

Nelson, M. E. 2001. *Strong Women, Strong Bones: Everything You Need to Know to Prevent, Treat, and Beat Osteoporosis.* New York: Perigee.

Von Der Lohe, E. 2003. *Coronary Heart Disease in Women: Prevention, Diagnosis, and Therapy.* New York: Springer-Verlag.

References

1. Statistical highlights. 2006. *Heart disease and stroke statistics—2005 update.* Dallas, TX: American Heart Association.
2. American Heart Association. 2006. *Women and cardiovascular diseases—statistics.* www.americanheart.org/downloadable/heart/1136818052118Females06.pdf (retrieved September 25, 2006).
3. National Library of Medicine. 2004. *Developmental process of atherosclerosis.* www.nlm.nih.gov/medlineplus/ency/imagepages/18020.htm (retrieved September 25, 2006); American Heart Association. 2003. *Atherosclerosis: A major cause of cardiovascular disease.* www.americanheart.org/downloadable/heart/1056719919740HSfacts2003text.pdf (retrieved February 6, 2006).

4. Cody, R. J., C. R. Conti, and P. Samet. 1993. Managing angina and concomitant disease. *Patient Care* 27:45–72.
5. American Heart Association. 2003. *Angina pectoris and heart attack*. www.americanheart.org/downloadable/heart/1056719919740HSfacts2003text.pdf (retrieved February 6, 2006).
6. Department of Health and Human Services, Office of Women's Health. 2002. *Women: Warning! It could be a heart attack!* www.womenshealth.gov/owh/pub/factsheets/heartattack.htm (retrieved September 25, 2006).
7. Ibid.
8. National Heart, Lung, and Blood Institute. 2005. *Congenital heart defects*. www.nhlbi.nih.gov/health/dci/Diseases/chd/chd summary.html (retrieved September 25, 2006).
9. American Heart Association. 2006. *Heart disease and stroke statistics—2006 update*. www.americanheart.org/downloadable/heart/1136308648540StatUpdate2006.pdf (retrieved February 6, 2006).
10. American Heart Association. 2002. *Genetic counseling for adults with congenital heart disease*. www.americanheart.org/presenter.jhtml?identifier_11083 (retrieved October 17, 2002).
11. National Heart, Lung, and Blood Institute. 2005. *Living with congenital heart defects*. www.nhlbi.nih.gov/health/dci/Diseases/chd/chd_living.html (retrieved September 25, 2006).
12. American Heart Association. 2005. *Arrhythmias originating in the atria*. www.americanheart.org/presenter. jhtml?identifier=10 (retrieved September 25, 2006).
13. Ibid.
14. Wood, M. A., and K. A. Ellenbogen. 2002. Cardiac pacemakers from the patient's perspective. *Circulation* 105:2136.
15. American Heart Association. 2003. *Heart and stroke facts*. www.americanheart.org/downloadable/heart/1056719919740HSFacts2003text.pdf (retrieved September 25, 2006).
16. Legato, M. J. 2002. *Eve's rib: The groundbreaking guide to women's health*. New York: Three Rivers Press, Random House.
17. American Heart Association. 2006. *Metabolic syndrome: Heart disease and stroke statistics—2006 update*. www.americanheart.org/downloadable/heart/1136308648540StatUpdate2006.pdf (retrieved September 25, 2006).
18. American Heart Association. 2005. *Heart disease and stroke statistics—2006 update*. http://circ.ahajournals.org/cgi/content/short/113/6/e8 (retrieved September 25, 2006).
19. American Heart Association, *Heart and stroke facts*.
20. National Heart, Lung, and Blood Institute. 2005. *Pregnancy*. www.nhlbi.nih.gov/issues/preg/preg.htm (retrieved September 25, 2006).
21. American Heart Association. 2005. *What are healthy levels of cholesterol?* www.americanheart.org/presenter.jhtml?identifier=183 (retrieved September 25, 2006); American Heart Association, 2005. *What's the difference between LDL and HDL cholesterol?* www.americanheart.org/presenter.jhtml?identifier=180 (retrieved September 25, 2006).
22. American Heart Association, *What are healthy levels of cholesterol?*
23. Gotto, A. M. 2002. Statins: Powerful drugs for lowering cholesterol. *Circulation* 105:1514.
24. American Heart Association, *Heart disease and stroke statistics—2006 update;* U.S. Department of Agriculture and U.S. Department of Health and Human Services. 2005. *Dietary guidelines for Americans 2005*. www.health.gov/dietaryguidelines/dga2005/document/html/chapter1.htm (retrieved September 25, 2006).
25. National Center for Health Statistics. 2002. National Health and Nutrition Examination Survey. Health. United States (Table 70). www.cdc.gov/nchs (retrieved September 25, 2006).
26. U.S. Department of Agriculture and U.S. Department of Health and Human Services, *Dietary guidelines for Americans 2005*.
27. Mosca, L. 2004. Heart disease prevention in women. *Circulation* 109:158–60.
28. American Heart Association. 2002. *Women, heart disease and stroke*. www.americanheart.org/presenter.jhtml?identifier_4786 (retrieved September 26, 2002).
29. American Heart Association. 2005. *Diabetes and Cardiovascular disease*. www.s2mw.com/heartofdiabetes/cardio.html (retrieved September 25, 2006).
30. American Heart Association, *What are healthy levels of cholesterol?*
31. Eaker, E. D., J. Pinsky, and W. P. Castelli. 1992. Myocardial infarction and coronary death among women: Psychosocial predictors from a 20-year follow-up of women in the Framingham Study. *American Journal of Epidemiology* 135:854–64.
32. Young, R. F., and E. Kahana. 1993. Gender, recovery from late life heart attack and medical care. *Women & Health* 20:11–31; Eysmann, S. B., and P. S. Douglas. 1992. Reperfusion and revascularization strategies for coronary artery disease in women. *Journal of the American Medical Association* 268:1903–7.
33. Mark, D. B., L. K. Shaw, et al. 1994. Absence of sex bias in the referral of patients for cardiac catheterization. *New England Journal of Medicine* 330:1101; Fiebach, N. H., C. M. Viscoli, and R. I. Horwitz. 1990. Differences between women and men in survival after myocardial infarction. *Journal of the American Medical Association* 263:1092–96.
34. Eysmann and Douglas, Reperfusion and revascularization strategies for coronary artery disease in women.
35. American Heart Association. 2006. *Heart disease and stroke facts—2006 Update*. www.americanheart.org/presenter.jhtml?identifier=4786 (retrieved October 4, 2006).
36. National Stroke Association. 2005. *Unique symptoms in women*. http://info.stroke.org/site/PageServer?pagename=WOMSYMP (retrieved September 25, 2006).
37. American Heart Association, *Heart disease and stroke facts—2006 Update*.
38. American Heart Association, *Heart disease and stroke facts—2006 Update*.
39. Kawachi, I., G. A. Colditz, M. J. Stampfer, et al. 1993. Smoking cessation and decreased risk of stroke in women. *Journal of the American Medical Association* 269:232–36.
40. Writing Group for the Women's Health Initiative Investigators. 2002. Risks and benefits of estrogen plus progestin in healthy postmenopausal women: Principal

results from the Women's Health Initiative randomized control study. *Journal of the American Medical Association* 288:321–33.

41. McBean, L. D., T. Forgac, and S. C. Finn. 1994. Osteoporosis: Visions for care and prevention—A conference report. *Journal of the American Dietetic Association* 94:668–71.
42. National Osteoporosis Foundation. 2005. *Disease facts.* www.nof.org/osteoporosis/disease facts.htm (retrieved January 15, 2006).
43. Jewish Women's Archive. *JWA–Lillian Wald–Henry Street Settlement.* www.jwa.org/exhibits/wov/wald/1w4.html (retrieved March 9, 2006); Krain, Jacob B. Lillian Wald. www.jewishmag.com/51/mag/wald/lillianwald.htm (retrieved March 9, 2006); Did You Know? *Did you know that Lillian Wald founded the Henry Street Settlement in 1893?* www.lowermanhattan.info/about/history/did-you-know/lillian_ward_henry_52706.asp (retrieved September 25, 2006).
44. National Osteoporosis Foundation, *Disease facts.*
45. Wolman R. L. 1994. Osteoporosis and exercise. *British Medical Journal* 309:400–3.
46. Ibid.
47. Rigotti, N. A., R. M. Neer, et al. 1991. The clinical course of osteoporosis in anorexia nervosa: A longitudinal study of cortical bone mass. *Journal of the American Medical Association* 265:1133–38.
48. Carr, B. R., B. Dawson-Hughes, and B. Ettinger. 1993. A real-world approach to osteoporosis. *Patient Care* 27:31.
49. Hollenbach, K. A., E. Barrett-Conner, et al. 1993. Cigarette smoking and bone mineral density in older men and women. *American Journal of Public Health* 83:1265.
50. International Osteoporosis Foundation. 2005. *Diagnosing osteoporosis.* www.osteofound.org/osteoporosis/diagnosis.html (retrieved September 25, 2006).
51. Wolman, Osteoporosis and exercise.
52. National Osteoporosis Foundation. 2002. *Recommended calcium intakes.* www.nof.org/prevention/calcium.htm (retrieved September 25, 2006).
53. International Osteoporosis Foundation. 2006. *Treatment of osteoporosis.* www.osteofound.org/osteoporosis/treatment.html (retrieved September 25, 2006).
54. Centers for Disease Control and Prevention. 2005. *National diabetes fact sheet, United States, 2005.* www.cdc.gov/diabetes/pubs/factsheet05.htm (retrieved September 25, 2006).
55. Centers for Disease Control and Prevention. 2005. *FAQs—Basics about diabetes.* www.cdc.gov/diabetes/faq/basics.htm (retrieved September 25, 2006).
56. Rimm, E. B., J. E. Manson, M. J. Stampfer, et al. 1993. Cigarette smoking and the risk of diabetes in women. *American Journal of Public Health* 83.211–14.
57. Centers for Disease Control and Prevention, *National diabetes fact sheet, United States, 2005.*
58. U.S. Food and Drug Administration. 2002. *Women and diabetes, take time to care about diabetes.* www.fda.gov/womens/taketimetocare/diabetes/fswomen.html (retrieved September 25, 2006).
59. Asthma and Allergy Foundation of America. *Asthma facts and figures.* www.aafa.org/display.cfm?id=8&sub=42#fast (retrieved September 25, 2006).
60. Ibid.
61. Ibid.
62. Ibid.
63. Centers for Disease Control and Prevention. *Asthma prevalence, health care use and mortality, 2002.* www.cdc.gov (retrieved September 25, 2006).
64. Asthma and Allergy Foundation of America, *Asthma facts and figures.*
65. U.S. Department of Health and Human Services. *Managing asthma during pregnancy: Recommendations for pharmacologic treatment (update 2004).* National Asthma Education and Prevention Program. www.nhlbi.nih.gov/health/prof/lung/asthma/astpreg.htm (retrieved September 25, 2006).
66. Ibid.
67. Department of Health and Human Services, Centers for Disease Control and Prevention 2005. *Third national report on exposure to environmental chemicals.* NCEH Publication No. 05-0570.
68. Asthma and Allergy Foundation of America, *Asthma facts and figures.*
69. Ibid.
70. Epilepsy Foundation of America. 2001–2005. *Women and epilepsy.* www.efa.org/answerplace/Life/adults/women/index.cfm (retrieved September 25, 2006).
71. Ibid.
72. Epilepsy Foundation of America. 2001–2005. *Health issues after your baby is born.* www.efa.org/answerplace/Life/adults/women/weiborn.cfm (retrieved January 14, 2006).
73. Ibid.
74. Arthritis Foundation. 2005. *The facts about arthritis.* www.arthritis.org/resources/gettingstarted/default.asp (retrieved January 26, 2006).
75. Arthritis Foundation. 2005. *AF Store: Start reading now.* www.arthritis.org/AFStore/StartRead.asp?idProduct=3328 (retrieved January 26, 2006); American College of Rheumatology. 2005. *Lose the gain, lessen the pain.* www.rheumatology.org/press/2005/bartlett.asp (retrieved January 26, 2006).
76. Laino, C. 1994. Rheumatoid arthritis: Rather than waiting months for a response to NSAIDs, rheumatologists are embracing an early, more aggressive use of second-line therapies at the first sign of clinical or functional deterioration. *Medical World News* 35:28–33.
77. Lupus Foundation of America, Inc. 2001. *Statistics about lupus.* www.lupus.org/education/stats.html (retrieved January 4, 2006).
78. Lupus Foundation of America, Inc. 2006. *Symptoms of lupus.* www.lupus.org/education/sympt.html (retrieved January 4, 2006).
79. American College of Rheumatology. 2006. *Patient education—systemic lupus erythematosus.* www.rheumatology.org/public/factsheets/sle_new.asp?aud=pat (retrieved January 4, 2006).
80. National Institute of Arthritis and Musculoskeletal and Skin Diseases, National Institutes of Health. *Questions and answers about fibromyalgia.* www.niams.nih.gov/hi/topics/fibromyalgia/fibrofs.htm (retrieved September 25, 2006); McCance, K. L., and S. E. Huether. 2006. *Pathophysiology: The biologic basis for disease in adults and children.* 5th ed. St. Louis: Mosby; Fibromyalgia Network. 2006.

Fibromyalgia basics: Symptoms, treatments and research. www.fmnetnews.com/pages/basics.html (retrieved September 25, 2006).

81. McCance and Huether, *Pathophysiology.*
82. National Institute of Arthritis and Musculoskeletal and Skin Diseases, National Institutes of Health, *Questions and answers about fibromyalgia.*
83. Fibromyalgia Network, *Fibromyalgia basics.*
84. National Multiple Sclerosis Society. 2005. *Who gets MS?* www.nationalmssociety.org/Who%20gets%20MS.asp (retrieved January 19, 2006).
85. National Multiple Sclerosis Society. 2003. *Sourcebook: Genetics.* www.nationalmssociety.org/Sourcebook-Genetics.asp (retrieved September 26, 2006).
86. National Multiple Sclerosis Society. 2003. *Sourcebook: Heat/temperature sensitivity.* www.nationalmssociety.org/sourcebook-Heat.asp (retrieved September 26, 2006); National Multiple Sclerosis Society. 2003. *Sourcebook: Exacerbation.* www.nationalmssociety.org/Sourcebook-Exacerbation.asp (retrieved September 26, 2006).
87. National Multiple Sclerosis Society. 2005. *Symptoms and symptom management.* www.nationalmssociety.org/Symptoms.asp (retrieved September 26, 2006).
88. National Multiple Sclerosis Society. 2005. *What is multiple sclerosis?* www.nationalmssociety.org/What%20is%20MS.asp (retrieved September 26, 2006).
89. National Multiple Sclerosis Society. 2005. *Treatments.* www.nationalmssociety.org/Treatments.asp (retrieved September 26, 2006).
90. Alzheimer's Foundation. 2002. *Causes and risk factors.* www.alz.org/AboutAD/causes.htm (retrieved September 26, 2006).
91. Deaths and percentage of total deaths for the 10 leading causes of death, by race: United States, 2002. March 7, 2005. *National Vital Statistics Reports* 53 (17).
92. Alzheimer's Foundation. 2005. *Ten warning signs of Alzheimer's Disease.* www.alz.org/AboutAD/Warning.asp (retrieved September 26, 2006).
93. Bloom, A., and A. Rulnick. 1994. AAHSA survey highlights similarities, variations in special care programs. *Brown University Long-Term Care Quality Letter* 6:1.

Reducing Your Risk of Cancer

Chapter Sixteen

CHAPTER OBJECTIVES

When you complete this chapter, you will be able to do the following:

- Identify the seven warning signs of cancer
- Describe the classifications of cancers
- Explain possible lifestyle and genetic causes of cancer
- Identify the risk and protective factors for each cancer
- Identify the primary cancers based on incidence and mortality
- Compare and contrast medical and complementary treatment options
- Explain the importance of social support in recovery from cancer

THE BIG "C"

One in three women today can expect to have cancer in her lifetime, and nearly 50 percent of these cases involve the female reproductive system. Many women will someday hear the words, "Your Pap smear was positive; we need to do further tests," or "You have a lump in your breast; we need to schedule a biopsy." Despite reassurance from the health care provider that there is no cause for concern at this time, a woman would probably experience a myriad of feelings. Two common reactions might be (1) to assume the worst, "It's CANCER and I'm going to die," or (2) to deny it, "There can't be anything wrong with me." The word "cancer" is so stigmatized that it evokes strong emotions.

This chapter provides information on the nature and sites of the most common cancers found in women, offers guidelines for early detection, suggests strategies for prevention and early intervention, and discusses various medical and complementary treatment protocols. This information can assist you to develop a realistic plan for cancer prevention and management.

DEFINING CANCER

Some women have the perception that all tumors are cancerous, that all cancers are the same, and that cancer is synonymous with death. However, most tumors are **benign** and are rarely life-threatening. Benign tumors are made up of cells that are encapsulated; they do not spread to other parts of the body and do not invade surrounding tissues. These tumors can usually be surgically removed and do not grow back. **Malignant tumors** are cancer and refer to numerous diseases characterized by abnormal cells that divide uncontrollably and have the ability to infiltrate and destroy normal cells. Cancer cells are not encapsulated, and they can break away from the primary tumor and **metastasize** (or travel) to other parts of the body through the bloodstream or the lymphatic system. Metastasized cancer cells can form new tumors and invade tissue and organs in the new area of the body.

The prognosis for a woman with cancer depends on a variety of factors, including the nature of the tumor, its location, and its stage. The key to survival of cancer is early detection. The earlier cancer is diagnosed, the better the

Health Tips 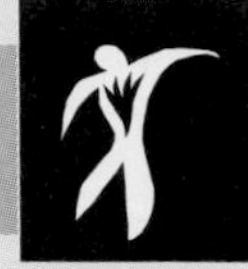

Seven Warning Signs of Cancer

The American Cancer Society has identified seven major warning signs of cancer:

- A change in bowel or bladder habits
- A sore that does not heal
- Unusual bleeding or discharge from any place
- A lump in the breast or other parts of the body
- Chronic indigestion or difficulty in swallowing
- Obvious changes in a wart or mole
- Persistent coughing or hoarseness

There are more warning signs for other kinds of cancer that are not as common as those listed above. To learn more about the warning signs of cancer, contact your local chapter of the American Cancer Society or the National Cancer Institute at 1-800-4-CANCER. Visit their Web sites at www.cancer.org and www.cancer. gov.

FYI 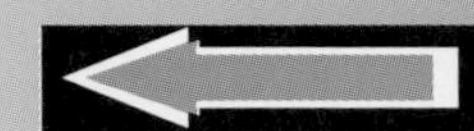

Cancer Incidence by Race and Ethnicity

The rate of cancer among women varies by race. Alaska Native women have the highest reported rates of cancer, followed by white women. The leading cancer sites among Alaska Native women are breast, colon and rectum, and lung. In fact, they have the highest rates of colorectal and lung cancer among all women. White women have the highest rates of breast cancer among all women, whereas African American women have the highest rates of lung and colon and rectum cancer of any group except Alaska Natives. The leading cancer sites among African American women are breast, colon and rectum, lung, uterus, and cervix. Asian women and Pacific Islander women experience higher rates of breast, lung, and colon and rectum cancer than any other cancer. However, the stomach is the leading cancer site for Japanese and Korean American women, and the cervix is the leading cancer site for Vietnamese American women. The leading cancer sites for Hispanic and Latino women are the breast, lung, and colon and rectum. Hispanic women are second only to Vietnamese women in the high rates of cervical cancer. Reported cancer rates are lowest for Native American women from New Mexico and for Korean American women. The data for Native American women from New Mexico, although showing the lowest overall reported cancer rates, are not known to be accurate. These women have been underrepresented in most studies.

TABLE 16.1 Leading Sites of New Cancer Cases and Death in Women, 2006 Estimates[1]

ESTIMATED NEW CASES	ESTIMATED DEATHS
Breast 212,920 (31%)	Lung & bronchus 72,130 (26%)
Lung & bronchus 81,770 (12%)	Breast 40,970 (15%)
Colon & rectum 75,810 (11%)	Colon & Rectum 27,300 (10%)
Uterine corpus 41,200 (6%)	Pancreas 16,210 (6%)
Non-Hodgkin's lymphoma 28,190 (4%)	Ovary 15,310 (6%)
Melanoma of skin 27,930 (4%)	Leukemia 9,810 (4%)
Thyroid 22,590 (3%)	Non-Hodgkin's lymphoma 8,840 (3%)
Ovary 20,180 (3%)	Uterine corpus 7,340 (3%)
Urinary bladder 16,730 (2%)	Multiple myeloma 5,630 (2%)
Pancreas 6,580 (2%)	Brain & other nervous system 5,560 (2%)
All sites 679,510 (100%)	All sites 273,560 (100%)

NOTE: Excludes basal and squamous cell skin cancer and in situ carcinoma except urinary bladder. Percentages may not total 100% due to rounding.

prognosis. The American Cancer Society (ACS) has identified seven warning signs of cancer. (See *Health Tips:* "Seven Warning Signs of Cancer.") If any of these signs are present, you should see your health care provider immediately. In 2006 the ACS estimated that 679,510 women would be diagnosed with cancer and 273,560 would die from it eventually.[2] (See Table 16.1.) The highest incidence and mortality rates for reported cancer cases in women are for cancers of the lungs, breast, and colon and rectum. (See *FYI:* "Cancer Incidence by Race and Ethnicity.")

CLASSIFICATIONS OF COMMON MALIGNANCIES

Each cancer is distinguished by the nature, site, or clinical course of the lesion. Generally, cancers are classified according to the part of the body in which they originate or by the type of cell as seen under the microscope. The World Health Organization has identified forty-six body

TABLE 16.2 Common Classifications of Cancer

Carcinoma
A malignant epithelial neoplasm that tends to invade surrounding tissue and to metastasize to distant regions of the body. Carcinomas develop most frequently in the skin, large intestine, lung, stomach, prostate gland, cervix, and breast. The tumor is firm, irregular, nodular, with a well-defined border.

Sarcoma
A malignant neoplasm of the soft tissues arising in fibrous, fatty, muscular, synovial, vascular, or neural tissue, usually first presenting as a painless swelling. About 40 percent of sarcomas occur in the lower extremities, 20 percent in the upper extremities, 20 percent in the trunk, and the rest in the head or neck. The tumor, composed of closely packed cells in a fibrillar or homogeneous matrix, tends to be vascular and is usually highly invasive.

Lymphoma
A neoplasm of lymphoid tissue that is usually malignant. Characteristically, the appearance of a painless, enlarged lymph node or nodes is followed by weakness, fever, weight loss, and anemia.

Leukemia
A malignant neoplasm of blood-forming tissues characterized by diffuse replacement of bone marrow with proliferating leukocyte precursors, abnormal numbers and forms of immature white cells in circulation, and infiltration of lymph nodes, the spleen, and the liver. Acute leukemia usually has a sudden onset and rapidly progresses from early signs, such as fatigue, pallor, weight loss, and easy bruising, to fever, hemorrhages, extreme weakness, bone or joint pain, and repeated infections. Chronic leukemia develops slowly, and signs similar to those of the acute forms of the disease may not appear.

TABLE 16.3 TMN Staging: Criteria for Stages Differ for Different Types of Cancer

STAGE	DEFINITION
Stage 0	Carcinoma in situ (early cancer that is present only in the layer of cells in which it began.
Stage 1, Stage II, Stage III	Higher numbers indicate more extensive disease: greater tumor size, and/or spread of the cancer to nearby lymph nodes and/or organs adjacent to the primary tumor.
Stage IV	The cancer has spread to another organ.

sites, with numerous types of cancer at many sites, totaling well over a hundred different cancers.

The four most common categories of cancer are carcinoma, sarcoma, lymphoma, and leukemia.[3] (See Table 16.2.) The reason for discussing these broad categories of cancers is to provide you with an understanding that *not* all cancers are the same. Carcinomas are by far the most common type of cancer found in the United States, representing 80–90 percent of all reported cancers. Carcinomas begin in the glandular or epithelial cells, which line the organs of the body. Sarcomas are cancers that begin in the connective tissues of the body, either the bone or soft tissues. Most tumors of bone and soft tissues are benign, and sarcomas are relatively rare in the United States. They account for less than 2 percent of all new cancer cases each year.

Lymphomas are cancers of the lymphatic system and can be broadly subdivided into Hodgkin's disease and non-Hodgkin's lymphomas (a number of diseases). Leukemia is a cancer of the blood-forming tissues and can be one of many types. Early symptoms may mimic other diseases, including mononucleosis, tonsillitis, mumps, and others. Therefore, blood tests and examination of the cells in the bone marrow are necessary for diagnosing leukemia.

In addition to the most common categories, it is important to understand the difference between in situ and invasive cancer. "In situ" refers to cancerous tumors that are usually early stage and localized. The survival rates are usually higher for in situ cancer than for *invasive* cancer, which has spread to other tissues. A variety of systems are used to determine the stage of cancer according to the major factors influencing prognosis. The most common system for determining the stage of cancer is the **TNM** staging system, developed by the American Joint Committee on Cancer and the International Union Against Cancer. In the TNM system, T represents the tumor size and level of invasion ranging from 1 to 4. N represents the nodal involvement, the size and number of the nodes, and degree of spread to lymph nodes ranging from 1 to 4. And M represents the absence or presence of distant metastases, denoted as X, 0, or 1. For example, Stage 0 for breast cancer refers to noninvasive or in situ cancers, whereas Stage 4 means the carcinoma extends beyond the breast to another part of the body such as bone, liver, or lung. Each cancer site has a different staging, unique to the site.[4] (See Table 16.3). Gynecologic cancers are frequently classified according to the guidelines of the International Federation for Gynecologic Oncology. This system divides the disease into five stages from Stage 0, a carcinoma in situ, to Stage IV, the metastasis to other sites. The stages were further subdivided into three grades with Grade 1 being well-differentiated with the best prognosis and Grade 3 being least-differentiated with the poorest prognosis.[5] For example, Stage I for endometrial cancer refers to carcinoma in situ, whereas Stage IV means the carcinoma extends beyond the pelvis and involves the bladder or rectum.

CAUSES OF CANCER

Scientists remain uncertain about the exact causes of cancer, although external (chemicals, radiation, and viruses) and internal (hormones, immune conditions, and inherited mutations) factors are recognized. Lifestyle and environmental factors account for most cancer risk, and a number of known **carcinogens** have been identified. Cigarette smoking, diet, exposure to carcinogenic chemicals, ionizing radiation, and ultraviolet rays account for more than 87 percent of all cancers. Researchers also study the patterns of cancer to determine the risk factors and protective conditions that increase or decrease the likelihood of getting cancer. Cancer is *not* caused by injuries, bruises, or bumps and is *not* contagious. Cancer develops over time. Still, most women who get cancer have no known risk factors. And many women who have risk factors do not get cancer. This section discusses some of the lifestyle and environmental factors contributing to cancer, and the biological changes that develop to increase the risk of developing cancer.

Lifestyle Factors Implicated in Cancer

Growing Older Perhaps the most important risk factor for cancer is aging. Most cancer occurs in people over the age of 65. However, people of all ages, even children, can develop cancer.

Cigarette Smoking Cigarette smoking is associated with cancers of the lung, larynx, pharynx, oral cavity, esophagus, pancreas, bladder, kidney, uterus, and cervix. Cigarette smoking accounts for 87 percent of lung cancer deaths and 30 percent of all cancer deaths. Passive (or secondhand) smoke causes disease, including lung cancer, in healthy nonsmokers. An estimated 45 million Americans are current smokers, which includes one in five U.S. women.[6] However, the per capita consumption of cigarettes continues to decline. Smoking cigarettes remains the most significant factor in premature death of women, particularly in the areas of cancer and heart disease. Lung cancer mortality rates are thirteen times higher for female smokers compared to females who have never smoked. In addition, secondhand smoke contributes to nearly 3,000 lung cancer deaths in nonsmoking adults each year.[7]

Diet Research suggests that approximately one-third of cancer deaths in the United States are due to dietary factors. The types of food consumed, the amount of fat consumed rather than the specific type of fat consumed, food preparation methods, and overall caloric balance are risk factors for some cancers in women, particularly cancers of the breast, colon, and rectum.

Scientific studies suggest that fruits and vegetables (especially green and dark yellow vegetables, cruciferous vegetables, soy products, and legumes) are protective factors for preventing some types of cancer, particularly for cancers of the gastrointestinal and respiratory tracts.[8] The 5-A-Day program, a partnership of grocers, produce suppliers, and federal and state health agencies, has undertaken a nationwide campaign to encourage people to eat five or more servings of fruits and vegetables each day as part of a low-fat, high-fiber diet.

Age Cancer deaths are certainly age-related. Even though the age-adjusted death rate from cancer has been rising, much of the increase can be attributed to a rise in lung cancer death rates. The death rates for most other age-related cancers have leveled off, and for people younger than 55 the cancer death rate has declined. Over 50 percent of all cancers occur in persons over the age of 65, and the age-related death rate for people aged 55 and older is still rising. Table 16.4 shows the probability of developing cancer for various age groups. You can see that the probability for all sites increases with age.

Viruses A number of viruses have been linked to an increased risk of cancer, including hepatitis B, human T-lymphotropic virus (HTLV-1), herpes simplex virus-2 (HSV-2), Epstein-Barr, and some types of human papilloma virus (HPV). Hepatitis B has been linked to liver cancer, whereas HSV-2 and HPV have been associated with an increase in cervical cancer.

Alcohol Consumption Heavy alcohol consumption, particularly in conjunction with cigarette use or chewing tobacco, contributes to an increased risk of cancer. These cancers include mouth, esophagus, liver, larynx, pharynx, breast, and stomach. Moderate alcohol use is associated with a slightly increased risk of breast cancer among women, but the reason is unknown. Some studies suggest that drinking alcohol is related to changes in hormonal levels, particularly an increase in estrogen levels in women.[9]

TABLE 16.4 The Probability of a Woman Developing Cancer

	BIRTH TO 39 (%)	40 TO 59 (%)	60 TO 69 (%)	BIRTH TO DEATH (%)
All sites*	1.99 (1 in 50)	9.06 (1 in 12)	10.54 (1 in 9)	38.09 (1 in 3)
Bladder†	.01 (1 in 9,513)	.12 (1 in 816)	.25 (1 in 104)	1.14 (1 in 88)
Breast	.48 (1 in 209)	4.11 (1 in 24)	3.82 (1 in 16)	13.22 (1 in 8)
Colon/rectum	.06 (1 in 1,567)	.70 (1 in 143)	1.16 (1 in 86)	5.55 (1 in 18)
Leukemia	.13 (1 in 788)	.14 (1 in 721)	.19 (1 in 513)	1.07 (1 in 93)
Lung/bronchus	.03 (1 in 3,103)	.80 (1 in 122)	1.68 (1 in 60)	5.72 (1 in 17)
Melanoma/skin	.21 (1 in 470)	.40 (1 in 248)	.26 (1 in 381)	1.30 (1 in 77)
Non-Hodgkin's lymphoma	.09 (1 in 1,158)	.31 (1 in 320)	.42 (1 in 77)	1.82 (1 in 55)
Uterine cervix	.15 (1 in 657)	.28 (1 in 353)	.15(1 in 671)	.74 (1 in 135)
Uterine corpus	.06 (1 in 1,641)	.72 (1 in 139)	.83 (1 in 74)	2.61 (1 in 38)

*All sites exclude basal and squamous cell skin cancers and in situ carcinomas except urinary bladder.
†Includes invasive and in situ cancer cases.
SOURCE: DEVCAN: Probability of Developing or Dying of Cancer Software, Version 6.0. Statistical Research and Applications Branch, National Cancer Institute, 2005. http://srab.cancer.gov/devcan.

Close Relatives with Certain Types of Cancer Some cancers (including melanoma and cancers of the breast, ovary, prostate, and colon) tend to occur more frequently in some families. It is unclear whether these cancers are related to heredity, factors in a family's environment, lifestyle patterns, or pure chance.

Hormone Replacement Therapy (HRT) Studies have shown that high cumulative exposure to estrogen increases the risk of endometrial cancer. Estrogen alone (ERT) may be prescribed for women who have had a hysterectomy because they are not at risk for uterine cancer. Progesterone and estrogen replacement therapy, (called hormone replacement therapy, or HRT) has been shown to largely offset the increased risk related to using only estrogen.[10]

Diethylstilbestrol (DES) DES is a synthetic form of estrogen that was used from the early 1940s to 1971 to prevent miscarriage. DES-exposed daughters are at increased risk for developing abnormal cells (dysplasia) in the cervix and vagina. Women who took DES during pregnancy may have a slightly higher risk of breast cancer. There does not appear to be an increased risk of breast cancer for DES daughters based on current knowledge.

Environmental Factors Implicated in Cancer

Exposure to Sun More than 1 million cases of basal cell or squamous cell cancers occur annually. The most serious form of skin cancer is melanoma. The ACS estimates that in 2007 there will be 59,940 new cases of melanoma and 8,110 people will die from it.[11] Ultraviolet rays (both UVA and UVB) have been linked to skin cancer. It is best to reduce exposure to the midday sun (10 A.M. to 3 P.M.) to avoid the sun when your shadow is shorter than you are. Wear a sunscreen with a protective factor of at least 15. Wear protective clothing when exposed to sunlight, and avoid artificial sources of UV light (such as sun lamps and tanning booths). UV radiation causes most cases of basal and squamous cell skin cancer and contributes significantly to skin melanoma. Levels of UV radiation may be increasing due to changes in the earth's ozone layer.[12]

Ionizing Radiation Ionizing radiation can include X-ray procedures, radioactive substances, rays from outer space, and other sources. High doses are related to increased risk of developing leukemia and cancers of the breast, thyroid, lung, stomach, and other organs. Low-dose levels have a negligible effect on cancer risk, but limiting exposure is prudent.

Therapeutic radiation (radiation received to treat existing cancer) can also damage normal cells, potentially increasing the risk for a second cancer. This risk depends on the person's age and the site that was treated. (See *FYI:* "Lifestyle, Environmental, and Hereditary Risk Factors Associated with Cancer.")

Chemicals and Other Substances Exposure to certain chemicals, metals, or pesticides can increase the risk of cancer. Asbestos, nickel, cadmium, uranium, radon, vinyl chloride, benzidene, and benzene are well-known carcinogens. Worksite rules should be followed closely to avoid or minimize contact with dangerous materials.

FYI

Lifestyle, Environmental, and Hereditary Risk Factors Associated with Cancer

- Tobacco
- Diet
- Alcohol
- Ultraviolet radiation
- Ionizing radiation
- Chemicals and other substances
- Age
- Close relatives with certain types of cancers
- Hormone replacement therapy (HRT)
- Diethylstilbestrol (DES)

CURRENT RESEARCH REGARDING CAUSES AND TREATMENT

Molecular and Cellular Causes of Cancer

Most carcinogens are introduced into the body through air, water, or diet and then deactivated by the body's immune system. However, some foreign substances become activated within the body and bind to the genetic coding material, DNA. Altered DNA may be responsible for the growth in cancer cells. Once scientists delineate the causes of cancer and the mechanisms contributing to abnormal cell growth, the possibility for a cure increases. Several theories elucidate the causes of abnormal cell growth and are discussed in the following sections. (See *Assess Yourself:* "What Is Your Cancer Risk?")

Cell Cycle Research

One avenue of cancer research is the study of the cell cycle. Cancer cells exhibit a loss of differentiation, increased invasiveness, and a decrease in responsiveness to drugs compared to normal cells. A normal cell cycle requires the coordination of a variety of macromolecular syntheses, assemblies, and movement. Hartwell and Kastan suggest that defects in the synthesis, assembly, or movement of DNA, the spindle, or spindle pole during cell replication may result in genetic instability that characterizes precancerous and cancerous cells.[13]

They conclude that if genomic instability contributes to cancer development, then finding procedures to reduce the instability may reduce the incidence and rate of cancer development. Cell biologists involved in cell cycle research are attempting to determine if the cell cycle is relevant to the development of novel anticancer agents.[14]

Gene Mutation Research

Oncogenes play a role in normal cell growth; however, when oncogenes mutate, they can cause rapid cell division. Ras oncogene mutation is found in 50 percent of all colon cancers and 90 percent of pancreatic cancers,[15] and it is a major factor in many epithelial cancers and myeloid leukemias.[16] Easton and colleagues found that the mutation of a *BRCA1* gene accounted for approximately 45 percent of families with significantly high breast cancer incidence and around 80 percent of families with increased incidence of both early-onset breast cancer and ovarian cancer.[17]

Duke University scientists are researching an enzyme that chops up DNA during the normal death and replacement of cells and confers a higher survival rate to cells even if they have harmful genetic mutations, such as in cancer.[18]

Some individuals may be more susceptible to mutations of genes, called suppressor genes. Although normal suppressor genes control cell growth, mutated ones allow rapid cell division. Researchers found mutations of the tumor suppressor gene *p53* were common in sarcoma patients who had a personal or family history of cancer, but not in patients without this background. The identification of these mutations may allow for genetic counseling.[19] Dr. Waun Hong, of the M. D. Anderson Cancer Center, is evaluating ways to restore normal *p53* function through gene therapy.[20]

Science is beginning to unravel the mechanism of some cancers, and genetic engineers hope to one day have the capacity to eliminate mutated genes and replace them with normal genes.

Adjuvant Treatment

Adjuvant therapy, such as radiation therapy or substances to enhance the action of drugs to treat the cancer, refers to the use of other forms of treatment to supplement or enhance the primary treatment. The use of drugs pre- and postoperatively improves the survival rate with certain cancers, including breast cancer and cervical cancer. **Neoadjuvant therapy** is a term used to describe the use of drugs to shrink the cancer before

Assess Yourself

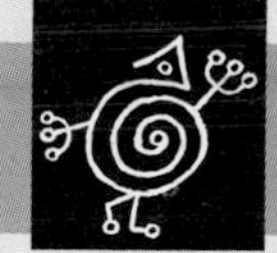

What Is Your Cancer Risk?

Check all of the following risk factors that apply to you.

Lung Cancer

____ 1. Cigarette smoking
____ 2. Living with a person who smokes
____ 3. Exposure to chemicals that are known carcinogens
____ 4. Radiation exposure
____ 5. Radon exposure
____ 6. Living in an area with heavy air pollution

Colon and Rectal Cancer

____ 1. Family history
____ 2. Physical inactivity
____ 3. High-fat diet
____ 4. Low-fiber diet

Breast Cancer

____ 1. Family history
____ 2. Early menarche—before age 12
____ 3. Late menopause—after age 50
____ 4. Lengthy exposure to cyclic estrogen (e.g., oral contraceptives)
____ 5. Never having children
____ 6. First birth of a child at a later age
____ 7. Obesity
____ 8. High socioeconomic status
____ 9. Higher education level

Cervical Cancer

____ 1. First intercourse at early age
____ 2. Multiple sex partners
____ 3. Cigarette smoking
____ 4. Low socioeconomic status

Endometrial Cancer

____ 1. Estrogen
____ 2. Tamoxifen (to prevent recurrence of breast cancer)
____ 3. Early menarche—before age 12
____ 4. Late menopause—after age 50
____ 5. Never having children
____ 6. History of infertility or failure to ovulate
____ 7. Diabetes
____ 8. Gallbladder disease
____ 9. Hypertension
____ 10. Obesity

Ovarian Cancer

____ 1. Age (over 50)
____ 2. Never having children
____ 3. Family history of ovarian cancer
____ 4. Breast cancer
____ 5. Living in an industrialized country

Skin Cancer

____ 1. Exposure to UV rays
____ 2. Fair complexion
____ 3. Family history
____ 4. Occupational exposure to coal tar, pitch, and so on

What measures can you take to reduce your risks?

surgical removal. This treatment is used with certain types of cancer, including late-stage breast cancer and brain tumors. **Chemotherapy,** chemical systemic treatment, can cure some cancers, keep others from spreading, cause remission, or reduce large tumors before surgery. Researchers continue to seek the most effective combinations of treatments to increase the survival rate.

Immunotherapy Research

Immunotherapy enhances the body's own immune system to fight a disease. When the body is functioning effectively, the immune system controls cancer cells. T-helper cells and **macrophages** use their own chemicals, tumor necrosis factor, interleukin, and interferon, to prevent tumor growth or attack cancer cells. Interferon, interleukin-2, and other biologic response modifiers are being tested for effectiveness in boosting the immune system's ability to counter malignant cell division. Gene therapy and vaccines are also being studied.

Stem Cell Transplantation

The transplantation of blood-forming *stem cells* helps patients to receive high doses of chemotherapy, radiation, or both. However, the high doses destroy both cancer cells and normal blood cells in the bone marrow. Once treatment is finished, patients can receive healthy, blood-forming stem cells via a tube placed into a large vein. The stem cells may be retrieved from the patient prior to treatment or harvested from another person. There can be serious side effects from stem cell transplantation such as infection and bleeding.[21] Now see *Viewpoint:* "Are We Winning the 'War on Cancer'?"

Viewpoint

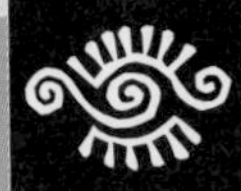

Are We Winning the "War on Cancer"?

The fear of cancer has increased proportionately to the risk of contracting the disease, from one in six persons in the 1960s to one in three in 2006. In 1971, President Nixon declared a "war on cancer" and Congress passed the National Cancer Act, which included funding for the creation of the National Cancer Institute (NCI). Although NCI had many responsibilities assigned to it, one of its primary roles was to find a cure for cancer. In 1992, more than 10 percent of the nation's entire health care budget was spent on treatment and research. The American public continues to receive mixed messages regarding the progress of cancer research. On one hand, NCI and the American Cancer Society suggest that we are winning the war on cancer. Officials point to the improvement of "five-year survival rates" for many cancers. On the other hand, some researchers point out that the incidence of many cancers, including breast cancer and lung cancer in women, continues to increase. They suggest that the survival rate of all cancers combined has risen only a few percentage points since the early 1970s. In fact, early detection accounts for most of the current success in treatment.

Some researchers suggest that we need to continue to spend our resources on finding a cure and better treatment for cancer. Others support more prevention, focusing primarily on lifestyle and environmental factors. What do you think? Which areas are most important to you?

Viewpoint

Cancer Rates Rising in China

China is the world's largest consumer of tobacco, and Chinese deaths from lung cancer continue to rise. Coincidentally, the Chinese government earns more tax revenue from tobacco than from any other industry. Three American tobacco companies have signed contracts to produce tobacco in China: Philip Morris, RJR Nabisco, and Rothmans.

Since 1987, U.S. cigarette exports have increased about 230 percent. This increase in exports to other countries includes Japan, South Korea, and the former Soviet Union.[23] What do you think about the American business involvement in the Chinese tobacco industry? What's the message to the people of China? What are your thoughts about the increase in tobacco exports to other countries?

CANCER AT SELECTED SITES: WHAT YOU NEED TO KNOW

Lung Cancer

Lung cancer surpassed breast cancer as the leading cause of cancer death in women in 1987. Seventeen years later, an estimated 81,770 women would be diagnosed and 72,130 women would die from lung cancer, many of them needlessly.[22] They are dying because they smoke cigarettes. Lung cancer is divided into two main types: non–small cell and small cell. The three main types of non–small cell lung cancer include squamous cell carcinoma, adenocarcinoma, and large cell carcinoma. Non–small cell lung cancer is more common and spreads more slowly. Small cell lung cancer grows more quickly and invades other organs. These two types of cancer spread in different ways and are treated differently. (Also see *Viewpoint:* "Cancer Rates Rising in China.")

Risk and Protective Factors The best advice for the prevention of lung cancer is "If you don't smoke, don't start." If someone close to you smokes, ask them to smoke somewhere else. If you smoke, QUIT! The incidence of lung cancer among women has continued to rise during the past 20 years, paralleling a previous increase in smoking. Passive or secondhand smoke is another primary risk factor for lung cancer. Avoiding smoke-filled areas, including the home of an indoor smoker and bars and restaurants where smoking is allowed, acts as a strong protective factor for avoiding lung cancer.

Teenage girls are being lured by the tobacco industry to assert their independence and charm by picking up the smoking habit. They also get the promise of weight control by smoking cigarettes. Advertisements push cigarettes by promising independence, weight control, adventure, and romance. Unfortunately, young women can look forward to premature aging, an increase in facial wrinkles, and becoming addicted to a powerful, cancer-causing product.

The overwhelming number of women who develop lung cancer are smokers or have lived with a smoker. However, some other factors have been implicated in increasing your risk of lung cancer, including having asbestos lung disease or obstructive airway disease, exposure to radon, and exposure to a variety of occupational substances

Women Making a Difference

Dana Reeve: Wife, Mother, and Activist

Dana Reeve, a nonsmoker, succumbed, at age 44, to lung cancer in March 2006, battling the disease with grace and defiant humor. This disease, however, does not define Dana Reeve! She was her husband's, Christopher Reeve, best friend and greatest support during the decade-long work of rehabilitation following a 1995 horseback riding incident that left him paralyzed. Dana Reeve bowed out of a singing and acting career to care for her husband. She worked with him in the Christopher Reeves Paralysis Foundation, which raised funds and supported research for new treatments for spinal cord injuries, working to improve the quality of life for people suffering from paralysis. Together they testified before Congress to help generate support for legislation that would expand funding for embryonic stem cell research; it passed the House last year, defying President Bush's veto threat.

In the months prior to her death, Reeve's busy schedule became even fuller: promoting a charity event in New York, speaking on Capitol Hill in support of paralysis research, promoting a children's book, and even performing her cabaret act at a Manhattan nightclub. The American Cancer Society issued a statement about Dana Reeve on March 7, 2006: "Ms. Reeve's strength and her work brought tremendous attention to two terrible disease conditions—spinal cord injuries and lung cancer." Grace, resolve, true love, and strong will describe the beautiful spirit of Dana Reeve—a woman who made a difference.

such as chromium, coal products, iron oxide, nickel, mustard gas, petroleum, and uranium. One of the most courageous and caring young women of this decade, Dana Reeve, wife of the late Christopher Reeve, succumbed to an aggressive form of lung cancer yet had never smoked cigarettes. (See *Women Making a Difference:* "Dana Reeve: Wife, Mother, and Activist.")

Early Detection The signs and symptoms a woman needs to recognize are a persistent cough, blood in the sputum, constant chest pain, recurring pneumonia or bronchitis, swelling in the neck and face, and a loss of appetite or weight loss. By the time these symptoms occur, lung cancer is often in its more advanced stages and has metastasized to other areas.

Screening and Diagnosis None of the many screening tests that have been used to detect lung cancer has provided a decrease in mortality, including X-ray films, fluoroscopy, tomography, bronchography, angiography, cytologic studies of sputum, bronchial washings, and needle **biopsy,** and more recently the **magnetic resonance imaging (MRI)** and **monoclonal antibodies.**[24] Newer screening tests, such as low-dose spiral computed tomography (CT) scans and molecular markers in sputum, provide some improved results in detecting lung cancer at earlier, more operable stages.[25] Because advanced-stage lung cancer causes such high mortality and screening has little effect on mortality rates, the best hope is prevention and better techniques for detection and treatment. More effective imaging methods and increased emphasis on smoking cessation are necessary for reducing lung cancer mortality. The presence of lung cancer is determined by examining tissue from the lung. A biopsy, the removal of a small sample of tissue, is done by bronchoscopy, needle aspiration, thoracentesis, or thoracotomy. If lung cancer is detected, it is then staged to determine the treatment plan.

Treatment Treatment depends on a number of factors, including the type of cancer, the size, the location, and the extent of the tumor. By the time a woman knows she has lung cancer, the cancer has likely metastasized to other areas of the body or to a greater portion of the lung. Epidermoid (squamous) cancers and adenocarcinomas account for 60 percent of lung cancers, 25 percent are small cell carcinomas, and 15 percent are large cell anaplastic (undifferentiated) cancers. Adenocarcinomas are by far the most common lung cancer in women. The prognosis for survival from lung cancer is poor, with only 15 percent of women diagnosed with lung cancer managing to survive 5 years or more.[26] Surgery is the most common treatment for non–small cell lung cancer. Cryosurgery (freezing and destroying cancer cells) may be used in later stages of cancer development. Small cell lung cancer spreads rapidly, and chemotherapy and radiation are the first treatments of choice. Photodynamic therapy (PDT), a type of laser therapy, may be used when the cancer cannot be removed through surgery. *Eriotinib* is an oral medication that targets the epidermal growth factor receptors involved in cell growth and proliferation. It has been approved for use in treating recurrent non–small cell lung cancers.[27] *Bevacizumab* is an injection used in combination with standard chemotherapy; it helps stop growth of blood vessels that supply nutrients to tumors.[28]

Breast Cancer

In the United States, breast cancer is the second leading cancer killer of all women and the leading cause of cancer death in African American women. Even though white women have the highest incidence rate of breast cancer, African American women have the highest death rate. Some researchers speculate that the higher death rate is probably due to diagnosis at a later stage of the disease. These women wait longer, are less likely to have clinical breast examinations, and have fewer mammograms. The incidence of breast cancer has declined since 1990 and accounts for 26 percent of all cancers in women. A woman's probability of developing breast cancer at some point in her lifetime is 1 in 8.[29] The cause for the continued rise in breast cancer remains speculative. Some of the recent rise in incidence has been attributed to increased emphasis on early detection, primarily through the use of mammograms. The American Cancer Society estimates that 178,480 women will get breast cancer and 40,460 women will die from it in 2007.[30]

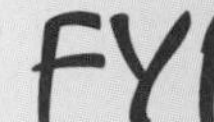

Abortion and Breast Cancer Not Associated

A study conducted by researchers in Denmark found that there is no overall increase in breast cancer for women who had abortions between the 7th and 14th weeks of gestation. Women who had later term abortions may face a greater risk of breast cancer; however, other factors may have contributed to the increased risk.

Risk and Protective Factors What do you think your risk for breast cancer is (high, medium, low)? Would you think it was low if your mother or grandmother didn't have breast cancer? Many women conclude that if their family history is free of breast cancer, they are free from risk. Not true! Although family history is a recognized risk factor, 85 to 95 percent of all women who develop breast cancer have no family history of the disease. In fact, 75 percent of all breast cancers occur in women with no known risk factors. All women are at risk because the two main risk factors are (1) being a woman and (2) getting older.

Age is a leading risk factor for breast cancer. Women 40 years and older account for 95 percent of new cases and 97 percent of breast cancer deaths. After age 40, non-Hispanic white women are more likely to be diagnosed with breast cancer than African American women, but African American women are more likely to die.[31] The average age of diagnosis for women is 61. Women aged 75 to 79 have the highest incidence of breast cancer.

Identifiable risk factors include family history, previous breast biopsy (with abnormal cell growth), previous breast exposure to radiation (from childhood cancer treatment), HRT (5 years or more after menopause), alcohol (two to five drinks daily), obesity and high-fat diets, personal history of breast cancer (mother, grandmother, or aunt), genetic alterations (BRCA1, BRCA2, and others), menarche at an early age (before age 12), late menopause (after age 50), never having children, use of DES during pregnancy, late childbearing (first child after age 30), dense breast tissue (more likely to occur in breasts with more lobular and ductal tissue). Identifiable protective factors include breast-feeding and having children. A recent study of 100,000 women found that for every 12 months of breast-feeding a woman reduces her risk of breast cancer by 4.3 percent.[32] For every birth, she reduces her risk by 7 percent. Recent studies have also explored the relationship between physical activity and breast cancer. There is continual evidence that exercise reduces the risk of developing breast cancer. The big unknown is how much exercise produces the best results. One study out of the Women's Health Initiative found that 1.25 to 2.5 hours per week of brisk walking reduced a woman's risk by 18 percent. However, walking 10 hours a week reduced the risk of developing breast cancer slightly more.[33]

Factors that have no proven relationship to breast cancer also should be recognized. Antiperspirants do not contribute to breast cancer. There is no evidence at this time that the chemicals used in antiperspirants are unsafe or that toxin buildup related to numerous chemicals, including those in antiperspirants, is related to carcinogenesis. Underwire bras do not cause breast cancer; there is no evidence that these bras obstruct lymph flow. There is no relationship between developing cancer and having had an induced or spontaneous abortion. (See *FYI:* "Abortion and Breast Cancer Not Associated.") There is no relationship between breast implants and breast cancer although silicone implants can cause scar tissue. Research does not currently show a link between breast cancer risk and exposure to environmental pollutants, such as the pesticide DDE (related to DDT) and PCBs (polychlorinated biphenyls).[34]

The best protection for a woman is early detection, that is, regular screening mammograms (see *FYI:* "Guidelines for Breast Cancer Detection"), breast exams by a health care provider, and monthly breast self-exams. A second protective factor is immediate treatment if breast cancer is diagnosed.

What to Look For The two most common warning signs are lumps or thickening in the breast. Most lumps are benign, particularly lumps that are soft, round, smooth, or movable. Generally, an irregular, hard lump that feels attached to breast tissue is more likely to be

FYI

Guidelines for Breast Cancer Detection

The American Cancer Society, the National Cancer Institute, and other medical groups recommend routine mammograms for all women over the age of 40. There is still some discrepancy for women in their forties. The American Cancer Society recommends mammograms *every year* for all women over the age of 40, and the National Cancer Institute recommends mammograms *every year or two* for all women over the age of 40. Both groups agree that mammograms should be conducted annually for women over age 50. Mammograms today can detect cancer in very early stages, well before physical symptoms can be detected by the woman or her health care provider. Studies show that women in their forties who had regular mammograms compared to those who did not have periodic mammograms were less likely to die of breast cancer and had more treatment options.

The American Cancer Society still recommends monthly breast self-examination (BSE) for women aged 20 and over. (See Chapter 8 for BSE instructions.) Clinical breast examinations are recommended every 3 years for women 20 and over and every year for women 40 and over.

malignant. Most breast cancers (70–80 percent) begin in the cells of the ducts, usually of the upper outer portion of the breast. In situ breast cancers are confined within the ducts or lobules; they have not spread beyond the area where they began. Lobular carcinoma in situ is sometimes believed to be a marker of increased risk for developing invasive cancer rather than a cancer itself. The seriousness of cancerous tumors that are invasive is determined by the staging at first diagnosis: local stage (confined to the breast), regional stage (spread to the lymph nodes), and distant stage (metastasized to other sites).

Additional warning signs include a change in the size or shape of the breast, discharge from the nipple, or a change in the color or texture of the skin of the breast or around the areola. Any discharge from the nipple should be brought to the attention of your health care provider!

Early Detection through Screening and Diagnosis

Early detection of breast cancer increases the likelihood of being cured. The best methods for detecting breast cancer are screening mammography, breast self-examination (BSE), and clinical breast examination (CBE). Ultrasonography, using high frequency sound waves, can also be used to determine whether a lump is a cyst or a solid mass. Lumps or changes discovered by BSE should be reported to your health care provider immediately. The American Cancer Society states that use of mammography, which can detect early changes in the breast, along with clinical breast exam and breast self-exam, offers women the best opportunity for reducing the breast cancer death rate through early detection.[35]

Mammography **Mammography** allows health care providers to detect breast cancer up to 2 years before a lump can be felt. Early detection increases the likelihood that the cancer hasn't metastasized. High-quality mammography, an X-ray technique to visualize the internal structure of the breast, helps health care providers identify very small lumps, areas of calcification, or other tissue changes. Mammography is the best method for detecting breast cancer, but it is not perfect. Dense breast tissue, common in younger women, reduces the mammographic image and makes early diagnosis of breast cancer more difficult. Young women in particular may experience more false positives, that is, suspicious lesions found through mammography that when biopsied are shown to be benign. One of the reasons for the controversy regarding mammography for young women is the additional monetary cost and emotional turmoil of false positives. False-negative results are rare, particularly with better imaging techniques. However, because they can occur, breast-self examination and clinical breast examination are important.

Women with breast implants should know that mammographic images have limited effectiveness. They should inform the technician before the mammogram is taken. The facility needs to use special techniques designed for women with implants, and technicians need to be familiar with doing mammograms for women with breast implants. Despite the known benefits of mammography, most women over the age of 40 have not had an initial screening mammogram and are unaware of its importance in early detection.

Biopsies What happens if a lump is detected on a manmogram? A second mammogram may be required if a positive result occurs. However, mammography cannot distinguish benign from malignant lesions with absolute certainty. A biopsy is the only method to determine if cancer cells are present. The health care provider may proceed with fine-needle aspiration, a procedure involving a very thin needle and a syringe. Fine-needle aspirations are most common in women who have large, palpable lesions. A needle is placed into the lump to determine if the lesion is solid or a fluid-filled **cyst.** If it is fluid-filled, the health care provider drains the fluid and the cyst collapses. If the cyst reappears, it can be drained again. No further treatment is necessary if the cyst does not reappear.

If the lesion is solid, the health care provider may attempt to draw out some cells for microscopic analysis. Fine-needle aspiration of a solid lesion requires great skill by the health care provider. If the lesion is malignant, it is important that cancerous cells be prevented from leaking out of the lesion into the body cavity.

Needle biopsy requires local anesthesia and uses a larger needle with a special cutting edge. A small core of tissue is removed, which may cause some bruising but rarely leaves a scar. This procedure is difficult, if not impossible, for hard or small lumps. Oftentimes, needle biopsies will be verified by surgical biopsies before further treatment is recommended.

A biopsy is the only method to determine if cancer cells are present. Whether surgical breast biopsy or needle aspiration is chosen by the health care provider depends on the nature and location of the lump. Surgical breast biopsy increases the tissue damage, is more costly, and is currently the only available method for women with nonpalpable or small lesions (less than an inch in diameter). An *excisional* biopsy removes *all* of the lump or suspicious tissue mass. This procedure is performed under a local anesthetic and typically on an outpatient basis; the woman goes home the same day. An *incisional* biopsy removes a portion or cross-section of the lump. This procedure is performed under a local anesthetic as well and is recommended for lumps larger than an inch in diameter. Fully 80 percent of women in the United States who undergo surgical breast biopsies do *not* have cancer.

A woman should consult her health care provider about the procedure being considered and ask whether there will be a change to the breast itself. Obviously, this depends on the type of procedure, the size of the lump, and the location of the lump. A woman needs to communicate effectively with her health care provider because she has a *right* to know what to expect. Remember, most lumps are benign.

Treatment Research has led to better treatment, a lower risk of death, and an improved quality of life for women who have breast cancer. The treatment prescribed by the **oncologist** should be based on the most current research. Treatment will be based on the stage of cancer and the woman's surgical preference.

Special lab tests help the oncologist learn more about the cancer. Hormone receptor tests can determine whether hormones help the cancer grow. Other tests help determine whether the cancer is likely to spread or to return after treatment. Additional tests of the bones, liver, or lungs may be ordered to determine if distant sites have been impacted.

In some instances, a second opinion may be required or wanted. A brief delay (3 to 4 weeks) does not reduce the effectiveness of treatment. Finding a doctor for a second opinion can be achieved in a variety of ways: through a referral from her primary physician, by calling 1-800-4-CANCER, through the local medical society directory or nearby medical school, or through the American Board of Medical Specialties directory found in the local library or online at www.certifieddoctor.org.

FIGURE 16.1 In lumpectomy, the surgeon removes the breast cancer and some normal tissue around it. (Sometimes an excisional biopsy serves as a lumpectomy.) Often, some of the lymph nodes under the arm are removed.

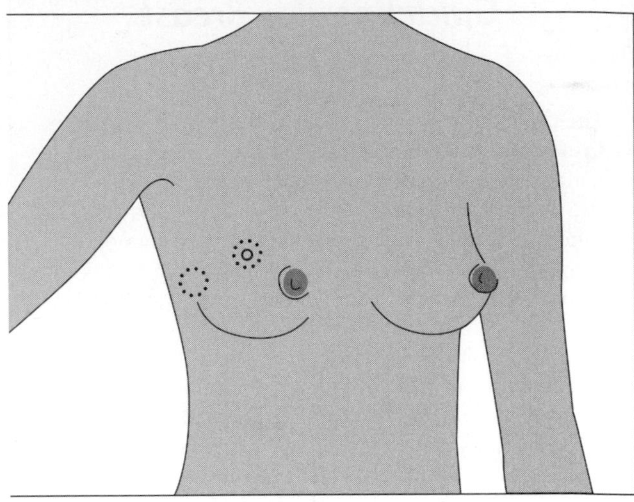

Breast cancer can be treated with local and/or systemic therapy. Local therapy (surgery or radiation therapy) is used to remove or destroy breast cancer at the site. Systemic treatments (chemotherapy, hormonal therapy, and biological therapy) are used to destroy or control cancer throughout the body. Surgery is the most common treatment for breast cancer. Breast-conserving surgery, an operation to remove the cancer but not the breast, includes **lumpectomy** (see Figure 16.1) and segmental mastectomy (partial mastectomy). At the time of surgery, some of the axillary (underarm) lymph nodes are often removed and examined under a mioroscope to see if the breast cancer has spread to the lymph nodes. After surgery, most women will receive **radiotherapy** (radiation treatment).

Mastectomy is surgery that removes the breast. In **total mastectomy** (see Figure 16.2), the whole breast is removed and some lymph nodes under the arm may also be removed. In **modified radical mastectomy** (see Figure 16.3), the whole breast, most of the lymph nodes under the arm, and often, the lining over the chest muscles, are removed. In radical mastectomy, the breast, both chest muscles, all of the lymph nodes under the arm, and some additional fat and skin are removed. Radical mastectomy is rarely used today although it was the standard procedure for many years; more effective, less invasive surgeries reduce potential risks of major surgeries. Mastectomy can be complemented by radiation

FIGURE 16.2 In total (simple) mastectomy, the surgeon removes the whole breast. Some lymph nodes under the arm may also be removed.

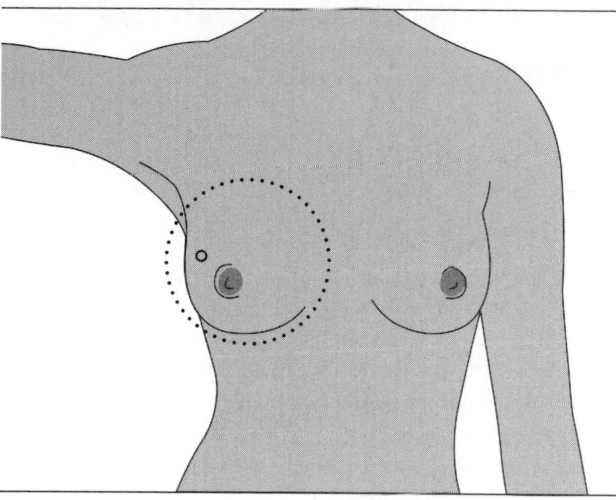

FIGURE 16.3 In modified radical mastectomy, the surgeon removes the whole breast, most of the lymph nodes under the arm, and often the lining over the chest muscles. The smaller of the two chest muscles also may be taken out to help in removing the lymph nodes.

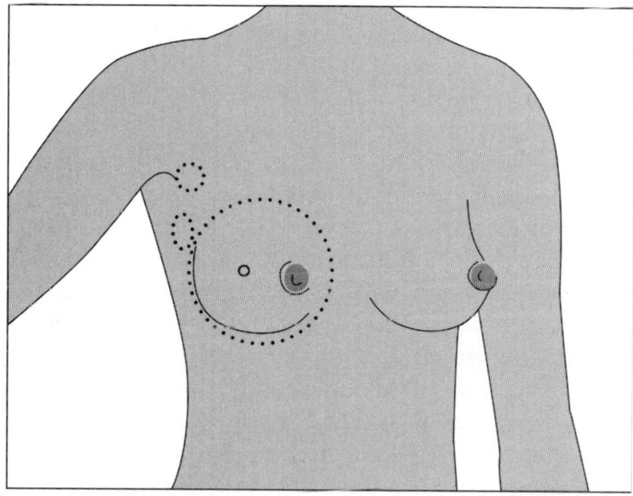

Viewpoint

Lumpectomy or Mastectomy?

Regaining control of your own life after the diagnosis of cancer is important. One of the first decisions facing a woman diagnosed with breast cancer is whether to have a lumpectomy or mastectomy. The literature regarding these procedures is mixed, and further study is needed. Researchers at the University of Pittsburgh conducted a large study of intraductal breast cancer and concluded that lumpectomy with radiation was an acceptable strategy. They assigned women to one of two treatments, surgery without radiation and surgery with follow-up radiotherapy. Women who had surgery alone had a recurrence rate of 16 percent, with half being invasive cancers. Women who had surgery with radiotherapy had a recurrence rate of 10 percent, with 3 percent being invasive cancers. The researchers concluded that lumpectomy with follow-up radiotherapy is effective.

Ninety-five percent of the women in this study who had the less aggressive lumpectomy did just as well as the women in the study who had a mastectomy. What information would you need to decide whether to have a lumpectomy or a mastectomy? What factors are most important to you?

therapy, chemotherapy, and hormonal therapy in combination or alone.

Researchers are studying other facets of cancer treatment. They are testing new anticancer drugs, doses, and treatment schedules. They are seeking ways to reduce the side effects of treatment, such as lymphedema (swelling under the arm caused by fluid buildup due to faulty lymphatic drainage) and the reduced ability of bone marrow to make blood cells. Procedures such as neoadjuvant chemotherapy (using chemo before surgery), sentinel lymph node biopsy, colony-stimulating factors, autologous bone marrow transplants, and peripheral stem cell transplants are being explored. Now see *Viewpoint:* "Lumpectomy or Mastectomy?" and *Her Story:* "Arlette: Surviving Breast Cancer."

Drug therapy is proving to be beneficial in reducing the risk of breast cancer reccurring. *Tamoxifen* is an antiestrogen drug, taken on a daily basis in pill form, that reduces the chances of the cancer coming back by about 50 percent for women with early breast cancer for cancers that had estrogen or progesterone receptors. *Aromatase inhibitors,* such as letrozole (Femara), anastrozole (Arimidex), and exemestane (Aromasin) work by blocking an enzyme responsible for producing small amounts of estrogen in postmenopausal women. Currently studies are comparing the use of tamoxifen and the aromatase inhibitors, both separately and in combination, and researchers are working to determine which of these strategies is more effective in preventing breast cancer from recurring.[36]

Rehabilitation Every effort is made to help a woman return to her normal routine as soon as possible. Exercising the arm and shoulder after surgery helps a woman regain her flexibility and strength. It also reduces pain and stiffness in the neck and back.

Her Story

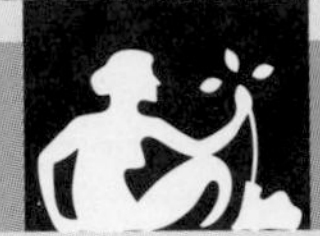

Arlette: Surviving Breast Cancer

Arlette is a healthy, active 52-year-old nurse practitioner. She discovered two breast masses on her routine mammogram. Nothing was noticeable on breast self-examination. Further testing including biopsies by her health care provider determined these to be ductal carcinoma. Arlette interviewed several surgeons, looking for one who would involve her in the decisions regarding treatment. After reviewing all the options, she and her surgeon agreed that bilateral modified radical mastectomies would be the treatment of choice for her. Having used relaxation tapes with several of her clients, Arlette asked a therapist friend to make an audiotape to use during the surgery. The tape was played during the surgery not only for Arlette but for the entire surgical team. The tape gave suggestions that she would relax and not subconsciously resist the surgery, that all would go smoothly, and that recovery would be rapid and without complications. This extensive surgery usually lasts about 5 hours, but Arlette's surgery was completed in 2½ hours with minimal bleeding. She recovered quickly and returned home within a few days after surgery. Her aftercare consisted of mild chemotherapy, physical therapy to assist with recovery of her range of motion, and psychotherapy to facilitate the changes she needed to make in her lifestyle. She was back to work in a few weeks. Five years later she is cancer-free. Arlette continues to use meditation, massage, and acupuncture; most of all, she has learned to listen to her body.

- What are your thoughts about Arlette's choices?
- Have you discussed treatment options with women who have survived cancer?
- What would you do if this had been you?

Lymphedema (swelling) can be prevented or reduced with certain exercises and by resting with the arm propped up on a pillow. If lymphedema occurs, other exercises or procedures will be necessary to drain the lymph. Any changes should be reported immediately, including pain, loss of appetite, changes in menstrual cycles, unusual bleeding, or blurred vision. Headaches, dizziness, shortness of breath, coughing or hoarseness, backaches, or digestive problems that don't go away or are unusual should also be reported.

Breast Reconstruction A woman who has a mastectomy has an additional choice to make. Should she have breast reconstruction surgery or wear a breast form or prosthesis? New methods and materials have made it possible for women to choose breast reconstruction. However, a number of factors should be considered. Breast reconstruction has some of the same risks and problems as breast implants (discussed in Chapter 2 on consumerism).

Breast reconstruction provides physical form to the breasts, but sensation is lost. If a woman is interested in breast reconstruction, she should inform her surgeon, who then consults with a plastic surgeon. She will need to discuss with the plastic surgeon which type of surgery would be best for her, expected recovery time, possible pain and scarring involved, and whether her insurance will cover the procedure. Insurance may pay the cost of reconstructive surgery that is due to breast cancer.

Breast reconstruction can be completed at the time of the mastectomy unless too little skin tissue or blood supply remains in the breast area. In that case, additional reconstruction will occur gradually until the skin is stretched enough to implant a permanent prosthesis. Breast reconstruction can be performed with *implants,* using bags filled with either saline (salt water) or silicone gel. The implant is placed under the chest muscle through an incision made by the surgeon. With a *flap procedure,* the woman's own tissue is used to reconstruct a breast. There are three types of flap procedures. The *TRAM flap,* the most common reconstructive choice, takes tissue from the abdomen and slides the tissue up a tunnel under the skin to the breast area. The *latissimus dorsi procedure* takes tissue from the shoulder area in the back and moves it to the breast area through a tunnel under the skin. In *free flap reconstruction,* tissue is taken from the buttocks or the rectus abdominis muscle and then transplanted to the breast area.[37]

Uterine and Cervical Cancer

The most common type of uterine cancer begins in the endometrium (the lining of the uterus) and is called endometrial cancer. Cancer that develops in the muscle (myometrium) is called uterine sarcoma, and cancer that begins in the cervix is called cervical cancer. Approximately 9,700 American women develop cervical cancer each year. Most cervical cancers are squamous cell carcinomas. Squamous cells are thin, flat cells that form on the surface of the cervix. Abnormal changes in the cells on the surface of the cervix are now classified according to the Bethesda System and include low-grade and high-grade squamous intraepithelial lesions (SIL). Low-grade SIL refers to early changes in the size, shape, and number of cells. Precancerous low-grade lesions may be called mild dysplasia or cervical intraepithelial neoplasia 1 (CIN 1). These changes most often occur in women between 25 and 35 years of age. High-grade SIL refers to a large number of precancerous cells that may be called moderate or severe dysplasia, CIN 2 or 3, or carcinoma in situ. These changes develop most often in women 30 to 40 years of age. Cervical cancer is nearly 100 percent curable, and endometrial cancer is nearly 94 percent curable when detected early. Deaths related to ovarian and uterine cancer, which comprise only 13 percent of the cancers of women, are exceeded only by deaths caused by lung, breast, and colon cancers. On January 1, 1993, the Centers for Disease Control and Prevention added cervical carcinoma to the case definition as one of the AIDS-defining illnesses.

Risk and Protective Factors Women who are at greatest risk for cervical cancer include those who have histories of early and continued sexual activity (with multiple partners); those with genital herpes; those infected with the human papillomavirus (transmitted from the male during intercourse and causing genital warts); those with frequent cervical infections; those who smoke cigarettes; women whose mothers were given DES; and women whose immune system is suppressed (e.g., HIV and organ transplant recipients). Endometrial cancer is most common in women over the age of 50.

The endometrium is the lining of the uterus. Women who are at higher risk for endometrial cancer include those with infertility problems or ovulation failure, family history of endometrial cancer, never having children, estrogen replacement therapy for 2 years without progesterone, or late menopause (after age 50). Women who have a combination of high blood pressure, diabetes, and obesity are also at higher risk. Tamoxifen-induced endometrial cancer tends to be more invasive and aggressive than endometrial cancer caused by any of the factors mentioned above.

Early Detection If a woman has a regular Pap test, most precancerous conditions will be detected and treated before cancer develops. Therefore, most invasive cervical cancers could be prevented. Early warning signs for cervical cancer include dysplasia (precancerous changes in the cells), detected only by the Pap test, and pelvic examination. Precancerous changes usually do not cause pain. Symptoms usually do not occur until the abnormal cells become cancerous and spread to nearby tissue. The most common symptom is abnormal bleeding in the middle of the regular menstrual cycle or after sexual intercourse, douching, or a pelvic exam. Bleeding after menopause and increased vaginal discharge are other symptoms. Only a health care provider can determine whether these changes are due to cancer or another health problem. The Pap test is rarely effective in detecting endometrial cancer. An annual pelvic exam by a health care provider is recommended for women age 40 and over. A biopsy may be required to collect samples of cells from inside the uterus to detect endometrial cancer.

Abnormal bleeding for young women is any change in their regular cycle. Abnormal bleeding for women going through menopause might include a heavier than normal flow or a period that lasts longer or comes sooner than expected. Most often, these symptoms do not indicate cancer but something less serious. Your health care provider should be contacted to diagnose the problem. Early detection is essential! The improved survival rates for women with uterine and cervical cancers reflect early diagnosis more than improved treatment.

Screening During a pelvic exam, a qualified health care provider examines the reproductive organs for possible problems. A visual exam explores for signs of infection or injury. A Pap test is performed to extract cells from the cervix to detect the presence of abnormalities. A Pap smear will detect abnormal cell changes (dysplasia) several years before cervical cancer occurs. Also, the uterus, vagina, fallopian tubes, ovaries, bladder, and rectum are palpated to search for growths or tenderness.

For endometrial cancer, there are no early detection tests or examination recommendations for women without symptoms. Most women are diagnosed due to certain symptoms. These include unusual bleeding or spotting, pelvic pain, a mass in the pelvic area, and weight loss. Women need to report any vaginal bleeding or spotting after menopause (or if they are still menstruating, any bleeding not related to a normal cycle) and pelvic pain to their gynecologist, who then may recommend a cynecologic oncologist, a specialist in treating cancers of the reproductive system. If cancer is suspected, endometrial tissue samples can be removed for observation under a microscope.

All women should begin cervical cancer screening about 3 years after they begin having vaginal intercourse, but no later than age 21. After age 30 and after three normal test results, the screening should be reduced to one screening every two to three years.[38]

Treatment Uterine and endometrial cancers are generally treated by surgery, radiation, hormones, and/or chemotherapy. As yet, the optimal therapy has not been defined. The main treatment for endometrial cancer is removal of the entire uterus, including cervix (hysterectomy), and ovaries and fallopian tubes. If the cancer has spread to the cervix or the parametrium (the connective tissue of the pelvic floor), the surgery may be a radical hysterectomy, the removal of the entire uterus. Hospital stay may be up to 7 days following this procedure. Vaginal hysterectomy, in which instruments are inserted into the vaginal and the uterus is removed through incisions in the vagina, usually requires a hospital stay of only 1 to 2 days and a 2- to 3-week recovery.[39] Lymph nodes near the tumor may be removed to determine if the disease has spread to other parts of the body. Two types of radiation treatment may also be used: external, in which a machine outside the body aims radiation at the tumor site, or internal, in which tiny tubes containing radioactive substances are inserted through the vagina and left in place for several days.

After a hysterectomy, it may take 4 to 8 weeks for a woman to return to normal activities. Sometimes nausea, vomiting, and bladder and/or bowel problems occur after surgery. When the ovaries are removed, menopause with more severe hot flashes and other symptoms than with natural menopause may occur. Health care providers prefer to avoid ERT to alleviate these symptoms because estrogen is a risk factor for uterine cancer. Follow-up checkups may include a physical exam, a pelvic exam, X rays, and lab tests.

The choice of treatment for cervical cancer depends on the location and size of the tumor, the stage, and the woman's age and general health. Because cervical cancer may spread to the bladder, rectum, lymph nodes, or lungs, the health care provider may order a number of tests. Most often, treatment involves surgery and radiation therapy. Chemotherapy and biological therapy (usually interferon) may also be recommended.

Ovarian Cancer

Ovarian cancer is a malignant tumor that begins in the ovaries. Epithelial carcinoma, cancer than begins on the surface of the ovary, is the most common type of ovarian cancer. Other types include germ cell tumors that begin in the egg-producing cells and stromal tumors, cancer that begins in the connective tissue surrounding the ovaries. Ovarian cancer is the seventh most common cancer in women, not including non-melanoma skin cancers. The American Cancer Society estimates that in 2007 there will be 22,430 new cases of ovarian cancer and 15,280 women will die from this cancer, accounting for the fourth leading cause of cancer death in women. This accounts for more deaths than any other cancer of the female reproductive system.[40] The rate of ovarian cancer has been slowly declining since 1991. Only 19 percent of all ovarian cancers are found before they spread outside the ovary. The overall 1-year survival rate for localized, regional, and metastasized ovarian cancers is approximately 76 percent, and the 5-year survival rate is 45 percent. Women over the age of 65 have a lower survival rate than younger women. The 5-year survival rate for ovarian cancer that has not spread outside the ovary is 93 percent.[41]

Risk and Protective Factors The risk factors for ovarian cancer include aging (one-half of all ovarian cancers develop in women over 63 years of age), obesity, a family history of ovarian cancer, a history of irregular menstrual periods, never having children, and previous breast, colon, or endometrial cancer. Current research suggests that women using fertility drugs, such as clomiphene citrate, may increase the risk of ovarian cancer. Other possible risk factors based on mixed research findings include the use of talcum powder and ERT. Talc, applied directly or found on sanitary napkins, has been shown to contribute to a slightly higher risk of ovarian cancer. In the past, talc was contaminated with asbestos, so it is difficult to determine if current use provides the same increased risk. Women who were on ERT longer than 10 years have twice the rate of ovarian cancer. Women are no longer encouraged to use ERT or HRT for an extended period of time.

Inheriting the BRCA1 and BRCA2 genes and several genes related to a hereditary type of colon cancer increases a woman's risk of ovarian cancer. However, most gene mutations occur during a woman's lifetime. Inherited mutations of oncogenes and/or tumor suppressor genes may result from radiation or cancer-causing chemicals. Research on tests to identify p53 tumor suppressor genes or HER2 oncogenes may help in predicting a woman's prognosis.

Pregnancy, breast-feeding, tubal sterilization, and birth control pills appear to *reduce* the risk of ovarian cancer in women.[42] Although no one is sure why oral contraceptives and tubal sterilization reduce the risk of ovarian cancer, reduction in the number of ovulations a woman has appears to be a protective factor.

Early Detection Hypertension is called the "silent killer." For women, ovarian cancer is also a "silent" killer. By the time the signs and symptoms appear, the ovarian cancer is usually in its later stages. Warning signs include a swollen abdomen (caused by fluid retention), abnormal vaginal bleeding, persistent digestive disturbances (indigestion or gas), leg pain, back pain, or long-term stomach pain. The generic nature of these symptoms makes diagnosis difficult.

Screening Transvaginal sonography, CA-125 radioimmunoassay (CA-125 is a tumor marker in the blood), and pelvic examinations are used to screen for ovarian cancer. The amount of protein in the blood is higher in many women who have ovarian cancer. A concern with using these tests for routine screening is the large number of false positives due to insensitivity; thus, screening is contraindicated in most women. Only women with hereditary cancer syndrome and a family history of ovarian cancer might benefit from routine screening.[43] There are currently no tests for germ cell or stromal tumors.

Treatment Ovarian cancer is the leading cause of death from gynecological malignancy in the United States. Since the death of comedian Gilda Radner in 1989, much attention and resources have gone into addressing this disease. Treatment options include surgery, radiation therapy, and drug therapy. Chemotherapy, using a variety of drugs, can be given by injection, by infusion, or by mouth. Caution with these powerful drugs is important because, along with killing cancer cells, the drugs will damage healthy body cells, including blood-producing cells of the bone marrow. Radiation therapy kills cancer cells with the use of high-energy X rays. It can be administrated by an external beam, which is similar to an X ray aimed directly on the area of the cancer. A type of monoclonal antibody therapy using the drug called trastuzumab (Herceptin) has been developed to interrupt growth-promoting action of the HER2 oncogene. Treatment with Herceptin has been approved for hormonal-related breast cancer, but clinical trials are still ongoing to determine its effectiveness with certain ovarian cancers. Biologic therapy, also called immunotherapy, is a treatment using the patient's immune system to fight cancer. Substances made by the body or in a lab are used to boost, direct, or restore the body's natural defenses against cancer. High-dose chemotherapy with stem cell transplant is being used not only to destroy cancer cells that have metastasized, but also to boost the body's own immune system. Stem cells are removed from the bone marrow of the patient, or a donor, and stored. Following chemotherapy, the stored stem cells are given back to the patient through an infusion in order to restore the body's blood cells.[44]

Skin Cancer

Skin cancer is the most prevalent and most curable type of cancer found in women. Each year, over 1 million persons (males and females) are diagnosed with basal and squamous cell skin cancer, and most, but not all, of these forms of skin cancer are highly curable.[45] Basal cell carcinomas are the most common type of malignancy in humans. They are usually raised, hard, reddish lesions with a pearly surface and rarely metastasize. Squamous cell carcinoma is most frequently found on the skin, but it is also located in the epithelium of the lungs, anus, cervix, larynx, nose, and bladder. These carcinomas are typically scaly and slightly elevated. They are a relatively slow-growing malignancy and the majority are localized, but a very small percentage can spread to other parts of the body.

Malignant **melanoma** is less common than other types of skin cancer but more dangerous. An estimated 26,030 women will be diagnosed with melanoma in 2007 and 2,890 will die.[46] Melanoma begins in melanocytes, the cells responsible for producing melanin. Melanin turns darker when exposed to sunlight, thus producing a suntan to protect the body from burning. Melanoma is ten times more prevalent in white women than in African American women.[47] It is usually found on the lower legs of white women and on the palms, skin under the nails, and soles of the feet of African American women. Skin cancers are the most frequent secondary lesions in patients with cancers in other sites.

Risk and Protective Factors Severe sunburning during early childhood and excessive exposure to sunlight during adolescence are known risk factors for skin cancer. Other risk factors include fair or lightly pigmented skin, occupational exposure to some products, and family history. The best protective factors to prevent skin cancer are adequate clothing, use of a proper sunscreen with solar protection (SPF 15 or higher), and limiting one's exposure to the sun (avoiding midday sun). Sunscreen should be applied at least 15 to 30 minutes before going in the sun, and applied frequently. Ninety percent of skin cancers occur on the parts of the body exposed most to the sun, such as the face, hands, forearms, and ears.

The National Weather Bureau, in cooperation with the Environmental Protection Agency and the Centers for Disease Control and Prevention, provides sun tanners with an Ultraviolet Index to determine the amount of safe time in the sun. The UV Index is a forecast of the peak amount of UV radiation to reach the earth's surface in a given location when the sun is at its highest peak, during the solar noon hour, from 30 minutes before and after 12 noon. Safeguards under the moderate range of the UV Index include minimizing exposure during peak times, using sunscreens of SPF 15 or higher, wearing clothing to cover the body, and wearing hats to shade the face and neck. (See *FYI:* "Ultraviolet [UV] Index.")

Early Detection To detect skin cancer, a woman needs to know how to recognize changes in skin and appearance of new skin growths. Basal cell cancers first appear as white or gray, small round or oval patches on the skin that are shiny and firm. Squamous cell cancers appear as small, round, and raised areas that are red and crusty.

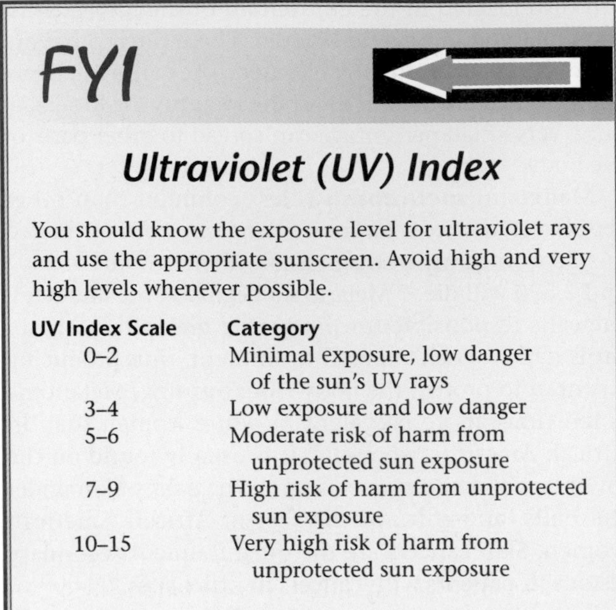

FYI

Ultraviolet (UV) Index

You should know the exposure level for ultraviolet rays and use the appropriate sunscreen. Avoid high and very high levels whenever possible.

UV Index Scale	Category
0–2	Minimal exposure, low danger of the sun's UV rays
3–4	Low exposure and low danger
5–6	Moderate risk of harm from unprotected sun exposure
7–9	High risk of harm from unprotected sun exposure
10–15	Very high risk of harm from unprotected sun exposure

A sore that won't heal may appear in the middle of a squamous cell cancer. The American Cancer Society recommends using the simple ABCD method as warning signs for the common type of melanoma: A is for *asymmetry*, where one part of the mole doesn't match the other part; B is for border *irregularity* such as ragged or notched edges; C is for color, where the *pigmentation*, or color, is not the same throughout the mole; and D is for *diameter* greater than 6 millimeters, or the size of a pencil eraser.[48]

Screening The best way to become familiar with your skin is to examine it regularly, every 6 to 8 weeks. If a health care provider thinks you may have skin cancer, a biopsy (a small sample of tissue) will be taken from the area.

Treatment Basal and squamous cell cancers are removed by several methods: surgical excision, electrodessication and curettage (electric current to destroy cancerous tissue and scraping to remove it), cryosurgery (freezing the affected tissue), or radiation therapy.[49] With malignant melanoma, the primary growth and surrounding lymph cells must be removed. When melanoma is at an advanced state, treatment will include immunotherapy or chemotherapy.[50]

Tanning Beds Most modern tanning beds emit predominantly UVA radiation, with small amounts of UVB. UVB rays are the harmful rays emitted by the sun, and they are becoming more of a hazard because of reduction in ozone layers. Tanning-salon operators point out that UVA rays are not harmful. They suggest that you should be concerned only with UVB rays. They use this difference as a selling point for the safety of tanning beds. They equate a suntan with good health. However, research demonstrates that exposure to UVA radiation leads to increased skin wrinkling, irregular pigmentation (including deeply pigmented freckles), and suppression of the immune system. And tanning by exposure to UVA rays does not prepare you for exposure to the UVB rays of the sun. Thus, tanning indoors before spring break does *not* prevent a sunburn. The best way to avoid premature wrinkling and aging of the skin and to prevent skin cancer is to stay away from tanning beds and out of the sun.

Colon and Rectal Cancer

The colon and rectum, together, form the large intestine (large bowel). The first 5 to 6 feet of the colon are the large intestine and the last 8 to 10 inches are the rectum. Cancer that affects both of these organs can be called colorectal cancer. In 2007, an estimated 74,630 new cases of colon and rectal cancer will be diagnosed in women and 26,180 women are estimated to die from the disease.[51]

Risk and Protective Factors Risk factors include a personal or family history of colorectal cancer, polyps in the colon, or ulcerative colitis. Polyps, masses of tissue that grow inward from the wall of the bowel, are known precursors to colorectal cancer. High-fat and low-fiber diets, physical inactivity, and low intake of fruits and vegetables are possible risk factors.[52] Although colorectal cancer is more common in adults over age 50, it can affect young adults and teens in rare instances. Familial polyposis, a rare inherited disease of hundreds of polyps, must be treated as it almost always leads to colorectal cancer. Women with a history of cancer of the ovary, uterus, or breast have an increased risk of colorectal cancer, as do women with a previous diagnosis of colorectal cancer. If numerous family members have had colorectal cancer, a woman's risk increases. Ulcerative colitis also increases a woman's risk of colorectal cancer.

Early Detection Five simple tests can be used to detect colorectal cancer: (1) fecal occult blood test (FOBT), (2) digital rectal examination by your health care provider, (3) sigmoidoscopy examination, (4) colonoscopy, or (5) a double-contrast barium enema (DCBE). The FOBT checks the stool for hidden blood, a possible sign of cancer or other problems in the colon. A woman prepares a special slide and gives it to her health care provider. A digital rectal examination, performed by a physician, determines the presence of a tumor. A fiber-optic sigmoidoscope (a flexible, hollow, lighted tube) is used to examine the rectum and lower colon. A colonoscopy examines the rectum and entire colon using a colonoscope. A DCBE is a series of X rays of the colon and rectum.

If a woman experiences any of the following, she should consult her health care provider immediately: a persistent change in bowel habits, diarrhea, constipation, feeling that the bowel does not empty completely, blood (bright red or very dark) in the stool, stools that are narrower than usual, general abdominal discomfort, unexplained weight loss, constant tiredness, or vomiting. Early detection of cancer when it is still in the polyp stage in polyps reduces the likelihood of metastasis to other body sites or the need for major surgery or a colostomy, an insertion in the abdomen for the elimination of body wastes.

Screening The American Cancer Society (ACS) has set the following guidelines for colon and rectal cancer detection for any woman without symptoms. A digital rectal examination is recommended for women every year after age 40. By age 50, the ACS recommends that women, as well as men, begin screening with one of the following examination schedules: (1) a fecal occult blood test (FOBT) or fecal immunochemical test (FIT) each year; (2) a flexible sigmoidoscopy (FSIG) every 5 years; (3) an FOBT or FIT each year and FSIG every 5 years; (4) a double-contrast barium enema every 5 years; (5) a colonoscopy every 10 years. Women who are at a moderate to high risk for colorectal cancer may have a different testing schedule.

Treatment There are three main types of treatment for colon and rectal cancers: surgery, which is the most common treatment; radiation; and chemotheapy.[53] If colorectal cancer is found, surgery with a possible follow-up of radiation therapy will occur. Chemotherapy may be effective after surgery in certain colon cancers if the tumor has penetrated the bowel wall. A new chemotherapy to combat colorectal cancer that has metastasized includes the drugs Oxaliplatin and 5-FU (fluorouracil) followed by leucovorin, which is given to prevent or treat toxicities of certain types of medication. Two new targeted therapies to treat metastatic colorectal cancer are Avastin, which blocks the growth of blood vessels to the cancer, and Erbitux, which blocks the effects of hormone-like substances that promote cancer growth.[54] Many women are afraid that colorectal cancer means living with a colostomy; however, the American Cancer Society states that it is rare that a permanent colostomy is needed even if the tumor can't be removed.[55] Thus, the fear of colostomies should not be a deterrent to early diagnosis.

Health Tips: "Protective Factors to Fight against Cancer" suggests ways to reduce your risk of cancer.

Health Tips

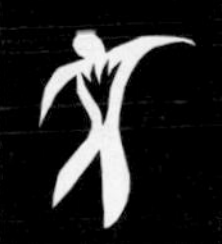

Protective Factors to Fight against Cancer

You can practice these protective factors to reduce your risk of cancer:

- Do not smoke.
- Live with a nonsmoker.
- Avoid smoke-filled areas.
- Maintain your desirable weight.
- Eat a wide variety of foods.
- Eat in moderation.
- Consume fresh fruits and vegetables daily (five servings daily).
- Eat plenty of high-fiber foods.
- Limit fat intake (under 20 percent of total calories).
- Limit alcohol consumption.
- Consume little or no salt-cured, smoked, or nitrite-cured foods.
- Limit exposure to sunlight.
- Limit exposure to industrial agents, asbestos, and radon.
- Limit exposure to both UV radiation and radiation from X rays.
- If you are 20 to 39 years old, get a cancer-related checkup every 3 years.
- If you are 40 years or older, get a cancer-related checkup annually.
- If you are 18 years or older, have an annual Pap test and pelvic exam.
- Practice monthly breast self-examination.

ACTIONS TO TAKE WHEN CANCER IS DIAGNOSED

When the diagnosis of cancer occurs, a common reaction is to feel like life is out of control. A woman can take a number of steps toward regaining control over her life. First, get more information about the particular cancer. As stated earlier, there are over a hundred different cancers, and each primary site could be one of several different kinds of cancers. Once a woman knows the type of cancer, she can call the National Cancer Institute (1-800-4 CANCER) or the American Cancer Society for more information. NCI provides booklets explaining the cancer, names of oncologists in the area, sites of clinical trials, and PDQ statements regarding the latest treatments.

Second, get a second opinion before deciding on a particular treatment protocol. Seeking confirmation is reasonable and common. The second oncologist should be informed about the initial diagnosis. She or he will likely be more direct and straightforward with recommendations, particularly because an expert opinion is being solicited rather than a request for involvement in the patient's progress.

Third, a woman should feel certain about her options. Any questions and responses that are not fully understood should be addressed. If an NCI-designated comprehensive or clinical cancer center is nearby, choose it. The specialists at these centers are most familiar with current treatment protocols and any recent research developments. The primary health care provider and surgeon should be board certified in cancer care, such as an oncologist or an oncology surgeon.

SOCIAL SUPPORT

Social support is a critical factor in recovery from a stressful event such as cancer. Support from family and friends plays a major role in the speed and level of recovery. Unfortunately, women with cancer seem to lose the level of support they enjoyed before the diagnosis of cancer. The fear of cancer causes some people to avoid contact with anyone or anything that reminds them of it. Cancer, compared to other chronic diseases, is a stigmatized condition. In fact, many people still believe that the diagnosis of cancer is a death sentence, and some may even believe cancer is contagious. Cancer support groups provide a confidential environment where patients and their families can discuss all aspects of the disease, such as managing side effects, sharing their feelings, and work-related concerns.[56]

Women who have undergone a modified radical mastectomy report that their most common concerns are the inability to engage in vigorous physical activity, the fear that the cancer will return, and resentment or worry regarding the quality of care received.[57] Women with chronic diseases such as heart disease feel some control over their destiny, such as when they can modify their diet and increase their physical activity level. This control provides them with a sense of doing something to improve their chance of survival. However, women living with cancer do not have the same opportunity to exhibit control.

The treatment for cancer may preclude women from continuing to engage in social activities. They may not have the same energy level as before and may focus their efforts on necessary tasks such as work and family. Outside activities may need to be curtailed during their period of recovery, and social contacts may be lost or less frequent. Cancer survivors who reported energy losses due to treatment also indicated a reduction in discretionary activities and social network size.[58] These reductions may lead to lower levels of emotional and physical support at a time when support is most needed. The American Cancer Society has recognized this need for support and provides several services for women and their families including the following: *Cancer Survivors Network,* an online community where persons with cancer can connect with other persons with cancer; *I Can Cope,* educational classes presented by health care personnel that provide practical knowledge and skills to help cancer patients cope with the disease; *Road to Recovery,* a program that provides transportation to get patients to and from treatment; *Reach to Recovery,* a program of breast cancer survivors who help women and their families deal with breast cancer; and *Look Good . . . Feel Good,* a service to help women deal with personal appearance during chemotherapy and radiation treatments.[59]

COMPLEMENTARY AND ALTERNATIVE TREATMENT IN CANCER MANAGEMENT

This chapter would not be complete without mention of the complementary and alternative therapies used to treat or cope with cancer. When medical therapies do not appear to provide the wanted results (whether by perception or in actuality), women often turn to complementary treatments to supplement the medical therapy. They have read about successes in popular magazines or heard about miracles from friends and family. The American Cancer Society continually reviews current practices, attempting to determine the benefit in the treatment of cancer in human beings. An explanation of a few complementary therapies follows. If you want information regarding the research on these and other therapies, check with the American Cancer Society or the National Institutes of Health for the most current findings.

Magnetic and Electronic Devices

Magnetic and electronic devices use cosmic rays, gamma rays, X rays, light waves, radio waves, and others to cure or slow the progression of cancer. Individuals using electronic devices in complementary therapies appeal to the balancing of life forces, the energy in the body.

Conventional therapies also use a variety of electronic devices, except these procedures have been accepted by the medical community. These devices are used for radiation therapy, magnetic resonance imaging, diagnostic X rays, and other therapies.

Radionic Devices Radionics theorize that radio-like frequencies emitted from pathogens can be used to diagnose and treat diseases. The first radionic device was called the Oscilloclast, which detected diseases by their vibratory rates. Many of the radionic devices used in cancer treatment today are imitations of this model.

Galvanic Devices Galvanic devices are being used by "Energy Medicine," a field using electrodes placed at acupuncture points to measure electrical resistance. Galvanic devices actually measure electrical resistance on the skin and can be influenced by skin moisture and the amount of pressure with which the probe is applied.

Low-Level Output Electrical Devices Low-level output electrical devices are used by some practitioners to treat cancer by passing currents through tumors or to actually diagnose cancer. Scientific experimentation using this procedure with cancer treatment is currently being conducted, and these legitimate experimental protocols are registered with the FDA. Fraudulent claims continue to surface with the FDA obtaining injunctions when possible.

Magnetic Devices Many makers of some permanent magnetic devices have been prosecuted by the FDA for false advertising. Electromagnetic devices differ in that they need a power source to activate the magnetism. These devices have not been proven to be effective in cancer treatment.

Color and Light Treatment Devices This therapy theorizes that shining colored light on the body can cure cancer. The FDA secured a permanent injunction against the use of spectrachrome devices, but they still find their way into some practitioners' offices. The use of full spectrum fluorescent light to prevent cancer has been proposed by some practitioners; however, full-spectrum light treatment includes UVB light, a known carcinogen for skin cancer.

Food Remedies

Vegetarian Diets A wide array of vegetarian diets have been tried by women with cancer in an effort to slow the progression of the disease. Vegetarians do not eat meat, fish, or poultry, but some will eat products with animal by-products. Vegans consume only foods with plant origin, whereas lacto-vegetarians consume foods with plant origin and dairy products. The Zen macrobiotic diet emphasizes cereals, such as rice. It is a low-fat, complex carbohydrate diet with no animal products, no refined sugar, and limited fluids. Miso, a soybean product believed to prevent cancer, is a staple of this diet.

Herbal and Vitamin Therapy An array of complementary treatments have been touted, including megavitamin therapy, enzyme therapy, shiitake mushrooms, shark cartilage, Essiac herbs, wheatgrass, coffee enemas, and others. Hoxsey therapy, a special herbal tonic, evolved when a farmer decided to collect herbs that had healed his cancerous horse. This therapy was banned by the FDA in 1960, but it is still available in Mexico. Shark cartilage therapy evolved because sharks are believed to seldom get cancer. Thus, proponents suggest that shark cartilage should be tested for its cancer-inhibiting ability. In 1970 Linus Pauling, a 1954 Nobel Prize–winning chemist, championed the use of vitamin C to treat a number of ailments, including cancer, flu,and cardiovascular disease. He recommended megadoses of vitamin C and suggested that current RDAs were much too low.

Spiritual and Meditation Practices

Relaxation A variety of relaxation techniques have been touted as beneficial for women with cancer, not so much as cures but rather as adjuvant therapy. Creative visualization, affirmations, biofeedback, self-hypnosis, humor, art and music therapy, and meditation were discussed in Chapter 5.

Acupuncture and Acupressure Acupuncture is an ancient Chinese form of healing that posits that all matter contains Yin/Yang energy. The balancing of life force (qi or "chee") must be maintained for harmony and health, and disease occurs when qi is blocked or flows unevenly. To rebalance qi, fine needles are placed in precisely determined sites to stimulate nerve impulses. These needles are manipulated to increase or decrease the flow of qi. Acupressure treats the whole body by using pressure points to stimulate the harmony of life forces. The points for these techniques are located along twelve meridians, related to the internal organs. Diseases can be diagnosed and cured by addressing the specific points on the meridians. Chapter 5 also discusses acupressure, providing further information regarding this technique. Now complete *Journal Activity:* "Complementary Cancer Therapy."

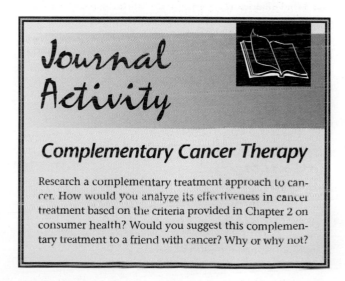

CHOOSING A TREATMENT PLAN

A woman diagnosed with cancer or a recurrence of cancer faces a myriad of decisions, including the choice of medical and complementary treatments. Complementary methods have been touted by too many individuals to be dismissed, yet grasping at straws does not provide a sense of control. Knowledge and accurate evaluation of the effectiveness of conventional therapy and alternative treatment protocols are the best methods to begin recapturing control. The first step for any woman is to focus on those things most within her control, including becoming more familiar with the treatment options available to her. Deciding whether to follow conventional therapy alone, or a combination of conventional and complementary/alternative therapies, depends on an accurate diagnosis by an oncologist and a clear picture of the prognosis for that particular type of cancer. A woman needs to be involved in the process of decision making throughout the treatment and recovery phase. Remember: Early detection is important to your well-being!

Chapter Summary

- Half of all cancers affecting women are cancers of the reproductive system.
- There are significant differences in benign and malignant tumors.
- The World Health Organization has identified forty-six body sites and numerous cancers at each site, over a hundred different cancers.
- The American Cancer Society has identified seven major warning signs of cancer.
- Lifestyle and environmental factors account for most cancer risks.
- The amount of fat a person consumes is a risk factor for some cancers.
- Cigarette smoking accounts for 85 percent of all lung cancer deaths and 30 percent of all cancer deaths.
- Lung cancer is the leading cause of cancer deaths in women.
- Breast cancer is the most prevalent type of cancer in women.
- If a woman has a diagnosis of cancer, she should get information about the cancer, get a second opinion from another physician, learn about all the treatment options for her type of cancer, and seek a support group to help her through the treatment and recovery.
- Screening mammography complemented by monthly breast self-examinations and clinical breast examinations are the best methods for early detection of breast cancer.
- Cervical and endometrial cancer are extremely curable if detected early.
- Skin cancer is the most prevalent and most curable type of cancer found in women.
- Melanoma can be detected by attention to asymmetry, border irregularity, color change, and diameter greater than 6 mm.
- Tanning beds emit UVA rays that contribute to skin wrinkling, irregular pigmentation, and immunosuppression.
- Social support is a critical factor in recovering from cancer.
- Many women explore complementary therapies as an adjunct to conventional health care.

Review Questions

1. What are the seven warning signs of cancer?
2. What are the definitions for the following terms: benign, malignant, metastasis, in situ, and invasive?
3. What are the four most common categories of cancer?
4. What are some of the lifestyle and environmental causes of cancer?
5. What are the leading cancer sites in women based on race and ethnicity?
6. What are the early signs and symptoms for each of the following cancers: lung, breast, uterine, and ovarian?
7. What are the five best preventive measures a woman can practice to reduce the risk of cancer? What criteria did you use to determine these choices?
8. Explain all treatment options for a woman who has been diagnosed with cancer.
9. What are the newer medications that are used for treatment of cancer?
10. What are some of the complementary therapies a woman might select to supplement conventional therapy?

Resources

Web Sites

American Cancer Society
800-ACS-2345
www.cancer.org/docroot/home/index.asp

American Institute for Cancer Research
www.aicr.org

Center for Complementary and Alternative Medicine
www.nccam.nih.gov

Corporate Angel Network, Inc.
914-328-1313
www.corpangelnetwork.org

Gilda's Club Worldwide
www.gildasclub.org
Intercultural Cancer Council
www.icc.bcm.tmc.edu
Mayo Clinic
www.mayoclinic.com
Memorial Sloan-Kettering Cancer Center
www.mskcc.org
National Breast Cancer Coalition (NBCC)
www.stopbreastcancer.org
National Cancer Institute
www.cancer.gov
NOAH: New York Online Access to Health
www.noah-health.org
Ovarian Cancer National Alliance (OCNA)
www.ovariancancer.org
Sisters Network, Inc.
www.sistersnetworkinc.org
The Susan G. Komen Breast Cancer Foundation
www.breastcancerinfo.com
Y-ME National Breast Cancer Organization, Inc.
www.y-me.org

Suggested Readings

Anastasia, P. J., F. J. Montz, and R. E. Bristow. 2005. *A Guide to Survivorship for Women with Ovarian Cancer.* Baltimore, MD: Johns Hopkins University Press.

Conner, K., and L. Langford. 2003. *Ovarian Cancer: A Guide for Women and Those Who Care about Them.* Sebastopol, CA: O'Reilly and Associates.

Delinsky, B. 2003. *Uplift: Secrets from the Sisterhood of Breast Cancer Survivors.* New York: Pocket.

Finkel, M. L. 2006. *Understanding the Mammography Controversy: Science, Politics, and Breast Cancer Screening.* Westport, CT: Praeger Publishers.

Goldberg, B. A., and M. A. Goldberg. 2002. *Alternative Medicine: The Definitive Guide.* Berkeley, CA: Ten Speed Press.

Love, S. M. 2005. *Dr. Susan Love's Breast Book.* 4th ed. Cambridge Press: DaCapo Publishers.

Lynn, C., L. C., Hartmann, C. L. Loprinzi, and B. S. Gostout, 2005. *Mayo Clinic: Guide to Women's Cancer.* Rochester, MN: Mayo Clinic Health Information.

Mayer, M. 2003. *After Breast Cancer: Answers to the Questions You're Afraid to Ask.* Sebastopol, CA: O'Reilly and Associates.

Olson, J. S. 2002. *Bathsheba's Breast: Women, Cancer & History.* Baltimore, MD: Johns Hopkins University Press.

Thompson, J. 2006. *Dear God, They Say It's Cancer: A Companion Guide for Women on the Breast Cancer Journey.* New York: Simon & Schuster.

Videotapes/DVDs

Titles from: Films for the Humanities & Sciences, P.O. Box 2053, Princeton, NJ 08543-2053, 1-800-257-5126, www.films.com

Breast Cancer: Prevention & Treatment, 2001
Cancer Self Defense, 2002
Early Breast Cancer: With Knowledge Comes Hope, 2003
Top Ten Cancer Myths, 2003

References

1. American Cancer Society. 2006. *Cancer facts and figures 2006.* Atlanta: American Cancer Society, p. 10.
2. Ibid., p. 4.
3. Ibid.
4. National Cancer Institute. 2004. *Staging: Questions and answers.* www.cancer.gov/cancertopics/factsheet/Detection/staging (retrieved October 2, 2006).
5. Ibid.
6. U.S. Department of Health and Human Services. 2004. *Women, tobacco, and cancer: An agenda for the 21st century.* Rockville, MD: U.S. Department of Health and Human Services, National Institutes of Health, National Cancer Institutes, p. 5.
7. American Cancer Society, *Cancer facts and figures 2006,* pp. 36–37.
8. Ibid., p. 42.
9. Ibid., p. 43.
10. Ibid., p. 21.
11. Ibid., p. 19.
12. Ibid.
13. Hartwell, L. H., and M. B. Kastan. 1994. Cell cycle control and cancer. *Science* 266:1821–27.
14. Wong, C. F., A. Guminski, N. A. Saunders, and A. J. Burgess. 2005. Exploiting novel cell cycle targets in the development of anticancer agents. *Current Cancer Drug Targets* 5 (2): 85–102.
15. American Cancer Society. 1994. *Cancer facts and figures 1994.* Atlanta, GA: American Cancer Society.
16. Karp, J. E., and S. Broder. 1994. Oncology and hematology. *Journal of the American Medical Association* 271:1693.
17. Easton, D. F., T. Bishop, D. Ford, and B. P. Crockford. 1993. Breast cancer linkage consortium. *American Journal of Human Genetics* 52:678.
18. Dukehealth.org. 2006. *Enzyme that digests DNA linked to increased genetic mutations, cancer susceptibility.* www.dukehealth.org/news/9452?from=RSS (retrieved October 2, 2006).
19. Toguchida, J., et al. 1992. Prevalence and spectrum of germlike mutations of the p53 gene among patients with sarcoma. *New England Journal of Medicine* 326:1301.
20. American Cancer Society. 2001. *A new century of cancer research is dawning.* www.cancer.org/docroot/NWS/content/NWS_1_1x_A_New_Century_of_Cancer_Research_is_Dawning.asp (retrieved October 3, 2006).
21. U.S. Department of Health and Human Services. 2005. *What you need to know about cancer.* NIH Publication No. 05-1566.
22. American Cancer Society, *Cancer facts and figures,* 2006, p. 4
23. American Cancer Society, *Cancer facts and figures 1994.*
24. McDougall, J. C. 1994. Lung cancer: To screen or not to screen? *Archives of Internal Medicine* 154:945; Flehinger, B. J., M. Kimmell, T. Polyak, and M. R. Melamed. 1993.

Screening for lung cancer: The Mayo Lung Project revisited. *Cancer* 72:1573.

25. American Cancer Society, *Cancer facts and figures 2006,* p. 14.
26. Ibid., p. 14–15.
27. MayoClinic.com. 2005. *Lung cancer.* www.mayoclinic.com/health/lung-cancer/DS00038 (retrieved October 2, 2006).
28. Ibid.
29. American Cancer Society, *Cancer facts and figures 2007*, p. 9.
30. Ibid., p. 10.
31. American Cancer Society. 2005. *Breast cancer facts and figures, 2005–2006.* www.cancer.org/downloads/STT/CAFF2005BrF.pdf (retrieved October 2, 2006).
32. Collaborative Group on Hormonal Factors in Breast Cancer. 2002. Breast cancer and breastfeeding: Collaborative re-analyses of individual data from 47 epidemiological studies in 30 countries, including 50,302 women with breast cancer and 96,973 women without the disease. *Lancet* 360:187–95.
33. American Cancer Society. 2006. *Breast cancer.* http://documents.cancer.org/104.00/104.00.pdf (retrieved October 2, 2006).
34. Ibid., p. 10.
35. Ibid., p. 15.
36. American Cancer Society, *Breast cancer*, pp. 40–41.
37. Susan G. Komen Breast Foundation. 2005. *Breast reconstruction and prosthesis.* www.komen.org (retrieved October 2, 2006).
38. American Cancer Society. 2005. *Endometrial (uterine) cancer.* www.cancer.org (retrieved October 2, 2006).
39. Ibid., pp. 14–15.
40. American Cancer Society. 2007. *Ovarian cancer*, p. 10. www.cancer.org (retrieved April 21, 2007).
41. Ibid., p. 16.
42. Ibid., pp. 8–9.
43. Ibid., p. 11.
44. National Cancer Institute. 2005. *Ovarian epithelian cancer (PDQ): Treatment patient version.* www.cancer.gov/cancertopics/pdq/treatment/ovarianepithelial/Patient (retrieved October 2, 2006).
45. American Cancer Society, *Cancer facts and figures 2007,* p.19.
46. Ibid., p. 4.
47. Ibid., p 19.
48. American Cancer Society. 2005. *Skin cancer prevention and early detection.* www.cancer.org/docroot/PED/content/ped_7_1_Skin_Cancer_Detection_What_You_Can_Do.asp? (retrieved October 2, 2006).
49. American Cancer Society, *Cancer facts and figures 2007,* p. 19.
50. Ibid.
51. Ibid., p. 4.
52. Ibid., p. 12.
53. Ibid.
54. American Cancer Society, *Cancer facts and figures 2007,* p. 12.
55. Ibid.
56. National Cancer Institute. 2002. *Cancer support groups: Questions and answers.* www.cancer.gov/cancertopics/factsheet/support/support-groups (retrieved October 2, 2006).
57. Zemore, R., J. Rinholm, L. Shepel, and M. Richards. 1990. Some social and emotional consequences of breast cancer and mastectomy: A content analysis of 87 interviews. *Journal of Psychosocial Oncology* 7:33–45.
58. Bloom, J. R., and L. Kessler. 1994. Emotional support following cancer: A test of the stigma and social activity hypotheses. *Journal of Health and Social Behavior* 35:118–33.
59. American Cancer Society, *Cancer facts and figures 2006,* p. 48.

Glossary

A

abortion—The termination of a pregnancy at any time before the fetus is capable of living outside the uterine cavity.

acquaintance rape—Sexual assault of a woman by a man she knows.

acquaintance violence—Violence or abuse committed by a parent, relative, coworker, neighbor, or friend.

acquired immune deficiency syndrome (AIDS)—All HIV-infected persons with less than 200 CD4+ T-lymphocytes/μL or a CD4+ percentage of less than 14.

acupressure—A relaxing natural therapy that teaches the body to identify and release patterns of holding tension.

acupuncture—Related to acupressure; utilizes fine needles inserted into acupressure points to stimulate relaxation and healing.

addiction—Compulsive, uncontrollable dependence on a substance, habit, or practice; withdrawal causes several mental, emotional, and physiological reactions.

adjuvant therapy—Treatment with substances that enhance the action of drugs to help the body produce antibodies.

adrenal glands—Located on top of the kidney and secrete corticoids.

adrenocorticotropic hormone (ACTH)—A hormone that stimulates the adrenal glands.

aerobic activity—Physical activities that require the heart and lungs to supply the increased demand of oxygen throughout the body.

agape love—A selfless and unconditional relationship between partners.

alcohol dehydrogenase (ADH)—An enzyme in the liver that metabolizes almost all of the alcohol consumed by an individual.

alcoholism—A chronic, progressive, and potentially fatal disease characterized by tolerance and physical and psychological dependence on alcohol.

alternative medicine—A method used in place of conventional medicine.

altruistic love—A relationship that places a partner's needs above one's own needs.

alveoli—Thin, saclike structures in the lungs in which gas exchange takes place between oxygen and blood.

Alzheimer's disease (AD)—A common dementia characterized by a gradual, progressive loss of brain cells.

amenorrhea—Absence of a monthly menstrual flow.

amnion—The membranes that contain the waters that surround the fetus in the uterus.

androgyny—Possessing a high number of attributes defined as masculine and a high number of attributes defined as feminine.

angina—Cluster of symptoms associated with oxygen deprivation.

angioplasty—Procedure that widens a narrow artery.

anorexia nervosa—Starving oneself, sometimes even to death, because of a personal belief that one is unattractive or unlovable.

anorgasmia—Condition resulting in the inability to experience orgasm; also called orgasmic dysfunction.

anterior cruciate ligament (ACL)—Support structure of the knee that can be injured due to contact with an object or when the leg is planted and then turned in another direction.

antioxidants—Compounds that reduce the destructive capacity of oxidizing compounds.

arteries—Blood vessels that carry oxygenated blood to the body and the heart.

arthritis—An inflammatory condition of the joints characterized by pain and swelling.

artificial insemination (AI)—Placing semen in the vagina or uterus by mechanical means rather than intercourse.

assertiveness—Standing up for personal rights and expressing oneself in direct, honest, and appropriate ways that do not violate another person's rights.

assertiveness training—One of the most common professional improvement programs currently offered; teaches the differences between assertive, aggressive, and nonassertive behavior and increase experience in applying reasonable assertive behavior.

assisted reproductive technology (ART)—Procedures used by infertile couples to achieve pregnancy.

atherosclerosis—Common disorder of arteries caused by a complicated process of injury to the vessel walls and buildup of fatty deposits.

atrial fibrillation—The most common heart rhythm abnormality.

autogenic phrases—Self-statements designed to calm the body and the mind.

autoinoculation—Self-spread of a disease from one part of the body to another.

autologous—Here, using one's own bone marrow for transplant.

autonomic nervous system(ANS)—Activated by the posterior section of your hypothalamus; excites and inhibits various bodily functions; stimulates motor functions, blood sugar production, and inhibitory functions.

autonomy—Maintaining an individual identity and self-direction.

avoidance addict—An unhealthy pattern of maintaining emotional distance from a partner to mask fear of intimacy.

B

ballistic stretching—Stretching a muscle by repeated bouncing, jerking, or swinging.

basal body temperature method—Natural family planning method that relies on monitoring decreases and increases in basal body temperature during the menstrual cycle.

basal metabolic rate—The minimum amount of energy expended to keep a resting person alive.

behavior change contract—A written agreement in a behavior change program that includes long-range and intermediate goals, target dates for completion, rewards, intervention strategies, and witnesses to the agreement.

benign—Not cancerous; harmless.

binge drinking—Consuming four or more drinks in a row for women (five or more for men).

binge eating disorder—Involves binge eating but not purging (vomiting and laxative abuse) afterward.

bioavailability—Rate and extent to which the active ingredient is absorbed from a drug product and becomes available at the site of action.

biofeedback—The use of electronic equipment to monitor the physiological state of the body while the individual learns techniques to voluntarily regulate the body's systems and reduce unwanted symptoms.

biopsy—Surgical removal of tissue for microscopic examination and diagnosis.

bipolar disorder—mixture of major depressive episodes and manic episodes.

birth control—Umbrella term for all the strategies used to prevent childbirth, including contraception.

blastocyst—A cluster of embryonic cells; the stage of development between the zygote and embryo.

body composition—The amount of lean and fat tissue in the body.

body dysmorphic disorder (BDD)—The classification of body-image disturbance reserved for the non–eating disorder population.

body mass index (BMI)—Numerical expression of body weight based on height (expressed in meters) to weight (expressed in kilograms) to help determine healthy body weight.

brand name—Patented name given to a drug by the manufacturer that developed the drug.

Braxton Hicks—Contractions or irregular tightening of the uterus during pregnancy, sometimes called false labor.

breast augmentation—Surgical method to increase the size of the breast by implanting synthetic materials into the chest wall behind the breast tissue.

breast reduction surgery—Surgery performed to reduce the size of the breasts.

bulimia nervosa—Eating and then vomiting soon afterward or using a laxative in order to avoid weight gain.

C

caffeinism—Chronic consumption of high levels of caffeine.

calipers—A device that measures the thickness of skin-folds taken at different sites on the body; the data are used to determine an individual's percent body fat.

capillaries—Blood vessels with thin membranes that allow for the exchange of carbon dioxide and waste by-products for oxygen and food.

carcinogenic—The ability to cause the development of cancer.

carcinogens—Substances that can cause the growth of cancer.

cardiorespiratory endurance—The ability to perform physical activities for long periods of time while oxygen is supplied to various tissues of the body.

cardiovascular system—Body system that includes the heart and blood vessels.

caveat emptor—Let the buyer beware; opposite of *caveat vendor,* or let the seller beware.

cervical cap—Small rubber cup fitted over the narrow lower end of the uterus to prevent sperm from entering the cervical canal.

cervical shield (Lea's shield)—A silicone cup with an air valve that fits tightly over the cervix to prevent sperm from entering the cervical canal; comes in one size.

cervicitis—Acute or chronic inflammation of the uterine cervix.

cervix—Part of the uterus that protrudes into the vaginal opening.

chemical name—The name that describes the molecular structure of a drug.

chemotherapy—Use of drugs to treat disease, most often cancer.

childhood abuse—Physical or mental injury, sexual abuse or exploitation, negligent treatment, or maltreatment of a child before age 18, by a person who is responsible for the child's welfare.

chlamydia—The most common sexually transmitted infection found in U.S. women; caused by microorganisms that live as parasites within cells.

cilia—Small, hairlike structures that produce motion to help clear the lungs.

clitoris—Pea-shaped projection made up of nerves, blood vessels, and erectile tissue.

closed adoption—Confidential and no contact between birth and adoptive parents.

codependency—A preoccupation with a particular individual and her problems to the point of self-neglect. This results from prolonged association with an addict who has an oppressive set of rules that prevent the open expression of feelings, concerns, and problems.

cognitive appraisal—The process of categorizing an encounter with respect to its significance for well-being.

cohabitation—Two people living together in a committed relationship without marriage.

coitus interruptus—An unreliable birth control method in which the penis is withdrawn from the vagina prior to ejaculation.

colostrum—The initial breast milk produced by the mother.

complementary medicine—A practice used in conjunction with conventional medicine.

comprehensive fitness program—A fitness program encompassing all components essential to overall fitness: cardiorespiratory endurance, muscle strength and endurance, flexibility, and body composition.

compulsive exercise—A compelling emotional drive to exercise excessively to achieve an ideal but unrealistic image rather than for health improvement.

computerized tomography (CT) scan—A beam that rotates around the body and provides a series of X-rays of a particular area of the body from various angles.

condom—A latex sheath designed to cover the erect penis and hold semen upon ejaculation.

congestive heart failure (CHF)— Circulatory congestion caused by heart damage that inhibits adequate blood flow to the body.
contraception—A variety of methods used to prevent fertilization of the ovum.
contraindications—Conditions adversely affected by specific actions.
coronary artery bypass grafting (CABG)—Any one of many types of surgery that allows blood to travel past or around a blockage.
corticoids—Hormones generated by the adrenal glands that influence the body's control of glucose, protein, and fat metabolism.
cosmetic surgeon—A physician who specializes in beauty-enhancing surgery such as face-lifts or breast augmentation.
cross-fiber friction massage—Massaging an area where injury or surgery has occurred to break up possible adhesions and scar tissue.
cycle-based method—Natural family planning method that relies on abstinence during the time of ovulation.
cyclothymic disorder—A chronic fluctuating mood disturbance involving numerous periods of mania and depression.
cyst—A closed sac in or under the skin containing liquid or semisolid material.

D

date rape—Sexual assault of a woman by a man she has agreed to see socially.
delirium tremens (DTs)—A condition resulting from withdrawal from chronic alcohol abuse and causing uncontrollable tremors, confusion, and vivid hallucinations.
democratic parenting style—A parenting style that seeks to raise a responsible child by setting limits for the child and giving the child choices within those limits.
Depo-Provera—Trademark name for a contraceptive method utilizing progestin injection into the gluteal or deltoid muscle once every 3 months.
depression—An emotional state of persistent dejection ranging from mild discouragement and gloominess to feelings of extreme despondency and despair.
detoxification—A period of time when an addict does not drink to rid the body of alcohol and its toxic chemicals.
diaphragm—Oval, dome-shaped device that covers the lower end of the uterus to prevent sperm from entering the cervical canal.
diaphragmmatic breathing—Slow, relaxed, deep breathing to calm emotions and fully oxygenate the body.
diastolic blood pressure—Amount of pressure the blood exerts against the arterties while the heart is relaxing.
Dietary Reference Intakes (DRIs)—Generic term that includes three types of reference values in the diets of particular age and gender groups.
dilation and currettage (D&C)—Medical procedure that dilates the cervix and scrapes the uterine lining to remove contents.
dilation and evacuation (D&E)—Medical procedure that dilates the cervix and aspirates the contents of the uterus.
disaccharide—A compound made up of two monosaccharides, or simple sugars; examples include sucrose, maltose, and lactose.
discouraged child—A child who feels she has no place of significance in the family.
distress—Stress that diminishes the quality of life, commonly associated with disease, illness, and maladaptation.
divorce—A legal dissolution to a marriage.
domestic abuse—Abuse committed in the home by an intimate associate, usually the spouse.
doula—A person who is trained to provide guidance and support to a woman during pregnancy and childbirth.
dysmenorrhea—Painful menstrual periods characterized by severe cramps, headaches, lower-back and/or leg pain; occasionally incapacitating pain.
dysrhythmia—Disturbances in the normal sequence of cardiac electric activity; sometimes referred to as arrythmia.
dysthymic disorder—Involves the presence of two of the following symptoms for most of the day for at least two years (1 year for adolescents and children): poor appetite or overeating, insomnia, low energy or fatigue, low self-esteem, poor concentration or difficulty making decisions, or feelings of hopelessness.

E

eclampsia—Acute toxemia of pregnancy characterized by convulsions and coma.
ectopic pregnancy—Implantation of the embryo in the fallopian tube, ovary, abdominal cavity, or cervix.
EDNOS (Eating Disorder Not Otherwise Specified)—Missing a diagnosis of anorexia or bulimia by only one criterion; afflicts 2 to 6 percent of the population.
effective communication—Components are appropriate body language, encouraging responses, paraphrasing, clarification, and summarization.
effective listening—Components are appropriate body language, encouraging responses, paraphrasing, clarification, and summarization.
ELISA test—Abbreviation for enzyme-linked immunosorbent assay, a screening test for the HIV antibody.
embryo—The developing egg from the time of implantation (about 2 weeks after conception) in the uterus until the 5th week of pregnancy.
emotional intelligence—The ability to recognize your emotions and those of the people around you and have the competence to work with those emotions to resolve problems, especially in the workplace.
emotional intimacy—A feeling of knowing and being known.
emphysema—Chronic shortness of breath caused by tissue deterioration characterized by increased air retention and reduced exchange of gases.
endocarditis—Inflammation or infection of the inside lining of the heart chambers and/or valves.
endocrine system—Bodily system that consists of endocrine glands in order to maintain and regulate body activities. It is activated by the anterior section of the hypothalamus.
endogenous factors—Events that occur within you.
endometriosis—Chronic growth of endometrial tissue outside the uterus; can be painful and debilitating.
endometrium—Mucous membrane lining the uterus.
epidemiology—The study of relationships of the various factors determining the frequency and distribution of diseases in a human community.
epilepsy—A group of nervous system disorders caused by uncontrolled electrical discharge from nerve cells of the surface of the brain marked by recurrent seizures.

epinephrine and norepinephrine—Powerful adrenal hormones whose presence in the bloodstream prepares the body for maximal energy production and skeletal muscle response.
episiotomy—Surgical procedure to widen the vaginal opening during childbirth.
erotic love—A relationship built on passion and sexual desire.
ethyl alcohol—A clear, somewhat tasteless liquid found in various types of beverages that produce intoxication; ethanol.
eustress—Stress that adds a positive, enhancing dimension to the quality of life.
exercise adherence—Consistent involvement in an exercise program to gain long-term health benefits.
exogenous factors—External events that influence you.
extreme obesity—A body mass index (BMI) greater than 39.

F

family planning—The ability to plan the number, spacing, and timing of births.
female condom—Thin, polyurethane pouch with two flexible rings; one covers the cervix and the other partially covers the vagina.
femininity—Possessing a high number of attributes defined as feminine and a low number of attributes defined as masculine.
feminist—A person who advocates for equal rights for all persons with a special focus on women's concerns.
feminist therapy—Also referred to as gender equity therapy; empowers women through an egalitarian (equity-based) relationship with the therapist.
fermentation—Process by which sugars are converted into grain alcohol through the action of yeast.
fetal alcohol effects (FAE)—A limited number of the characteristic birth defects associated with fetal alcohol syndrome such as below normal IQ, learning disabilities, hyperactivity, short attention span, and often similar physical malformations as with FAS; completely preventable.
fetal alcohol syndrome (FAS)—A cluster of birth defects including irreversible mental and physical disabilities that develop as a result of expectant mothers consuming excessive amounts of alcohol.
fibrocystic breast condition—Catchall phrase for any signs or symptoms not related to breast cancer.
fibromyalgia—A common and chronic musculoskeletal syndrome characterized by fatigue, widespread pain in the muscles, ligaments, and tendons, and multiple "tender points" on the body where there is increased sensitivity to touch or slight pressure.
fight-or-flight response—The body's innate response to stress by either confrontation or avoidance.
five stages of grief—A grief process model that includes the stages of denial, anger, sorrow/despair/depression, bargaining, and acceptance.
flexibility—The range of motion of a particular joint.
follicular phase—First stage of a woman's menstruation and ovarian cycle.
Food and Drug Administration (FDA)—The federal agency charged with approval and control of drug-related products in the United States.
free radicals—Toxic chemicals in the body that cause damage to body cells and can lead to serious illnesses such as cancer.

G

gamete intrafallopian transfer (GIFT)—Use of a laparoscope to guide the transfer of unfertilized eggs and sperm into the woman's fallopian tubes through an incision in the abdomen.
gender-relations theory—originally began as self-in-relation theory; a response to traditional Western psychology that emphasizes separation and individuation, but neglects the intricacies of human interconnection.
gender-role socialization—The tendency to interact with a child or to limit the experiences of a child in ways that seem more suitable to traditional roles relative to the child's gender.
general adaptation syndrome (GAS)—A pattern of responses in reaction to life demands or threats.
generic name—Common name for a drug.
glamorization—Basing the desirability of a woman on her body shape, mainly thinness in the arms, legs, face, and waist, and largeness of the breasts and hips (the hourglass figure). Thought to have begun in the 1830s when the camera was invented.
glycemic index—Measures the speed by which foods raise the blood glucose level.
gonorrhea—A sexually transmitted infection caused by the bacterium *Neisseria gonorrhoea*.
grief—The emotional experience of loss.
grief process—Different methods of examining the ways in which people deal with the loss of loved ones, usually defined as having different stages or processes.
gynecology—The study and treatment of medical concerns specific to women.

H

health care maintenance—The continuation of what one is doing to maintain one's current health status.
health education—Involves research and study in the causes, prevention, and treatment of disorders. Also involves the publication and distribution of this information to the public.
health intervention—The act or fact of interfering so as to modify.
health maintenance organization (HMO)—A type of health insurance that provides a full-range of health care services using specific physicians and specialists for a prepaid amount of money.
health promotion—(a) Dissemination through literature and workshops of information regarding healthy lifestyles, enhancement of life quality, and illness prevention; (b) includes the idea that health is something to be nurtured and by doing so we prevent the onset of illness and disease.
health-related components of fitness—Cardiorespiratory endurance, muscular strength and endurance, flexibility, and body composition.
heme iron—Iron found in animal tissue in the form of hemoglobin and myoglobin.
hemodialyis—A medical procedure that removes impurities or wastes from the blood.
hemoglobin—The iron-bearing molecules found in red blood cells that carry oxygen to and carbon dioxide away from body cells.
hepatitis A virus (HAV)—A disease of the liver caused by the hepatitis A virus.

hepatitis B virus (HBV)—A viral infection causing inflammation of the liver; may be severe and result in prolonged illness or death.

hepatitis C virus (HCV)—A disease of the liver caused by the hepatitis C virus.

herpes simplex virus (HSV)—A viral infection that attacks the skin and nervous system, usually producing short-lasting, fluid-filled blisters on the skin and mucous membranes.

heterosexism—A belief or attitude that results in bias or discrimination toward anyone who is not heterosexual.

HIPAA—Policy that requires health care providers to develop procedures that protect the privacy of patients' health care information and records.

homeostasis—Relative balance in the internal environment of the body; naturally maintained by adaptive responses that promote healthy survival.

homophobia—The fear or dislike of someone who is homosexual.

hormone replacement therapy (HRT)—Treatment of menopausal symptoms with a series of drugs designed to boost hormone levels.

hot flashes—Short periods of extreme warmth experienced by some women around the time of menopause; also called hot flushes.

human immunodeficiency virus (HIV)—The organism that causes AIDS.

human papilloma virus (HPV)—A group of more than one hundred viruses including genital warts; some types increase the risk of cancer.

hymen—Fold of mucous membrane, skin, and fibrous tissue covering the vaginal opening.

hypertension—Common disorder marked by high blood pressure; divided into stage 1 and stage 2.

hypothalamus—Activates the endocrine system and the autonomic nervous system.

hysterectomy—An operation to remove a woman's uterus and, sometimes, the fallopian tubes, ovaries, and cervix.

I

infant mortality—Statistical rate of infant death during the first year of birth expressed as the number per 1,000 live births.

intracytoplasmic sperm injection (ICSI)—A type of in vitro fertilization (IVF) in which a single sperm is injected into the center of an egg; can be used with sperm that are less mobile or weaker.

intrauterine device—Contraceptive method made of plastic or other material that is inserted into the uterus to prevent pregnancy.

intrauterine growth retardation—Abnormal process in which the development and maturation of the fetus is impeded or delayed by a number of factors, including genetics, drugs, and malnutrition.

in vitro fertilization (IVF)—Surgical retrieval of eggs, fertilization in the laboratory, and transfer of the embryo into the uterus.

ischemia—Lack or absence of oxygen.

isokinetic—Exercise in which muscular force is exerted at a constant speed against an equal force that is exerted by a strength-training machine.

isometric—Exercise that increases muscle tension by applying pressure against stable resistance; accomplished by opposing different muscles.

isotonic—Muscle contraction in which force is generated while the muscle changes in length.

J

jaundice—Yellowing of the skin, mucous membranes, and eyes caused by too much bilirubin in the blood.

K

Kegel exercises—Exercises in the genital area that help strengthen the muscles of the pelvic floor.

ketones—Chemical by-products resulting from the incomplete breakdown of fats.

L

labia majora—Two folds of skin, one on each side of the vaginal opening.

labia minora—Two folds of skin between the labia majora, from the clitoris to the vaginal opening.

liberal feminism—A philosophy that sees the oppression of women as a denial of equal rights, representation, and access to opportunities.

lightening—The descent of the uterus and fetus into the pelvic cavity, which occurs 2 to 3 weeks before the onset of labor.

love addict—An unhealthy pattern of becoming involved with a partner to mask fear of abandonment.

ludic love—A relationship built on game playing and maintaining distance.

lumpectomy—Surgical removal of breast cancer and some normal tissue surrounding it.

lupus—Systemic lupus erythematosus is a chronic, autoimmune disease of connective tissue that causes inflammation and affects vital organs.

luteal phase—Part of the menstrual cycle that includes the development of the corpus luteum.

M

macrominerals—Nutrients required in the body in amounts exceeding 100 mg/day.

macrophage—Any large cell that can surround and digest foreign substances in the body.

magnetic resonance imaging (MRI)—Magnetic fields that absorb radio waves to produce images of organs and processes inside the body.

main-stream smoke—Smoke drawn through the cigarette and inhaled and exhaled by the smoker.

major depressive disorder—Typically the recurrence of a major depressive episode.

major depressive episode—The presence of at least five of the following symptoms for most of the day for at least a 2-week period: feelings of sadness or emptiness, diminished interest or pleasure, weight loss, insomnia, feelings of worthlessness or inappropriate guilt, diminished ability to think or concentrate, recurrent thoughts of death or suicide.

malignant tumors—Cancerous tumors; characterized by abnormal cells that divide uncontrollably and have the ability to infiltrate and destroy normal cells.

mammography—Imaging of the breast produced by low-dose X ray.

manic love—A consuming or obsessive relationship built on a strong need for love and affection.
marital rape—Sexual assault of a woman by her husband.
masculinity—Possessing a high number of attributes defined as masculine and a low number of attributes defined as feminine.
massage— Systematically stroking, kneading, and pressing the soft tissues of the body to induce a state of total relaxation.
maternal mortality—Death of a woman while pregnant or within 42 days of termination of the pregnancy.
meditation—A technique to calm the mind and body through a conscious mental process that induces a relaxation response.
melanoma—Any of a group of skin cancers made up of melanocytes.
menarche—The first menstrual cycle for a female.
menopause—The end of ovulation and menstruation.
menstruation—The sloughing off of the endometrium.
metabolic rate—Rate or intensity at which the body produces energy.
metastasis—The process by which cancer is spread to distant parts of the body.
methylxanthines—A family of chemical compounds that function as mild central nervous system (CNS) stimulants, includes caffeine.
midwife—A person who is trained to assist a woman during pregnancy and childbirth delivery.
misogyny—An attitude or behavior of hatred toward women.
mitral valve prolapse (MVP)—Condition in which one or both flaps of the mitral valve are enlarged and fail to close properly.
modified radical mastectomy—Surgical removal of the whole breast, most of the lymph nodes under the arm, and often, the lining of the chest muscles.
monoamine oxidase inhibitors (MAOIs)—Antidepressant drugs that work by increasing the levels of numerous neurotransmitters in the body.
monoclonal antibodies—A group of identical antibodies made from a single antibody.
monosaccharides—Simple sugar molecules; examples include glucose, fructose, and galactose.
mons pubis—The triangular, mounding area of fatty tissue that covers the pubic bone.
mourning—The actual expression of loss, or the behaviors that take place as a result of the grief experience.
multiple sclerosis (MS)—Chronic, debilitating disease that affects the central nervous system and causes damage to or loss of myelin.
muscular endurance—The ability for a muscle to generate force over a period of time or for a number of repetitions.
muscular strength—Ability of a muscle to generate force against some type of resistance.
myocardial infarction (MI)—A heart attack.

N

negative reinforcer—Removal of something uncomfortable to increase the likelihood that a behavior will be repeated.
neoadjavant therapy—The use of drugs to shrink a cancer before surgical removal.
neurotherapy—Training the brain waves to enhance cognitive performance or recover from emotional or physical trauma or drug addiction.
nicotine—Physically and psychologically addictive stimulant substance found in tobacco.
nonheme iron—Iron found in plant sources and tissues in animals other than heme iron tissues.
nonoxynol-9 (N-9)—A lubricant that is no longer recommended for the prevention of HIV or other STIs.
nutrient density—The ratio of nutrients to energy in a food product; high-density means the food has more nutrients than calories. Soda pop has low nutrient density.

O

obesity—A body mass index greater than 30.
omnivorous—Consuming both plant and animal food sources.
oncogenes—Genes that may cause a cell to be changed to cancer.
oncologist—A physician who specializes in cancer care.
ongoing mindfulness—The process of exploring the impact that sociocultural influences have on you and your life development.
open adoption—Contact between birth and adoptive parents occurs as the child is being raised; contact can be occasional to regular depending on the agreement.
oral contraceptives—Pills that contain estrogen and/or progestin and inhibit ovulation through suppressing follicle stimulating and lutenizing hormones.
osteoarthritis (OA)—A degenerative joint disease.
osteoporosis—A bone-weakening disorder in which normal bone density is lost; marked by thinning of bone tissue and growth of small holes in bone.
ovaries—Reproductive organs found on each side of the lower abdomen beside the uterus.
overweight—A body mass index (BMI) of 25 or greater.
ovulation—The release of the mature egg from the ovary.
ovulatory phase—Part of the menstrual cycle that includes the release of the mature egg from the ovary.
oxidation—Any process in which the oxygen content of a compound is increased.

P

pacemaker—A medical device implanted to treat slow heart rate (bradycardia).
patellofemoral knee pain—An injury to the knee that is characterized by nonspecific pain under the kneecap.
patent medicines—Those medicines available to the general public without a prescription; information pertaining to the drug is usually available on the drug label.
peer marriage—Egalitarian partnership between two people.
pelvic inflammatory disease (PID)—Any inflammation of the female reproductive tract, especially one caused by bacteria.
perimenopause—A decline in monthly hormonal cycles before menopause.
perineum—Part of muscle and tissue located between the vaginal opening and the anal canal.
physical dependency—Body cells dependent upon a chemical substance to maintain homeostasis.
phytochemicals—Nonnutrient substances found in plant foods that have a positive effect on the body's physiology phytonutrients.
pituitary gland—A gland of the brain that releases adrenocorticotropic hormone as part of the stress response.

placenta—The structure inside the uterus that provides the communication between the mother and the fetus.
plastic surgeon—A physician who specializes in reconstructive surgery and also performs beauty-enhancing procedures.
PNF—Contraction and relaxation of a muscle prior to stretching it; allows for longer stretches and faster development of joint flexibility.
polycystic ovarian syndrome (PCOS)—Occurs when the ovaries produce excessive amounts of male hormones (androgens) and multiple small cysts develop.
polysaccharides—Compounds composed of numerous saccharide units; complex carbohydrates.
positive reinforcer—Presentation of a reward to increase the likelihood that a behavior will be repeated.
postmenopause—Begins when menstruation has ceased for 1 year.
posttraumatic stress disorder (PTSD)—A variety of symptoms (for example, irritability, insomnia, anxiety) that result from viewing or being involved in a traumatic event.
pragmatic love—A relationship built on practical needs between partners.
preeclampsia—A disorder encountered early in the pregnancy characterized by hypertension or swelling.
preferred provider organization (PPO)—Physicians who agree to provide their services for a reduced rate to insurance companies.
premenopause—Period of time when menstrual periods are irregular but the classic symptoms of menopause, hot flashes and vaginal dryness, have not occurred.
premenstrual dysphoric disorder (PMDD)—Bouts of marked premenstrual depressed mood, anxiety, sadness, or anger that occur a few days before menstruation; the most severe type of menstruation related mood distress.
premenstrual syndrome (PMS)—Nervous tension, irritability, and so forth that occur a few days before menstruation.
preventive health action—Measures serving to avert the occurrence of illness or disease.
primary infertility—Inability of a couple to conceive a pregnancy after at least 1 year of unprotected intercourse
primary infertility—Inability to conceive after a year of unprotected sexual intercourse.
primary prevention—An extension of health education.
proactive care—Designing and living a lifestyle that reduces the risk of illness and also improves one's current health status.
problem solving—Step-by-step approach of planning and negotiating and involves all parties to be affected.
progressive relaxation—A technique that involves alternately tensing and releasing the muscles of the body and resulting in greater relaxation.
proof—Measurement of ethyl alcohol content found in beverages; stated in terms of percentages.
psychological abuse—Use of children, intimidation, threats, and economic domination to control, manipulate, and cause anxiety in one's partner.
psychological dependence—Dependence on the feeling produced by the presence of the drug in the body; an emotional or psychological desire to continue using the drug; habituation.
psychosomatic disorders—Physical illnesses generated by the effects of stress.
punishment—Presentation of something uncomfortable to reduce behavior.

Q

quackery—The promotion of a medical remedy that does not work or has not been proven to work.
quickening—A mother's first perception of fetal movement.

R

radiotherapy—High-energy radiation therapy using X rays or gamma rays to treat cancer; also called radiation therapy.
reactive care—The treatment of any illness, disorder, or disease that may develop.
rebound deficiencies—High doses of vitamins administered to a pregnant woman resulting in her fetus overexcreting excess vitamins; causes the newborn to continue excreting after birth.
Recommended Dietary Allowances (RDAs)—Recommended nutrient intakes that meet the needs of healthy people of similar age and sex based on current knowledge.
reflexology—The use of compression massage on designated areas on the hands and feet.
relaxation response—A brief technique to quiet the body and the mind that involves slow, deep breathing combined with muscle relaxation.
resiliency—The ability to recover, overcome adversity, and bounce back following difficult situations.
rheumatoid arthritis (RA)—An autoimmune, chronic inflammatory disease of unknown cause that involves the joints and/or internal organs.
RICE—Rest, ice, compress, elevate; temporary care of a minor injury that does not need a physician's attention.
ring—Clear, flexible, thin polymer ring that provides a continuous low dose of etonogesterel (progestin) and ethinyl estradiol (estrogen) to prevent pregnancy.
RU-486—Trademark name for a drug therapy used to induce abortion.

S

saline implant—A pouch filled with salt water used to reconstruct or increase the size of the breast.
sandwich generation—Women in middle adulthood.
secondary infertility—Difficulty conceiving after already having conceived and carried a normal pregnancy.
secondary prevention—Identifies persons who are in the early stages of "unhealth," which may lead to the development of disorders or illnesses.
secondary reinforcer—A less obvious reinforcer that may be contributing to resistance to change.
selective reuptake inhibitors (SSRIs)—Among the most prescribed and profitable drugs on the antidepressant market; they include Zoloft and Prozac.
self-caring—Taking care of one's own personal physical, emotional, and spiritual needs.
self-efficacy—The conviction that one can successfully execute the behavior or behaviors required to produce desired outcomes.

self-esteem—How good one feels about oneself, measured by the distance between the perceived self and the ideal or preferred self.

sexism—An attitude or act of bias or discrimination against a person because of the person's gender.

sexual assault—Sexual improprieties or sexual violence directed toward another person, including rape.

sexual discrimination—Discrimination (usually in employment) that excludes one sex (usually women) to the benefit of the other sex.

Sexual function—The ability to experience desire, arousal, orgasm, and satisfaction.

sexual harassment—Unwanted sexual advances, requests for sexual favors, and other verbal or physical conduct of a sexual nature that negatively affects the work environment.

shin splints—Strains of the muscles that move the foot and ankle at their attachment point to the shin; can result in a stress fracture to the long bone in the leg.

side effects—Undesirable, uncomfortable, or unsafe reactions when using any type of drug in which the effects are unexpected.

side-stream smoke—Smoke from the lit end of the cigarette; contains more tar, nicotine, and carbon monoxide than mainstream smoke.

silicone gel–filled implant—A pouch filled with silicone gel used to reconstruct or increase the size of the breast.

smoking cessation program—A program to quit smoking that includes behavioral modification techniques, group support, program meetings, and occasionally includes nicotine substitutes.

sociocultural influences (SCIs)—Include (but not limited to) family members, family history, family values, religious doctrine, media, school activities and personnel, community events, national events, world events, historical events, friends, famous persons, and significant others.

spermicide—A chemical substance that kills or immobilizes sperm.

spina bifida—Congenital birth defect in which the spine fails to enclose the spinal cord; usually occurs within the first month of pregnancy.

static stretching—Stretching muscles in a slow and gentle manner and holding that position for 10–30 seconds.

storgic love—A relationship built on security and friendship.

stress—A physiological and psychological state of arousal caused by the perceived presence of a challenging or threatening event.

stress amenorrhea—Cessation of the mentrual flow caused by stress.

stressors—Factors or events, real or imagined, that elicit a state of stress.

stroke—A vascular disease caused when a blood vessel bursts or becomes clogged in the brain; a brain attack.

sudden infant death syndrome (SIDS)—Sudden and unexpected death of an apparently normal and healthy infant that occurs during sleep, and with no physical or autopsy evidence of disease.

support network—Resources consisting of three systems that focus on clarifying how you define meaning from life through your beliefs and values, how you access support from those around you, and how you draw upon your own personal strengths and abilities.

surrogacy—A woman, other than the partner, who agrees to become pregnant and carry the fetus to full term.

symptothermal method—Natural family planning method that combines basal body temperature and the cycle-based method.

syphilis—A sexually transmitted infection caused by the bacterium (spirochete) *Treponema pallidum*.

systolic blood pressure—Amount of pressure the blood exerts against the arteries while the heart is contracting.

T

tar—Sticky black particulate matter in tobacco.

tertiary prevention—The application of an intervention to treat an existing disorder or illness.

tetrahydrocannabinol (THC)—The active ingredient in the hemp plant *Cannabis sativa;* found in marijuana, hashish, and ganja.

thought stopping—An important technique for altering negative self-suggestions.

TNM—A staging system for determining the stage of cancer.

total mastectomy—Surgical removal of the whole breast and possibly some lymph nodes under the arm.

toxemia—Presence of bacterial toxins in the blood; also called blood poisoning.

toxic shock syndrome (TSS)—A disease caused by a toxin produced by the bacterium *Staphylococcus aureus,* most commonly found in menstruating women using high-absorbent tampons.

transdermal patch—A contraceptive patch that releases progestin and estrogen through the skin into the bloodstream.

trans fat—The fatty acids formed when hydrogen is pumped into liquid vegetable oils to make them more firm.

transient ischemic attacks (TIAs)—Small strokes that produce strokelike symptoms that are temporary.

treatment interventions—Actions that are taken to halt the progress of a discomfort, disorder, or disease and, if possible, move the individual away from the discomfort and toward increased health.

trichomoniasis—An STI that commonly infects the vagina.

tricyclic antidepressants—Drugs that have little effect on psychotic symptoms; however, they have been found to elevate the mood of persons who have depression.

trigger-point massage—Placing pressure on a muscle where the ligaments or tendon is attached.

tubal ligation—Sterilization process in women in which the fallopian tubes are blocked to prevent pregnancy.

type 1 diabetes—A disease in which the pancreas produces little or no insulin; once called insulin-dependent or juvenile diabetes.

type 2 diabetes—A disease in which the pancreas produces insulin but the body is resistant or cannot utilize it.

U

United States Pharmacopeia (USP)—Describes the properties of medicines and ensures the purity of the drug.

urethritis—Inflammation of the urinary opening often caused by infection in the bladder or kidneys.

uterine fibroids—Common tumors of the uterus composed of muscle and fibrous tissue.

uterus—Pear-shaped female organ of reproduction in which the ovum implants and develops.

V

vacuum aspiration—Suction method by which the fetus and placenta are removed up to the 14th week.

vagina—Part of female genitals that form a canal from the vaginal opening to the cervix.

vaginitis—An inflammation of the vaginal area; often characterized by discharge or itching.

vasectomy—Sterilization process in men in which the vas deferens are blocked to prevent pregnancy.

vasoconstrictors—Substances that constrict the blood vessels of the body causing an elevation in blood pressure and heart rate.

vasovasostomy—Microsurgical procedure used to reverse a vasectomy.

veins—Blood vessels that carry deoxygenated blood and waste by-products to the heart and lungs.

vulva—The pudendum; the outer genitals of a female.

W

Western blot test—Laboratory test used to detect the presence of HIV antibodies; regarded as more accurate than the ELISA.

withdrawal symptoms—Unpleasant symptoms such as tremors, insomnia, and seizures when drug use is discontinued.

Y

Yasmin—A low-dose oral contraceptive.

yoga—Body postures and poses to improve health.

Z

zygote—The developing egg from the time it is fertilized until implantation in the uterus.

zygote intrafallopian transfer (ZIFT)—Fertilization of the eggs in the laboratory and use of the laparoscope to transfer the fertilized eggs (zygote) into the woman's fallopian tube.

Credits

Chapter 2

p. 21 (photo): Courtesy of James Robinson; **p. 36 (photo):** Keith Brofsky/Getty Images.

Chapter 3

p. 65 (Fig. 3.1): Reprinted from *Journal of Counseling and Development,* 71 (2):171, © 1992 ACA. Reprinted with permission. No further reproduction authorized without written permission of the American Counseling Association; **p. 70 (Fig. 3.3):** Adapted from Maslow, Abraham H., Frager, Robert D., and Fadiman James, *Motivation and Personality,* 3rd ed., 1997, Pearson Education, Inc., Upper Saddle River, NJ.

Chapter 5

p. 104 (photo, top): Eric Audras/Photoalto/PictureQuest; **p. 104 (photo, bottom):** Photodisc/Getty Images; **p. 107 (Fig. 5.2):** From Payne, W., Hahn, D., and Lucas, E., *Understanding Your Health,* 9th ed., New York: McGraw-Hill, 2007; **p. 114 (Assess Yourself):** From Chandler, C. and Kolander, C., Quick and effective stress screening. *Human Stress: Current Selected Research,* 5:203–206, 1997 (AMS Press). Reproduced with permission; **p. 123 (photo):** Duncan Smith/Getty Images; **p. 127 (photo):** Digital Vision/Getty Images.

Chapter 6

p. 138 (Her Story): Reproduced with permission; **p. 143 (Health Tips):** From Payne, W., Hahn, D., and Lucas, E., *Understanding Your Health,* 9th ed., New York: McGraw-Hill, 2007; **p. 145 (photo):** © PhotoDisc/Getty Images; **p. 148 (FYI):** From *Behind Closed Doors: Violence in the American Family,* © 1988 by Murray A. Strauss, Richard J. Gelles, and Suzanne Steinmetz. Reprinted with permission; **p. 154 (poem):** © 1993 Portia Nelson from the title *There's a Hole in My Sidewalk,* Hillsboro, OR: Beyond Words Publishing, Inc. (800) 284-9673.

Chapter 7

p. 160 (Assess Yourself): Modified from Payne, W., Hahn, D., and Lucas, E., *Understanding Your Health,* 9th ed., New York: McGraw-Hill, 2007; **p. 165 (FYI) and p. 166 (Health Tips):** Evans, P. (1996). *The Verbally Abusive Relationship.* (Holbrook, MA: Adams Media), p. 36. Copyright © 1992, 1996 by Patricia Evans. Used by permission of Adams Media. All rights reserved.

Chapter 8

p. 184 (Fig. 8.1): From Wardlaw, G. M., *Contemporary Nutrition: Issues and Insights,* New York: McGraw-Hill, 1997; **p. 186 (Fig. 8.2):** Reprinted by permission of the American Cancer Society, Inc., from www.cancer.org. All rights reserved; **p. 198 (Fig. 8.4):** Modified from Payne, W., Hahn, D., and Lucas, E., *Understanding Your Health,* 9th ed., New York: McGraw-Hill, 2007.

Chapter 9

pp. 206, 207, 208, 210, 215, 224, 225 (Figs. 9.1, 9.2 bottom, 9.3, 9.7, 9.8 bottom, 9.10, 9.11, 9.12): From Payne, W., Hahn, D., and Lucas, E., *Understanding Your Health,* 9th ed., New York: McGraw-Hill, 2007; **p. 208 (Fig. 9.4):** Laura J. Edwards; **p. 209 (Fig. 9.5):** Courtesy of Wisconsin Pharmacal Company. Photo by Diana Linsley; **p. 209 (Fig. 9.6):** Laura J. Edwards; **p. 210 (Fig. 9.8 top):** Laura J. Edwards; **p. 215 (Fig. 9.9 top):** Courtesy of Alza Corporation; **p. 217 (FYI):** © May 1992 Elaine Lissner, Male Contraception Information Project. Statistics in this chart are referenced in *Frontiers in Nonhormonal Male Contraceptive Research,* available from MCIP, P.O. Box 8483, Santa Cruz, CA 95061. Enclose three stamps. This chart may be duplicated and distributed without permission; **pp. 221, 222 (Tables 9.2, 9.3):** American College of Obstetricians and Gynecologists, *You and Your Baby: Prenatal Care, Labor and Delivery, and Postpartum Care* (Patient Education Pamphlet No. AB005), Washington, DC. © ACOG, April 1994. Used with permission; **p. 227 (FYI):** WHO. Used with permission; **p. 234 (Fig. 9.14):** Guttmacher Institute, Facts on induced abortion in the United States, *In Brief,* New York: Guttmacher Institute, 2006, www.guttmacher.org/pubs/fb_induced_abortion.html (retrieved October 4, 2006); Guttmacher Institute. *Get "In the Know": Questions About Pregnancy, Contraception, and Abortion,* New York: Guttmacher Institute, 2006, www.guttmacher.org/in-the-know/pregnancy.html (retrieved October 4, 2006); **p. 241 (Assess Yourself):** Adapted from Kazak, A. and Linney, J. A., Stress, coping, and life change in the single parent family, *American Journal of Community Psychology,* 11:207–220.

Chapter 10

p. 249 (photo): © PhotoDisc/Getty Images; **p. 270 (photo):** © PhotoDisc/Getty Images; **p. 276 (Fig. 10.3):** Copyright 2002 Tufts University.

Chapter 11

p. 286 (Fig. 11.1): Courtesy of James Robinson; **p. 286 (Fig. 11.2):** Courtesy of James Robinson; **p. 286 (Fig. 11.3):** Courtesy of James Robinson; **p. 288 (Fig. 11.4):** Photos courtesy of James Robinson; **p. 288 (Table 11.2):** From THE ACTIVE WOMAN'S HEALTH AND FITNESS HANDBOOK by Nadya Swedan, copyright © 2003 by Nadya Swedan. Used by permission of Perigee Books, an imprint of Penguin Group (USA) Inc.; **p. 291 (Fig. 11.5):** From Payne, W., Hahn, D., and Lucas, E., *Understanding Your Health,* 9th ed., New York: McGraw-Hill, 2007, artwork by Jeanne Robertson; **p. 293 (Journal Activity):** Adapted from Fahey, T. D., Insel, P. M., and Roth, W. T., *Fit & Well,* 7th ed., New York: McGraw-Hill, 2007.

Chapter 13

p. 329 (photo): Ryan McVay/Getty Images; **p. 336 (photo):** PhotoDisc/Getty Images.

Chapter 14

p. 368 (photo): Reproduced with permission of Clement Communications, Inc. (1998).

Color Insert

Color Plates 1–7: From Payne, W., Hahn, D., and Lucas, E., *Understanding Your Health,* 9th ed., New York: McGraw-Hill, 2007; **Color Plates 8–9** Courtesy American Academy of Dermatology, artwork by Don O'Connor.

Index